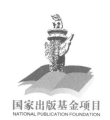

National Key Book Publishing Planning Project of the 13th Five-Year Plan
"十三五"国家重点图书出版规划项目
International Clinical Medicine Series Based on the Belt and Road Initiative
"一带一路"背景下国际化临床医学丛书

Psychiatry

精神病学

Chief Editor Li Youhui
主编 李幼辉

U0339685

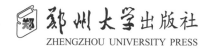
郑州大学出版社
ZHENGZHOU UNIVERSITY PRESS

图书在版编目(CIP)数据

精神病学 = Psychiatry：英文／李幼辉主编. — 郑州：郑州大学出版社，2020. 12
("一带一路"背景下国际化临床医学丛书)
ISBN 978-7-5645-5992-2

Ⅰ. ①精…　Ⅱ. ①李…　Ⅲ. ①精神病学 – 英文　Ⅳ. ①R749

中国版本图书馆 CIP 数据核字(2019)第 006071 号

精神病学 = Psychiatry：英文

项目负责人	孙保营　杨秦予		策 划 编 辑	杨秦予
责 任 编 辑	张　霞 董　珊		装 帧 设 计	苏永生
责 任 校 对	陈文静		责 任 监 制	凌　青　李瑞卿

出版发行	郑州大学出版社有限公司		地　　址	郑州市大学路 40 号(450052)
出 版 人	孙保营		网　　址	http://www. zzup. cn
经　　销	全国新华书店		发行电话	0371-66966070
印　　刷	河南文华印务有限公司			
开　　本	850 mm×1 168 mm　1 / 16			
印　　张	29.75		字　　数	1 157 千字
版　　次	2020 年 12 月第 1 版		印　　次	2020 年 12 月第 1 次印刷

书　　号	ISBN 978-7-5645-5992-2		定　　价	176.00 元

Staff of Expert Steering Committee

Chairmen

Zhong Shizhen   Li Sijin   Lü Chuanzhu

Vice Chairmen

Bai Yuting   Chen Xu   Cui Wen   Huang Gang   Huang Yuanhua
Jiang Zhisheng   Li Yumin   Liu Zhangsuo   Luo Baojun   Lü Yi
Tang Shiying

Committee Member

An Dongping   Bai Xiaochun   Cao Shanying   Chen Jun   Chen Yijiu
Chen Zhesheng   Chen Zhihong   Chen Zhiqiao   Ding Yueming   Du Hua
Duan Zhongping   Guan Chengnong   Huang Xufeng   Jian Jie   Jiang Yaochuan
Jiao Xiaomin   Li Cairui   Li Guoxin   Li Guoming   Li Jiabin
Li Ling   Li Zhijie   Liu Hongmin   Liu Huifan   Liu Kangdong
Song Weiqun   Tang Chunzhi   Wang Huamin   Wang Huixin   Wang Jiahong
Wang Jiangang   Wang Wenjun   Wang Yuan   Wei Jia   Wen Xiaojun
Wu Jun   Wu Weidong   Wu Xuedong   Xie Xieju   Xue Qing
Yan Wenhai   Yan Xinming   Yang Donghua   Yu Feng   Yu Xiyong
Zhang Lirong   Zhang Mao   Zhang Ming   Zhang Yu'an   Zhang Junjian
Zhao Song   Zhao Yumin   Zheng Weiyang   Zhu Lin

专家指导委员会

Staff of Editor Steering Committee

Chairmen

Cao Xuetao   Liang Guiyou   Wu Jiliang

Vice Chairmen

Chen Pingyan   Chen Yuguo   Huang Wenhua   Li Yaming   Wang Heng

Xu Zuojun   Yao Ke   Yao Libo   Yu Xuezhong   Zhao Xiaodong

Committee Member

Cao Hong	Chen Guangjie	Chen Kuisheng	Chen Xiaolan	Dong Hongmei
Du Jian	Du Ying	Fei Xiaowen	Gao Jianbo	Gao Yu
Guan Ying	Guo Xiuhua	Han Liping	Han Xingmin	He Fanggang
He Wei	Huang Yan	Huang Yong	Jiang Haishan	Jin Chengyun
Jin Qing	Jin Runming	Li Lin	Li Ling	Li Mincai
Li Naichang	Li Qiuming	Li Wei	Li Xiaodan	Li Youhui
Liang Li	Lin Jun	Liu Fen	Liu Hong	Liu Hui
Lu Jing	Lü Bin	Lü Quanjun	Ma Qingyong	Ma Wang
Mei Wuxuan	Nie Dongfeng	Peng Biwen	Peng Hongjuan	Qiu Xinguang
Song Chuanjun	Tan Dongfeng	Tu Jiancheng	Wang Lin	Wang Huijun
Wang Peng	Wang Rongfu	Wang Shusen	Wang Chongjian	Xia Chaoming
Xiao Zheman	Xie Xiaodong	Xu Falin	Xu Xia	Xu Jitian
Xue Fuzhong	Yang Aimin	Yang Xuesong	Yi Lan	Yin Kai
Yu Zujiang	Yu Hong	Yue Baohong	Zeng Qingbing	Zhang Hui
Zhang Lin	Zhang Lu	Zhang Yanru	Zhao Dong	Zhao Hongshan
Zhao Wen	Zheng Yanfang	Zhou Huaiyu	Zhu Changju	Zhu Lifang

编审委员会

主任委员

    曹雪涛   梁贵友   吴基良

副主任委员（以姓氏汉语拼音为序）

    陈平雁   陈玉国   黄文华   李亚明   王 恒

    徐作军   姚 克   药立波   于学忠   赵晓东

委　　员（以姓氏汉语拼音为序）

曹　虹	陈广洁	陈奎生	陈晓岚	董红梅	都　建
杜　英	费晓雯	高剑波	高　宇	关　颖	郭秀花
韩丽萍	韩星敏	何方刚	何　巍	黄　艳	黄　泳
蒋海山	金成允	金　清	金润铭	李　琳	李　凌
李敏才	李洒昶	李秋明	李　薇	李晓丹	李幼辉
梁　莉	林　军	刘　芬	刘　红	刘　晖	路　静
吕　滨	吕全军	马清涌	马　望	梅武轩	聂东风
彭碧文	彭鸿娟	邱新光	宋传君	谈东风	涂建成
汪　琳	王慧君	王　鹏	王荣福	王树森	王重建
夏超明	肖哲曼	谢小冬	徐发林	徐　霞	许继田
薛付忠	杨爱民	杨雪松	易　岚	尹　凯	余祖江
喻　红	岳保红	曾庆冰	张　慧	张　琳	张　璐
张雁儒	赵　东	赵红珊	赵　文	郑燕芳	周怀瑜
朱长举	朱荔芳				

Editorial Staff

作者名单

主　审
　　黄旭枫　　澳大利亚卧龙岗大学
主　编
　　李幼辉　　郑州大学第一附属医院
副主编
　　况　利　　重庆医科大学附属第一医院
　　王艺明　　贵州医科大学附属医院
　　朱　刚　　中国医科大学附属第一医院
　　孙　黎　　北京大学第六医院
编　委（以姓氏汉语拼音为序）
　　陈　策　　西安交通大学第一附属医院
　　陈　宏　　温州医科大学附属第一医院
　　邓　红　　四川大学华西医院
　　郭　鑫　　武汉大学人民医院
　　李　静　　重庆医科大学附属第一医院
　　连　楠　　郑州大学第一附属医院
　　刘　芳　　昆明医科大学第一附属医院
　　牛琪惠　　郑州大学第一附属医院
　　史利民　　大理大学第一附属医院
　　王亚丽　　新乡医学院第二附属医院
　　王　媛　　中国医科大学附属盛京医院
　　杨　磊　　郑州大学第一附属医院

Preface

At the Second Belt and Road Summit Forum on International Cooperation in 2019 and the Seventy-third World Health Assembly in 2020, General Secretary Xi Jinping stated the importance for promoting the construction of the "Belt and Road" and jointly build a community for human health. Countries and regions along the "Belt and Road" have a large number of overseas Chinese communities, and shared close geographic proximity, similarities in culture, disease profiles and medical habits. They also shared a profound mass base with ample space for cooperation and exchange in Clinical Medicine. The publication of the International Clinical Medicine series for clinical researchers, medical teachers and students in countries along the "Belt and Road" is a concrete measure to promote the exchange of Chinese and foreign medical science and technology with mutual appreciation and reciprocity.

Zhengzhou University Press coordinated more than 600 medical experts from over 160 renowned medical research institutes, medical schools and clinical hospitals across China. It produced this set of medical tools in English to serve the needs for the construction of the "Belt and Road". It comprehensively coversaspects in the theoretical framework and clinical practicesin Clinical Medicine, including basic science, multiple clinical specialities and social medicine. It reflects the latest academic and technological developments, and the international frontiers of academic advancements in Clinical Medicine. It shared with the world China's latest diagnosis and therapeutic approaches, clinical techniques, and experiences in prescription and medication. It has an important role in disseminating contemporary Chinese medical science and technology innovations, demonstrating the achievements of modern China's economic and social development, and promoting the unique charm of Chinese culture to the world.

The series is the first set of medical tools written in English by Chinese medical experts to serve the needs of the "Belt and Road" construction. It systematically and comprehensively reflects the Chinese characteristics in Clinical Medicine. Also, it presents a landmark achievement in the implementation of the "Belt and Road" initiative in promoting exchanges in medical science and technology. This series is theoretical in nature, with each volume built on the mainlines in traditional disciplines but at the same time introducing contemporary theories that guide clinical practices, diagnosis and treatment methods, echoing the latest research findings in Clinical Medicine.

As the disciplines in Clinical Medicine rapidly advances, different views on knowledge, inclusiveness, and medical ethics may arise. We hope this work will facilitate the exchange of ideas, build common ground while allowing differences, and contribute to the building of a community for human health in a broad spectrum of disciplines and research focuses.

Nick Lemoine

Foreign Academician of the Chinese Academy of Engineering

Dean, Academy of Medical Sciences of Zhengzhou University

Director, Barts Cancer Institute, London, UK

6th August, 2020

Foreword

Mental illness and mental health are the major health problems facing human beings in the 21st century. Psychiatry becomes more and more important in clinical medicine because of the changes of global disease spectrum and disease burden. Centering on the training objectives including the essential theory, science, new knowledge, enlightenment and applicability. Guided by the bio−psycho−social medical model, this book emphasizes to view mental disorders as a whole, focusing on cultivation of basic theories, basic knowledge and basic skills as well as on the developments of thinking, practical, analytical and problem−solving abilities. Drawing the materials from the latest development of psychiatric discipline, this book endeavor to reflect the new progresses and achievements in international psychiatric field. We have adopted the classification and diagnostic criteria for mental and behavioral disorders in the 10th edition of the International Classification of Diseases (ICD−10) of the World Health Organization as the main theme, the book endeavors to provide rich, novel, and practical content.

The book consists of twenty−three chapters, including traditional psychiatry and mental health problems. To meet the requirements of training clinicians, this book covers psychosomatic disorder, psychophysiological disorder, stress disorder, suicidal behavior and crisis intervention, rehabilitation and prevention of mental disorders, drug therapy, psychotherapy of mental disorders, and legal issues of mental disorders. Therefore, this book provides those details about the obvious changes in the spectrum of mental disorders and mental health problems with considerations of fast changing of worldwide social and economic conditions.

We have invited the experts from the clinical fields of psychiatry and mental health in China to contribute chapters of this book. We do realize, given the limited time and the depth and breadth of our knowledge, some pitfalls maybe inevitable. We kindly encourage readers to help us by putting forward valuable suggestions in order to improve this book.

We would like to give our special thanks to Professor Huang Xufeng, MD, PhD and DSc from School of Medicine, University of Wollongong, Australia. He has meticulously reviewed and annotated all chapters of this book, and strictly reviewed the the oretical aspects and contents of clinical diagnosis and treatment. Also, we would like to thank all contributing writers for their enthusiasm and dedication. We would like to express our sincere gratitude to our leaders and colleagues of the First Affiliated Hospital of Zhengzhou University for their support and help.

Authors

Contents

Chapter 1 Introduction ·· 1
  1.1 Concept and development of psychiatry ································ 1
  1.2 Biological basis of psychiatric disorders ······························ 4

Chapter 2 Classification and Diagnosis System of Psychiatric Disorders ······ 11
  2.1 Introduction ·· 11
  2.2 Diagnosis system of psychiatric disorders ···························· 13

Chapter 3 Psychiatric Symptomatology ································ 15
  3.1 Introduction ·· 15
  3.2 Disturbances of consciousness ·· 17
  3.3 Memory disorder ·· 20
  3.4 Disorders of intelligence ·· 22
  3.5 Disorders of perception ·· 23
  3.6 Disturbance of thoughts ·· 26
  3.7 Disorders of emotion ·· 29
  3.8 Disorder of psychomotor ·· 31

Chapter 4 Assessment and Diagnosis of Mental Disorders ········ 33
  4.1 Introduction ·· 33
  4.2 General principles and procedures for psychiatric assessment ······ 34
  4.3 The psychiatric history ·· 38
  4.4 Examination of mental condition ····································· 43
  4.5 Physical examination and special examination ······················ 45
  4.6 Diagnosis of mental disorders ··· 47
  4.7 Application of standardized psychiatric assessment and rating scale ······ 48
  4.8 Writing of psychiatric records ·· 50

Chapter 5 Organic Mental Disorders ································ 56
  5.1 Introduction ·· 56
  5.2 Brain organic mental disorders ·· 63

Chapter 6 Mental Disorders due to Physical Diseases ············ 74
  6.1 Introduction ·· 74
  6.2 Mental disorders due to systemic infectious diseases ·············· 75
  6.3 Mental disorders due to endocrine diseases ························ 77
  6.4 Mental disorder due to connective tissue disease ·················· 81

6.5　Mental disorders due to disease of internal organs ……………………………………… 83

6.6　Mental disorders due to diabetes mellitus ………………………………………………… 85

Chapter 7　Mental and Behavioral Disorders Caused by Psychoactive Substance
Use ………………………………………………………………………………… 86

7.1　Introduction ………………………………………………………………………………… 86

7.2　Mental and behavioral disorders due to use of opioids …………………………………… 90

7.3　Mental and behavioral disorders due to use of alcohol …………………………………… 92

7.4　Mental and behavioral disorders due to use of barbiturates and benzodiazepines ………… 99

7.5　Mental and behavioral disorders due to use of CNS stimulants ………………………… 100

7.6　Mental and behavioral disorders and tobacco …………………………………………… 102

7.7　Prospects …………………………………………………………………………………… 103

Chapter 8　Schizophrenia and Other Psychotic Disorders ……………………………… 105

8.1　Introduction ………………………………………………………………………………… 105

8.2　Schizophrenia ……………………………………………………………………………… 105

8.3　Paranoid mental disorders ………………………………………………………………… 119

8.4　Acute delusional disorder ………………………………………………………………… 120

8.5　Acute transient psychosis ………………………………………………………………… 122

Chapter 9　Mood Disorders ………………………………………………………………… 123

9.1　Introduction ………………………………………………………………………………… 123

9.2　Overview …………………………………………………………………………………… 123

9.3　Etiology ……………………………………………………………………………………… 126

9.4　Clinical features …………………………………………………………………………… 133

9.5　Diagnosis and differential diagnosis ……………………………………………………… 136

9.6　Course and prognosis ……………………………………………………………………… 142

9.7　Treatments ………………………………………………………………………………… 144

Chapter 10　Neurosis ………………………………………………………………………… 156

10.1　Introduction ……………………………………………………………………………… 156

10.2　Pathogenesis of neurosis ………………………………………………………………… 156

10.3　Clinical features,diagnosis and treatments of neurosis ………………………………… 158

10.4　Phobia ……………………………………………………………………………………… 162

10.5　Panic disorder …………………………………………………………………………… 165

10.6　Generalized anxiety disorder …………………………………………………………… 168

10.7　Obsessive-compulsive disorder ………………………………………………………… 171

10.8　Somatoform disorders …………………………………………………………………… 173

10.9　Neurasthenia ……………………………………………………………………………… 178

10.10　Neuroses rehabilitation ………………………………………………………………… 181

Chapter 11　Dissociative Disorders ……………………………………………………… 183

11.1　Introduction ……………………………………………………………………………… 183

11.2　Etiology and pathogenesis ……………………………………………………………… 183

11.3　Clinical features ………………………………………………………………………… 185

11.4　Diagnosis and differential diagnosis …………………………………………………… 188

11.5　Treatments ………………………………………………………………………………… 189

11.6　Prevention and healthcare of dissociative disorders …………………………………… 191

Chapter 12 Stress Related Disorders ·· 192
  12.1 Introduction ·· 192
  12.2 Acute stress disorder ··· 195
  12.3 Post traumatic stress disorder ··································· 199
  12.4 Adjustment disorder ·· 204
Chapter 13 Physiological Disorders Related to Psychological Factors ········ 207
  13.1 Introduction ·· 207
  13.2 Eating disorders ·· 207
  13.3 Sleep disorders ·· 217
  13.4 Sexual dysfunctions ·· 229
Chapter 14 Psychosomatic Illnesses ·· 234
  14.1 Introduction ·· 234
  14.2 Etiology and pathogenesis ··· 235
  14.3 Types of psychosomatic disease ································· 238
  14.4 Diagnosis and differential diagnosis ···························· 241
  14.5 Treatments ·· 243
  14.6 Prevention ·· 245
Chapter 15 Consultation-liaison Psychiatry ································· 246
  15.1 Introduction ·· 246
  15.2 Working scope ·· 247
  15.3 Clinical application ··· 250
Chapter 16 Child and Adolescent Psychiatry ······························ 260
  16.1 Disorders of psychological development ························· 260
  16.2 Behavioral and emotional disorders ····························· 279
Chapter 17 Personality and Personality Disorders ······················ 309
  17.1 Introduction ·· 309
  17.2 Classification of personality disorders in ICD-10 ············· 310
Chapter 18 Psychosexual Disorders ·· 328
  18.1 Introduction ·· 328
  18.2 Overview ·· 328
  18.3 Epidemiology ·· 329
  18.4 Etiology and pathogenesis ··· 331
  18.5 Clinical features ·· 334
  18.6 Diagnosis and differential diagnosis ···························· 340
  18.7 Course and prognosis ·· 343
  18.8 Treatments ·· 344
Chapter 19 Suicide and Crisis Intervention ································· 349
  19.1 Introduction ·· 349
  19.2 Risk factors ··· 352
  19.3 Assessment of patients with suicidal behaviors ·············· 355
  19.4 Suicide prevention ·· 362
  19.5 Crisis intervention ··· 365

Chapter 20   Somatotherapy for Mental Disorders ·· 369
    20. 1   Introduction ··· 369
    20. 2   Psychotropic drugs treatment ··· 369
    20. 3   Electroconvulsive therapy ··· 407
    20. 4   Transcranial magnetic stimulation ·· 410
Chapter 21   Psychotherapy ·· 413
    21. 1   Introduction ··· 413
    21. 2   Clinical psychotherapy ·· 413
Chapter 22   Rehabilitation and Prevention of Mental Disorders ····················· 428
    22. 1   Inroduction ··· 428
    22. 2   Mental rehabilitation ·· 429
    22. 3   Prevention of mental disorders ·· 433
Chapter 23   Mental Illness and Legal Issues ··· 438
    23. 1   Introduction ··· 438
    23. 2   The crimes and assessments of offenders with mental disorder ··············· 439
    23. 3   The association between mental disorder and crime ····························· 448
References ··· 457

Chapter 1

Introduction

Psychiatry is a branch of clinical medicine. Psychiatric disorders refer to the disturbance of structure and brain function under the influence of various biological, psychological and environmental factors which will lead to the abnormalities of psychiatric activities such as cognition, affection, will and behavior. Psychiatry is the performance of the unity of biology–psychology–social. This chapter introduces some basic concepts, history, development and biological basis of psychiatry.

1.1 Concept and development of psychiatry

1.1.1 Psychiatry and related concepts

Psychiatry: it is a medical specialty that studies the etiology, pathogenesis, clinical manifestation, diagnosis and treatment of mental disorders which began from 18th century. At first it was a part of neurology, with its development, it was separated from the neurology in mid 20th century. However, the boundary is not clear because they have common fundamental pathological system (neural system) and overlapped patient population.

Psychopathology: it is a subject that studies mental illness or emotional disorders which can be divided into descriptive psychopathology and explanatory psychopathology. Descriptive psychopathology is the description of symptoms of abnormal mental or emotional state and direct appearance of behavioral change. Through this kind of description, psychiatrists should have the ability to differentiate, identify the symptoms of mental illness. So it is also called "the fundamental professional skill of a psychiatrist". Explanatory psychopathology means using experimental methods to verify the causes of symptoms.

Mental illness: it can also be called mental disorder or psychiatric disorder, which is characterized by different kinds of abnormalities in emotion, cognition, behaviors and have an effect on daily life and work.

1.1.2 The history and future of psychiatry

In ancient times, since lack of knowledge of psychiatry, patients with psychiatric disorders were often seen as ridden by devil and would be abused and executed. With the development of culture and technology, there are changes in people's view on psychiatric disorders. From 5th century B. C. to 4th century

B. C. ,Hioopcrates who was an Ancient Greek physician suggested that brain was the organ of mind and proposed the psychiatric humoral pathology theory. After the French Revolution in 18th century,Pinei proposed to treat psychiatric patient with humanitarianism which improved the management of mental patients. From 18th century to 19th century,psychiatry was included into medicine. At the end of 19th century,Kraepelin summarized the results of previous study,determined the distinction between early-onset dementia,mannia-depression and organic dementia,classified the psychiatric disorders from the point of clinical and pathological anatomy which laid the foundation of biological psychiatry. At the same time,Freud set up the Psychoanalysis theory,discussed the etiology from the area of pathological psychology. Bleuler in Switzerland who was a famous psychiatrist in the early 20th century proposed the name of "schizophrenia" in 1911 which replaced Kraepelin's "early-onset dementia". Lately,Meyer set up psycho-biological theory,emphasized the role of factual social environment factor in forming personality or psychiatric disorders. After 1950s,psychiatric drugs began to be widely used in psychiatry which promoted the development of psychiatry. With the advance of therapy,the closed-off management had been replaced by open management which would benefit the recovery of patient.

Comparing with other specialties,the mechanism,and etiology of the most psychiatric disorders are still not clear. There are several areas in psychiatry that are waiting to be explored. Nowadays,some study trends are formulated that need to be discovered further.

First is the early discovery,early diagnosis and early treatment. Since the specialties of psychiatric disorders,the public don't have enough aware of some relative performance which is actually the symptom of a mental illness. They may treat it as a simple disturbed mood state which could recover with time. This kind of thought will delay their seeking for help from professional psychiatrist. This is the reason why early discovery is important. Furthermore,since the diagnosis standard of psychiatric disorder is not accuracy enough and have more subjective factors,many misdiagnosis have occurred.

Second is genetic discovery of psychiatric disorders which will lead to the new treatment thought that aiming to molecular pathophysiology and biotechnology but not the treatment just aiming to control the symptoms. In recent years,many researches have suggested the genetic influence on psychiatric disorders such as depression,anxiety,schizophrenia,Alzheimer's disease and Parkinson disease.

Third is neuroplasticity which has become a new cellular and molecular level impairment that may lead to symptoms of some psychiatric disorders such as depression,mania,schizophrenia. It enriches the knowledge that symptoms are not only due to the chemical imbalance. And it also offers us a strategy to reverse the neuron degeneration and impairment in brain.

Forth is the new treatment agents of psychiatric disorders in neural level,such as caspase inhibitors,neurogenesis stimulators,neurotrophic enhancers(nerve growth factor,brain-derived neurotrophic factor,vascular endothelial growth factor),antioxidants,glia proliferation enhancers,tumor necrosis factor alpha inhibitor.

Fifth is the treatment therapy of chemical neural stimulation such as ECT,repetitive transcranial magnetic stimulation,vagus nerve stimulation and deep brain stimulation.

Sixth is the importance of pharmacogenomics. It can determine the therapy doses individually and play an important role in decreasing the drug side effect.

Seventh is collaborative model. It can help us know more about the fact that different physical system disease can increase the susceptibility to psychiatric disorders,and some psychiatric disorders also can increase the susceptibility to other physical disease.

1.1.3 The branches of psychiatry

(1)Clinical psychiatry

It generally represents the total of psychiatry. In large-scale psychiatric organization, it can be divided into several small specialties.

(2)Child and adolescent psychiatry

It aims to study the psychiatric disorders in childhood of different age and psychological development disorder problems. It particularly emphasizes the prevention of psychiatric disorders.

(3)Geriatric psychiatry

It focus on the diagnosis, treatment and prevention of organic and non-organic psychiatric disorders in old age.

(4)Forensic psychiatry

It aims to solve the problems between the law and psychiatric disorders and focus on the problem between capacity for criminal responsibility and capacity in civil disputes.

(5)Consultation-liaison psychiatry

It means dealing with the diagnosis and therapy of the psychiatric disorders that induced by diseases of other departments in general hospital.

(6)Social psychiatry

It focus on the etiological analysis of psychiatric disorders and social culture. It aims to study the social etiology of psychiatric disorders and the influence of social factor to prevalence rate, clinical manifestation and prognosis of disease. And meanwhile it tries to propose prevention method.

(7)Community psychiatry

It is the diagnosis, therapy, prevention and recovery of psychiatric patient in community or outside the hospital under the theoretical direction of community psychiatry.

(8)Addiction psychiatry

It is the study of etiology, mechanism, effective therapy, effective discovery of drug dependence and the regularity of psychiatric disorders accompanied with drug dependence.

1.1.4 Related disciplines of psychiatry

(1)Medical psychiatry

The study of psychological factor's function on health, the onset and development of disease. It emphasizes the bio-psycho-social medical model.

(2)Behavior medicine

It is a combination of behavioral scientific technology and the biomedical technology. And apply these technologies to the diagnosis, therapy, prevention and recovery of disease.

(3)Psychosomatic disease

It refers to the organic disease that its onset and development can be influenced by social psychological factors, such as primary hypertension. And the functional disorder that can be influenced by social psychological factors is called psychosomatic disorders.

(4)Psychosomatic medicine

It studies the situation that happens due to mental factor but performing as somatic diseases.

(5)Neuroscience

It is the study of the physiological basis of human nervous system, brain, perception, sensation, memory and learning.

　(6) Medical anthropology

　It is the applying of anthropology to health, disease, medicine and therapy. It is also the study of human disease, health care problems and their relationship with biology, social culture factors.

　(7) Medical sociology

　It is the applying of sociology to study health problems which are related with social structure or social process from the perspective of population and the social psychology factors which are related with disease.

　(8) Medical humanities

　It is the inter-discipline of medicine and humanities that aims to understand health, disease and medicine from the perspectives of history, philosophy, literature and art.

1.2　Biological basis of psychiatric disorders

1.2.1　The structure and function of brain

　The brain integrates the affects of genetic, environmental and psycho social and then promotes the development of emotion, cognition and behavior.

1.2.1.1　Structure

　In brain, there are a number of about 10^{11} neurons and a more large amount of glial cells. Among them there are complex connections to transmit signals through synapses that help to maintain the basic function of human body.

　(1) Neuron types

　Almost all the neurons can be divided into two forms: projection or local circuit neurons (inter-neurons). The projection neurons can transmit signal or stimulus from peripheral to brain (sensory neurons), from brain to peripheral (motor neurons) and from one brain region to another. The local circuit neurons can only transmit signal or stimulus inside the brain region.

　(2) Glial types

　The glial cells can be divided into astrocytes, oligodendrocytes and Schwann cells, microglias. Astrocytes have functions of composing the blood-brain barrier, removing neurotransmitters in synaptic cleft such as glutamate and GABA, buffering the concentration of potassium in extracellular fluid. Oligodendrocytes and Schwann cells participate in forming the myelin sheath through wrapping their processes on the axons which will benefit the conduction of chemical signals along the axons. Microglia has function of eliminating the debris generated by the neurons' damage or death.

1.2.1.2　Function of different brain regions

　The function of brain depends on several neuron circuits. The connection between neurons or neuron circuits is complex. It can be divergent or convergent, and it can also be organized in rank way or parallel way. One neuron can participate in several neuron circuits and the connection between different brain regions can be reciprocal.

　Different brain regions have different functions. The cerebral cortex is mainly to modulate the sensory and motor function, and it also can manage memory, learning and conscious. The hippocampus plays an important role in the formation, reorganization and consolidation of memory. The striatum is important to habitual learning through a kind of feedback−guided learning. Reward−based learning is associated with mid brain(substantia nigra and ventral tegmental area). The amygdala plays a role in not only the emotional learning but also the modulation between declarative and nondeclarative memory. The prefrontal cortex is seen as helping to access memory more strategically and retrieve the information most related with current goal,so it is important to working memory. Memory and learning function depends on the intact state of brain. For example,patient with frontal lobe damage have deficiency in memory.

1.2.2   Neurobiological basis of psychiatry

The signal transmission can be divided into chemical transmission and electrical transmission. Among them,the neurotransmitter plays an important role. In central nervous system,there are mainly three kinds of neurotransmitter:monoamines,aminoacids and neuropeptides.

1.2.2.1   Monoamines

Monoamines neurotransmitter system participates in many psychiatric disorder's pathology and treatment. Neurotransmitter needs to combine with special receptors. There are several kinds of receptor sub−types for each monoamines neurotransmitter which can act in different ways. We can find that to one certain monoamines,sometimes it can lead to the activation of a cell and sometimes it may lead to inhibition. This phenomenon is due to the different distribution of receptor sub−types on the cells surface. Neurotransmitter receptors can be divided into 2 types:ligand−gated channel and G protein−linked receptors. Ligand−gated channel is an ion channel. When it combines with receptor,ion channel opens and ion will enter into cells and change the potential of intracellular and extracellular and then according the ions are positive or negative,it can generate action potential or make it more difficult to generate action potential. Except for HT3 receptor,all the monoamines neurotransmitter receptors belong to G protein−linked receptors. Different kinds of monoamines neurotransmitter receptors can integrate with diverse G protein,activate diverse second signal messenger and then generate different responses. Monoamines neurotransmitter receptors distribute on both presynaptic and postsynaptic membranes.

(1)Dopamine

Dopaminergic neuron mostly distributes in hypothalamus arcuate nucleus,substantia nigra pars compacta and ventral tegmental area. From the substantia ventral−tegmental area complex,dopaminergic neuron can generate three signal pathways. One projects to cerebral cortex,especially the frontal lobe cortex,which is called mesocortical pathway. The other one projects to nucleus accumbens,amygdaloid nucleus and hippocampus which is called mesolimbic pathway. Due to the relationship of these two pathways' function,they are defined as the meso−corticolimbic system. It plays an important role in emotional reaction,motivation, reward,addiction and learning. It also has a function on the pathology of schizophrenia,depression,anxiety and drug abuse. The third pathway projects to striatum which is called nigrostriatal pathway. This pathway integrates the neuron circuits in basal ganglia which is associated with the pathology of Parkinson disease.

Dopamine receptors have 5 types: D_1R, D_2R, D_3R, D_4R and D_5R(Pierce et al. ,2006). D_1 receptor can couple with Gs protein and stimulate adenylate cyclase activity and further facilitate the synthesis of cyclic adenosine monophosphate(cAMP),while D_2 receptor can couple with Gi protein and inhibit adenylate cyclase activity. There is study found increase density of D_2 receptors in schizophrenia brain. D_2 receptors have a high affinity for antipsychotic drugs. The extra−pyramidal side effects of antipsychotic drugs are associated with the blockade of D_2 receptors in striatum. D_3 and D_4 receptors are like D_2 receptor,both inhibit adenylate cyclase activity. D_5 receptor is like D_1 receptor.

(2) Serotonin

Serotonin has an effect on many brain functions including the regulation of emotion, fear responses, appetite, sleep and sexual behavior. Serotonergic pathway originates from the raphe nuclei and projects to almost every region of brain. The projection to the hippocampus has been seen as an important factor in development and treatment of depression. The hypofunction of 5-HT is related with depression and the hyperfunction of 5-HT is related with mania.

When serotonin is released to the synaptic cleft, it can combine with nearly 20 receptors. These receptors can be divided into seven families. 5-HT1A, 5-HT1B, 5-HT1D and 5-HT2B are autoreceptors distributed on the serotonin-containing raphe neurons which means they can regulate serotonin release themselves through negative feedback mechanisms. A large amount of evidence suggests that the 5-HT1A is important to depression and antidepressant activity. Its activation will lead to the inhibition of serotonin release. However there was evidence suggested that the long term stimulation of 5-HT1A would make it desensitize or downregulate and after a period of time it will no longer inhibit serotonin release. It explains the time needed for antidepressant drug such as SSIRs to take effect (Pierz et al., 2014).

(3) Norepinephrine

Adrenergic receptors can be divided into three subfamilies: α_1, α_2, and β. The function is well known in peripheral nervous system such as the regulation of smooth muscle contraction and blood pressure. However their function in brain is less known. In the brain, these three receptors are distributed in the cerebral cortex, the hippocampus, septum, amygdala, and thalamus. α_2 receptors are distributed on both presynaptic as an autoreceptor and postsynaptic membrane, and both has a function of inhibiting cAMP formation and activating potassium channels that leads to membrane hyperpolarization and inhibits the noradrenergic neurons. This mechanism leads to the sedative effects just like α_2 receptor agonist-clonidine. Moreover, the activation of α_2 receptors in brainstem can reduce sympathetic but enhance parasympathetic nervous system. This can explain clonidine's function in lowering blood pressure and restraining the sympathetic hyperactivity. β_1 and β_2 receptors play an important role in the consolidation of memory. Propranolol (nonspecific antagonist of both β_1 and β_2 receptors) is used as the treatment of hypertension, arrhythmia, social phobia and post-traumatic stress disorder.

(4) Histamine

Histamine has the functions of modulating arousal, wakefulness, feeding behavior, body temperature, motion, attack behavior and neuroendocrine. There are four types of histaminergic receptors: H_1, H_2, H_3, and H_4. In central nervous system, H_1 receptors are distributed in the thalamus, the cortex and cerebellum. H_1 receptor couples with Gq protein, activates phosphoinositide turnover and leads to the increase of excitatory neuronal responses. So the blockade of H_1 receptor can explain the effect of the sedation and weight gain generated by antipsychotic and antidepressant drugs. Conversely, there are evidence suggested that H_1 receptor agonists could stimulate arousal and inhibit food intake. Within the central nervous system (CNS), H_2 receptors are distributed in the neocortex, hippocampus, amygdala, and striatum. H_2 receptors can couple with Gs protein, activate adenylate cyclase and produce excitatory effects on hippocampus and thalamus. Within the CNS, H_3 receptors have been found distributed in the frontal cortex, striatum, amygdaloid complex and substantia nigra. H_3 receptors can couple with Gi/o protein, inhibit denylate cyclase and voltage-activated Ca^{2+} channels. Blockade of H_3 receptors have functions of suppressing appetite, promoting arousal, and enhancing cognition.

(5) Acetylcholine

Cholinergic receptors include two types: muscarinic receptors (G-protein-coupled receptors) and nicotinic receptors(ligand-gated ion channels). Within the CNS, muscarinic receptors have an effect on learning and memory, sleep, sense of pain, motor control and the regulation of seizure susceptibility.

The most abundant muscarinic receptors in the forebrain is M1 receptors which are distributed in the cortex, hippocampus, and striatum. Evidence suggested their function in memory and synaptic plasticity. M2 receptors have an effect on mediating tremor and hypothermia. The muscarinic agonists' analgesia effect also depends on M2 receptors. M4 receptors are distributed in the hippocampus, cortex, striatum, thalamus, and cerebellum. M4 receptors in striatum have an opposite effect to D_1 dopamine receptors and antiparkinsonian agents also take anticholinergic effect on this kind of receptors. Nicotinic acetylcholine receptors are a kind of ligand-gated ion channel receptors which can mediate rapid, excitatory signaling. After combining with acetylcholine, the ion channel will open and the outflow of Na^+, K^+, and Ca^{2+} ions will lead to membrane depolarization. Nicotinic receptors have an effect on cognitive function, especially working memory, attention, and processing speed. In Alzheimer's disease, the nicotinic acetylcholine receptors in cortex and hippocampus will significantly decrease, and the utility of nicotine can improve attention deficits. In the treatment of Alzheimer's disease, through the use of cholinesterase inhibitors that aims to improve cholinergic function and decrease normal degradation of acetylcholine, cognitive dysfunction and behavioral disturbances have been improved.

1.2.2.2　Amino acid neurotransmitter

(1)Glutamine

Within the CNS, there are several glutamatergic pathways. The thalamocortical projections and the corticolimbic projections are glutamatergic. The temporal lobe circuit's mechanism of developing new memories also includes 4 series of glutamatergic synapses.

The glutamate receptors can be divided into three types: α-amino-3-hydroxy-5-methyl-4-isoxazole propionic acid(AMPA) receptors, kainic acid(KA) receptors and N-methyl-D-aspartic acid(NMDA) receptors. AMPA receptors can take an excitatory neurotransmission effect through excitatory postsynaptic currents. The AMPA receptor family is consisted of four sub-units: GluR1, GluR2, GluR3 and GluR4.

There is evidence suggested that the long-term activation of AMPA/KA receptors and NMDA receptors can lead to a large amount of influx of Na^+ and Ca^{2+} ions and further cause the influx of H_2O. The process can result in acute cellular edema which will lead to the death of narcotic cells. Furthermore, the persistent elevation of Ca^{2+} can also induce apoptosis by disrupting the mitochondria. This kind of phenomenon is called excitotoxicity which has an effect on Alzheimer's disease. Memantine, a weak noncompetitive inhibitor of NMDA receptors has been proved to have treatment effect on Alzheimer's disease. It reduces the NMDA receptors relating excitotoxicity effect but does not influence normal neurotransmission, thereby can suppress the neuronal degeneration in Alzheimer's disease.

(2)GABA

GABA is a kind of inhibitory amino acid transmitter. GABAergic control has functions of regulating the cognition, memory and learning, motor function, circadian rhythms, neural development, adult neurogenesis and sexual maturation. The dysfunction of GABAergic neurotransmission has been confirmed of relating with several kinds of psychiatric disorders such as anxiety disorders, schizophrenia, alcohol dependence and seizure disorders. The GABA receptors can be divided into 2 types: GABAA/C receptors which are ionotropic and GABAB receptors.

When activating the GABAA complex, it will cause a change in potential. In the mature neuron, the activation of it will cause an influx of Cl^- ions which will lead to membrane hyperpolarization. Hyperpolarization is inhibitory because it makes it more difficult to generate an action potential. However In immature neurons, which have unusually high levels of intracellular Cl⁻, activating the GABAA receptor can conversely cause depolarization. Because of this, anticonvulsants may actually exacerbate seizures in the neonatal period because of its effect of enhancing GABAA receptor activity. There is evidence suggested that the Aβ−induced disruption of GABAergic inhibitory neurotransmission could be the mechanism of Alzheimer's disease. The disruptions in GABAergic signaling can lead to the impairment of glutamatergic and cholinergic excitatory signaling and further have an effect on excitatory/inhibitory balance disruptions that lead to early cognitive deterioration in Alzheimer's disease(Govindpani et al. ,2017).

1.2.2.3   Neuropeptides

Neuropeptides have been suggested that have relationship with the regulation of locomotion, learning and memory, thermo regulation, food and water consumption, responses to stress and pain, emotion, sex, sleep and social cognition. Because of this, neuropeptidergic systems may also related with some psychiatric disorder such as psychosis, mood disorders, dementias, and autism spectrum disorders. Neuropeptides can have an effect not only on neurons, but also on partial neural organs, its main function is to integrate the respective system function of the brain and body. Neuropeptides can play a role as an neurotransmitter, neuromodulator, or neurohormone.

1.2.3   Neuroendocrine basis of psychiatry

Neuroendocrine has a close relationship with mental activities. In the CNS the brain is not only responsible for regulating the release of hormone, but also has secretory function and acts as a target of some hormone. Many psychiatric disorders have abnormalities in endocrine system such as depression, PTSD and schizophrenic. Meanwhile, some endocrine system illness are also with psychiatric symptoms such as Cushing syndrome, Addison's disease, hyperthyroidism and hypothyroidism.

1.2.3.1   Hypothalamic−pituitary−adrenal axis

Hypothalamic−pituitary−adrenal(HPA) axis is composed of corticotropin releasing hormone(CRH) released by hypothalamus, adrenocorticotropic hormone(ACTH) released by pituitary and cortisol released by adrenal cortex. These three kinds of hormones can play a role in arousal, sensory processing, pain, sleep, and memory storage and retrieval. Abnormalities in HPA function have been proved of having relationship with several kinds of psychiatric disorders such as mood disorders, PTSD, dementias and substance use disorders.

The concentration of these hormones can change with the stress factor. Persistent chronic stress can increase CRH and arginine vasopressin(AVP) in the paraventricular nucleus of the hypothalamus and further reduce the number of CRH receptor in the anterior pituitary. In acute stress, ACTH will increase butin chronic stress, it will decrease.

The release of glucocorticoid is controlled by serotonergic and cholinergic regulation and is inhibited by GABA and opioids. Dopaminergic activity in certain areas of the brain can increase in acute addition of glucocorticoids but decrease in chronic hypercortisolemia. There are researches suggested that in Cushing syndrome which has an increase level of cortisol concentration, more than 50% of patients had a disturbances of mood and more than 10% of study cases appeared psychosis or suicidal thought. In major depressive disorder, cognitive impairment is common and are decided by the degree of the increase of cortisol and the possible reduction in hippocampal size. This explains the fact that the reduction in cortisol levels can have a treatment effect on mood and mental status. For example, Mifepristone(RU486) which is used as a treatment of Cushing syndrome has been reported to anesis psychosis and depression and it can even take effect on psychosis or depression of psychotic disorder that has no relationship with Cushing syndrome. In Addison's disease(characterized by decrease level of concentration of glucocorticoid), there are symptoms such as apathy, social withdrawal, impaired sleep and fatigue which can be seen as the result of reduction of glucocorticoid. There are findings suggested that corticosteroids also have regulatory effects on serotonergic function, especially 5-HT1A receptor. In schizophrenia, clozapine which is a kind of treatment of schizophrenia can improve cognitive functioning possibly through preventing hippocampal damage reduced by corticol, and reverses the impairment of long-term potentiation(an important synaptic plasticity for memory) induced by stress.

1.2.3.2 Hypothalamus-pituitary-gonadal axis

Gonadotropin releasing hormone(GnRH) can lead to the release of luteinizing hormone(LH) and follicle stimulating hormone(FSH) from the pituitary. The gonadal hormones include progesterone, androstenedione, testosterone, estradiol(E_2), and others which can be secreted by the ovary and testis, but androgens can also be released by the adrenal cortex. The prostate gland and adipose tissue also participates in the synthesis and storage of dihydrotestosterone. Some studies suggested that there were connections between the increase of testosterone and aggression. Abnormal testosterone levels have been proved of relating with a variety of disorders such as schizophrenia, PTSD, depression, andanorexia. Within the premenstrual, post menstrual and postpartum period, the hormone change in women is more likely to induce mood disorder or some other psychiatric disturbances. Mood changes in premenstrual and postpartum mood disturbances is related with these hormones with serotonin. Women with depression history have higher level of FSH, LH and lower E_2 levels and have a higher risk of a younger perimenopause period.

Estrogens can influence neural activity in the hypotha-lamus and limbic system and regulate the synthesis and release of dopamine. Evidence suggested that some psychiatric drugs may change the menstrual cycle. And the estrogen concentrations have an effect on the risk of tardive dyskinesia. And lower level of estrogen is related with acute psychosis in both women and men and often displays more severe negative symptom and poorer cognitive function. There is evidence that gonadal steroids can influence spatial cognition and verbal memory and have an effect on improving age-related neuronal degeneration. There is also evidence that in postmenopausal women, estrogen addiction may decrease the risk and postpone the onset of dementia of the Alzheimer's disease. Some animal studies suggested that estrogen could inhibit monoamine oxidase and increase sensitivity to serotonin. Long-term utilities of estrogen can lead to a decrease in 5-HT1 and an increase in 5-HT2 receptors.

Progesterone itself and the metabolites of progesterone both have an anxiolytic and hypnotic properties via GABAA agonistic activity. Since progesterone which has anti-estrogen effects can decrease the number of estrogen receptors and increase MAO activity, it has been seen as related with dysphoric mood. The ratio of progestin to estrogen in oral contraceptives has been suggested to have a relationship with the negative mood change and can perform differently depending on depression history.

1.2.3.3 Hypothalamic-pituitary-thyroid axis

Hypothalamic-pituitary-thyroid(HPT) axis is composed of thyrotropin releasing hormone(TRH) released by hypothalamus, thyroid stimulating hormone(TSH) released by pituitary and thyroid hormone released by thyroid including T_3 and T_4. The central noradrenergic systems can sti-mulate the secretion of TSH, while the central dopamine neurons inhibit the release of TSH. TRH can influence the neuronal excitability, behavior, and neurotransmitter regulation such as the septo hippocampal band's cholinergic system and the mesolimbic and nigrostriatal's dopamine system.

Thyroid hormones have an important function of regulating central adrenergic receptor. It can decrease the release of presynaptic noradrenaline and increase the number of postsynaptic β-adrenergic receptor. Hypothyroidism is related with decreased number of β receptor. Thyroid hormones can also make a change in serotonin. T_3 can increase 5–HT in frontal cortex and decrease the number of 5–HT1A auto–receptors. There are evidence suggested that mania symptom could occur if the thyroid status in hypothyroid individuals is normalized rapidly. Hyperthyroidism has symptoms of fatigue, irritability, insomnia, anxiety, restlessness, weight loss, emotional ability, difficulties in focusing on concentration and memory problems.

In hyperthyroid states, using MAO inhibitors or tricyclic antidepressant drugs should be cautious because it may lead to synergistic cardiotoxicity. There are reports suggested that haloperidol(a kind of antipsychoitic drug) can result in increasing thyrotoxicosis and hyperthyroidism can play a role in enhancing the neurotoxicity effects of antipsychotic drugs. A transient hyperthyroxinemia has been found in many psychiatric disorders such as eating disorders, panic disorder, alcoholism, schizophrenia, and major depressive disorder just because of decreasing level of response of TSH to TRH. Most antidepressant therapies have influence on the concentration of thyroid hormone. There are reports suggested that among patients who used lithium as a treatment, about 30% of patients had an elevated TSH level and approximately one–sixth of patients developed frank hypothyroidism.

1.2.3.4 Growth hormone and somatostatin

Somatotropin or growth hormone(GH) is synthesized by the pituitary gland. The release of it mainly depends on dopamine, serotonin(5–HT1D receptor), and norepinephrine(α_2–adrenergic receptor). GH can stimulates lipolysis and ketogenesis which play an important role in the stress adaptation and prevent hypoglycemia. There is report suggested that in anxious subjects, the level of GH increased due to the psychological stress maybe through increasing the activity of noradrenergic system. There is quite a large number of GH deficient patients with depression, using GH as a therapy can improve their depression score.

Somatostatin(SRIF)can inhibit the secretion of ACTH, thyrotropin, GH, and prolactin by pituitary and affect the release of catecholamine neurotransmitters and serotonin. SRIF can be associated with various cognitive dysfunction disorders such as Huntington's disease, Parkinson disease, multiple sclerosis, and Alzheimer's disease.

1.2.3.5 Prolactin

The secretion of prolactin can be inhibited by dopamine neurons of the hypothalamus tuberoinfundibular section(Sadock et al. ,2009), therefore, it can also be increased by classical antipsychotic drugs which is a kind of side effect. Hyperprolactinemic patients often have symptoms of depre-ssion, libido reduction, low stress tolerance, anxiety, and increased irritability. There are associations between the seve-rity of tardive dyskinesia and the concentrations of prolactin especially those tardive dyskinesia that led by antipsychiatric drug in females.

In addition, AVP, oxytocin, neuropeptide Y, galanin, insulin, leptin, cholecystokinin, gastrin and gastrin–releasing peptide(GRP), neurotensin and parathyroid hormone also have important physiological function and have relationship with many kinds of neuropsychiatric system disease.

Zhu Gang

Chapter 2

Classification and Diagnosis System of Psychiatric Disorders

The diagnosis and classification is to classify the mental symptoms according to the diagnosis standard. Classification is needed in psychiatry because it can enable clinicians to communicate with one another about the diagnoses given to their patients. The most widely used disease classification systems are International Classification of Diseases(ICD system) published by the World Health Organization(WHO) and Diagnostic and Statistical Manual of Mental Disorders(DSM system) published by the American Psychiatric Association(APA). In China, there is also Classification and Diagnostic Criteria of Mental Disorders in China(CCMD system) published by Chinese Medical Association. In this chapter, we review the history and development of these classification systems.

2.1 Introduction

2.1.1 The history of classification

In 1967, Henry Brill firstly discussed the purpose of classification in Comprehensive Textbook of Psychiatry(CTP), reviewed the problems of previous classification method, and proposed the problems of applying diagnosis criterion into clinical issues.

Classification aims to classify psychiatric disorders into different categories according to the symptom characteristic which will help us have a more logical understand of psychiatry and benefit the diagnosis and therapy. The classification should concern about the etiology or pathophysiology. A suitable classification should have three characteristics: communication, control, and comprehension.

Communication: the classification should be able to provide a suitable, effective way to name the categories so that the clinicians could describe a serious of symptoms into one name, so the name of categories should reach a high level of agreements among clinicians.

Control: it refers to the prevention and therapy of mental illness. A classification should provide knowledge of mental illness that could benefit the control of it.

Comprehension: classification should provide the understanding of etiology and development process of a mental illness which can lead to more effective treatment.

Classification is needed for several purposes.

To enable clinicians communicate and discuss the diagnosis given to patients with other clinicians.

To understand the implications of the diagnosis in forms of their symptoms, prognosis and etiology.

To relate the findings of clinical research to patients seen in everyday practice.

To facilitate epidemiological studies and the collection of reliable statistics.

To ensure that research can be conducted with comparable groups of subjects.

In 1840, the first official mental illness system appeared but was just used for the decennial census which only had one category combining the idiotic and insane people together. In 1880, mental illness was firstly divided into different categories although only had seven categories. In 1889, the International Congress of Mental Science in Paris adopted the 11 categories proposed by a commission. In 1923, the Bureau of the Census cooperated with the American Psychiatric Association and the National Committee for Mental Health and proposed a classification system consisted of 22 disorders. It was revised and published into the first edition of the American Medical Association's Standard Classified Nomenclature of Disease in 1953. However, this classification system was just designed for chronic disorders, but didn't include acute disorder, psychosomatic disorders and personality disorders which occurs frequently in the period of World War II. So just after the World War II, the Veterans Administration and the military developed their own systems. In 1948 WHO revised the International List of Causes of Death into the Manual of the International Classification of Diseases, Injuries, and Causes of Death (ICD−6) which was the first time including the classification of mental illness. However, it didn't include the categories of dementias, many personality disorders, and adjustment disorders, so it was not widely accepted. In 1952, APA published the first version of Diagnostic and Statistical Manual of Mental Disorders (DSM−I) including 106 diagnoses. Considering the unsatisfactory of ICD−6, the World Health Organization cooperated with the United States Public Health Service and published ICD−8 in 1968. Since ICD−8 didn't have an accompanying glossary, in 1972 the APA published the glossary based on ICD−8. In 1967, the draft of the second version of DSM was adopted by the APA which had 182 disorders in 10 major categories. It allowed clinicians to make diagnosis to every disorders that appeared, unlike DSM−I discouraged multiple diagnosis. In 1975, the ninth version of the ICD (ICD−9) classification of mental disorders with a glossary was published which had no obvious difference from ICD−8. The DSM−III was published in 1980 which was the first official diagnosis system that specified inclusion and exclusion diagnostic criteria, included some diagnosis method into clinical use and expanded the number of disorders into more than 200. And it was also the first official diagnosis system that proposed the multiaxial evaluation system. The DSM−IV was ultimately published in 1994. The DSM−IV−TR was published in 2000.

2.1.2   The Multi−axial diagnosis system

The multi−axial diagnosis system refers to two or more sets of information (such as symptoms, etiology and personality type) in determining a diagnosis scheme. Erik Essen−Möller was the first to propose it in psychiatry in 1971 by considering the clinical syndrome as one axis and aetiology as another. Multi−axial classification is integral used in DSM−IV and ICD−10. But there are some voice suggested that it might be too complex and cost too much time to use as a daily diagnosis method.

2.1.3   The five−axial system

Axis I : all the clinical disorders except for the personality disorders and mental retardation.

Axis II : the personality disorders and mental retardation.

Axis Ⅲ : general medical condition that may related with mental disorders such as physical disorders.

Axis Ⅳ : psychosocial and environmental problems.

Axis Ⅴ : the assessment of the whole function such as symptom severity, social functioning, and occupational functioning.

2.2   Diagnosis system of psychiatric disorders

2.2.1   International Classification of Diseases

International Classification of Diseases(ICD system) is an international disease classification method that published by the WHO. It originated from the International List of Causes of Death which aimed to make a unified registration of death in 1891. It was revised several times later. In 1940, it first included mental disease into classification of disease and became the first comprehensive disease classification, which is called ICD-6. The latest version is ICD-10 published in 1992, this version considered the etiology, pathology and symptomatology classification discipline, and was broadly used in several countries.

It is consisted of 10 major categories, and each categories included 10 subclasses. The 10 major categories are as follows.

F00-F09, organic, including symptomatic, mental disorders.

F10-F19, mental and behavioral disorders due to psychoactive substance use.

F20-F29, schizophrenia, schizotypal and delusional disorders.

F30-F39, mood(affective) disorders.

F40-F48, neurotic, stress-related and somatoform disorders.

F50-F59, behavioral syndromes associated with physiological disturbances and physical factors.

F60-F69, disorders of adult personality and behaviour.

F70-F79, mental retardation.

F80-F89, disorders of psychological development.

F90-F98, behavioral and emotional disorders with onset during occurring in childhood and adolescence.

2.2.2   Diagnostic and Statistical Manual of Mental Disorders

Diagnostic and Statistical Manual of Mental Disorders(DSM system) is based on symptomatology classification discipline. The first version of Diagnostic and Statistical Manual of Mental Disorders was published by the American Psychiatric Association(APA) in 1952. And then it was constantly revised and expanded the disease classification and categories later. In 1968, DSM-Ⅱ was published and made some changes on the basis of ICD-8 according to American situation. This version regarded homosexuality as a kind of mental illness, this point was lately removed by psychiatric vote in 1973. DSM-Ⅲ which was published in 1980 proposed the multi-axis diagnosis system and provided operational criteria for each diagnosis. In 1994, DSM-Ⅳ was published, and lately the revised version DSM-Ⅳ-TR was published in 2000 which used the five-axis diagnosis system. The latest version is DSM-5 published in 2003.

DSM-Ⅳ divides psychiatric disorders into 17 major categories as follows. ①Disorders usually first diagnosed in infancy, childhood, or adolescence. ②Delirium, dementia, and amnestic and other cognitive disorders. ③Mental disorders due to a general medical condition not elsewhere classified. ④Substance-related disorders. ⑤ Schizophrenia and other psychotic disorders. ⑥ Mood disorders. ⑦ Anxiety disorders. ⑧Somatoform disorders. ⑨Factitious disorders. ⑩Dissociative disorders. ⑪Sexual and gender identity disorders. ⑫Eating disorders. ⑬Sleep disorders. ⑭Impulse—control disorders not elsewhere classified. ⑮Adjustment disorders. ⑯Personality disorders. ⑰Other conditions that may be a focus of clinical attention.

The latest version expands the 17 major categories of DSM—5 into 22 major categories as follows. ①Neurodevelopmental disease. ②Schizophrenia spectrum and other psychotic disorders. ③Bipolar and associated disorders. ④Depressive disorders. ⑤Anxiety disorders. ⑥Obsessive—compulsive and related disorders. ⑦Trauma and stressor related disorders. ⑧Dissociative disorders. ⑨Somatic symptom and related disorders. ⑩Feeding and eating disorders. ⑪Elimination disorders. ⑫Sleep—wake disorders. ⑬Sexual dysfunctions. ⑭Gender dysphonia. ⑮Disruptive, impulse—control, and conduct disorders. ⑯Substance—related and addictive disorders. ⑰Neurocognitive disorders. ⑱Personality disorders. ⑲Paraphilic disorders. ⑳Other mental disorders. ㉑Medication—induced movement disorders and other adverse effects of medication. ㉒Other conditions that may be a focus of clinical attention.

2.2.3　Classification and Diagnostic Criteria of Mental Disorders in China

Classification and Diagnostic Criteria of Mental Disorders in China(CCMD system) takes account of both etiology,pathology classification and Symptomatology classification discipline. The first version of Classification and Diagnostic Criteria of Mental Disorders in China was published in 1978,it summarised psychiatric disorders into 10 categories. Later Chinese psychiatry association established Chinese psychiatric disorders classification scheme and diagnosis criterion formulation working community in 1987,after two years, CCMD-2 was published. The revised version(CCMD-2-R) was published in 1995. The latest version is CCMD-3 published in 2001. It is similar to ICD-10 but makes some changes according to the situation of our country.

CCMD-3 divides psychiatric disorders into 10 major categories as follows. ① Organic mental disorders. ②Mental disorders due psychoactive substances or non—addictive substances. ③Schizophrenia and other psychotic disorders. ④ Mood (affective) disorders. ⑤ Hysteria, stress—related disorders, neurosis. ⑥Physiological disorders related to psychological factors. ⑦Personality disorders,habit and impulse disorders,psychosexual disorders. ⑧Mental retardation,and disorders of psychological development with onset usually occurring in childhood and adolescence. ⑨Hyperkinetic,conduct,and emotional disorders with onset usually occurring in childhood and adolescence. ⑩Other mental disorders and psychological health conditions.

Zhu Gang

Chapter 3

Psychiatric Symptomatology

3.1 Introduction

The study of psychiatric symptoms or syndromes is called symptomatology. Morbid mental activity may manifest itself as a variety of syndromes. At present, the etiology and pathogenesis of many psychiatric diseases are unclear, precise identification of the syndromes of mental illness is the first necessary step in clinical diagnosis and treatment.

In physical medicine, syndromes existed long before the etiology of these illnesses were known. Some of these syndromes have subsequently been shown to be true disease entities because they have one essential cause, such as smallpox and measles. With each new step in the progress of medicine, such as microscopy, immunology, electrophysiology. Some syndromes have been found to be true disease entities, while others have been split into more discrete entities. We must not forget that syndromes may or may not be true disease entities, and the multifactorial etiology of psychiatric disorder, related to both constitutional and environmental vulnerability, may make the goal of identifying psychiatric syndromes as discrete diseases.

In psychiatry, as in other branches of medicine, many syndromes began as one specific and striking symptom. Later, the recognition that certain other signs and symptoms co-occurred simultaneously led to the establishment of true syndromes.

This chapter introduces the most common psychiatric symptoms in clinical practice according to the classification of normal mental processes, cognition (including consciousness, memory, intelligence, sensation, thought), emotion, volition and psychomotor.

3.1.1 The nature of psychiatric symptoms

The first major classification of mental illness was based on the distinction between disorders arising from disease of the brain and those with no such obvious basis, i. e., organic versus functional states. These terms are still used, but as knowledge of the neurobiological processes associated with psychiatric disorders has increased, their original meaning has been lost. Schizophrenia and manic depression are the typical examples of functional disorders, but the increasing evidence of the role of genetics and neuropathological abnormalities shows that there is at least some organic basis for these disorders.

The organic syndromes due to brain disorders can be classified into acute, subacute and chronic. The acute organic syndromes are characterized as alteration of consciousness, which can be dream-like, depressed or restricted. This gives rise to four subtypes, i. e. , delirium, subacute delirium, organic stupor or torpor, and the twilight state. In subacute delirium there is a general lowering of awareness and marked incoherence of psychic activity, so that the patient is bewildered and perplexed. Isolated hallucinations, illusions and delusions may occur. The level of awareness varies, and is lower at night-time. The chronic organic states include various dementias, generalized and focal, as well as the amnestic disorders.

The functional syndromes refer to those with no readily apparent brain disease, although increasingly it has been recognized that some finer variety of brain disease may exist, often at a cellular level. For many years, it was customary to divide these functional mental illnesses into neuroses and psychoses. The person with neurosis was believed to have insight into his illness, with only part of his personality involved in the disorder, and to have intact reality testing. The individual with psychosis, on the other hand, was believed to lack insight, had the whole of his personality distorted by the illness and constructed a false environment out of his distorted subjective experience. However, such differences are an over simplification, since many individuals with neurotic conditions have no insight, and far from accepting their illness, may minimize or deny it totally, while people with schizophrenia may seek help willingly during or before episodes of relapse. Moreover, personality can be changed significantly by non-psychotic disorders such as depressive illness, while it may be intact in some people with psychotic disorders such as persistent delusional disorder. Over time the use of the terms neurotic and psychotic changed and instead of describing symptoms, particularly symptom types such as hallucinations or delusions, in the psychotic person they were used to distinguish mild and severe disorders or to distinguish those symptoms that were ego-syntonic(i. e. , creating no distress for the person or compatible with the individual's self-concept or ego) or ego-dystonic(i. e. , causing distress and incompatible with the person's self-concept).

3. 1. 2   Identification of psychiatric symptoms

To determine whether a person's mental activity or behavior is a symptom of psychiatric disorder, should be based on the following. ①The form and content of symptoms is clearly inconsistent with the surrounding objective environment. ②The appearance and disappearance of symptoms can be controlled by that patient. ③Symptoms bring painful experience and varying degree of social functional damage to that patient. We can differentiate by the following methods. ①Vertical comparison, which means to explore whether mental state of the person changes obviously by comparing with the past consistent performance. ②Horizontal comparison, refers to compare mental state of the person with most health, whether the difference is coarse, last long beyond the general limit. ③Conduct a specific analysis based on psychological background and the constitutional and environmental vulnerabilityin episode.

Main means of mental state examination are conversation and observation in the diagnostic interview. Skilled interviewing and good therapeutic relationships generally play acritical role in the recognition of psychiatric symptoms, especially for the psychiatric symptomshidden.

In the observation of psychiatric symptoms, not only the presence or absence of psychiatric symptoms, but also the frequency, duration and severity all need to be noted. In general, psychiatric symptoms are not manifested at all time and must be carefully and repeatedly observed. It is easy to cause missed diagnosis and misdiagnosed according to short-term, one-sided observation.

There are four steps in the mental state examination. First, identify psychiatric symptoms, determine whether there are psychiatric symptoms, and what kinds of psychiatric symptoms they are. Second, learn about the intensity, duration and severity of these psychiatric symptoms. Third, analyze the relationship among different psychiatric symptoms. Fourth, pay attention to the identification between the "functional" psychiatric symptoms and psychiatric symptoms caused by organic brain diseases, to avoid misdiagnosis. For example, flat expression could occur in depressive symptom, negative symptom of schizophrenia, and also in "mask face" of extrapyramidal syndrome. Fifth, explore the possible cause or influencing factors of psychiatric symptoms, including biological, social, and psychological factors. Eliminating these factors is helpful for patients to reduce psychiatric symptoms.

3.1.3 The classification of psychiatric symptoms

There are several ways to classify psychiatric symptoms, according to psychological processes, such as consciousness, memory, intelligence, perception, thought, emotion, volition, and psychomotor. The human mental activity is a whole, a variety of psychological processes which are closely coordinated, collaborative activities. In order to facilitate the description of the process of mental activity, psychiatrists artificially separated mental activity. In general, psychiatric symptoms can be classified as four psychopathology as follow.

3.1.3.1 Consciousness, memory and intelligence

Consciousness, memory and intelligence are basis of individual cognitive activities. Which are refered to how individuals learn about and understand themselves and the world. Serious abnormalities in this area suggest that patients possibly have organic mental disorders.

3.1.3.2 Perception and thought

Perception and thought are the core of individual's cognitive process, such as perceiving themselves and the world, thinking, reasoning, learning and expressing of ideas. The patient has no disorder of consciousness, memory and intelligence but has serious abnormalities of perception and thought, like hallucination and delusion, is likely to refer to a severe psychosis, such as schizophrenia.

3.1.3.3 Emotion

Emotion can be defined as a positive or negative experience that is associated with a particular pattern of physiological activity. Abnormalities of emotion can be seen in a variety of mental disorder, severe emotional abnormalities are more common in mood disorder.

3.1.3.4 Volition and psychomotor

Volition and psychomotor reflect how individuals respond to internal and external stimuli. Abnormalities in this area can also be seen in a variety of mental disorder, especially severe mental disorders.

3.2 Disturbances of consciousness

Different scientific disciplines define consciousness from different perspectives. In philosophy, consciousness refers to the subjective world compared with the objective existence, and includes all the mental activities of human beings. In psychology, consciousness is regarded as the function of the brain and refers to the reflection of the objective reality. In medicine, consciousness is awareness of the self and the environment, which describes that sets of neural processes that allow an individual to perceive, comprehend, and act upon the internal and external environments.

Although psychiatry is a branch of medicine, the understanding of consciousness has its own particularity. The awareness in psychiatry is classified into environmental – consciousness and self – consciousness based on the individual's understanding of the objective reality and their own conditions. Environmental-consciousness includes the understanding of the content and nature of various external things, and self-consciousness includes understanding of their own thinking, emotion, behavior, function and self-concept, and ability to conduct self-evaluation and self-adjustment.

3.2.1 Definition of consciousness disorder

Disorders of consciousness are medical conditions that inhibit consciousness. Consciousness disorder is defined as any change from complete self-awareness and arousal to inhibition or absent.

3.2.1.1 Environmental-consciousness disorder

The environmental-consciousness disorder in psychiatry is roughly equivalent to the consciousness disorder in general medicine, which includes lowering and restriction of consciousness, and change of consciousness content. Disorders of environmental-consciousness are generally associated with disorders of perception, attention, attitudes, thinking, registration and orientation. As mentioned earlier, serious environmental-awareness disorder can be accompanied by an disorder of self-consciousness.

3.2.1.2 Self-consciousness disorder

Serious environmental-consciousness disorder often accompanied by the disorder of self-consciousness, which is the main characteristic of organic mental disorder, is more common in clinical departments rather than psychiatric. The simple disorder of self-consciousness is mainly found in non-organic mental disorders such as schizophrenia. The environmental awareness is generally normal.

3.2.2 Classification of consciousness disorder

3.2.2.1 Dream-like change of consciousness

With dream-like change of consciousness, the level of consciousness is lowered, which is the subjective experience of a rise in the threshold for all incoming stimuli. The patient is disoriented for time and place, but not for person. The main feature in this state is often the presence of visual hallucinations, usually of small animals and associated with fear or even terror. The patient is unable to distinguish between their mental images and perceptions, so that their mental images acquire the value of perceptions. As would be expected, thinking is disordered as it is in dreams and shows excessive displacement, condensation and misuse of symbols.

(1) Clouding of consciousness

Clouding of consciousness known as brain fog or mental fog, is a term used in medicine denoting an abnormality in the regulation of the overall level of consciousness that is mild and less severe than a delirium. The sufferer experiences a subjective sensation of mental clouding described as feeling "foggy". Clouding of consciousness differs from normal delirium by being overall less severe, lacking acuteness in onset and duration, having a relatively stable sleep-wake cycle, and having relatively stable motor alterations.

(2) Delirium

Delirium also known as acute confusing state, is an organically caused decline from previously baseline level of mental function. It often has a fluctuating course, attentional deficits, and disorganization of behavior. It typically involves other cognitive deficits, changes in arousal (hyperactive, hypoactive, or mixed), perceptual deficits, altered sleep-wake cycle, and psychotic features such as hallucinations and delusions. Delirium itself is not a disease, but rather a set of symptoms.

3.2.2.2 Lowering of consciousness

With lowering of consciousness the patient is psychologically benumbed and there is a general lowering of consciousness without hallucinations, illusions, delusions and restlessness. The patients are apathetic, generally slowed down, unable to express themselves clearly, and may persistent. There is no accepted term for this state that is best designated as "torpor". In the past, this type of consciousness was very often the result of severe infections such as typhoid and typhus. Nowadays, it is more commonly seen in the context of arteriosclerotic cerebral disease following a cerebrovascular accident.

(1) Somnolence

Somnolence is a state of strong desire for sleep, or sleeping for unusually long periods. It has distinct causes. It refers to the usual state preceding falling asleep, the condition of being in a drowsy state due to circadian rhythm disorders, or a symptom of other medical problems. It can be accompanied by lethargy, weakness, and lack of mental agility.

(2) Sopor

Sopor is a condition of abnormally deep sleep or a stupor from which it is difficult to rouse. It involves a profound depression of consciousness, which is manifested by drowsiness, while maintaining coordinated defensive reactions to stimuli such as pain, harsh sound, and bright light, and preserving vital functions. Sopor may be caused by a drug; such drugs are deemed soporific. A stupor is worse than a sopor.

(3) Coma

Coma is a state of unconsciousness in which a person can not be awakened; fails to respond normally to painful stimuli, light, or sound; lacks a normal wake-sleep cycle; and does not initiate voluntary actions.

3.2.2.3 Restriction of consciousness

With restriction of consciousness, awareness is narrowed down to a few ideas and attitudes that dominate the patient's mind. There is some lowering of the level of consciousness, so that in some cases the patient may only appear slightly bemused and uninformed bystanders without realizing they are confused. Disorientation for time and place occurs. Some patients are relatively well-ordered in their behavior and may wander, but usually they are not able to fend for themselves, like the patient with a hysterical twilight state.

(1) Twilight state

The term "twilight state" describes the condition which there was a restriction of the morbidly changed consciousness, a break in the continuity of consciousness, and relatively well-ordered behavior. If one keeps strictly to these criteria, then the commonest twilight state is the result of epilepsy. However, this term has been used for any condition in which there is a real or apparent restriction of consciousness, so that simple, hallucinatory, perplexed, excited, expansive, psychomotor and orientated twilight states have been described.

(2) Hysterical twilight state

In severe anxiety the patient may be so preoccupied by their conflicts that they are not fully aware of their environment and find that they have only a hazy idea of what has happened in the past hour or so. This may suggest to the patient that amnesia is a solution for their problems, so that they "forget" their personal identity and the whole of their past as a temporary solution for their difficulties. This restriction of consciousness resulting from unconscious motives has been termed a "hysterical twilight state". It may be difficult to decide how much the motivation of a hysterical twilight state is unconscious because in some cases the subject seems to be deliberately running away from his troubles.

(3) Fugues

Wandering states with some loss of memory have also been called fugues, but not all fugues are hysterical. For example, some individuals with depression may commit suicide and wander about indecisively for days before finding their way home. Hysterical fugue may be more common in subjects who have previously had a head injury with concussion, possibly because they are familiar with the pattern of amnesia from their past experience of concussion and can therefore present it as a hysterical symptom.

3.2.3   Disturbances of attention and concentration

Attention can be active when the subject focuses on some internal or external event, or passive when the same events attract the subject's attention without any conscious effort on their part. Active and passive attention are reciprocally related to each other, since the more the subject focuses their attention the greater must be the stimulus that will distract them(i. e. , bring passive attention into action).

Disturbance of active attention shows itself as distractibility, so that the patient is diverted by almost all new stimuli and habituation to new stimuli takes longer than usual. It can occur in fatigue, anxiety, severe depression, mania, schizophrenia and organic states. In abnormal and morbid anxiety, active attention may be made difficult by anxious preoccupations, while in some organic states and paranoid schizophrenia, distractibility may be the result of a paranoid frame of mind. In other individuals with acute schizophrenia, distraction may be regarded as the result of formal thought disorder because the patient is unable to keep the marginal thoughts(which are connected with external objects by displacement, condensation and symbolism) out of their thinking, so that irrelevant external objects are incorporated into their thinking.

(1)Inattention is described as a failure to attention.

(2)Aprosexia is an abnormal inability to pay attention, characterized by a near-complete indifference to everything.

(3)Hyperprosexia is a abnormal state in which a person concentrates on one thing to the exclusion of everything else.

(4)Distractibility is a condition in which the attention of the mind is easily distracted by small and irrelevant stimuli.

3.2.4   Disorder of orientation

Orientation is normally described in terms of time, place and person. When consciousness is disturbed it tends to affect these three aspects in that order. Orientation in time requires that an individual maintain a continuous awareness of what goes on around them and recognize the time mark. When the customary events that mark the passage of time are missing, it is very easy to become more or less disoriented of time. Everybody who has been in a strange place has experienced this. Orientation for place is retained more easily because the surroundings provide some clues. Orientation for person is lost with greatest difficulty because the persons themselves provide the information that identifies them.

3.3   **Memory disorder**

Memory is consisted of three types: sensory, short-term and long-term. Sensory memory is registered for each of the senses and its purpose is to facilitate the rapid processing of incoming stimuli so that comparisons can be made with material already stored in short-term and long-term memory. Short-term memory, it also called working memory, allows for the storage of memories for much longer than the few seconds available to sensory memory. Short-term memory aids the constant updating of one's surroundings. When memories have been rehearsed in short-term memory, they are encoded into long-term memory. Encoding is the process of placing information into memory reservoir, which can occur for specific stimuli as well as for the general me-mory. The storage of material in long-term memory allows for recall of events from the past and for the utilization of information learned through the education system.

The process of remembering includes 4 parts: registration, retention, retrieval and recall. For the purposes of discussion, we can classified memory impairments into amnesias (loss of memory) and paramnesias (distortions of memory).

3.3.1 The amnesias

Amnesia is defined as partial or total inability to recall past experiences and events. The origin may be organic or psychogenic.

Failure to recall may also occur due to normal memory decay, so that if an item is not rehearsed the memory fades and thereafter can not be retrieved. A further cause of normal memory failure is interference from related material. In proactive interference old memories interfere with new learning and hence with recall, while in retroactive interference new memories interfere with the retrieval of old material. Proactive interference explains why learning Chinese this year will make it difficult to learn French next year, while retroactive interference explains why learning Chinese this year makes it difficult to recall the French learned last year.

3.3.1.1 Organic amnesias

(1) Retrograde amnesia

In organic brain diseases, memory is poor owing to disorders of perception and attention. Hence there is a failure to encode material in long-term memory. In acute head injury, there is an amnesia, known as retrograde amnesia, that embraces the events just before the injury. This period is usually no longer than a few minutes but occasionally may be longer, especially in subacute conditions.

(2) Anterograde amnesia

Anterograde amnesia is amnesia for events occurring after the injury. These occur most commonly following accidents and are indicative of failure to encode events into long-term memory.

(3) Blackouts

Blackouts are circumscribed periods of anterograde amnesia experienced particularly by those who are alcohol dependent during and following bouts of drinking. They indicate reversible brain damage and vary in length but can span many hours. They also occur in acute confusing states (delirium) due to infections or epilepsy.

(4) Korsakoff's syndrome

Korsakoff's syndrome is the amnestic syndrome caused by thiamine deficiency, patients with amnesia or those with Korsakoff's syndrome usually have a loss of memory extending back into the recent past for a year or so.

3.3.1.2 Psychogenic amnesias

(1) Dissociative or hysterical amnesia

Dissociative or hysterical amnesia is the sudden amnesia that occurs during periods of extreme trauma and can last for hours or even days. The amnesia will be for personal identity such as name, address and history as well as for personal events, while at the same time the ability to perform complex behaviors is maintained.

（2）Katathymic amnesia

Katathymic amnesia is also known as motivated forgetting, which is the inability to recall specific painful memories, and is believed to occur due to the defense mechanism of repression. Katathymic amnesia is more persistent and circumscribed than dissociation in that there is no loss of personal identity.

（3）Anxiety/depressive amnesia

Anxiety amnesia occurs when there is anxious preoccupation or poor concentration in disorders such as depressive illness or generalized anxiety. Initially it may wrongly suggest dissociative amnesia. More severe forms of amnesia in depressive disorders resemble dementia and are known as depressive pseudodementia. Amnesias in anxiety and depre-ssive disorders are generally caused by impaired concentration and resolve once the underlying disorder is treated.

3.3.2　Distortions of memory or paramnesia

This is the falsification of memory by distortion and can be conveniently divided into distortions of recall and distortions of recognition.

3.3.2.1　Distortions of recall

（1）Retrospective falsification

Retrospective falsification refers to the unintentional distortion of memory that occurs when it is filtered through a person's current emotional, experiential and cognitive state. It is often found in those with depressive illness who describe all past experiences in negative terms due to the impact of their current mood.

（2）False memory

False memory is the recollection of an event (or events) that did not occur but which the individual subsequently strongly believes did take place.

3.3.2.2　Distortions of recognition

（1）Déjà vu

Déjà vu is not strictly a disturbance of memory, but a problem with the familiarity of places and events. It comprises the feeling of having experienced a current event in the past, although it has no basis in fact.

（2）False reconnaissance

False reconnaissance is defined as false recognition or misidentification and it can occur in organic psychoses and in acute and chronic schizophrenia. It may be positive when the patient recognizes strangers as their friends and relatives.

3.3.3　Hyperamnesia

Flashbacks are sudden intrusive memories that are associated with the cognitive and emotional experiences of a traumatic event such as an accident. It is regarded as one of the characteristic symptoms of post-traumatic stress disorder (PTSD).

3.4　Disorders of intelligence

Intelligence is the ability to think and act rationally and logically. The measurement of intelligence is complex and controversial. In practice, intelligence is measured with tests of the ability of the individual to solve problems and form concepts by using words, numbers, symbols, patterns and non-verbal material.

The most common way of measuring intelligence is in terms of the distribution of scores in the population. The person who has an intelligence score on the 75 percentile has a score that is such that 75% of the appropriate population scoreless and 25% score more. Some intelligence tests used for children give a score in terms of the mental age, which is the score achieved by the average child of the corresponding chronological age.

3.4.1   Intellectual disability

Intellectual disability is also known as general learning disability, and mental retardation (MR), is a generalized neurodevelopmental disorder characterized by significantly impaired intellectual and adaptive functioning. It is defined by an IQ score under 70, and deficits in two or more adaptive behaviors that affect daily life. Down syndrome and fragile X syndrome are examples of syndromic intellectual disabilities.

3.4.2   Dementia

Dementia is a loss of intelligence resulting from brain disease, characterized by disturbances of multiple cortical functions, including thinking, memory, comprehension and orientation. The most common type of dementia is Alzheimer's disease, which makes up 50% to 70% of cases. Other common types include vascular dementia (25%), Lewy body dementia (15%), and frontotemporal dementia.

3.5   Disorders of perception

Disorders of perception includes sensory distortions and sensory deceptions. In distortions there is a constant real perceptual object, which is perceived in a distorted way, while in sensory deceptions a new perception occurs that may or may not be in response to an external stimulus.

3.5.1   Sensory distortions

These are changes in perception that are the result of a change in the intensity and quality of the stimulus or the spatial form of the perception.

3.5.1.1   Changes in intensity (hyper- or hypo-aesthesia)

Increased intensity of sensations (hyperaesthesia) may be the result of intense emotions or a lowering of the physiological threshold. Anxiety and depressive disorders as well as hangover from alcohol and migraine are all associated with increased sensitivity to noise (hyperacusis) so that even day-to-day noises such as washing crockery are magnified to the point of discomfort.

Hypoacusis occurs in delirium, where the threshold for all sensations is raised. This highlights the importance of speaking to the delirious patient more slowly and louder than usual. Hypoacusis is also a feature of other disorders associated with attentional deficits such as depression and attention-deficit disorder.

3.5.1.2   Changes in quality

It is mainly visual perceptions that are affected by this, brought about by toxic substances. Colouring of yellow, green and red have been named xanthopsia, chloropsia and erythropsia.

3.5.1.3   Changes in spatial form (dysmegalopsia)

This refers to a change in the perceived shape of an object. Micropsia is a visual disorder in which the patient sees objects as smaller than they really are. The opposite kind of visual experience is known as macropsia or megalopsia. Dysmegalopsia can result from retinal disease, disorders of accommodation and convergence but most commonly from temporal and parietal lobe lesions.

3.5.1.4 Distortions of the experience of time

From the psychopathological point of view there are two varieties of time: physical and personal. It is the latter that is affected by psychiatric disorders. We are all aware of the influence of mood on the passage of time, so that when we are happy "time flies", and when we are sad it passes more slowly. By contrast the manic patient feels that time speeds by and that the days are not long enough to do everything. Distortions of the experience of time is also seen in acute organic states and schizophrenia.

3.5.2 Sensory deceptions

These can be divided into illusions(misinterpretations of stimuli arising from an external object) and hallucinations(perceptions without an adequate external stimulus).

3.5.2.1 Illusions

In illusions, stimuli from a perceived object are combined with a mental image to produce a false perception. Illusions can occur in delirium when the perceptual threshold is raised and an anxious and bewildered patient misinterprets stimuli.

3.5.2.2 Hallucinations

A hallucination is a false perception which is not a sensory distortion or a misinterpretation, but which occurs at the same time as real perceptions. It differs from an illusion in being experienced as originating in the outside world or from within the person's body(rather than as imagined). Most of the statements are derived from the work of Jaspers (1962), who first distinguished between true perceptions and mental images. Perceptions are substantial; appear in objective space; are clearly delineated, constant and independent of the will; and their sensory elements are full and fresh. Mental images are incomplete; are not clearly delineated; are dependent on the will; exist in subjective space; are inconstant and have to be recreated.

(1)Types of hallucination

1)Anditory hallucinations

Auditory hallucination may be elementary and unformed, and experienced as simple noises, bells, undifferentiated whispers or voices. Elementary auditory hallucinations can occur in organic states and noises, partly organized as music or completely organized as hallucinatory voices, in schizophrenia. Patients explain the origin of the voices in different ways. They may insist that the voices are the result of witchcraft, telepathy, radio, television, and so on. Sometimes they claim that the voices come from within their bodies such as their arms, legs, stomach, etc.

Hallucinatory voices vary in quality, ranging from those that are quite clear and can be ascribed to specific individuals to those that are vague and which the patient can not describe with any clarity. Patients are often undisturbed by their inability to describe the direction from which the voices come or the sex of the person speaking. This is quite unlike the experience of the healthy individual. The voices sometimes give instructions to the patient, these are termed "imperative hallucinations". In some cases the voices speak about the person in the third person and may give a running commentary on their actions. These are among Schneider's first-rank symptoms, and although this was one thought to be diagnostic of schizophrenia, this is no longer the case since these symptoms have also been described in mania.

The effect of the voices on the patient's behavior is variable. Some patients(becoming fewer in number with advances in treatment) have continuous hallucinations that do not trouble them.

Sometimes the voices seem to speak the patients thoughts as he is thinking them, or to repeat them immediately after he has thought them.

2) Visual hallucinations

Visual hallucination may be elementary in the form of ashes of light, partly organized in the form of patterns, or completely organized in the form of visions of people, objects or animals. Figures of living things and inanimate objects may appear against the normally perceived environment or scenic hallucinations can occur in which whole scenes are hallucinated rather like a cinema film. Visual hallucinations are more common in acute organic states with clouding of consciousness than in functional psychosis. All varieties of visual hallucination are found in acute organic states but small animals and insects are most often hallucinated in delirium. Scenic hallucinations are common in psychiatric disorders associated with epilepsy. Visual hallucinations are extremely rare in schizophrenia, so much so that they should raise a doubt about the diagnosis. Some patients with schizophrenia describe visions and these appear to be pseudo-hallucinations, but on occasion others will insist that their hallucinations are substantial.

3) Olfactory hallucinations

Hallucinations of odor can occur in schizophrenia and organic states and, uncommonly, in depressive psychosis. It may be difficult to be sure if there is a hallucination or an illusion. There may also be a problem distinguishing olfactory hallucination from delusion, since there are some people who insist that they emit a smell. It is important to ascertain if they actually smell this odor, since many seem to base their belief on the behavior of other people who, they say, wrinkle their noses or make reference to the smell. Some patients with schizophrenia claim that they can smell gas and that their enemies are poisoning them by pumping gas into the room.

4) Gustatory hallucinations

Hallucinations of taste occur in schizophrenia and acute organic states. It is not always easy to know whether the patient actually tastes something odd or if it is a delusional explanation of the effect of feeling strangely changed. Depressed patients often describe a loss of taste or state that all food tastes the same.

5) Tactile hallucinations

This may take the form of small animals crawling over the body, so-called formication. This is not uncommon in acute organic states. In cocaine psychosis this type of hallucination commonly occurs together with delusions of persecution and is known as the "cocaine bug".

(2) Special kinds of hallucination

1) Functional hallucinations

An auditory stimulus causes a hallucination but the stimulus is experienced as well as the hallucination. In other words the hallucination requires the presence of another real sensation. For example, a patient with schizophrenia first heard the voice of God as her clock ticked.

2) Reflex hallucinations

Synaesthesia is the experience of a stimulus in one sense modality producing a sensory experience in another. For example, one patient described hearing his own reflection and said that when attempting to carry out some action he could hear himself doing so.

3) Extracampine hallucinations

The patient has a hallucination that is outside the limits of the sensory field. For example, a patient sees somebody standing behind them when they are looking straight ahead or hear voices talking in Beijing when they are in Wuhan.

4) Hypnagogic hallucinations

Hypnagogic hallucinations occur during drowsiness, are discontinuous, appear to force themselves on the subject and do not form part of an experience in which the subject participates as they do in a dream.

5) Organic hallucinations

Organic hallucinations can occur in any sensory modality and they may occur in a variety of neurological and psychiatric disorders. Organic visual hallucinations occur in eye disorders as well as in disorders of the central nervous system and lesions of the optic tract. Complex scenic hallucinations occur in temporal lobe lesions.

3.6 Disturbance of thoughts

3.6.1 Classification of thought disorders

Any classification of thought disorders is bound to be arbitrary, at least to a certain extent. Thus it has been customary to divide thought disorders into disorders of content and disorders of form; or to put it into more familiar language, disorders of belief and disorders of reasoning. It is obvious that this division is somewhat artificial because belief and reasoning can not be sharply separated. Realizing that any division is bound to be arbitrary, it is suggested that we divide thought disorders into those of the stream of thought, the possession of thought, the content of thought and the form of thought.

3.6.1.1 Disorders of thought stream

Disorders of thought stream can be further divided into disorders of tempo and disorders of continuity.

(1) Disorders of thought tempo

1) Flight of ideas

In flight of ideas thoughts follow each other rapidly; there is no general direction of thinking; and the connections between successive thoughts appear to be due to chance factors which, however, can usually be understood. The patient's speech is easily diverted to external stimuli and by internal superficial associations. Flight of ideas is typical of mania.

2) Inhibition or slowing of thinking

With inhibition or slowing of thinking, the thought is slowed down and the ideas and mental images is decreased. Slowing of thinking is seen in both depression and the rare condition of manic stupor. The apparent cognitive deficits in individuals with slowing of thinking in depression may lead to a mista-ken diagnosis of dementia.

3) Circumstantiality

Circumstantiality occurs when thinking proceeds slowly with many unnecessary and trivial details, but finally the point is reached.

(2) Disorders of the continuity of thinking

1) Perseveration

Perseveration occurs when mental operations persist beyond the point at which they are relevant and thus prevent progress of thinking. Perseveration may be mainly verbal or ideational.

2) Thought blocking

Thought blocking occurs when there is a sudden arrest of the thought, leaving a "blank". An entirely new thought may then begin. When thought blocking is present, it is highly suggestive of schizophrenia.

3) Obsessions and compulsions

It is customary to distinguish between obsessions and compulsions. Obsessions occur in obsessional states, depression, schizophrenia, and occasionally in organic states; compulsive features appear to be particularly common in post-encephalitic parkinsonism. Compulsions are, in fact, merely obsessional motor acts.

4) Thought insertion

In pure thought insertion the patient knows that thoughts are being inserted into their mind and they recognize them as being foreign and coming from without; this symptom, although commonly associated with schizophrenia.

5) Thought deprivation

The patient finds that as they are thinking, their thoughts suddenly disappear and are withdrawn from their mind by a foreign influence.

6) Thought broadcasting

The patient knows that as they are thinking, everyone else is thinking in unison with them.

3.6.1.2   Disorder of thought form

The term "formal thought disorder" is a synonym for disorders of conceptual or abstract thinking that are most commonly seen in schizophrenia and organic brain disorders. Schneider (1930) suggested there were three features of healthy thought.

Constancy: this is characteristic of a completed thought that does not change in content unless and until it is superseded by another consciously-derived thought. Organization: the contents of thought are related to each other in consciousness and do not blend with each other, but are separated in an organized way. Continuity: there is a continuity of the sense continuum, so that even the most heterogenous subsidiary thoughts, sudden ideas or observations that emerge are arranged in order in the whole content of consciousness.

Schneider claimed that individuals with schizophrenia complained of three different disorders of thinking that correspond to these three features of normal or non-disordered thinking. These were: a peculiar transitoriness of thinking, the lack of normal organization of thought, and desultory thinking. There were three corresponding varieties of objective thought disorder, as follows.

(1) Transitory thinking

Transitory thinking is characterized by derailments, substitutions and omissions. The grammatical and syntactical structures are both disturbed in transitory thinking.

(2) Drivelling thinking

Withdrivelling thinking, the patient has a preliminary outline of a complicated thought with all its necessary particulars, but loses preliminary organization of the thought, so that all the constituent parts get muddled together.

(3) Desultory thinking

In desultory thinking speech is grammatically correct but sudden ideas force their way in from time to time. Each one of these ideas is a simple thought that, if used at the right time would be quite appropriate.

3.6.1.3   Delusion

A delusion is a belief that is firmly held on inadequate grounds, that is not affected by national argument or evidence to the contrary, and that is not a conventional belief that the person, might be expected to hold given their educational, cultural and religion background. The fact that a delusion is false makes it easy to recognize, but this is not its essential quality. A common delusion among married persons is that their spouses are unfaithful to them. In the nature of things, some of these spouses will indeed have been unfaithful; the delusion will therefore be true, but only by coincidence. Delusion needs to be differentiated with other items, such as:

Delusion-like ideas: delusion-like idea is secondary and can be understandably derived from some other morbid psychological phenomenon, while true delusions are the result of a primary delusional experience that can not be deduced from any other morbid phenomenon.

Overvalued idea: this is a thought that, because of the associated feeling tone, takes precedence over all other ideas and maintains this precedence permanently or for a long period of time.

(1) Types of delusion

1) Primary delusions

The essence of the primary delusional experience(also termed apophany) is that a new meaning arises in connection with some other psychological event. Primary delusional experiences tend to be reported in acute schizophrenia but are less common in chronic schizophrenia.

2) Secondary delusions and systematization

Secondary delusions can be understood as arising from some other morbid experience.

(2) The content of delusions

The content of delusions of schizophrenia is dependent, to a greater or lesser extent, on the social and cultural background of the patient. Common general themes include persecution, jealousy, love, grandiosity, guilt, and poverty.

1) Delusions of persecution

Delusions of persecution may occur in the context of primary delusional experiences, auditory hallucinations, bodily hallucinations or experiences of passivity. Delusions of persecution can take many forms. In delusions of reference the patient knows that people are talking about him, slandering him or spying on him. Ideas and delusions are not confined to schizophrenia and can occur in depressive disorder and other psychotic illnesses. Delusions of influence are a "logical" result of experiences of passivity in the context of schizophrenia. These passivity feelings may be explained by the patient as the result of hypnotism, witchcraft, radio waves, atomic rays or television.

2) Delusions of infidelity

Delusions of infidelity may occur in both organic and functional disorders. The patient often has been suspicious, sensitive and mildly jealous before the onset of the disorder. Delusions of infidelity may develop gradually, as a suspicious or insecure person becomes more and more convinced of their spouse's infidelity and finally the idea reaches delusional intensity. For example, a jealous husband, may insist that his wife has sexual intercourse with someone else, or may search his wife's underclothes for stains and claim that all stains are due to semen.

3) Delusions of love

The patients are convinced that someone is in love with them although the alleged lover may never have spoken to them.

4) Grandiose delusions

There is considerable variability in the extent of grandiosity associated with grandiose delusions in different patients. Some patients may believe they are God, or famous movie star. Others are less expansive and believe that they are skilled sportspersons or great inventors.

5) Delusions of guilt

In severe depressive disorder, self-reproach may take the form of delusions of guilty, when the patients believes that they are evil and have ruined their family. They may claim to have committed an unpardonable sin and insist that they will rot in hell for this.

6) Delusions of poverty

The patients with delusions of poverty are convinced that they are impoverished and believe that destitution is facing them and their family.

7) Insight

Insight is a multidimensional concept referring to awareness of illness, specific symptoms and their consequences, as well as need for treatment. Insight refers to the patient's ability to understand that some of his or her non-reality based experiences (usually hallucinatory experiences and delusional representations) are secondary to having psychosis rather than reality. Awareness and attribution of current and past symptoms represent specific aspects of insight. Additional dimensions of insight include a more global understanding of the diagnosis and need for treatment.

3.7   Disorders of emotion

Emotion is a stirred-up state caused by physiological changes as a response to some event, which tends to maintain or abolish the causative event. A feeling can be defined as a positive or negative reaction to some experience or event and is the subjective experience of emotion. The feelings may be depression, anxiety, and fear. Mood is a pervasive and sustained emotion. Descriptions of mood should include intensity, duration and fluctuations as well as adjectival descriptions of the type. Affect, meaning short-lived emotion, is defined as the patient's present emotional responsiveness. Doctor infers affect of patients from their body language including facial expression and it may or may not be congruent with mood. It is described as constricted, blunt or flat.

Some emotional reactions are normal responses to events, take an example, the grief reaction that follows the death of a loved one or the response of a previously healthy person to a life-threatening diagnosis. Unfortunately, in practice there has been little attempt to distinguish these understandable and non-morbid reactions from those are abnormal. Many of the symptoms complained of are present both in the normal responses and in those that are abnormal; for example, following a bereavement it is expected that tearfulness, sleep disturbance, anorexia and poor concentration will occur most intensely in the initial days and will diminish over time. When the grief reaction is prolonged or becomes a depressive episode, a similar constellation of symptoms is also present.

Abnormal emotional reactions are understandable in the context of stressful events but are associated with more prolonged impairment in functioning. Functional incapacity is present in abnormal states but absent in the normal reactions.

3.7.1   Depressed mood/depression

Depressed mood means that the patient experiences a negative and unpleasant affect, and in English "depressed" "anguished" "mournful" "sad" "anxious" "blues" are used. The word "depressed" is increasingly used because of the higher information (partially because of the internet) the public has today on depression. The way patient uses describes this experience depends on his/her cultural and educational background, and can focus on bodily function or on existential and interpersonal dysphoria and difficulties. Somatic complaints are more prominent in milder cases usually seen in the primary care setting, particularly in patients with anxious depression. These patients were considered to suffer from "masked" depression.

3.7.2 Anhedonia

Anhedonia refers to the inability to experience normal emotions. Usually, patients with anhedonia are incapable of even feeling depressed and they can't even cry. The patient abandons activities, which in the past were a source of joy and gives up interest in life. Patients with more severe depression are indifferent even concerning their children or spouse and isolate themselves. The difference from the flat (blunted) affect seen in schizophrenia is that anhedonia is itself painful. As depression starts remitting, anhedonia is one of the first symptoms to remit.

3.7.3 Elation

Elation refers to a state of exaltation, over-confidence, and enjoyment, with the person feeling cheerful, laughing and making happy and expressive gestures. It is not always pathological.

3.7.4 Irritability

Irritability mood is a state which the person is easily annoyed by external stimuli and expresses anger and hostility at a low threshold. The presence of an irritable is often the cause for misdiagnosis of the patient, especially in combination with lability and mixed states.

3.7.5 Anxiety

Anxiety is an unpleasant affective state and a simple definition is fear for no adequate reason. Descriptive terms such as tension and stress are often used by the patient. Sometimes anxiety is accompanied by physical symptoms such as palpitations, sweating, difficulty breathing, dizziness, etc. , and if the physical symptoms occur suddenly, and in combination, the result is overwhelming fear, and the term panic attack is used.

Patients often use the word anxiety to describe worry or, if asked directly if they are anxious, they may reply "I have nothing to be anxious about". Some of these patients, however, may admit on further questioning that they feel frightened for no reason, while others do not make the connection between the cause and their symptom.

3.7.6 Phobia

When the fear is restricted to one object, situation or idea, the term phobia is used. Phobias are associated with physical symptoms of anxiety and with avoidance. Most fears are learned responses, such as the person who develops a fear of dogs after being bitten. Some phobias are secondary to morbid states, most commonly depressive illness, and others, such as fear of contamination, are regarded as obsessional symptoms.

3.7.7 Parathymia

Some patients with schizophrenia completely lost all emotional so that the patient is indifferent to their own well-being and that of others. It shows itself as insensitivity to the subtleties of social intercourse and is known as inadequacy or blunting of affect and was called "parathymia" by Bleuler. Parathymia manifests itself as social awkwardness and inappropriateness, for example the patient who took visitors to the yard in his house to show them a dead dog.

3.7.8 Lability of affect

Lability of affect is defined as rapid and abrupt changes in emotion largely unrelated to external stimuli. These shifts occur without warning. It is found in some people with no psychiatric disorder. For example, those who are soft may easily cry. Those with personality disorder of the borderline type may also exhibit lability of affect. However, it is most common in mixed affective states (dysphoric mania) and in mania where short bursts of weeping are present. It may also be a feature in organic brain disease following damage to the frontal lobe or following cerebrovascular accidents.

3.7.9 Affective incontinence

Affective incontinence refers to a total loss of control and this is particularly common in cerebral atherosclerosis and in multiple sclerosis, where spontaneous outbursts of laughter or crying occur. In its most severe form the terms "forced laughing" and "forced weeping" are used to describe this, but there is a mismatch between the emotional expression and the subjective feelings since there is an absence of concomitant feelings of happiness or sadness.

3.8 Disorder of psychomotor

Psychomotor is relating to the psychological processes associated with muscular movement and to the production of voluntary movements. Normally humans experience their actions as being their own and as being under their own control, although this sense of personal control is never in the forefront of consciousness, except when a particular effort is made to overcome the effects of fatigue or toxic substances that are clouding our consciousness and making it difficult for us to control our bodies. In obsessions and compulsions the sense of possession of the thought or act is not impaired, but the patient experiences the obsession as appearing against their volition, so that although they have lost control over a voluntary act, they still retain personal possession of the act.

3.8.1 Psychomotor acceleration

Acceleration is considered to be the hallmark of mania, characterized by excessive activity (which is goal directed, high energy and endurance) as well as rapid, pressured speech.

3.8.2 Psychomotor slowing

Psychomotor slowing means that the patient is inert and slow, both physically and mentally. It does not always have an effect on overall performance although everything is done with much effort.

3.8.3 Psychomotor retardation

When psychomotor slowing is excessive, then psychomotor retardation appears and it includes reduction or disappearance of spontaneous motor activity, slumped posture and gaze, reduced and slow speech, and great fatigue.

3.8.4　Stupor

Stupor is a state of more or less complete loss of activity where there is no reaction to external stimuli; it can be regarded as an extreme form of hypokinesia. Psychomotor inhibition and obstruction may produce a general slowing down of activity, and as these disorders become more severe, the patient's condition approaches stupor. Completely stuperose patients are mute, but in sub−stuperose states, patients may reply questions in muttered monosyllables. Stupor may occur in shock, dissociative or conversion disorders, depression, psychosis, catatonia and organic brain disease.

3.8.5　Catatonia

Catatonia is defined as a complex condition, which can include diverse symptoms and signs such as motoric immobility or on the contrary excessive purposeless motor activity not influenced by external stimuli, motiveless negativism, mutism, peculiar or stereotyped movements, mannerisms, grimacing and sometimes echolalia or echopraxia.

3.8.6　Waxy flexibility

In perseveration of posture the patient tends to maintain for long periods postures that have arisen fortuitously or which have been imposed by the examiner. The patient allows the examiner to put their body into uncomfortable positions and maintains such postures for at least one minute and usually much longer. Sometimes there is a feeling of plastic resistance as the examiner moves the patient's body, which resembles the bending of a soft wax rod, and when the passive movement stops the final posture is preserved.

3.8.7　Movement disorders associated with antipsychotic medication

Antipsychotic medication has been associated with a range of movement disorders, including, extra-pyramidal side−effects. Some of them (for example, tardive dyskinesia) are associated with mental illness (for example, schizophrenia) prior to the prescription of any medication.

In summary, movement disorders associated with antipsychotic medication include acute akathisia (restlessness or inability to keep still), chronic akathisia, acute dystonia (involuntary sustained muscle contraction or spasm), tardive dystonia, and acute and tardive dyskinesia (repetitive, purposeless movements, usually of the mouth, tongue and facial muscles). In addition to the externally observable signs associated with these extrapyramidal side−effects, it is important to elicit the psychological or subjective components of these effects. Akathisia, in particular, may be associated with subjective restlessness, tension and general unease. Tardive dyskinesia may lead to significant additional stigmatization and social disability.

Guo Xin

Chapter 4

Assessment and Diagnosis of Mental Disorders

4.1 Introduction

The human spirit is the reflection of the objective world in the human brain. The brain is the organ of all mental activities, and the mental activity is the function of the highly differentiated material of the brain. People's spiritual activitiescan not exist without the brain. Similarly, human spiritual activities cannot develop without social practice. In fact, the diagnosis of mental disorders has its has its strict standards, patients or family member of patients feel wrong, it is necessary to timely psychiatric doctors to a diagnosis.

4.1.1 Establish a therapeutic relationship

(1) The psychiatric must ensure that the patient feels able and willing to give an accurate and full victory.

(2) Do not judge the patients' value and attitudes towards life and respect their personality, beliefs and culture.

(3) The psychiatrist needs to have sufficient information about the patient's life history, current circumstances, and personality.

4.1.2 Psychiatric assessment

It includes two parts: medical history and psychiatric assessment. It is the basis of diagnosis. How to collect medical history and conduct psychiatric assessment is a basic skill that must be mastered by psychiatrist. Psychiatric themselves are both reliable diagnostic tools and therapeutic tools.

4.2 General principles and procedures for psychiatric assessment

Psychiatric assessment is a process of checking the mental state of a patient through observation and interview. By observing the general expression, emotional responses, actions and behaviors of the patients, those symptoms can be found, such as delusions, hallucinations, delusions. Through the body check, doctors can make judgments whether those signs are positive, and whether there is resistance or waxy flexion. In order to know whether the patients exist the tendency of imitating or not, the doctor must make some commands as well as some actions, and observe the patient's responses respectively.

The purpose of psychiatric interview is to establish a therapeutic relationship; to collect the necessary information in order to make a diagnosis; to understand personal development history and personality characteristics, including major life events, interpersonal relationship and coping style, etc. A psychiatric assessment to obtain necessary information to make a diagnosis; to understand the patient from the perspective of the whole person; to carry out preliminary mental health education to the patient.

4.2.1 General principles of psychiatric assessment

4.2.1.1 Therapeutic relationship

The establishment of a therapeutic relationship refers to a special interpersonal relationship established by medical personnel in the medical process with patients and their families. The importance of therapeutic relationship is reflected mainly in two aspects: first, therapeutic relationship is an important prerequisite for carrying out medical work; second, good therapeutic relationship has positive psychological support. Good therapeutic relationship is very important in medical practice and even has direct therapeutic effect. It is believed that the more doctors and patients understand each other, the more easily the therapeutic relationship will be established. Pure biomedical thinking mode, the therapist has absolute authority, is in the position of the director, the command, the controller, actively controls the process and the progress of the treatment. This puts patients on the location of the completely passive obedience, only requires patients to answer the question and don't want to listen to, interpretation of conversational style not conducive to the establishment of the therapeutic relationship, effectively meeting influence physicians, to obtain useful information, to make the right diagnosis, formulate and implement effective treatment plan. Efforts to build a good therapeutic relationship often result in more than half the effort.

4.2.1.2 Principle of trust

Respect for the principle of trust should be an equal relationship between patients and physicians, and their personalities, rights and privacy should be respected. Establishment of a therapeutic relationship is also essential if the patient is engaging fully in discussions about management , and adhering to any treatment decision which are agreed upon.

In the process of psychiatric assessment, we should start from establishing a trusting relationship with patients so as to ensure the smooth operation of the diagnosis and treatment and achieve satisfactory results. The doctor should treat patients with respect and trust, and should not allow patients to feel their own diseases. The doctor should listen attentively to the patient's history, use sympathy, understanding, encouragement and heuristic questions to guide the patient to pour out the depression, annoyance and pain in the heart. Through psychiatric examination, the patient feels that the doctor is sure of the treatment of the disease and increases the patient's confidence in the treatment.

4.2.1.3   Principle of confidentiality

Confidentiality is the most important ethical principle and professional ethics that clinicians should follow to keep confidential the patient's name, occupation, illness and treatment process. Without the consent of the patient, the healer may not disclose the confidential information obtained during the treatment to the third party. At the beginning of the diagnosis and treatment process, the patient should be shown the confidentiality principle, so that the patient's trust can be obtained, and the good doctor—patient relationship can be promoted to obtain reliable information about the disease.

In some special cases the principle of confidentiality may be broken: patients may harm to themselves or others; the patient disclaims confidentiality or agrees to disclose relevant information; the patient is evaluated and treated according to the law. These three conditions require the minimum level of information disclosure and disclosure of the necessary information.

4.2.1.4   Comprehensive principles

(1) Integration of the mind and body

The human spirit and physiology interact cohesively. Mental disorders are often accompanied by somatic manifestations, and physical conditions are often the cause of mental disorders. As a result, this will require a doctor to the patient's body and mind in the process of mental examination and influence each other, maintain a high level of sensitivity to the dialectical unity of thinking to analyze and look at problems, rather than in isolation one of them.

(2) Synthesis of causes

Each person is a complex of physiology, psychology and society. Therefore, it is also the result of the interaction of these three factors that causes the mental disorders of visitors or patients. Therefore, the analysis, evaluation, diagnosis and treatment of patients should also be taken from these three perspectives.

4.2.2   Basic skills of psychiatric assessment

4.2.2.1   The basic training that a psychiatrist should have

(1) Receptive attitude

The receptive attitude psychiatrist faces a particular group of patients. Talk, behavior, way of life, and even life habits are influenced by the mental symptoms and deviate from the conventional patterns, mental disorders always become the object of discrimination, exclusion, isolated and ignored. In the whole process of psychiatric diagnosis and treatment, the doctor must have close contact with the patient to complete the psychiatric diagnosis and treatment. So psychiatrists need a higher level of professionalism. To be a good psychiatrist, you should sympathize with and care for the patient, and tolerate the sick behavior of the patient. Whatever the patient is, the doctor must accept it faithfully, without any rejection, disgust, disgust, or impatience.

(2) Keen observation

Accurate diagnosis and treatment should be based on observing the patient's facial expressions, eyes, posture, movement, dressing, general state and consciousness. By observing the attitude of the patient to the company, we can judge the advantages and disadvantages of the social support system. Analyze the attitude and response of the patient to the doctor. Acute observation helps to establish a better diagnosis, to judge the prognosis, and to establish a therapeutic relationship.

(3) Good introspective ability

When dealing with patients, a good introspective psychiatrist should try not only to observe the patient's inner world, but also to observe his inner heart. In the psychiatrists' daily life, they may encounter various patients behaved pathologically. Doctors, they are not saints, they may also be irritated by the patients' weird behaviors, especially those with the intention of attack, or insult, which in return have negative effects on doctors, such as: anger, resentment, hatred, jealousy, and so on. If this negative emotion accumulates, it will not only harm the health of the doctor, but also harm the medical behavior. In addition to mastering the skills of negative emotions, psychiatrists should also be aware that analyzing their inner feelings calmly may also help to make the right diagnosis. As a red-faced, brawny man calls to the doctor to tell him about his physical ailments, the boredom of the doctor can prompt the diagnosis of a "hypochondriac". When the doctor take dozens of minutes after talking with a patient, still without a clue, nor to the jaw, the doctor do his own confusion and anxiety patients there are communication barriers, and communication barrier is one of the characteristic symptoms of schizophrenia.

(4) Rich experience and knowledge

People with mental disorders in young and old, learning has high and low, cultural background, family environment, growth experience is different, to do to deal with the "people" rather than dealing with "disease" is not easy. This needs the doctor with medical knowledge outside of all kinds of knowledge and rich experience, can communicate with all kinds of patients, to understand the spirit of the living in the big world patients complicated inner experience.

4.2.2.2　Communication skills that a psychiatrist should possess

Good communication skills are the cornerstone of good medical practice. Its importance is manifested in the following aspects: effective communication is an essential part of diagnosis; effective communication can improve the patient's adherence to treatment; effective communication helps to improve doctors' clinical skills and self-confidence; effective communication helps to improve patient satisfaction; effective communication can improve the efficiency of health resources and improve the quality of health services. Therefore, in a broad sense, communication skills should be a required course for all clinicians.

(1) Listening

Listening is the most effective way to establish a doctor-patient relationship and conduct a mental examination. Doctors must spend as much time as possible listening to patients with patience, concentration and care. If the patient is far away from the topic, the doctor can help the patient return to the subject by reminding him. The doctor should allow the patient to have ample time to describe his physical symptoms and internal pain, and the abrupt interruption of the patient's trust may be lost in an instant. It can be said that listening is the most important step in developing a good relationship between doctors and patients.

(2) Affirmation

Affirmation is the "personal authenticity" of the patient's experience and feelings. We do not agree with the patient's pathological beliefs or hallucinations, but we can show the patient that the doctor understands the feelings he describes. Acceptance, rather than a simple negative attitude, is conducive to communication between doctors and patients. Such as anxiety depression patients with somatic symptoms as complaint always feel uncomfortable in all parts of the body, although various physical test results were negative, but patients still can not dispel fear or doubt, because uncomfortable feeling is real. At this point, we should first affirm that the patient's feelings have "individual authenticity", and express understanding and sympathy. Of course, the physician must also confirm the "objective reality" of the results and use communication skills to explain why. For this kinds of the patient, agreeing with his uncomfortable feeling is the basis for confidence building.

(3) Clarification

Clarification is to analyze the nature of symptoms, the process of events and the emotional experience of patients. Try not to ask questions in a way that avoids patients accusing or doubting the doctor's motive. It is best to let the patient fully describe the event and understand how the patient feels at all stages of the event.

(4) Be good at asking questions

The purpose of the question is to clarify symptoms and guide the conversation. If the patient is too repetitive, use questions to give guidance, pay attention to this question should be a patient care about most, the most important problems in communication, then naturally turn to other issues need to be further clarified. There are two ways to ask questions: open conversation and closed-door conversation.

(5) Refactoring

Retell or summarize the patient's words in different words and sentences without changing the meaning and purpose of the patient's speech. Refactoring can highlight key topics and show patients that doctors can fully understand the patient's feelings.

(6) Representative

Some thoughts and feelings are not to be said, but they are important to the patient. At this point, the doctor can talk about it. This requires a keen observation of the doctor. For example, for people with sexual dysfunction who are ashamed to talk about the topic, the doctor starts "I think people are in your situation, and there are some problems…" The technique can promote communication between doctors and patients.

(7) Encourage patients' expression

There are many ways to encourage patient expression. In addition to the non-verbal communication mentioned above, doctors can use sentences to encourage patients to go on. The use of an example can even lead to a patient's empathy with his or her own experience, thereby communicating with the patient.

The training of communication skills needs to be improved through a lot of clinical practice.

4.2.3　The basic steps of psychiatric assessment

4.2.3.1　Start

The patient comes into the psychiatric department with an extremely complicated mood, such as fear, restlessness, helplessness, shame. So at the beginning of the psychiatric examination, the first task of the physician is to relax the patient. After the patient relaxed, the doctor began to talk with the patient, to understand the general condition of the patient and the main problems of medical treatment.

The following should be noted.

(1) Interviews should be conducted only by doctors and patients, and the conversation will not be heard by others, making patients feel that their privacy is respected. Conversations can't be interrupted by frequent interruptions (such as ringing phones, other people entering the office), which can make patients feel uneasy.

(2) If the conditions permit, multiple chairs should be placed in different places, and the patients should choose their own seats. Doctors can speculate on the patient's attitude towards treatment, such as rejection or acceptance.

(3) For the first time, the doctor needs to give a brief introduction of his basic situation, such as his own work experience and expertise, and set an equal tone for the doctor-patient relationship. At the same

time, according to the age of the patient, the title of the patient is determined, and the patient may be asked to call the doctor directly.

(4) If the patient is still nervous, the examiner should carefully understand the situation and find the cause of the patient's tension. Such as when a patient is very worried about the conversation will be leaked to others, or the patient is with very reluctant to see a doctor(e. g. , patients with alcohol dependence) , then you need a doctor for patients with solemn commitment.

(5) If the patient is confused in the initial contact, the doctor should consider whether the patient is out of anxiety, mental retardation, mental retardation or dementia. If there are serious cognitive function in patients with confirmed damage or disturbance of consciousness, you should consider to the people familiar with the history, at the same time use other ways to complete the examination of mental patients(see mental health check).

4.2.3.2   In-depth

After the general contact is over, the mental examination enters the substantive content. The doctor should understand the patient's mental state, the mental symptoms, the causes and the evolution of the mental symptoms. Deep conversation lasts between 20 and 45 minutes. Attention should be paid during the deep conversation.

(1) To be open and open to the mind, the partner can ask open-ended questions such as, "can you tell me more about your illness?" "what's the matter with you?" "How is your mood?". Open questions can inspire patients to talk about their inner experiences. At this stage, we can understand the patient's main pathological experience and its development process, and observe the patient's expression, mood changes, and abnormal posture, action, behavior and intention requirements.

(2) If necessary, the doctor can interrupt the patient's conversation and ask the key question directly, but it should be used sparingly.

(3) Doctors can use non-verbal communication to encourage or stop a patient's conversation. For example, a doctor may lean forward and stare. Frequent nodding and other gestures encourage the patient to talk about what the doctor wants to know. It can also be used to indicate that the doctor is not interested in what the patient is saying now. For many patients, the physical contact between patient and physician will help ease the tension of anxiety in the patients, such as effectively hold patients' hands, shoulders, or patted patients can shorten the interpersonal distance.

4.2.3.3   Conclusion

At the end of the conversation, the doctor should make a brief summary and ask the patient if there are any important questions not mentioned. The patient's questions should also be explained and guaranteed. If there is an arrangement for further treatment of the patient, it should be explained to the patient. Finally, politely say goodbye.

4.3   The psychiatric history

The correct diagnosis of mental disorders depends on detailed medical history and adequate psychiatric examination. The medical history of the patients is mainly based on requiring the patient in person and discussing with the informants. But patients' self-reported history is often not comprehensive, or because of the patients' lack of understanding of diseases and concealing the fact that or because nervous at home, missing is very important for psychiatric diagnosis of events, or patients have no cooperation, keep silent. Therefore, to the informant(including the relatives of the patient, such as spouse, parents and children; students, colleagues and leaders who study and work with them), it is often necessary to have close friends, neighbors, and medical staff who have previously worked with patients.

4.3.1 Methods of collecting psychiatric history

Unlike most of other clinical medicine, some serious mental disorder exists obvious behavior disorder in the state of illness, often denied his sickness, effectively to talk. Sometimes, they prevent the patient himself from providing an accurate medical history. In this case, the medical history is mainly derived from various sources, including family members, relatives, colleagues, classmates, friends, neighbors, and medical staff who have been treated before. For some light mental disorders, the relevant information provided by friends and relatives can be helpful for the diagnosis, comprehensive evaluation and treatment of patients. Clinical history is generally taken as follows.

(1) The subjective medical history is collected from the patient, which mainly refers to the medical history only provided by the patient. It is the main way to collect relevant information for outpatient patients, especially the psychological consultation outpatient. For some patients with severe mental disorders, during the period of onset, may be "objective history" than the history of "subjective" more reliable, but most of psychiatric symptoms can be subjective, because these symptoms are inner experience of person, the only person who could have described.

(2) The objective history from mainly by a person other than the insider information provided, are usually based on two or more people to an event or some kind of behavior consistent with the description, but in principle should get the consent of the patient himself, special circumstances should be their guardian's consent. People who know can supplement the information we can't get from patients. In particular, we can learn about the patient's past personality through the informed person, and the elderly relatives know more about the family history than the patients.

In general, the doctor should first talk to the patient, followed by the family. In some cases, we can first understand the patient's recent mental state, but first observe the general physical condition of the patient, such as whether the vital signs are stable or not. The patient's consent should be obtained before talking to the family members so that the patient feels respected. When talking with family members, whether the patient is present can be decided by the patient himself. Communication with family members can help doctors better understand the relationship between patients and their families. At the same time, doctors should strive to establish a therapeutic alliance with their families, so that the guardian recognizes the importance of systematic treatment of mental disorders.

When collecting an objective history, the physician should tell the history person the importance of collecting the history, obtain their cooperation, and then patiently listen to them to introduce the history. Due to the lack of professional knowledge, making history of contact with patients may have limitations, some subjective or may have some prejudice, so they provide medical history may be incomplete and inaccurate, often have the following kinds: ①introduced the emphasis on mental factors and ignore the body when tell the history. ②To provide more positive symptoms, but to ignore the early symptoms and less obvious abnormal manifestations. ③It provides an unusually large number of emotions and behaviors, ignoring the patient's mental and inner experience. Therefore, in the collection of medical history, the physician is not only the listener, but also should observe the psychological state of the donor, and be good at guiding, so as to obtain the relatively objective and comprehensive real material.

Supplement 1: check the patient firstly or ask the family firstly?

The history of data collection has always been different. Chinese psychiatrists are used to collecting medical history first for family members or other insiders, and some textbooks explicitly state that. There is a historical reason for this. Over the years, our country occupies the overwhelming majority of hospitalized patients with involuntary, patients hospitalized from don't want to and the psychiatric hospitals and doctors take resistance, this will encourage doctors to family members or people first to understand the history. The psychiatrists in the developed countries, especially in Europe and the United States, often choose to interview patients first, and ask the patient's permission before asking the family and the source. This will fully demonstrate respect for the patient. With the occurance of mental health and the raising awareness of mental health in China, the proportion of involuntary hospitalizations is steadily declining, and we would have thought that the well-reasoned practice faced new challenges, requiring serious reflection and adaptation.

Some clinicians believe that it is difficult for patients with severe psychosis to accurately describe their illness, and some doctors even believe that patients are prone to false statements and incoordination. These ideas come from the practical effects of clinical work. Due to the disturbance of consciousness, severe psychomotor excitement or inhibition, obviously uncooperative patients do need first to family members or people know the history, it prompted physicians in the face of the other patients also habitually do, thus formed the traditional idea for a long time. But they ignored another clinical fact: more patients, including some of the more serious psychiatric patients, were able to tell the whole story, and to tell the story.

Past history collection and mental examination of young physicians training is insufficient, lack of experience of young physicians feel and talk to patients' families is relatively easy, virtually to strengthen the collection history consciousness and the ability of the family members. First understand the history of the family members can provide spiritual check with emphasis, to quickly determine whether symptoms exist within the given time, in order to fulfill the task of definite diagnosis and formulating treatment in a timely manner. But it is also easy to make young resident relying on medical history information, loss of power to discover new problems, in the spirit when check with rules have access to information from the history, learned to talk with patients, which affects and patient communication. New lines of resident in mental check when I do not know where laid a hand on him, if the lack of empathy, acceptance and clinical communication consciousness, for a limited time to complete the implementation of the symptoms of task, tend to patients with closed questions way to check the information from family members. It is not only difficult to obtain the patient's trust, but also leads to the patient's aversion, hostility and unwillingness to cooperate. Such a vicious cycle makes young doctors more reluctant to engage in deep communication with patients, and the development of mental examination skills quickly meets the bottleneck and it is difficult to improve further. If in training consciously take the way of talking first and patients can be "forced" trained physicians note taking the initiative to communicate with patients, make full use of clinical communication skills from patients get the history data and other clinical information accurately. Therefore, it is better to combine these two methods from the perspective of training young physicians. For newly trained residents who have just received training, it is appropriate to take a medical history and then conduct a psychiatric examination. Then in-depth training, should be increased gradually to do mental examination way, focus on training of physicians and patients with different types of communication, so that residents in the future independent engaged in clinical work, able to cope with the actual situation of different. In the eyes of development, it is very helpful to have a talk before the patient.

4.3.2　Outline of the psychiatric history

Contents of medical history collection include general information, chief complaint, current history, past history, personal history, family history.

4.3.2.1　The general information

Including name, gender, age, marriage, nationality, occupation, educational level, address, telephone number or e-mail address, and the estimate of the history data reliability.

4.3.2.2　Main complaint

They are main mental symptoms and course of illness(cause of medical treatment). The reasons for this visit should be fully expressed, with the aim to be concise and focused, and to use the language of the history speaker as far as possible, without the use of technical terms.

4.3.2.3　History of present condition

It's an important part of the history. In general, the onset of disease and its clinical manifestations are described. It mainly includes the following contents.

(1)Conditions and causes of the disease

Understand the condition of the patient under the circumstances, namely the background of the patient's onset and the biological, psychological and social factors related to the patient. If there are social psychological factors, we should know the relationship between their contents and mental symptoms. It is the cause of the disease or the cause. Whether there is infection, poisoning, somatic disease and other factors.

(2)The onset time and form, course

The occurrence or urgency of mental disorders may be calculated in days or hours, even in the form of sudden onset, while some insidious patients are often difficult to determine the date of onset, but the approximate period of time and age should be determined. The clinical mental state from normal to obvious mental symptoms, the time within 2 weeks is called acute onset, 1－2 months for sub－acute onset, more than 1 months for chronic onset. Some diseases, early symptoms may be personality changes(such as Alzheimer's disease, schizophrenia), onset should be based on the time of personality change. The longitudinal description includes normal mental activity before onset; first symptom; the specific manifestations and duration of the symptoms; the interrelationship between symptoms; the evolution of symptoms and their relationship with life events, psychological conflicts and drugs used; function changes that have occurred in comparison with previous social functions; the course of disease are progressive, paroxysmal, and ductility. If the course of the disease is long, it can focus on the social function of the last year and the situation of life self－care.

(3)Any treatment received

The time and place of the medical treatment, the diagnosis(the changing reason should be understood) and the treatment, especially the drug name, dose, time, curative effect, side reaction, and the form of relieving symptoms, should be understood and recorded in detail for the reference of diagnosis and treatment.

(4)General conditions of the disease

The work, study, sleep, diet, life care, contact with the surrounding environment, attitude to the understanding of the disease, all have great significance for disease diagnosis. There are no negative thoughts, self－injury, suicide, injury, impulsive behavior and so on, so as to prevent the disease.

4.3.2.4　Past psychiatric and medical history

It refers specifically to the history of diseases of the past, including organ diseases, neurological diseases and so on. Including general health, after this clinic has no direct relation with the history of diseases, such as fever, convulsions, coma, history of drug allergy, infection, poisoning, body disease history, especially about presence of nervous system diseases such as encephalitis, brain injury, we should pay attention to these diseases and in time for connection between mental disorders, whether there is a causal relationship. There is no alcohol, drug, venereal disease, suicide or other psychiatric history.

4.3.2.5   Personal history

Generally refers to the whole life experience from the mother's pregnancy to the onset of the disease. However, the patient should be asked according to the age of onset.

Targeted inquiries should also be made according to different age characteristics. For adelescents, we should focus on their childhood conditions, such as the formation of diet and sleep habits, the phenomenon of picky food, anorexia, dream eating, sleepwalking, molars, bed wetting, general contact and behavior characteristics with others; whether emotion is stable, shyness, fear and so on; relationship with parents. The experience of separation between parents and school achievements and conduct. The process of puberty should also be understood. For adults and elderly patients, we should know their occupational status, work history, marriage and childbearing history, and family atmosphere. Sexual life, such as sexual development, attitudes and feelings towards sex, have an impact on the occurrence and development of mental disorders and should not be ignored. For women, the menstrual cycle should be asked in detail.

4.3.2.6   Family history

Including the age, occupation and personality characteristics of parents, current state of health or date and cause of death, family structure, economic status, social position, family members, especially quality of relationship with patients. Parent—child relationship and special events in family have great influence on the formation of personality and the occurrence and development of disease. Family history of psychosis, including mental disorders, personality disorders, epilepsy, alcohol and drug dependence, mental retardation, suicide, and non—consanguineous marriages. A positive family history of mental illness suggests that the cause of the disease may be hereditary.

4.3.3   Matters needing attention in collecting medical history

(1) How to collect information about personality characteristics is a difficult problem for beginners. It can be inquired from the following aspects.

1) Relationships: relationships with family, friendships(few or many, superficial or close, with own or opposite sex), relationships with work colleagues, superiors and subordinate relations.

2) Habit: have special diet, sleeping habits; Have a special hobby or pain; Smoking, drinking, drug use and other habits;

3) Interests and hobbies: the use of leisure time, whether there is interest and hobbies, hobbies are widespread; whether there is no special preferences;

4) Predominant mood: anxious, despondent, optimism, pessimistic, overconfident , self-deprecating, stable or fluctuating, controlled or demonstrative.

5) The attitude and standards , ask patients about their own views and other people´s evaluation of him. Understanding the behavior of patients in specific situations and their performance in work and social activities can also help to understand the personality characteristics of patients.

(2) The patient and the family are most concerned about the present medical history, and the time limit, generally first from the present medical history to ask. The family history, personal history, and previous history of hospitalization are more conducive to the collection of the present medical history in the context of

full understanding of the background. However, it can be handled flexibly according to the specific situation.

(3) The history should be accurately described, and reflect the development process of the disease and the characteristics of various psychiatric symptoms. Some important symptoms can be recorded in the patient's original words, and avoid medical terms. The medical history should be kept confidential, not as a small talk.

4.4　Examination of mental condition

Mental status examination refers to the examination method of all aspects of the patient's mental activity through the conversation and direct observation of the patient. The attention is focused on what the patient sees and what the patient feels, and the attention is focused on what the doctor sees and heard. The 2 methods are usually intertwined, inseparable, and equally important, but focus on the patients in a different state of disease.

4.4.1　Examination of the mental status of the cooperative patients

4.4.1.1　Appearance and behavior

(1) Appearance

Includes physical constitution, physical condition, hairstyle, outfits. Severe self-neglect, such as squalor, slovenliness, hints of schizophrenia, alcohol or drug dependence, and the possibility of dementia; manic patients tend to be overblown. In addition to serious physical illness, anorexia should also be considered in young female patients.

(2) Facial expression

The facial expression can provide a person's emotional state at present, such as a tight brow, helpless eyes showing depressed mood.

(3) Posture and movement

Manic patients are overactive and restless. Depressed people are less active and slow. Anxious patient shows motor agitation or tremor. Some patients show involuntary movements such as twitching and dancing.

(4) Social behavior

Understand the contact between patients and surrounding environment, whether they care about things around them, whether they are active or passive, and how cooperative they are. Manic patients tend to break social norms and cause problems of interpersonal communication. Patient with schizophrenia may be withdrawn and preoccupied. The patient's social situation should be carefully described and illustrated with examples.

(5) Activities of daily living

Can patients take care of their daily life, such as eating, changing clothes, cleaning?

4.4.1.2　Speech and thoughts

(1) Rate and quantity of speech, whether there are thoughts of thinking, slow thinking, poor thinking and interruption of thinking.

(2) Flow of speech and logical thinking logic structure, whether there is loose thinking, broken, symbolic thinking, logic error or new words. Whether the patient's speech belongs to the pathologic tautology,

whether there is persistent speech.

(3) Whether the content of speech is delusional. Delusion of the type, content, nature, time, is a primary or secondary, development trend, content, scope, whether as a system it is ridiculous or reality, the relationship with other mental symptoms and so on.

4.4.1.3　Mood

Emotional activity can be evaluated by subjective inquiry and objective observation. Objective performance can be judged according to the patient's facial expression, posture, movement, speech, autonomic nervous response(such as breathing, pulse, sweating). The subjective experience can be talked about, trying to understand the patient's inner world. According to the intensity, duration and nature of the emotional response, the dominant emotion is determined, including high emotion, low emotion, anxiety, fear, and apathy. whether emotions are prone to fluctuation and emotional fragility; there is no such thing as an unadaptable emotion. If the patient is depressed, be sure to ask the patient if he or she has a suicidal idea for emergency risk intervention.

4.4.1.4　Perceptions

There is no illusion, the type of illusion, the content, the occurrence time and frequency, the relationship with other mental symptoms; whether there are hallucinations, types of hallucinations, content, whether it is true or false, conditions, time and frequency, relationships and effects of other psychiatric symptoms.

4.4.1.5　Cognitive funtion

(1) Orientation force includes self-orientation, such as name, age, occupation, and orientation of time (especially the time period estimation), location, character and surrounding environment.

(2) Attention is assessed whether there is a decrease in attention or lack of attention and difficulty in concentration.

(3) The state of consciousness depends on orientation, attention(especially the ability to focus attention) and other mental states, and to determine whether there is a degree of consciousness disorder and consciousness.

(4) Memory evaluation of immediate memory, close memory and remote memory, whether there is amnesia, dislocation, fiction and other symptoms.

(5) According to the patient's culture education level, the smart question is appropriate. Including general knowledge, professional knowledge, computational power, understanding, analysis of comprehensive ability and abstract generalization ability. Special intelligence tests can be carried out if necessary.

(6) Self-knowledge: after the medical history of the collection and mental state examination, the doctor should also have a general understanding of the patient's mental state. Patients' individual symptoms can ask patients, this understanding degree, as the doctors should ask patients about their overall mental symptoms to judge, can extrapolate the self-knowledge of patients, and further conclude that patients in the diagnosis and treatment in the process of cooperation.

4.4.2　Psychiatric examination of uncooperative patients

4.4.2.1　Unconsciousness cooperation

Patients may be excessively excited or overly inhibited(such as silence or stupor) or hostility and do not cooperate with the examination. Only by careful observation of the following aspects can doctors draw the correct diagnosis.

(1) General appearance can be used to observe the patient's state of consciousness, appearance, con-

tact,cooperation,diet,sleep and self-care.

（2）Whether the speech has spontaneous,that is completely silent;whether or not to imitate speech, continuous speech;a silent patient can express his thoughts in words.

（3）Facial expressions are dull,euphoric,happy,anxious. The presence of gaze,the listening,closed eyes,the expression of fear;attitudes and reactions to medical personnel,relatives and friends.

（4）Whether there is a special position in the action,whether the action is increased or decreased; whether there is a rigid action,imitate action;whether the action has a purpose;whether or not to disobey, passive obedience;no impulse,hurt,self-injury. Patients with aggressive behavior should avoid a positive conflict with the patient and,if necessary,restrain the patient properly,which will help the patient to calm down.

4.4.2.2　Patients with disturbance of consciousness

If a patient presented with a trance,incoherent speech,aimless behavior,and disturbed sleep rhythm, the patient was highly suggestive of an awareness disorder. It should be evaluated from the perspective of orientation,immediate memory and attention. To estimate the severity of the disorder,and to speculate on the cause of the disorder,it is necessary to urgently adopt measures that may retain the patient's life.

4.4.2.3　Risk assessment of patients with mental disorders

When the patient has a hurtful or self-injury behavior,it require an emergency risk assessment. The purpose of risk assessment is to determine the possible adverse consequences of the patient;determining factors that may induce dangerous behavior in patients;determining factors that may prevent a patient from developing dangerous behavior;it determines which measures can be taken immediately.

Good risk assessment is based on a comprehensive history of acquisition and carefully check,other sources of information,including the people familiar with the situation,always of medical records,public security bureau of archives,etc. ,can be used as important reference material. Generally speaking,severe depression patients,elderly men,poor support system,low socio-economic status,and previous self-injury history are all high risk factors for self-injury or suicide. And schizophrenia,imperative hearing,male,previous history of violence,suggest higher risk.

Measures can be taken to reduce the risk in different situations. If the patient's guardian is warned in advance,he or she may take precautions against the possible behavior of the patient. Notify the police when personal safety is threatened;strictly inspect the belongings carried by the patient before admission. In case of emergency,the patient should be hospitalized.

4.5　Physical examination and special examination

Somatic symptoms involve various systems of the body,which can have multiple symptoms simultaneously,presenting discomfort or pain. Patients may have been seeking medical attention for a long time,failing to find evidence of organic disease,and even surgery to find nothing. But it can not dispel the patient's doubt,often accompanied by obvious anxiety and depression,can lead to the social function defect.

4.5.1　Physical examination and neurological examination

Many somatic diseases are accompanied by psychotic symptoms,and somatic diseases occur in people with mental disorders. Therefore,both in the outpatient and in the emergency room,the patient should be subjected to comprehensive physical and neurological examination.

4.5.2 Laboratory inspection

Laboratory examinations can provide the basis for a diagnosis of mental disorders caused by physical illness, by psychoactive substances, and poisoning. With the in-depth study of etiology and pathogenesis of mental illness, many psychiatric diseases that have been considered "functional" in the past have been found to have pathological changes detected by objective means. The results of these laboratory tests will likely be part of the diagnostic criteria for mental illness in the near future.

4.5.3 Brain imaging examination

Modern technology not only provides a means of examining brain morphology, but also checks the level of functional activity in different regions of the brain. CT, and MRI can understand the structural changes of the brain. FMRI(functional magnetic resonance imaging), SPECT(single photon emission computed tomography imaging), and PET(positron emission tomography) can make us qualitative and quantitative analysis of the functional level of brain tissue. These will help us further understand the neurophysiological basis of fewer obstacles.

As mentioned above, the so-called "functional" disease must have pathophysiological basis. With the development of technology, it is quite possible to achieve these pathophysiological changes, and relevant indicators are likely to become part of the diagnostic criteria in the future. Because of the nonoriginality of functional brain imaging, the current work is one of the hotspots and focuses of "functional" diseases. But given the complexity of the brain, a single objective test is limited in the value of diagnosing a particular mental disorder. It is likely to be a combination of inspection indicators, forming a multi-dimensional diagnostic system to help us diagnose or identify mental disorders.

4.5.4 Neuropsychological assessment

Neuropsychological assessments need to be done by specially trained neuropsychologists. The assessment includes intelligent screening of patients suspected of having a mental disorder, an assessment of reading and writing in children with learning difficulties, and an assessment of personality.

A well-designed neuropsychological test can assess the function of certain parts of the brain, such as a test for the function of a fixed leaf. These tests can be combined with neuroimaging to track changes of brain lesions.

Supplement 2:biomarkers in the field of mental illness.

Emil Kraepelin, the father of modern biological psychiatry, has opened a laboratory biomarker for biological research in major psychiatric disorders. He asked his student, Alois Alzheimer, to describe the pathological changes in the brains of people with schizophrenia. Alzheimer's became the discoverer of Alzheimer's disease, named after him. Until recently, in the face of the latest progress in the biological markers, not only may help diagnose disease in preclinical stage, can also evaluate the efficacy of the treatment, and can provide a new treatment to prevent disease progression.

The pursuit of laboratory testing dates back to the Hippocratic era. Modern times began in the 19th century when Willlterirn Griesinger predicted that "mental illness is a disease of the brain". More recently, during the period 1990—1999, Dr. Ginerin Jiredid worked at the national institute of mental health for 10 years, also known as the "decade of the brain". Over the past decade, despite painstaking efforts to find biological markers for so-called functional mental disorders, little has been achieved. A few years ago, advances in the biological testing of mood disorders were encouraging. For example, in the absence of Cushing disease, adrenal enlargement is a relatively specific indication of depression. Similarly, the dexamethasone depression test has good sensitivity and specificity to the diagnosis of depression. But it doesn't apply to generalized depression. In addition, studies have found that shortening the incubation period is a meaningful finding for depression in a broad sense, including dysthymia. When the clinical diagnosis is ambiguous, it is very important to find the laboratory test method with diagnostic value. For example, in the early stages of the disease, schizophrenia and bipolar disorder have a lot of overlap in symptoms, and emotional symptoms can be seen in schizophrenia spectrum disorders, and vice versa. Laboratory tests with diagnostic value are more necessary for patients with unclear diagnosis than those with typical clinical symptoms. It is clear that schizophrenia and bipolar disorder have heterogeneity in phenotype and genotype, and depression is more heterogeneous. Therefore, the biological examination of the main mental diseases will play an important role in predicting the curative effect of the treatment methods including physical therapy, drug therapy and psychological treatment.

The era of application of biomarkers in the field of mental illness has come. Due to its repeatability, reliability, specificity, and diseases such as schizophrenia, bipolar disorder, depression, and the correlation of subtypes, biological marker is quite broad prospects and the need for more in-depth research.

4.6　Diagnosis of mental disorders

After detailed mental examination, physical and neurological examination, laboratory examination, brain imaging examination and neuropsychological assessment, the doctor can make a preliminary judgment on the current mental status of patients. Further combination with complete medical history data, related to personal life history, especially the social psychological factors, analysis of induction, it is concluded that the diagnosis. In the process of psychiatric diagnosis, the following factors should be considered.

4.6.1　Transverse diagnosis process

The horizontal diagnosis includes two aspects: psychiatric status examination and dynamic observation of mental activity. The purpose of psychiatric examination is to discover the dominant mental activity. A depression in patients with clinical manifestation of the dominance of usually is "depression, loss of interest, energy and happy experience". If we find the main syndrome, it is easy to make a diagnosis. Similarly, if one always complains suffering persecution of the experience of others, but not based on facts, and is equally to any different opinion, or even doubt to dissent, should first consider the diagnosis of "paranoid state". However, it is certainly not enough to observe the mental state of patients with cross-section and static observation. As one patient motion performance behavior disorder in the night, and there is no purpose, staring vacantly, reply is not to the point, and has a relatively normal during the day, if you don't understand delirium itself has volatility, especially at night is aggravating features, clinicians are likely to cause confusion to the diagnosis of the patients. Another example, one of the children at school is always silent, can talking and laughing in the home, on the basis of different locations and different clinical phase, will make us easier to make the diagnosis of "selective mutism".

4.6.2　Longitudinal diagnosis process

The diagnosis should be considered in combination with the patient's age, gender, occupation, living environment, previous personality characteristics, history of disease, disease form and pathogenesis. For example, the first case of old age should consider the brain organic mental disorder; The toxic workers should be considered for toxic mental disorders; The patients with obsessive-compulsive disorder have the characteristics of being too stereotyped, pursuing perfection and being cautious in their behavior. Alzheimer's disease has a high family history and so on. It has been mentioned in the previous article that the onset of disease is acute, subacute and chronic, and the course of disease is characterized by seizures, periodicity, intermittency, and progressive. The acute onset is often the mental disorder caused by infection and poisoning, as well as separatist and stress disorders; the multiple onset of schizophrenia, progressive progress, paroxysmal recurrent disease, and visibility mental disorder.

4.6.3   Matters needing attention during the diagnosis process

(1) The diagnosis is a process of doctors know illness, through the patient's medical history collection, physical examination and necessary laboratory examination, obtain first-hand information, through the analysis, synthesis, analogy, judgment, reasoning, make the nature of disease, rational, abstract judgment, it is concluded that the rational knowledge for disease diagnosis, then take the corresponding treatment measures according to the diagnosis, observe the course of development and treatment, in turn, to verify the original diagnosis, further affirm or modify or even deny it. So the doctor's understanding of the disease is gradually deepened. This is a process from sensibility to reason, from theory to practice.

Some inexperienced doctors are only used to finding evidence to prove their first impression, and they are easily predisposed. Diagnosis, generally speaking, includes 3 stages: the clinical data collection, analysis, diagnosis, and by observing the disease diagnosis and by observing the development of the disease and treatment to the diagnosis of fulfilled or revision process.

(2) The diagnosis process should be based on the grade diagnosis, first to determine whether the patient has the organic factor, and only when the organic matter is eliminated, the "functional" mental disorder is considered. In the diagnosis of "function" in the process of the disorder, that wants to consider is psychotic (such as hallucinations, delusions, reality testing disabilities), or non psychosis (neuropathic, without the heavy mental characteristics), should also consider the personality and psychological stress factors and the relationship of the disease.

4. 7   Application of standardized psychiatric assessment and rating scale

Psychological rating scale method has been in research in recent years, clinical, education, justice, sports and business management in areas such as widely used, for psychiatric examination and treatment effect in the diagnosis of the psychological development of clinical medicine scale is also growing. The following are some of the standardized psychological psychiatric common mental checking and rating scale.

4.7.1   Standardized diagnostic mental examination tools

The world health organization has studied the reliability and consistency of diagnosis of mental disorders in different social and cultural backgrounds, and foundthere are differences in the diagnosis among clinicians. The reasons for the differences include the sources of data collected are different; the understandings of the term and different; the methods of the interview are different and the disease classification and diagnostic criteria are different. This tool is by psychiatrist with clinical experience on diagnosis and(or) diagnostic criteria for design, it includes a series of items, each entry represents a symptoms or clinical variables, inspection procedures, ask questions and grading standard, with entry of this tool. It is a pattern or semi-structured procedure of interview inspection tool, doctors or researchers in strict accordance with the provisions of inquiry and check, define the obtained results are following entry score coding, determine the existence and judging the severity of symptoms. The same diagnosis can be obtained by different doctors using this standardized inspection tool, which greatly improves the consistency of the diagnosis. Currently, the commonly used diagnostic psychodiagnostic tools include the composite international diagnostic interview-core version, which is the composite international diagnostic interview table and SCID(structured clinical interview for DSM-5). The former can be diagnosed by ICD-10 and DSM-5 respectively(note: compared with DSM-IV, DSM-5 epitaxy widens and content becomes thinner). Depressive disorder and bipolar disorder are all mood disorders in DSM - IV, while DSM - 5 divides them into two types of mental disorders. Depressive disorders in DSM-IV include 3 types of typical depression, dysthymia, and other unspecified depressive disorders. Depressive disorders in DSM-5 include disruptive mood disorders, typical depressive disorders, persistent depression, premenstrual dysthymia, material and drug induced depressive disorders, depressive disorders caused by other physical problems, other specific depressive disorders, and non specific depressive disorders 8 subtypes. DSM-5 also adds a number of associated symptoms to typical depressive disorders, such as anxiety symptoms, mixed characteristics, melancholy characteristics, atypical characteristics, and psychosis with the same mood as the mood), and the latter can only be diagnosed by DSM-5, which can be operated by a non-psychiatrist, who must be used by a trained psychiatrist. In recent years, in some epidemiological studies, there has been a simpler diagnostic tool, the mini-international neuropsychiatric interview.

The main purpose of DSM-5 is to help the trained clinicians to diagnose mental disorder as part of the case formulation assessment, for each individual to make comprehensive treatment plan. Each diagnosis standard can not cover the whole content of conform to the disease definition, there are far more complex than the brief description of cognition, emotion, behavior and physiological processes. Diagnostic criteria, therefore, is the purpose of the signs and symptoms of the disease is summarized as pointing to the characteristic of a disease syndrome, and the history of these diseases have a characteristic, biological and environmental risk factors, neural psychological and physiological factors and typical clinical course.

4.7.2   Mental symptom rating scale

At present, the rating scales in mental health, psychiatry research and play an increasingly important role in clinical practice, international, professional magazines seldom does not scale for assessment of application research papers published.

Psychiatric symptoms rating scale is generally used in psychiatric patients, and the evaluators are mainly trained psychiatrists. Commonly used psychiatric symptoms rating scale:

(1)The Hamilton rating scales for depression is mainly used to assess the severity of depression.

(2)The Hamilton rating scales for anxiety(HRSA) is mainly used to assess the severity of anxiety.

(3)Brief psychiatric rating scale(brief informed rating scales, BPRS) contains 18 symptoms entries, level 7 score, it is mainly used for rating the severity of scale disorders, especially before and after the clinical symptoms and treatment of patients with schizophrenia.

(4)Positive and negative symptoms scale(PANSS), developed on the basis of BPRS, and used for the existence and severity of symptoms in different types of schizophrenia patients.

4.7.3 Psychological measurement scale

Psychological measurement scale is mainly used in the general population, can be a health group, also can be in the mood, personality deviation on or have a certain difficult groups, environmental adaptation evaluator mainly psychologists, mental health workers. Commonly used mental health rating scale:

(1) The SCL-90 (symptom self-assessment scale, Symptoms Checklist-90): this scale includes 90 items, can comprehensive evaluation of the evaluation of mental state, such as thinking, emotion, behavior, interpersonal relationship, living habits and psychotic symptoms. There are 10 factors, such as somatic, compulsive symptoms, interpersonal sensitivity, depression, anxiety, hostility, paranoia, and psychosis. The scale is widely used to assess the mental health of different groups, such as the mental health status of the family members of patients with dementia, and the influence of examination stress on students' psychological state.

(2) The life quality comprehensive evaluation questionnaire (Generic Quality of life Inventory-74), a total of 74 entries from physical function, psychological function, social function and material life state four dimensions to assess the evaluation of health related quality of life. The scale is a self-rating scale. quality of life appraisal for the use of questionnaire gradually increased, reflects the transformation of medical model, allowing people to promote and maintain the individual physical, psychological and social function in terms of "good" state gave more attention.

(3) Minnesota Multiphasic Personality Inventory (MMPI) is one of the world's most widely used psychological test. It is consisted of a total of 566 questions, including some subscales, such as hypochondriacal (Hs), hysteria (Hy), depressed (D), personality disorder (Pd), the male-female tendency (Mf), delusion (Pa), breakdown psychasthenia (Pt), schizophrenia (Sc), hypomania (Ma), social inner (Si), can understand the evaluation of personality traits, also can give psychiatric diagnosis of hints.

(4) The evaluation scale of cognitive activities is used to assess the level of infants, the intelligence level of children and adults, the memory and intelligence of the elderly, etc. The commonly used scales include children's Wechsler intelligence scale, clinical memory scale, and simple mental state examination (MMSE). MMSE is simple and easy to use, and can be used as the screening and evaluation of patients with moderate and severe dementia.

In short, each tool contributes to an individual's comprehensive assessment, which helps to develop a diagnosis and treatment plan based on the individual's clinical presentation and condition. Cultural factors are particularly important for diagnostic evaluation, and the formal interview of culture is considered as a useful tool for communication with individuals. Across the symptoms of diseases and the severity of the specific diagnostic evaluation provides a quantitative rating of important clinical field, it is designed for both the assessment, to establish a rating compared to baseline and subsequent clinical treatment, and used for monitoring, change, and help to develop treatments. At the same time, digital applications will undoubtedly facilitate the use of these assessment tools, including the assessment tools that provide further assessment and development possibilities.

4.8 Writing of psychiatric records

Psychiatric records reflect the overall diagnosis and treatment of the patient in the hospital, which is important for both the medical staff and the patient. If the course of illness is long, multiple attacks should be written from the beginning of the disease; if the course of disease is episodic, periodical and circulatory, it should be described in the corresponding level. Pay attention to whether there are residual symptoms in the intermittent periods, and the patient's social abilities. The unsafe behaviors of the patients should be emphasized. It is said to be unified and written in the third person.

4.8.1　Principles of writing medical records

Medical record writing principle is a basic requirement to guide clinicians written records, also is the fundamental basis of evaluation of clinical medical records quality. The writing of medical records should follow the principles of objective, true, accurate, timely and complete.

(1) Objective refers to the objective existence of the patient's disease, not the human will to transfer all phenomena. In the case of medical history, it should be written according to the original meaning of the patient's description. From the signs, should be examined in person and checked all the negative result of positive and important, is can't listen to or according to the arbitrary, or copying others writing.

(2) Authenticity is the result of the analysis of the patient's history and the significance of the examination after the medical history and examination of the patient. Statement on the patients medical history, symptoms and detected signs, through the analysis of doctor comprehensive judgment, so that the doctor written records can truly reflect the patient's disease occurrence, development and evolution process.

(3) The physician has to find out the contents related to the disorder from a large number of language, and to process and refine them accurately. The diagnosis of the disease is also accurate.

(4) Timely means that the physician must finish the medical records within the prescribed time. For example, hospital records should be completed within 24 hours of admission to the hospital.

(5) Integrity refers to the medical history and physical examination required by the physician to be detailed and comprehensive, and all information in the medical records shall not be lost.

It is important to note that mental symptoms should not be used in the medical history to describe the mental state of the patient as much as possible. While the recording of psychiatric examination can be used in terms, it must describe the specific content. In order to accurately reflect the mental symptoms, the current use of the answer type records. A good psychiatric medical record should give a person a sense of urgency, and even if the physician who has never seen the patient re-read the medical record, he will be more objective to understand the clinical situation of the patient.

Supplement 3: Chinese psychiatrist's moral and ethical standard.

(1) Psychiatrists should respect the basic human rights and dignity of patient.

(2) Psychiatrists can not use their own privileges to exploit patients in their interactions outside medical activities and medical activities.

(3) Psychiatrists should keep secrets for the patient's clinical data.

(4) The psychiatrist should obtain informed consent of the patient before taking any treatment.

(5) Psychiatrists should not abuse their professional knowledge and skills to provide services for activities other than medical services.

(6) Psychiatrists should be responsible for all their medical problems.

(7) If a psychiatrist is engaged in research work, he or she should observe accepted ethical standards.

(8) Psychiatrists should provide the best services available to patients.

(9) Psychiatrists should constantly seek to provide their own professional level and share it with their peers.

(10) Psychiatrists should work to improve the quality of mental health services, improve accessibility, promote equitable distribution of health resources, and promote community awareness of mental health and mental illness.

4.8.2　Requirements for medical records

The medical records need to be finished within 24 hours after admission. The medical history and physical examination should be conducted under the guidance of the resident physician. The medical records must be reviewed by the superior physician in time and modified or supplemented.

Hospital medical record content includes the general information, the main complaint, HPI, past medical history, personal history, family history, physical examination, specialized subject, auxiliary examination, medical records, preliminary diagnosis and physician signature.

(1) General information including name, gender, age (chronological age), nationality, marital status, place of birth (province, city and county), occupation (indicating the position and the specific type of work), date of admission, history of record date, the presenter (indicate the relationship with the patient).

(2) The main complaint is the main symptom and duration of the patient's visit. The main complaint should be about the main disease description, and the text should be concise, with a high generality, generally not more than 20 words. A good main complaint can reflect the nature of the disease, such as "sensitive and suspicious, a year in the air, and two weeks of aggravation" suggesting schizophrenia.

Complained of a description to give an accurate, not vague, symptoms listed as long as you write the main characteristics, as far as possible triggers, evolution, and has been used for the treatment of such as described in the HPI. When the main complaint is more than 1, it should be listed in chronological order, but not more than 3. When describing time, try to be as specific as possible and avoid the vagueness of the concept of "days". In the case of acute onset, the time limit should be calculated in hours and minutes.

(3) The present medical history refers to the details of the occurrence, evolution, diagnosis and treatment of the disease, and should be written in chronological order. Content including the main symptoms change situation, the characteristics and development through after accompanying symptoms, diagnosis and treatment and results, sleeping and eating, such as general conditions change, related to the differential diagnosis and the positive or negative information. The present history should be consistent with the main complaint. When writing, you should pay attention to the logic, use proper words, so as to objectively and truthfully record without subjective speculation or comment. Although it is no close relationship with this disease, other diseases that still need to be treated can be recorded in another paragraph after the present medical history. The incidence of the disease includes the onset time, the location, the onset of the disease, the early symptoms, the symptoms and severity of the disease, the possible causes or causes of the disease.

Main symptoms, the change of the characteristics and development must be written, including the main symptoms of the location, nature, extent and duration, the development and evolution of symptoms or intensifying factor, etc. The accompanying symptoms should describe the salient features, the association between the main symptoms, and subsequent evolution.

The diagnosis and treatment process and the result refer to the examination and treatment after the onset, including examination, time, result, diagnosis and treatment method, effect and adverse reaction. The history of the present medical history is still a medical history, such as the present medical history of patients with recurrent depression, which should be described in the first episode.

General conditions include mood, mental state, life habit, sleeping, appetite, urine, weight and labor capacity.

(4) The previous history is about the patient's health condition and disease condition before hospitalization. Generally, it is not directly related to the disease. Contents include past general health status, history of disease, history of infection, vaccination history, history of surgical trauma, history of blood transfusion, drug(food) allergy history. Review system, the hospital medical records also calls the sequential to write the respiratory system, circulatory system, digestive system, urogenital system, blood system, endocrine metabolism, bone road system, nervous system and immune system nine symptoms or disease, diagnosis and treatment.

(5) Personal history, menstrual history and personal history of marital history including birth place, place to place, residence time; professional nature, working conditions, living habits, hobbies(with alcohol and alcohol addiction, should indicate the time and quantity); a history of contact with poison and water; there is a history of major trauma.

The history of menstruation includes the age of first menstruation, period of menstruation/cycle, and age of amenorrhoea. The unamenorrhea recorded the duration of the last menstrual period, the amount, color and character of the menstrual period, whether there were dysmenorrhea, blood clots, leucorrhea(quantity, odor, traits), etc.

The history of marriage includes marriage age, initial pregnancy, pregnancy and childbirth, miscarriage, premature birth, dystopia and death.

Birth, postpartum hemorrhage history, whether there is puerperal fever, birth control and sterilization condition, spouse health condition.

The above contents should be recorded in detail, and the contents related to diagnosis and differential diagnosis should not be missed. In the case of the diagnosis of "alcohol induced mental disorder", the amount and duration of alcohol consumption should be described in detail; clinically, early pregnancy is sometimes misdiagnosed as other diseases, mainly due to the omission of the last menstrual history.

(6) Family history includes the health status of parents, brothers, sisters, spouses and children, a history of infectious diseases, genetic diseases or similar diseases; if death indicates the cause of death and date. If necessary, ask your grandparents, grandparents, uncle, and cousins. For important genetic diseases, a family map should be drawn after full investigation.

(7) Physical examination is one of the basic skills of a clinician and should be written in a systematic way. Contents include vital signs(temperature, pulse, respiration, blood pressure), general(mind, body posture, gait, features, development, nutrition), skin, mucous membrane, superficial lymph nodes, the head and its organs, the neck, chest(thoracic and lung, heart, blood vessels), abdomen(liver, spleen), anal rectum and genitalia, spine, limbs, nervous system. Physical examination should be written in accordance with the system, and the results of each part, especially the chest and abdomen, should be recorded in the order of sight, touch, tapping and listening. The positive signs should be recorded in detail, and should be recorded for negative signs(such as undetected lung disease in patients with respiratory diseases, and in patients with liver disease).

(8) The specialized situation should record the special situation of the specialized subject according to the specialized subject.

(9) Auxiliary examinations are the main examinations and results related to the disease before admission. The date of examination shall be indicated. The name of the institution shall be indicated if it is examined by other medical institutions.

(10) The summary of medical records is a part of the medical records(large medical records). A concise summary of the main complaint, present(past) medical history, physical examination, laboratory or spe-

cial examination results is required.

(11) The preliminary diagnosis is the diagnosis of the comprehensive analysis based on the patient's admission to the hospital. If the initial diagnosis is multiple, it should be distinct.

(12) A physician who signs a medical history and makes a physical examination of the patient, should sign it after completing the medical record. The medical records written by the intern shall be reviewed, modified and signed by the medical personnel who are in the legal practice of this medical institution.

4.8.3 Psychiatric assessment and writing

Psychiatric assessment can be divided into two categories: cooperation and non-cooperation.

4.8.3.1 Psychiatric assessment of cooperative patients

General performance: describe the state of consciousness of the patient (awareness, etc.), orientation (peripheral orientation such as time, place and character orientation); ego orientation (such as name, age, occupation), the contact situation (active or passive, conditions and degree of cooperation, attitude towards the environment, etc.), daily life (including instrument, diet, urine and sleep); the menstrual situation of female patients; contact with other patients, participate in the group activities of the ward and work and entertainment.

Consciousness obstacle: describe patients with and without consciousness obstacle, including the illusion (type, time and frequency, and its relationship with other psychiatric symptoms and effects, etc.), hallucinations (type, time and frequency, and its relationship with other psychiatric symptoms and effects, etc.), comprehensive perception disorder (type, time and nature, etc.).

Attention: whether the concentration, lack of concentration, possible influence factors.

Thought disorder: including the form of thinking disorder (describe the amount and speed of the patients with abnormal, interruption of flight of slow thinking and poverty of thought, etc.), the thought content disorders (if there is a delusion, describes the type, content, nature, occurrence, development trends, range, whether fixed or system, absurd degree or the degree of reality, relationships with other psychiatric symptoms, etc.; if there is a compulsion concept, describe the relationship between its kind, content, development dynamics and emotional intention activities).

Memory: describes whether the patient has memory loss (including immediate memory, close memory and distant memory), memory enhancement, and whether or not to forget, construct and make up.

Intelligence: including general knowledge, professional knowledge, computational power, understanding, analytical synthesis and abstract generalizationability.

Self-knowledge refers to the analysis of disease symptoms, critical cognition ability and attitude towards treatment. Including self-knowledge, some self-knowledge and self-knowledge is almost complete.

Affective disorder: including emotional upsurge, depression, anxiety, apathy, emotion, emotional retardation. Patients should be paid attention to when to observe expression, posture, tone of voice, inner experience and emotional strength, stability, emotion and other mental activities whether to cooperate, to the things around if there is a corresponding emotional reaction, etc.

Volition and behavioral activity: the decrease or enhancement of natural activity (such as appetite and libido), including the decrease or enhancement of the will, whether it is exciting, rigid, or strange. Pay attention to its stability and impulsivity, and the degree of cooperation with other mental activities.

4.8.3.2 Psychiatric examination of patients without cooperation

Of excitement, restlessness and stupor state uncooperative patients, such as inspection, although there are some difficulties, but should be timely observed the condition changes, must be patient and meticulous, repeatedly observe the patient's words and deeds and expression. Pay special attention to changes in time and environment. Mental examination of non-cooperative patients should be described as follows.

State of mind: it is very difficult to examine an uncooperative patient, but it is very important. It can be judged from the patient's spontaneous speech, facial expression, lifeself-care situation and behavior. In particular, the expression is excited restlessness patient, especially the speech motor sexual excitement state should examine the consciousness obstacle carefully.

Orientation: the directional barrier is often associated with the state of consciousness. There is no obstacle to the general analysis of the orientation force through spontaneous speech, living and the response to regular contact with the medical staff.

Posture: whether the posture is natural, there are all comfortable positions, whether the posture is long time invariable or more dynamic. What happens to the body when it oscillates, how the muscle tone is.

Daily life: whether the diet and urine can be self-care, female patients can take the initiative to take care of menstrual health. If the patient refuses to eat, to nasal feeding, infusion and other attitudes, how sleep is.

Speech: the coherence and content of the speech of the excited patient, whether or not the words are imitated, whether the words are clear, the pitch is high and low, whether to use gestures or facial expressions. Whether a silent patient can express his or her inner experience and requirements in words without aphasia.

Facial expressions and emotional reactions: facial expressions such as rigid, euphoric, happy, sad, anxious, whether or not, how to respond to staff and relatives and friends. It should also be noted that the patient is closed, staring or alert to changes in the surroundings when no one is present. When asked about the patient's content, there is no emotional disclosure. And observe whether the patient showed a trance, dazed and aimless movement.

Phenomenon of hyperthyroidism, actions and behavior: presence of instinct activities have preserved the buckling, increase or decrease, with or without rigid motion, mimicry and repetitive movements, with or without impulse self-injury suicide behavior, whether to command obedience. Observe whether the patient has resistance, obstinacy, avoidance, attack and passive obedience.

Wang Yali, Liu Fang

Chapter 5

Organic Mental Disorders

5.1 Introduction

This chapter discusses those conditions in which mental disorder arises as a result of demonstrable structural disease of the brain or a physiological disturbance affecting cerebral function.

5.1.1 Basic concepts

At the interface between psychiatry and neurology lies a range of disorders that have been traditionally termed organic in order to differentiate them from functional psychiatric disorders such as schizophrenia. Scientific advances have rendered this distinction an anachronism as few would dispute that organic changes in the brain underpin the psychopathology of those disorders previously regarded as functional. Therefore, "organic" is just a relative term. Based on the development of medical science, some functional mental disorders will be discovered certain organic changes in the brain.

This chapter broadly follows the ICD-10 classification. In relation to other mental disorders due to brain damage and dysfunction and to physical disease(F00-F09), we have described the cognitive and psychological consequences of common neurological disorders that the psychiatrist is likely to encounter. For the clinical practice purpose, we describe them based on the known psychological and behavioural correlates of damage to different parts of the brain, and the psychological and social factors associated with the subsequent disability and handicap.

5.1.2 Common clinical syndromes

5.1.2.1 Delirium

Delirium is an organic syndrome of non-specific cause characterised by rapid onset and associated with concurrent disturbances of consciousness and attention, perception, thinking, memory, psychomotor behaviour, emotion and sleep/wake cycle. There are multiple underlying etiological factors, common causes including head injury, stroke, alcohol withdrawal and infection. The condition usually runs a fluctuating course and may resolve spontaneously. Delirium has also been described using other terms including "acute confusional state" "acute brain syndrome" and "acute organic reaction".

(1) Etiology

There are various causes of delirium(Table 5-1), the commonest of which are peripheral infections, drugs, alcohol withdrawal, cerebral hypoxia and head injury.

Table 5-1   Some causes of delirium

Vascular	Transient ischaemic attacks, cerebral infarcts(often secondary to hypertension), subarachnoid haemorrhage, transient global amnesia
Trauma	Head injury
Epilepsy	Psychomotor seizures and postictal states
Vitamin deficiencies	Particularly B_1, B_{12} and nicotinic acid
Metabolic abnormalities	Hepatic or renal failure, water and electrolyte disturbances, acute intermittent porphyria
Endocrine abnormalities	Thyroid, parathyroid and adrenal disorders, hypo- and hyperglycaemia, hypopituitarism, phaeochromocytoma
Cerebral hypoxia	May be secondary to cardiorespiratory failure or severe anaemia, leading to reduced arterial oxygen concentration; also post-anaesthesia
Toxins	Alcohol(excessive consumption or acute withdrawal), carbon monoxide poisoning, industrial metals such as lead, mercury or manganese, drugs-illicit substances or prescribed medication
Space occupying(cerebral lesions)	Brain tumors, subdural hematoma, cerebral abscess
Infections	Cerebral(meningitis, encephalitis) or peripheral(respiratory, urinary tract)

(2) Clinical features

Case report:

A general practitioner was called to the home of one of his elderly patients by the police, after they had received a call from her requesting help. On arrival, he found the woman hiding in her garden shed, insisting that she had seen Vietnamese Boat People climbing out of the lavatory bowl and overrunning her house. A history obtained from a neighbour confirmed that the woman had appeared perfectly well when she was seen 2 days before hand. The patient was too distraught to examine further, as she kept screaming that she could see "the invaders" standing behind the doctor. In view of the absence of any previous psychiatric history, and the apparently rapid onset of symptoms, the doctor suspected that the most likely cause of her hallucinations and persecutory beliefs was a delirium. He arranged for the woman to be admitted to the local psychogeriatric unit, which she readily agreed to in order to escape from the horde she believed was occupying her home. On admission, she was found to be febrile and a urine sample which she provided was noted to be bloodstained and foul-smelling. Culture later confirmed the presence of an Escherichia coli infection. Antibiotic treatment resulted in the resolution of her urinary and psychiatric symptoms within 7 days.

There are 4 cardinal clinical features of delirium(DSM-IV).

1) Disturbance of consciousness with reduced ability to focus sustain or shift attention.

2) Altered cognition or the development of a perceptual disturbance.

3) The disturbance develops over a short period of time and is fluctuating.

4) History examination and laboratory investigation reveal delirium to be a physiological consequence of an underlying general condition or to being caused by intoxication or medication or by more than one of

these etiologies.

The neuropsychological hallmark of delirium is marked abnormalities of attention. This is often accompanied by a generalised cognitive impairment affecting orientation, memory and planning skills. A fluctuating level of consciousness and awareness of the surrounding environment is almost invariable. Accompanying disturbances of the sleep−wake cycle, affect perception and psychomotor performance are also highly clinally relevant both in terms of diagnosis and management. The symptoms of delirium are usually worse at night.

The onset is typically acute, impairment of consciousness being associated with confusion, disorientation, poor concentration and distractability. The subject tends to be restless, emotionally labile, anxious and perplexed especially when he fails to comprehend either his surroundings or what is happening to him. Delirium characteristically has a fluctuating course, with periods of clouded consciousness interspersed with lucid intervals. Symptoms are often worse at night, when darkness or poor lighting exacerbate misinterpretation of sensory stimuli. Delirium is associated with gross disturbance of perception, namely illusions and hallucinations, as a result of which delusional ideas may develop. Following recovery, the individual frequently has little or no recollection of events during his illness.

(3) Diagnosis

According to the ICD−10, for a definite diagnosis of delirium, symptoms (mild or severe) should be present in each one of the following areas.

1) Impairment of consciousness and attention (on a continuum from clouding to coma; reduced ability to direct, focus, sustain, and shift attention).

2) Global disturbance of cognition (perceptual distortions: illusions and hallucinations, most often visual; impairment of abstract thinking and comprehension, with or without transient delusions, but typically with some degree of incoherence; impairment of immediate recall and of recent memory but with relatively intact remote memory; disorientation for time as well as, in more severe cases, for place and person).

3) Psychomotor disturbances (hypoactivity or hyperactivity and unpredictable shifts from one to the other; increased reaction time; increased or decreased flow of speech; enhanced startle reaction).

4) Disturbance of sleep−wake cycle (insomnia or, in severe cases total sleep loss or reversal of the sleep−wake cycle, daytime drowsiness; nocturnal worsening of symptoms; disturbing dreams or nightmares, which may continue as hallucinations after awakening).

5) Emotional disturbances, e. g., depression, anxiety, fear, irritability, euphoria, apathy, or perplexity.

The onset is usually rapid, the course diurnally fluctuating, and the total duration of the condition much less than 6 months. The above clinical picture is so characteristic that a fairly confident diagnosis of delirium can be made even if the underlying cause is not clearly established.

(4) Management

The basic principle of management involves the identification and treatment of the underlying cause. Nursing care should include reassuring the patient during periods of confusion, and maintaining a well−lit and uncluttered environment to avoid increasing his disorientation. Simple measures, such as regularly reminding him of the time, his whereabouts and who is caring for him, can considerably reduce distress. Similarly, unnecessary noise should be kept to a minimum, and the patient is best cared for in a single room, ideally being attended by the same nurse on each shift.

Disturbances of fluid and electrolyte balance will need to be corrected, whilst the administration of psychotropic drugs is preferably kept to a minimum, as they may increase the level of confusion. However, if the patient is very restless and disturbed by day, sedation may be needed, in which case small doses of haloperidol can be given. Benzodiazepines or chlormethiazole are often used as sedatives in delirium tremens and as a general measure to help induce sleep. The prognosis will to an extent depend on the underlying cause, and although in most cases recovery is complete, some acute organic syndromes progress to a chronic phase or have a fatal outcome.

5.1.2.2   Dementia

Dementia is an acquired global impairment of cerebral function, which occurs in a setting of clear consciousness. Characteristically, the syndrome has a gradual onset and tends to run a progressive, irreversible course. Structural brain damage is frequently present. Impairment of intellect is the central feature(resulting in defects of memory, attention, thinking and comprehension), although other mental functions(mood, personality and social behaviour) are usually affected simultaneously, and may sometimes be the prominent or presenting features. The commonest causes are Alzheimer's disease and vascular dementia.

(1) Etiology

A large number of conditions can cause dementia, of which the most important are listed in Table 5-2.

Table 5-2   Some causes of dementia

Degenerative conditions	Alzheimer's disease with early onset and with late onset, Pick's disease, Huntington's chorea, Creutzfeldt-Jakob Disease, Parkinson disease
Vascular	Multi-infarct dementia, cerebrovascular accident, systemic lupus erythematosus, subarachnoid hemorrhage, subcortical vascular dementia
Trauma	Severe head injury, punch-drunk, syndrome
Epilepsy	Dementia more likely when epilepsy is chronic and severe or where there is underlying brain damage
Vitamin deficiencies	Vitamin B_1, B_{12} and folate, nicotinic acid
Metabolic abnormalities	Wilson's disease, chronic uraemia endocrine abnormalities hypothyroidism, parathyroid disorders, hypopituitarism, hypoglycaemia, diabetes
Cerebral hypoxia	Post-cardiac arrest, respiratory failure, severe anaemia
Toxins	Prolonged alcohol consumption, carbon monoxide poisoning, exposure to heavy metals such as lead mercury, silver or aluminium
Space-occupying	Brain tumors, cerebral abscess, subdural haematoma cerebral lesions
Infections	Encephalitis, neurosyphilis, meningitis, human immunodeficiency virus(AIDS)
Miscellaneous causes	Multiple sclerosis, normal pressure hydrocephalus, non-metastatic cancer

(2) Clinical features

Case Report:

A 76-year-old woman was found by the police walking along the road in the early hours of the morning, wearing only a nightdress and slippers. She told the patrolman that she was going shopping and seemed oblivious to the fact that it was still the middle of the night. She was able to give her name and address, and was taken home. Her husband had been unaware that she had got up and left the house, but he told the policeman that he had become increasingly concerned about his wife's behaviour and forgetfulness during the past few months, and was finding it hard to cope. She had always been a neat and fastidious person, and although she still attempted to do the housework, their home had become progressively untidy despite his efforts to maintain some sense of order. Although she was generally pleasant and cheerful, he had noticed that whenever she found herself unable to perform simple tasks around the house, she would become very emotional, and once or twice when he had tried to help her, she had reacted explosively, screaming and sobbing uncontrollably for some time afterwards. On numerous occasions she had left things burning on the stove, and only the day before had left the gas unlit, until the smell had alerted him to the danger. He had suggested to his wife that she should go and see the doctor, but she said she felt quite well, and he assumed her forgetfulness was just part of growing old.

Later that morning she was visited by her general practitioner, who had not seen her for many months, since she was an infrequent attender at surgery. Although he noted that the woman was apparently bright and alert, she failed to recognise him, and was unable to remember any of the events that had taken place in the early hours, insisting that she had slept well throughout the night. She did not know the day of the week, and thought the month was February, even though it was midsummer and very warm. Cognitive testing showed that her short—term memory was clearly impaired, although her husband confirmed that events she recalled from the past were accurate.

Because of the difficult domestic situation, and the need to carry out further assessment, it was decided to admit the woman to the local psychogeriatric unit, which she agreed to with some persuasion. She became ex-tremely agitated shortly after admission, and that night broke the fire alarm on the ward in an effort to get help, insisting that she was being held in prison. With considerable effort, the nurses managed to calm her down and persuaded her to stay. During the next week, it was apparent to the nursing staff that she was inca-pable of finding her way around the ward, although she was able to dress and feed herself with some assistance. Results of investigations excluded any treatable cause for her condition, and in view of the overall findings, she was diagnosed as suffering from senile dementia.

Dementia usually has an insidious onset, and characterized by the following main features.

1) Impairment of cognitive functions.

2) Impairment of social life function.

3) Deterioration of behavioral and psychological symptoms.

In the initial stages there might be little evidence of disability other than the occasional lapse of recent memory which is often interpreted as normal forgetfulness. Premorbid personality traits are sometimes exag-gerated; e. g. , the person who has always been "set in his ways" may become increasingly rigid and inflexi-ble in his manner. Insight is often retained during this early phase, so that the sufferer can become anxious and depressed at the realisation of his failing mental faculties. As further deterioration develops, diminishing intellectual capacity and memory loss are more apparent. This can sometimes lead to the development of persecutory delusions, particularly if misplaced articles are assumed to have been stolen.

Wandering(especially at night) and neglect of personal hygiene, diet and clothing are often major cau-ses for concern for relatives and other care givers. Other changes which occur in speech and behavior in-clude perseveration(the inappropriate repetition of words or actions), confabulation(a falsification of memo-ry), nominal aphasia(the inability to name objects) and catastrophic reactions(explosive displays of emo-tion in response to demands beyond the subject's capabilities). Thinking becomes slow and restricted, and is associated with a diminution of the range of activities in which the subject engages.

In the later stages of the illness, there is a progressive deterioration of the personality, associated with a lack of emotional response, apathy and loss insight. Hallucinations can occur in all sensory modalities. So-cially unacceptable behaviour, such as aggressiveness, sexual disinhibition and incontinence, often increases and is eventually accompanied by a general deterioration in physical health. Ultimately, the subject becomes bed—ridden, with death frequently resulting from intercurrent physical illness.

It is important when contemplating a diagnosis of dementia to distinguish the condition from a depressive episode. This can sometimes be difficult especially if depressed mood is denied or the patient is uncommunicative. Furthermore, the psychomotor retardation and poor concentration occasionally found in affective disorders may be interpreted as being due to memory impairment, personality deterioration and intellectual deficit(depressive pseudodementia). It is estimated that 10% of individuals in whom a diagnosis of dementia is initially made, have later been shown to suffer from a depressive disorder. A correct diagnosis is more likely where a history is obtained from a relative or friend, behavior is observed over a period of time on the ward or in the home, and information is recorded concerning sleep pattern, weight change and eating habits. Psychometric testing may be useful in confirming or refuting the provisional diagnosis, but where doubt persists, a trial of antidepressant medication or ECT might help resolve the dilemma. It must also be remembered that depression and dementing illnesses are not mutually exclusive and may coexist. Indeed, there is evidence that depression is a not infrequent component of early dementia.

(3)Diagnosis

The diagnosis of dementia is based on clinical manifestation. Although the ancillary laboratory investigations may help in elucidating the etiology, they do not help in diagnosing dementia. According to the ICD-10, the following features are required for the diagnosis.

1)Evidence of decline in both memory and thinking, sufficient enough to impair personal activities of daily living.

2)Memory impairment typically affects the registration, storage, and retrieval of new information(recent memory), but previously learned material(remote memory) may also be lost, particularly in later stages.

3)Thinking is impaired, the flow of ideas is reduced, and the reasoning capacity is also impaired.

4)Presence of clear consciousness(consciousness can be impaired if delirium is also present).

5)Duration of at least 6 months.

The following conditions must be kept in mind in the differential diagnosis of dementia.

1)Normal aging process

Although the impairment of memory and intellect are common in the old, their mere presence does not justify a diagnosis of dementia. Dementia is diagnosed only when there is demonstrable evidence of memory and other intellectual function impairment which is of sufficient severity to interfere with social or occupational functioning. The normal memory impairment in old age is called as benign senescent forgetfulness.

2)Delirium

The syndromes of delirium and dementia may overlap.

3)Depressive pseudodementia

Depression in the elderly patients may mimic dementia clinically. It is called depressive pseudodementia. The identification of depression is very important as it is far more easily treatable than dementia. The depressed patients themselves complain of memory impairment, difficulty in sustaining attention and concentration, and reduced intellectual capacity. In contrast, patients with dementia do not complain of those disturbances.

(4)Management

If possible, the cause should be treated. For example dementia caused by head injury or by a stroke. The plan of treatment should seek to improve functional ability as far as possible, relieve distressing symptoms, make practical provisions for the patient, and support the family. There is no established specific drug treatment for dementia. Medication is mainly used to alleviate certain symptoms, such as anxiety and agitation, or depression. If the patient is over-active, deluded, or hallucinated, a phenothiazine may be appropriate but care is needed to find the optimal dose. If the patient has depressive symptoms, a trial of anti-depressant medication is worthwhile even in the presence of dementia.

The primary aim of management in a case of irreversible dementia is to maintain the quality of the subjects life and his standard of functioning at an optimal level for as long as possible. The patient should preferably be kept at home. So as to minimise the confusion and disorientation which is likely to occur if he is placed in an unfamiliar environment. The maintenance of good physical health is important to prevent accelerated deterioration.

5.1.2.3 Amnesic syndrome

It's a syndrome which associated with chronic prominent impairment of recent memory, with relative preservation of other cognitive functions, in the absence of generalized intellectual impairment. Remote memory is sometimes impaired, while immediate recall is preserved. Time sense and the sequencing of events is usually disturbed, along with difficulties in learning new material. Confabulation may be present but is not essential to the diagnosis. Korsakoff's psychosis due to alcohol abuse is an example of this condition.

(1) Etiology

Alcohol abuse, the most frequent cause, seems to act by causing a deficiency of thiamine. Several other causes also seem to act through thiamine deficiency, for example gastric carcinoma and severe dietary deficiency. Other causes involve the brain directly may be damaged by vascular lesions, carbon monoxide poisoning, or encephalitis; and by tumours in the third ventricle. Another cause is bilateral hippocampal damage due to surgery.

(2) Clinical features

Case Report:

A 45-year-old housewife has been drinking in secret for several years. She started with one or two small glasses of Irish Cream per night to "help her sleep", but, with time, her nightly intake has increased to 4-5 hard liquor shots. Now she needs a few glasses of wine in the early afternoon to prevent shakiness and anxiety. During the past year, she could not remember her husband's new mobile phone number, and missed several important family events, including her son's high school graduation. Because she was too ill or she did not want to risk missing her nightly drinking. She is ashamed of her "secret" and has tried to limit her alcohol intake but without success.

The central feature of amnestic disorder is a profound impairment of recent memory. New learning is grossly defective, but remote memory is relatively preserved. One consequence of this profound disorder of memory is an associated disorientation in time. Gaps in memory are often filled by confabulating. The patient may give a vivid and detailed account of recent activities, all of which, on checking, turn out to be inaccurate. Other cognitive functions are relatively well preserved. However, the disorder is not limited entirely to memory; some emotional blunting and lack of volition are often observed as well.

(3) Diagnosis

According to the ICD-10, the following features are required for the diagnosis.

1) Recent memory impairment; anterograde and retrograde amnesia.

2) No impairment of immediate retention and recall, attention, consciousness, and global intellectual functioning.

3) Historical or objective evidence of brain disease or injury (occurs particularly with bilateral involvement of diencephalic and medial temporal structures).

（4）Differential diagnosis

Amnestic syndrome should be differentiated from delirium, dementia, non-organic mental disorders and psychogenic amnesia. Differentiation from the first three is relatively easy on the basis of the pattern of memory loss.

（5）Management

Treatment of the underlying cause, e. g. , thiamin(high doses) in Wernicke-Korsakoff syndrome. However, usually the treatment is of not much help, except in prevention of further deterioration and the prognosis is often poor.

Supportive care and rehabilitation training for general condition and the associated medical illness should be carried out as early as possible.

5.1.2.4　Organic personality

The organic personality disorder is characterized by a significant alteration of the premorbid personality caused by an underlying organic cause without major disturbance of consciousness, orientation, memory or perception.

The personality change may be characterized by poor impulse control, emotional lability, apathy, accentuation of earlier personality traits, or hostility.

According to the ICD-10, the following features are required for the diagnosis of organic personality disorder, in addition to the general guidelines for the diagnosis of other organic mental disorders, described earlier.

In addition to an established history or other evidence of brain disease, damage, or dysfunction, a definitive diagnosis requires the presence of two or more of the following features.

（1）Consistently reduced ability to persevere with goal-directed activities, especially those involving longer periods of time and postponed gratification.

（2）Altered emotional behavior, characterized by emotional lability, shallow and unwarranted cheerfulness(euphoria, inappropriate jocularity), and easy change to irritability or short-lived outbursts of anger and aggression; in some instances apathy may be a more prominent feature.

（3）Expression of needs and impulses without consideration of the consequences or social convention (the patient may engage in dissocial acts, such as stealing, inappropriate sexual advances, or voracious eating, or may exhibit disregard for personal hygiene).

（4）Cognitive disturbances, in the form of suspiciousness or paranoid ideation, and/or excessive preoccupation with a single, usually abstract, theme(e. g. , religion, "right and wrong").

（5）Marked alteration of the rate and flow of language production, with features such as circumstantiality, over-inclusiveness, viscosity, and hypergraphia.

（6）Altered sexual behavior(hyposexuality or change of sexual preference).

Treatment of the underlying cause of organic personality disorder should be applied as etiological treatment.

5.2　Brain organic mental disorders

5.2.1　Definition

Brain organic mental disorders are defined as mental disorders arise as a result of demonstrable structural or functional disease of the brain. The most common causes are cerebral degenerative disease, cerebrovascular disease, intracranial infection, craniocerebral trauma and cerebral tumor. The category of "organic disorders" has been retained in ICD-10(F00-F09) and CCMD-3, but discarded in DSM-Ⅳ. Consequently, we use it here.

The diagnosis of brain organic disorder should based on following conditions.

(1) Presence of confusion, disorientation, memory impairment or neurological symptoms or signs, like seizures, impairment of consciousness, head injury, sensory or motor disturbance.

(2) In terms of timing, the first episode of psychiatric symptoms is very closed related to the development of brain disorder.

(3) Recovery of brain disorder will result in relieving of psychiatric symptoms.

(4) The psychiatric symptoms should not be resulted in other causes such as genetic diseases, or stress responses.

The treatment strategy for brain organic disorder:

(1) Protopathy treatment should be the first consideration.

(2) Psychiatric symptoms required symptomatic treatment which based on the indications and usage of psychoactive medications.

(3) Management of complications: such as accompanying infections, increased intracranial pressure, pressure sores. Intensive nursing care should give to those with self-injury or violence.

5.2.2   Alzheimer's disease

Alzheimer's disease(AD), also referred to senile dementia, is a chronic neurodegenerative disease that mainly manifests dementia syndrome. It starts slowly and worsens progressively and irreversibly. Malnutrition, pneumonia and dehydration are the most frequent immediate causes of death brought by AD.

5.2.2.1   Neuropathology

AD is characterised by loss of neurons and synapses in the cerebral cortex and certain subcortical regions. This loss results in gross atrophy of the affected regions, including degeneration in the temporal lobe and parietal lobe, and parts of the frontal cortex and hippocampus. Degeneration is also present in brainstem nuclei like the locus coeruleus. Studies using MRI and PET have documented reductions in the size of specific brain regions in people with AD as they progressed from mild cognitive impairment to AD, and in comparison with similar images from healthy older adults.

Both amyloid plaques and neurofibrillary tangles are clearly visible by microscopy in brains of those afflicted by AD. Plaques are dense, mostly insoluble deposits of beta-amyloid peptide and cellular material outside and around neurons. Tangles(neurofibrillary tangles) are aggregates of the microtubule-associated protein tau which has become hyperphosphorylated and accumulate inside the cells themselves. Although many older individuals develop some plaques and tangles as a consequence of aging, the brains of people with AD have a greater number of them in specific brain regions such as the temporal lobe. Lewy bodies are not rare in the brains of people with AD.

5.2.2.2   Pathogenesis

Molecular biology study on AD has made great progress in recent years. Several competing hypotheses exist trying to explain the cause of the disease.

(1) Genetic factor

The genetic heritability of AD, based on reviews of twin and family studies. Most of autosomal dominant familial AD can be attributed to mutations in one of three genes: those encoding amyloid precursor protein

（APP）and presenilins 1 and 2. Most mutations in the APP and presenilin genes increase the production of a small protein called Aβ42, which is the main component of senile plaques. Some of the mutations merely alter the ratio between Aβ42 and the other major forms（particularly Aβ40）, without increasing Aβ42 levels. The best known genetic risk factor is the inheritance of the ε4 allele of the apolipoprotein E （APOE）. The APOEε4 allele increases the risk of the disease by three times in heterozygotes and by 15 times in homozygotes.

（2）Amyloid hypothesis

The amyloid hypothesis postulated that extracellular amyloid beta（Aβ）deposits are the fundamental cause of the disease. A specific isoform of apolipoprotein, APOE4, is a major genetic risk factor for AD, which leading to excess amyloid buildup in the brain. The primary pathogenic form of Aβ, could bind to a surface receptor on neurons and change the structure of the synapse, thereby disrupting neuronal communication. The updated theory holds that an amyloid-related mechanism that prunes neuronal connections in the brain in the fast-growth phase of early life may be triggered by ageing-related processes in later life to cause the neuronal withering of AD.

（3）Tau protein hypothesis

In this model, hyperphosphorylated tau protein begins to pair with other threads of tau. Eventually, they form neurofibrillary tangles inside nerve cell bodies.

The microtubules disintegrate, destroying the structure of the cell's cytoskeleton which collapses the neuron's transport system. This may result first in malfunctions in biochemical communication between neurons and later in the death of the cells.

（4）Cholinergic hypothesis

This model proposes that AD is caused by reduced synthesis of the neurotransmitter acetylcholine. Acetylcholine deficiency will result in memory loss, but medications intended totreat have not been very effective. Other cholinergic effects have also been proposed.

5.2.2.3　Clinical feature

Case Report:

A 78-year-old man, is seen by his GP after his wife expresses concern about his condition. He has gradually become very forgetful over the last 1-2 years. His wife says that he recently got lost when out shopping, even though they had lived in the same place for years, and that at a recent family gathering he had not been able to remember the names of some of the younger family members. He has always managed the household bills, but recently his wife has taken over, as he complains that "things are getting too complicated". He complains that he can not find things around the house because his wife keeps moving them, which she denies.

He has had no significant medical problems in the past, and his physical examination is normal. He looks fit and he takes no medication. He speaks fluently but makes frequent errors, either using incorrect words or substituting made-up words instead. He can name three objects but can not recall them later. When asked the name of the current Prime Minister, he says "I've never met him." His wife is very anxious and asks the doctor any treatment that could help him and slow down his mental decline.

AD gradually progresses over 7-10 years. There are no remissions, although the rate of decline may vary. Most patients present with insidious anterograde memory impairment, which may be moderately severe before it is recognized.

Other cognitive impairments ensue, especially agnosia and disorders of executive function. A striking clinical feature in many cases is the patient's lack of appreciation（insight）into the nature and severity of cognitive problems. Another striking clinical feature is the sparing of motor function and of primary touch, hearing, and sight.

With insidious onset, AD starts slowly and worsens progressively and irreversibly. The average course is 8-10 years. It characterized clinically by memory loss and other disorders of cognitive function, other enduring personality changes.

In the early stage, people with AD present the increasing impairment of learning and memory. Language problems are mainly characterised by a shrinking vocabulary and decreased word fluency, leading to a general impoverishment of oral and written language. Patient with AD is usually capable of communicating basic ideas adequately. While performing fine motor tasks such as writing, drawing or dressing, certain movement coordination and planning difficulties (apraxia) may be present, but they are commonly unnoticed. As the disease progresses, people with AD can often continue to perform many tasks independently, but may need assistance or supervision with the most cognitively demanding activities.

In the moderate stage, progressive deterioration eventually hinders independence, with subjects being unable to perform most common activities of daily living. Speech difficulties become evident due to an inability to recall vocabulary, which leads to frequent incorrect word substitutions (paraphasias). Reading and writing skills are also progressively lost. Complex motor sequences become less coordinated as time passes and AD progresses, so the risk of falling increases. During this phase, memory problems worsen, and the person may fail to recognise close relatives. Long-term memory, which was previously intact, becomes impaired. Behavioural and neuropsychiatric changes become more prevalent. Sundowner syndrome may present.

Common manifestations are wandering, irritability and labile affect, leading to crying, outbursts of unpremeditated aggression, or resistance to caregiving. Approximately 30% of people with AD develop illusionary misidentifications and other delusional symptoms. Subjects also lose insight of their disease process and limitations (anosognosia). Urinary incontinence can develop.

During the final stages, the patient is completely dependent upon caregivers. Language is reduced to simple phrases or even single words, eventually leading to complete loss of speech. Despite the loss of verbal language abilities, people can often understand and return emotional signals. Although aggressiveness can still be present, extreme apathy and exhaustion are much more common symptoms. People with AD will ultimately not be able to perform even the simplest tasks independently; muscle mass and mobility deteriorates to the point where they are bedridden and unable to feed themselves. The cause of death is usually an external factor, such as infection of pressure ulcers or pneumonia.

5.2.2.4 Diagnosis and differential diagnosis

AD is usually diagnosed based on the patient's medical history, history from relatives, and behavioural observations, by exclusion of all other causes of dementia. The presence of characteristic neurological and neuropsychological features and the absence of alternative conditions is supportive. Advanced medical imaging with computed tomography(CT) or magnetic resonance imaging(MRI), and with single-photon emission computed tomography(SPECT) or positron emission tomography(PET) can be used to help exclude other cerebral pathology or subtypes of dementia. Moreover, it may predict conversion from prodromal stages (mild cognitive impairment) to AD. A definitive diagnosis ultimately requires both the characteristic dementia in life and the characteristic pathology after death.

American National Institute of Neurological and Communicative Disorders and Stroke-Alzheimer's Disease and Related Disorders Association(NINCDS-ADRDA) criteria for the clinical research and diagnosis of Alzheimer's disease, which were proposed in 1984.

(1) Dementia established by clinical examination and standardized brief mental status.

(2) Examination and confirmed by neuropsychological tests.

(3) Deficits in two or more areas of cognition.

(4) Progressive worsening of memory and other cognitive function.

(5) No disturbance of consciousness.

(6) Onset between 40-90 years.

(7) Absence of other systemic or neurologic disorders sufficient to account for the progressive cognitive defects.

(8) Progressive deterioration of specific cognitive functions such as language(aphasia), motor skills (apraxia), and perception(agnosia).

(9) Impaired activities of daily living and altered patterns of behavior.

(10) Family history of a similar disorder, especially if confirmed neuropathologically.

(11) Normal lumbar puncture.

(12) Normal pattern or nonspecific changes in electroencephalogram.

(13) Evidence of cerebral atrophy on computed tomography, with progression on serial observation.

Features against diagnosis of AD:

(1) Sudden onset.

(2) Focal neurologic findings such as hemiparesis, sensory loss, visual field deficits, and incoordination early in the course of the illness.

(3) Seizures or gait disturbance at the onset or very early in the course of the illness.

5.2.2.5   Treatment and rehabilitation

There is no cure for AD; available treatments offer relatively small symptomatic benefit. Current treatments can be divided into pharmaceutical, psychosocial and caregiving.

Five medications are currently used to treat the cognitive problems of AD: four are acetylcholinesterase inhibitors(tacrine, rivastigmine, galantamine and donepezil) and the other(memantine) is an NMDA receptor antagonist.

Reduction in the activity of the cholinergic neurons is a well-known feature of AD. Acetylcholinesterase inhibitors are employed to reduce the rate at which acetylcholine(ACh) is broken down, thereby increasing the concentration of ACh in the brain and combating the loss of ACh caused by the death of cholinergic neurons. There is evidence for the efficacy of these medications in mild to moderate AD, and some evidence for their use in the advanced stage. The most common side effects are nausea and vomiting. These side effects arise in approximately 10%-20% of users, are mild to moderate in severity, and can be managed by slowly adjusting medication doses.

Psychosocial interventions are used as an adjunct to pharmaceutical treatment and can be classified within behaviour-, emotion-, cognition- or stimulation-oriented approaches. Since AD has no cure and it gradually renders people incapable of tending for their own needs, caregiving is essentially the treatment and must be carefully managed over the course of the disease.

As the disease progresses, different medical issues can appear, such as oral and dental disease, pressure ulcers, malnutrition, hygiene problems, or respiratory, skin, or eye infections. Careful management can prevent them, while professional treatment is needed when they do arise.

5.2.3   Vascular dementia

Vascular dementia, also known as multi-infarct dementia(MID) and vascular cognitive impairment (VCI), is a group of disorders mainly caused by thromboemboli(originating in extracranial vessels damaged by atherosclerosis) producing numerous cerebral infarcts, in association with cystic necrosis and gliosis, leading to worsening cognitive decline that occurs step by step. The term refers to a syndrome consisting of a complex interaction of cerebrovascular disease and risk factors that lead to changes in the brain structures due to strokes and lesions, and resulting changes in cognition. The temporal relationship between a stroke and cognitive deficits is needed to make the diagnosis. Vascular dementia is the second most frequent cause of dementia following AD with late onset, with a peak onset between 60−70 years, and is slightly more prevalent in males.

Unlike dementia in AD, in which impairment of cerebral function is both insidious and progressive, deterioration in MID tends to occur in a stepwise fashion, correlating with repeated episodes of cerebral infarction over a length of time. As a result, periods of relative stability may be observed, during which no significant decline of mental function occurs.

The mood is often labile and nocturnal confusion is a common feature, although characteristically, personality and insight are preserved until the later stages of the illness. There may be evidence of arteriosclerotic changes elsewhere in the body and hypertension is a common finding. Focal neurological signs are frequently present, and there may be a history of headaches, dizziness, epileptic seizures, cerebral ischaemic attacks or strokes.

The ICD−10 criteria for vascular dementia:

(1) Unequal distribution of deficits in higher cognitive functions with some affected and others relatively spared. Thus, memory may be quite markedly affected while thinking, reasoning, and information processing may show only mild decline.

(2) There is evidence for focal brain damage, manifest as at least one of the following unilateral spastic weakness of the limbs, unilaterally increased tendon reflexes, an extensor plantar response, pseudobulbar palsy.

(3) There is evidence from the history, examination, or rest of significane cerebrovascular disease, which may reasonably be judged to be etiologically related to the dementia(history of stroke, evidence of cerebral infarction).

In addition to general aspects of management, treatment should be directed towards the control of hypertension, although this needs to be cautiously handled in the elderly to avoid causing further cerebral ischemia if the blood pressure falls too low. The prognosis is generally poor, death occurring within 5 years of diagnosis, usually from other complications such as ischemic heart disease or cerebrovascular accident.

5.2.4　Intracranial infection and mental disorders

It's a group of disorders mainly caused by intracranial infections of virus, bacteria, spirochaeta, and other pathogens. Notably encephalitis, cerebral abscess, meningitis and neurosyphilis.

5.2.4.1　Encephalitis

Encephalitis can follow viral infections, such as herpes simplex, HIV, influenza and measles(including vaccination), or occur secondary to bacterial meningitis, cerebral abscess and blood−borne infections. Clinical features include a rapid onset of headache, pyrexia and vomiting, often associated with photophobia, neck stiffness, and sometimes papilloedema. An acute organic syndrome can develop and may be accompanied by seizures. Those who survive the initial infection may be left with residual neurological deficits, personality changes and cognitive impairment. Following resolution of the acute phase, which was marked by daytime drowsiness and visual disturbance, many sufferers were left with residual features of Parkinsonism, as well as undergoing personality changes or deveoping schizophrenic−like disorders. Anti−virus treatment should be applied at early stage apart from symptomatic treatment.

5.2.4.2 Creutzfeldt–Jakob disease

The rates of Creutzfeldt–Jakob disease(CJD, also known as a human prion disease) range from 0.25 to 2.00 cases per million persons a year worldwide. This transmissible, rapidly progressive disorder occurs mainly in middle age or older and is manifest early on by fatigue, flu–like symptoms, and aphasia or apraxia. Subsequent psychiatric manifestations include mood lability, anxiety, euphoria, depression, delusions, hallucinations, or marked personality changes. Progression of disease occurs over months leading to dementia, akinetic mutism, coma, and most patients die within 2 years. Other common neurological findings are generalized startle myoclonus, cortical blindness, and extrapyramidal and cerebellar signs.

Pathological changes includ the classic triad of spongiform vacuolation, loss of neurons, and glial cell proliferation. An immunoassay for Creutzfeldt–Jakob disease in the CSF is currently under development, showing promise in supporting the diagnosis of Creutzfeldt–Jakob disease in patients with dementia. EEG abnormalities, although not specific for Creutzfeldt–Jakob disease, are present in nearly all patients. CT and MRI studies may reveal cortical atrophy later in the course of disease; SPECT and PET reveal heterogeneously decreased uptake throughout the cortex. There is no known treatment for Creutzfeldt–Jakob disease.

5.2.4.3 Neurosyphilis

Neurosyphilis is now a rare complication of spirochaetal infection. Three types are recognised; meningovascular syphilis produces inflammation of the meninges and cerebral arteries, resulting in irritability, headaches, lethargy and labile mood. Tabes dorsalis involves atrophy of the dorsal roots and posterior columns of the spinal cord, and is characterised by ataxia, pain andparaesthesia of the lower limbs. The most important type from the psychiatric viewpoint is general paresis, which may develop up to 25 years after the initial infection. Pathological changes comprise thickening of the dura mater, cerebral atrophy (particularly of the frontal lobe), as well as inflammatory and degenerative changes of the cerebral cortex. Psychiatric manifestations include depression, mania, personality changes of a frontal lobe type(apathy and disinhibition), paranoid psychosis and a slowly progressive dementia. Serological testing of the blood or cerebrospinal fluid should be considered in all individuals who show evidence of organic brain disease or any unexplained psychiatric disorder.

5.2.5 Traumatic brain injury and mental disorders

In China, thousands of people are admitted to hospital with traumatic brain injuries each year, mostly as a result of road traffic accidents. In the minority of cases where more severe brain injuries are sustained, long–term organic, psychiatric or social sequelae can develop, many of them result in permanent disability. The degree of impairment will depend on many factors: the circumstances of the accident, the site and extent of any brain damage, the age and personality of the individual, and the social dysfunction which results from the injury.

The acute stage of traumatic brain injury is characterised by disturbance of consciousness, even delirium or coma, and follow with post–traumatic(anterograde) amnesia(PTA), the most useful prognostic indicator after a head injury is the duration of, this being the interval of time between the head injury and the return of normal, continuous memory. Unlike retrograde amnesia, the duration of PTA does not usually diminish with time. Furthermore, it can extend beyond the return of clear consciousness, and is likely to be prolonged in the elderly. As a general rule, PTA of less than 12 hours indicates the likelihood of a full recovery. When it exceeds 24 hours in duration, there is an increased risk of residual disability such as brain damage, epilepsy, psychiatric disorder or intellectual deficit. PTA is an unreliable prognostic indicator in the case of penetrating head injuries, where serious complications can occur even though loss of memory is minimal or non-existent.

The length of retrograde amnesia represents the time between the moment of injury and the last clear memory before the incident. Although it frequently occurs, it is a poor prognostic indicator. Irrespective of its initial length, retrograde amnesia invariably shrinks over a period of time, so that its final duration is usually less than a minute.

The chronic stage of traumatic brain injury is characterised by psychiatric complications. The development of mental disorder following a head injury is more likely when trauma is severe, especially if it is associated with brain damage or epilepsy. Other risk factors include an abnormal premorbid personality, or a personal/family history of psychiatric disorder. Personality changes and neurotic symptoms occur in about one-fifth of severe head injuries, whilst 10% of cases develop schizophrenic-like, paranoid or affective psychoses. Cognitive impairment is seen in a small proportion of subjects, especially if the PTA is of more than 24 hours' duration.

A postconcussional syndrome can occur following head injury, which is not attributable to severe brain damage. The symptoms include headache, dizziness, fatigue, irritability, poor concentration, insomnia and reduced tolerance to stress. Anxiety and depression may also be present. The cause of these symptoms is not always clear and both organic and psychological factors have been implicated.

Both organic and psychiatric impairment may result in time off work following a head injury, and this can extend to long-term sick leave or redundancy. Relationship difficulties may also develop, and sometimes lead to marital breakdown and social isolation. Those are the frequent social complications.

5.2.6   Intracranial tumors and mental disorders

Brain tumors characteristically produce focal neurological disturbances by occupying space within the skull and often invade the brain tissue, tends to cause a rise in intracranial pressure. Primary and metastatic intracranial tumors produce direct and indirect effects on brain functions that could result in behavioral alterations. Intracranial tumors account for approximately 10% of all malignant neoplasms in humans and for about 2% of all cancer-related deaths. Benign tumors are 12 times as prevalent as primary malignant tumors; metastatic tumors (from lung, breast, stomach, thyroid, or kidney) about three times as prevalent. Before neuroimaging and modern neurosurgical techniques became available it was well recognized that some patients with tumors would first present with neurobehavioral or psychiatric manifestations.

Many brain tumors cause psychological symptoms at a certain stage in their course, and a significant proportion present with such symptoms. Psychiatrists are likely to see patients with slow-growing tumors in "silent" (especially frontal) areas. These produce psychological effects, but few neurological signs, for example, subfrontal meningioma or glioma of the corpus callosum. The nature of the psychological symptoms is influenced by the global effects of raised intracranial pressure, in addition to the tumor location. The rate of tumor growth is also important; rapidly expanding tumors with raised intracranial pressure can present as delirium, whereas slower-growing tumors are more likely to cause chronic cognitive deficits. Focal lesions give rise to a variety of specific neuropsychiatric syndromes; those near the frontal poles typically manifest initially as personality change. Craniopharyngiomas and otic tumors around the hypothalamus are also often associated with personality changes and apathy.

When subdivided by location, 70% of intracranial tumors in the adult are supratentorial and 30% are infratentorial(in the posterior fossa); the ratio is reversed in children. In adults, 22% of tumors are located in the frontal lobe,22% in the temporal lobe; in both locations, tumors are relatively silent. Parietal tumors account for 12%, occipital for 4%; 10% are pituitary tumors, and 30% are in the posterior fossa.

Intracranial tumors have a high incidence of mental symptoms, consisting of personality changes, emotional disturbances, and intellectual defects. General symptoms of intracranial tumors include the classical triad of headache(the initial symptom in a third of cases), vomiting(sometimes projectile in nature), and papilledema(relatively rare despite its traditional inclusion as a member of the triad). Other general symptoms are visual field defects, seizures(with few exceptions, the EEG shows increasing focal abnormality), aphasia, vertigo, slowed pulse and increased blood pressure, coma, confusion, and progressive dementia. Psychiatric symptoms are frequent, occurring in 40%–100% of patients depending on the type and location of tumor. Meningiomas are particularly likely to produce symptoms such as depression, anxiety, or personality change. Tumors in certain locations, the prefrontal or temporal lobes, third ventricle, or limbic system, may mimic the "functional" psychoses and other primary psychiatric disorders.

Patients with brain tumors typically present with headaches, seizures, nonspecific cognitive or personality changes, or focal neurological signs. The subtlety of presentation of brain tumors should be aware for efficient and expeditious diagnosis. A single seizure, loss of interest in usual activities, or loss of hearing for high frequencies may all signal a suspicion of tumor. As a result of the widespread availability of sensitive imaging techniques such as MRI, tumors are being detected at an earlier stage, and patients with subtle clinical signs and symptoms are being diagnosed.

The course and ultimate prognosis for a patient with an intracranial tumor depend upon the tumor's histological type, rate of growth, invasiveness, and response to treatment. Given the early diagnosis of brain tumors and their surgical treatment will be necessary. Most patients with neuropsychiatric symptoms after brain tumors were treated with drugs frequently used among patients with functional psychiatry symptoms, such as neuroleptics, anticonvulsants, antidepressants, and lithium. These drugs should be used empirically with care in patients with brain tumors due to their adverse effects, such as excessive sedation and lowered seizure threshold.

5.2.7   Epilepsy and mental disorders

Epileptic seizures affect approximately one in every 200 people and can be generalised or focal(particularly of the temporal lobe). One quarter or more patients with epilepsy have schizophreniform psychoses, depression, personality changes, or hyposexuality. Mental disorder is especially common in those with temporal lobe epilepsy, where convulsions are rare, the seizures being characterised by complex psychomotor manifestations such as automatisms, fugues, mood changes, hallucinations and other phenomena.

The reasons for the increased rate of psychiatric disturbance amongst epileptics remain unclear, although possible causes include undetected "brain damage", abnormal mental functioning during the interictal period(between seizures), the side-effects of anticonvulsant drugs, and the stigma associated with the condition. Psychiatric disturbance amongst epileptics could divided into 4 subtypes: before, during, after the seizure, and between seizures.

5.2.7.1   Pre-ictal phenomena(before the seizure)

Certain individuals have a tendency to develop prodromal moodiness and iritability for several hours or days prior to a seizure. An aura is often experienced immediately before the epileptic attack, and may involve hallucinations or illusions, mood changes and feelings of unreality, including the phenomenon of déjà vu. This is a sudden feeling of familiarity with a place or situation which the individual knows he has not previously encountered.

5.2.7.2   Ictal and post-ictal phenomena(during and after the seizure)

These are most commonly associated with temporal lobe seizures, usually in the absence of aconvulsion. Automatisms involve the performance of simple or complex actions in a state of clouded consciousness, so that the subject is unaware of his behaviour. Episodes rarely last for more than a few minutes, and often commence with the individual seeming dazed and staring vacantly ahead. This may be followed by complex facial movements, such as repetitive blinking, chewing or lip-smacking. Sometimes, the subject wanders about in an apparently purposeful manner, and might pick up objects or move items of furniture around. Once the automatism is completed, he may appear confused and suspicious, since he has no memory of the incident. Very rarely, criminal acts are judged in court to have taken place during an automatism, as a result of which the defendant is not considered fully responsible for his behavior.

Fugues involve wandering behavior during a seizure, and are associated with amnesia for the episode. There is clouding of consciousness and those affected have been known to travel great distances from their point of origin. Fugues can also occur in the setting of a depressive or dissociative disorder.

Twilight states involve a subjective alteration of awareness, so that emotionally significant experiences and perceptions have a dream-like quality. The episode usually lasts for several hours, during which time psychomotor retardation and perseveration of movements or speech occur.

Transient hallucinatory experiences are quite common in temporal lobe epilepsy, and may involve any of the sensory modalities.

5.2.7.3   Interictal phenomena(between seizures)

Psychiatric disturbance is common during the interictal period(especially between temporal lobe seizures), with neurotic disorders such as anxiety, minor depressive and phobic states being the most frequently encountered forms of mental disorder. By comparison, psychoses are relatively rare; illnesses which are clinically indistinguishable from schizophrenia have been reported as occurring in the interictal phase in those with temporal lobe epilepsy of the dominant lobe, and are said by some authorities to be more common when the frequency of seizures is diminished. This may explain why psychotic symptoms develop, or are sometimes exacerbated, when fits are well controlled with anticonvulsant drugs. Interictal affective disorders, which are most commonly depressive, are thought to be associated with nondominant temporal lobe seizures.

Epileptics do not differ from the general population with regard to intelligence, but in a small proportion of cases, a dementia develops involving diffuse cerebral atrophy and personality deterioration. This seems to be more likely where there is underlying brain damage, or where the epilepsy is chronic and severe. It has also been proposed that the dementia is related to long-term administration of anticonvulsant drugs, but so far this theory remains unproven.

There is no definite link between epilepsy and criminal behaviour, although the prevalence of the disorder amongst prisoners is slightly greater than in the general population. The reasons for this are undetermined.

In the treatment of psychiatrically disturbed patients with epilepsy, a first consideration is the use of psychoactive anticonvulsant medications. Carbamazepine, valproate, gabapentin(Neurontin), and lamotrigine (Lamictal) have significant antimanic and modest antidepressant properties, probably through mood-stabilization effects. They have some efficacy in the long-term prophylaxis of manic or depressive episodes. Gabapentin also decreases anxiety and improves general well-being in some epilepsy patients.

A second consideration is the seizure-threshold lowering effect of psychotropic medications. This is usually not a problem but can occasionally reach clinical significance in poorly controlled epilepsy. Psychotropic drugs are most convulsive when the drug is introduced rapidly and in high doses. For example, clozapine has induced seizures.

A third treatment consideration is the potential for interaction of anticonvulsant and psychotropic medications. Most commonly, an anticonvulsant drug increases the metabolism of a psychotropic drug with a consequent decrease in its therapeutic efficiency. Conversely, withdrawal of anticonvulsant drugs can precipitate rebound elevations in concentrations of the psychotropic medication. Compared to older drugs, the new anticonvulsant medications have fewer potential interactions with psychotropic medications. Gabapentin, lamotrigine, vigabatrin, and tiagabine are relatively free of enzyme-inducing or enzyme-inhibiting properties.

Epilepsy surgery is a fourth treatment consideration and is limited to patients with medically intractable seizures. Over 80% of temporal lobectomy patients experience some reduction in their seizure frequency and over 50% are entirely seizure-free. Removal of the amygdala and most of the hippocampus may have postoperative behavioral effects.

Shi Limin

Chapter 6

Mental Disorders due to Physical Diseases

6.1 Introduction

This chapter is concerned with those conditions in which mental disorder arises as a result of a physiological disturbance affecting cerebral function.

Mental disorders due to physical diseases are defined as any brain dysfunction which is clearly caused by various systemic disturbances outside the brain, such as infection, endocrine disturbance, nutritional and metabolic disorders. Clinical manifestation mainly presents acute brain syndrome — delirium, or chronic brain syndrome — cognitive impairment and personality changes. Depression, elation, delusion, hallucination, psychomotor agitation and stupor may present. In any specific case, one or more of the characteristic symptoms may predominate. The signs of organicity include:

(1) Disturbances in orientation.

(2) Impairment of memory.

(3) Impairment in the maintenance of the level of consciousness and attention.

(4) Impairment of all intellectual functions (comprehension, calculation, knowledge, learning, etc.).

(5) Defective judgment.

(6) Lability, shallowness, and similar instabilities of the affect.

(7) Overall changes in the personality, with the appearance of conduct foreign to the patient's natural or usual behavior.

Common clinical features of mental disorders due to physical diseases include:

(1) Psychiatric symptoms usually appear in the peak of the physical diseases.

(2) Psychiatric symptoms usually fluctuate with physical disease.

(3) The symptoms are less severe in daylight and severe at night or vary with physical disease.

(4) Course and prognosis mainly depend on the treatment of primary diseases.

(5) The prognosis is better if psychiatric symptom lasts for a shorter period; in severe case, patients may leave behind personality change and intellectual disturbance.

(6) Commonly associated with physical and NS signs and positive laboratory results.

With regard to diagnosis of mental disorders due to physical diseases, three key core features should be based on:

(1)Evidence of physical disease.

(2)Evidence indicates that physical disease cause mental disorders.

(3)Presence of atypical symptom of mental disorders.

According to CCMD-3, the following 4 criterias are required for the diagnosis.

(1)Symptom criteria

1)Presence of a systemic disease as evident in the clinical history, physical examination and lab investigation results.

2)Onset and course of the mental disturbance follow that of the underlying systemic disorder with one of the following clinical features: ①cognitive impairment; ②amnesic syndrome; ③personality change; ④disorder of consciousness(e. g. , delirium) ; ⑤psychotic symptoms(e. g. , hallucination, delusion, or catatonic syndrome) ; ⑥affective disorder; ⑦neurosis-like symptoms; ⑧mixed or atypical presentation.

3)When there is no evidence of mental disorders due to other causes such as psychosocial stressors or use of psychoactive substances.

(2)Severity criteria

The condition has resulted in impairment in activities of daily living and social functioning.

(3)Course criteria

The onset and clinical course follow that of the underlying physical problem.

(4)Exclusion

Excluding schizophrenia, mood disorder. The therapeutic principles of mental disorders due to physical diseases include:

1)To treat primary diseases firstly.

2)To use antipsychotic drug appropriately.

3)To improve nursing care and psychological care.

6.2　Mental disorders due to systemic infectious diseases

Systemic infectious diseases are caused by extracranial invasion of infectious agents including viruses, viroids, prions, bacteria, and other pathogens. Those impairments of body function, metabolic disorders, and the toxins the pathogens produced, often result in mild mental disturbances, such as disorder of consciousness(e. g. , delirium) , cognitive impairment, psychotic symptoms(e. g. , hallucination, delusion, or catatonic syndrome) , and neurosis-like symptoms. Onset and course of the mental disturbance follow that of the underlying systemic disorder. Psychiatric symptoms usually fluctuate with physical disease.

6.2.1　Mental disturbance due to influenza

Influenza, commonly known as "the flu", is an infectious disease caused by an influenza virus. Symptoms can be mild to severe. The most common symptoms include: a high fever, runny nose, sore throat, muscle pains, headache, coughing, and feeling tired. These symptoms typically begin 2 days after exposure to the virus and most last less than a week. Mental disturbance due to influenza include dizziness, confusion, fatigue, headache, insomnia and somnolence. During the hyperpyrexia stage, anxiety and depression may present.

6.2.2   Mental disturbance due to pneumonia

During the hyperpyrexia stage of pneumonia, disturbance of consciousness (e. g. , clouding of consciousness) , delirium may present. Time of disturbance of consciousness duration will be ended after the pneumonia takes a turn for the better.

6.2.3   Mental disturbance due to infectious endocarditis

Infective endocarditis is an infection of the inner surface of the heart, usually the valves. Symptoms may include fever, small areas of bleeding into the skin, heart murmur, feeling tired, and low red blood cell count. Complications may include valvular insufficiency, heart failure, stroke, and kidney failure. The cause is typically a bacterial infection and less commonly a fungal infection. Risk factors include valvular heart disease including rheumatic disease, congenital heart disease, artificial valves, hemodialysis, intravenous drug use, and electronic pacemakers. The bacteria most commonly involved are streptococci or staphylococci. Diagnosis is suspected based on symptoms and supported by blood cultures or ultrasound.

During the hyperpyrexia stage of infectious endocarditis, mild psychiatric symptoms may present. Severe cases usually present delirium, agitated symptoms, behavior change, and focal nervous system signs.

6.2.4   Mental disturbance due to typhoid

Typhoid, is a bacterial infection due to *Salmonella typhi* that causes symptoms. Symptoms may vary from mild to severe and usually begin six to thirty days after exposure. Often there is a gradual onset of a high fever over several days. Weakness, abdominal pain, constipation, and headaches also commonly occur. Diarrhea is uncommon and vomiting is not usually severe. Some people develop a skin rash with rose colored spots. Severe cases may present neuropsychiatric symptoms(described as "muttering delirium" or "coma vigil") , with picking at bedclothes or imaginary objects at peak time. Delirium and confusion are frequent, often calm, but sometimes agitated. This delirium gives to typhoid the nickname of "nervous fever". Apathy, slow response, fragmentary hallucination and delusion of reference may occur.

6.2.5   Mental disturbance due to Sydenham's chorea

Sydenham's chorea(SC) or chorea minor(historically and traditionally referred to as St Vitus' dance) is a disorder characterized by rapid, uncoordinated jerking movements primarily affecting the face, hands and feet. Sydenham's chorea results from childhood infection with Group A beta−hemolytic streptococcus and is reported to occur in 20% −30% of patients with acute rheumatic fever(ARF). The disease is usually latent, occurring up to 6 months after the acute infection, but may occasionally be the presenting symptom of rheumatic fever. Sydenham's chorea is more common in females than males and most patients are children, below 18 years of age.

Sydenham's chorea is characterized by the abrupt onset(sometimes within a few hours) of neurologic symptoms, classically chorea, usually affecting all four limbs. Other symptoms include behavior change, dysarthria, gait disturbance, loss of fine and gross motor control with resultant deterioration of handwriting, headache, slowed cognition, facial grimacing, fidgetiness and hypotonia. Also, there may be tongue fasciculations("bag of worms") and a "milk sign", which is a relapsing grip demonstrated by alternate increases and decreases in tension, as if hand milking.

6.2.6   Mental disturbance due to infection of HIV

Acquired immune deficiency syndrome(AIDS) is a spectrum of conditions caused by infection with the human immunodeficiency virus(HIV). Following initial infection, a person may not notice any symptoms or may experience a brief period of influenza-like illness. Typically, this is followed by a prolonged period with no symptoms. As the infection progresses, it interferes more with the immune system, increasing the risk of developing common infections like tuberculosis, as well as other opportunistic infections, and tumors that rarely affect people who have working immune systems. These late symptoms of infection are referred to as acquired immunodeficiency syndrome. This stage is often also associated with unintended weight loss.

The neuropsychiatric complications of AIDS are various according to different stages of disease.

(1) Affective disturbance

Early in the course of disease, patients may present shock — numbness, denial — this is not true, anger—why have I got it, bargain—I will do anything, acceptance—how can I live with this. Other syndromes commonly occur—shock, fear and anxiety, depression, anger and frustration, guilt, shame, stigma, suicide ideation.

(2) Psychotic symptoms

Usually occur at middle and late of the course. Schizophrenic syndrome, acute paranoid disorder, and transient mental disorder may present.

(3) Disturbance of consciousness

Delirium is frequent, clouding of consciousness, disorientation, excited agitation, auditory or visional hallucination may present.

(4) Dementia symdrome

HIV infection of the CNS results in a progressive subcortical dementia, the AIDS dementia complex. Cognitive impairments associated with HIV occur in the domains of attention, memory, verbal fluency, and visuospatial construction. Specifically for memory, the lowered activity of the hippocampus changes the basis for memory encoding and affects mechanisms such as long-term potentiation. Confabulation, paramnesia and withdrawal behavior are frequent.

6.3   Mental disorders due to endocrine diseases

The endocrine system is a network of glands that produce and release hormones that help control many important body functions, including the body's ability to change calories into energy that powers cells and organs. Each gland of the endocrine system releases specific hormones into the bloodstream. These hormones travel through the blood to other cells and help control or coordinate many body processes. It plays a vital role in general chemical changes or the activities of other organs at a distance. Any defects or excess in the internal secretions of the different glands could result in various endocrine diseases, include mental disorders. Hyperthyroidism, hypothyroidism, hyperfunction of pituitary gland, adrenocortical hyperactivity, sexual hormone imbalance frequently be associated with psychiatric organic syndromes.

6.3.1   Mental disorder due to hyperthyroidism

Hyperthyroidism is excessive activity of the thyroid gland. It is a common disorder affecting between 2% and 5% of all females at some time in their lives. Most cases are the result of disease of the thyroid gland. The commonest cause is Graves disease, also called thyrotoxicosis. Single or multiple adenomas or nodules in the thyroid also cause hyperthyroidism. There are several other rare causes, including inflammation caused by a virus, autoimune reactions and cancer. The symptoms of hyperthyroidism affect many of the body's system as a consequence of the much increased metabolic rate: these include the cardiovascular, nervous, alimentary and musculoskeletal systems.

Psychiatric features include nervousness, fatigue, insomnia, mood lability, and dysphoria. Speech may be pressured, and patients may demonstrate a heightened activity level. Cognitive symptoms include a short attention span, impaired recent memory, and an exaggerated startle response. Patients with severe cases may exhibit visual hallucinations, paranoid ideation, and delirium. While some symptoms of hyperthyroidism resemble those of a manic episode.

Treatments for Graves disease are antithyroid drugs, radioactive iodine (RAI), and surgical thyroidectomy.

For patients with psychotic symptoms, medium-potency antipsychotics are preferable to low-potency drugs, as the latter can worsen tachycardia. Similarly, tricyclic drugs should be used with caution, if at all, in these patients. In general, the psychiatric symptoms resolve with successful treatment of the hyperthyroidism.

6.3.2   Mental disorder due to hypothyroidism

Psychiatric complications of hypothyroidism are common and the condition may be mistaken for a primary mental disorder. Features include depressed mood, fatigue, apathy, poorconcentration and psychomotor retardation. Severe hypothyroidism may result in the development of "myxoedema madness", in which delirium is sometimes associated with a psychosis. Epilepsy, ataxia and coma can also occur, whilst dementia may develop in chronic cases.

For patients presenting with severe psychiatric symptoms (e. g. , psychosis or suicidal depression), urgent psychiatric treatment is necessary. Psychotropic agents should be given at low doses initially, as the reduced metabolic rate in hypothyroid patients may produce reduced breakdown and therefore higher blood concentrations of medications.

6.3.3   Mental disorder due to hypercortisolism

Hypercortisolism (Cushing syndrome) may result from overactivity of the adrenal cortex or the prolonged use of steroid drugs. For patients with psychotic symptoms, depression is common, but sometimes the mood is elevated. Delirium or a paranoid psychosis can also occur.

Psychiatric symptoms are myriad. Most patients experience fatigue, and approximately 75% report depressed mood. Of these, approximately 60% experience moderate or severe depression. The severity of depression does not appear to be influenced by the underlying cause of the Cushing syndrome. Depressive symptoms occur more commonly in female patients than in male patients with Cushing syndrome.

Manic and psychotic symptoms occur much less frequently than depression, in approximately 3%-8% of patients, but reach 40% in patients with adrenal carcinomas. In iatrogenic hypercortisolism and adrenal carcinomas, however, mania and psychosis may predominate. The psychiatric disturbances in prednisone-treated patients tend to appear within the first 2 weeks of treatment and occur more commonly in women than men.

6.3.4   Mental disorder due to adrenocortical insufficiency

Adrenocortical insufficiency results from inadequate production of three major steroid hormones, glucocorticoids, mineralocorticoids, and sex steroids, by the adrenal gland. In primary adrenal insufficiency, adrenal hypofunction results from adrenal gland disease (e. g. , autoimmune disease, infection, idiopathic atrophy, metastatic tumor). ACTH and CRH concentrations increase in response to low concentrations of adrenal steroids. Because ACTH is metabolized to a-melanocyte-stimulating hormone, which promotes melanocyte activity.

Acute adrenal insufficiency can be life threatening, particularly in cases of acute adrenal insufficiency. Symptoms include weakness, hypoglycemia, hyponatremia, hyperkalemia, nausea, diarrhea, fever. Psychotic symptoms include delirium, stupor and coma.

Chronic adrenal insufficiency produces more-subtle symptoms, including fatigability, salt craving, weight loss, vitiligo, nausea, hyperpigmentation, loss of body hair, muscle cramps, apathy, irritability, and mild-to-severe depression. Symptoms develop insidiously over months or years. The substitution therapy could relief patient's physical and mental symptoms rapidly.

6.3.5   Mental disorder due to parathyroid diseases

Parathyroid hormone(PTH) is an endocrine factor having effects on calcium and phosphorus homeostasis. If for any reason there is a excess(hyperparathyroidism) or deficiency(hypoparathyroidism) parathyroid hormone secretion of the parathyroid glands, the calcium and phosphorus homeostasis will be broken. The commonest neuropsychiatric changes include anxiety, depression, fatigue or apathy. With very high or low serum calcium levels, great restlessness, impairment of consciousness, learning and memory problems, and seizures may occur.

The commonest cause of hypoparathyroidism, is accidental injury to or removal of the glands during the operation of thyroidectomy for the treatment of Graves disease. This is one of the hazards of thyroidectomy in view of the very close relationship of the parathyroid glands to the thyroid gland. Psychiatric symptoms could be dilirium, impairment of memory and personality changes.

6.3.6   Mental disorder due to dysequilibrium of gonadal hormone

This section is concerned with psychiatric disorders which are associated with menstruation, pregnancy and childbirth, menopause, or gonadal dysgenesis.

6.3.6.1   Premenstrual syndrome(PMS)

Many women feel tense, irritable and mildly depressed for 5-7 days prior to the onset of a period, and there may be accompanying symptoms of breast tenderness and abdominal distension. In most cases, the symptoms resolve rapidly once menstruationbegins, but in some women they are sufficiently distressing for medical help to be sought. Premenstrual syndrome is correlated with the menstrual cycle, typically beginning soon after ovulation and building to a peak about 5 days before the menstrual period. Psychological symptoms include anxiety, crying spells, depression, and fatigability; physical symptoms include weight gain, breast tenderness, swelling of the legs, and bloating. The syndrome has been attributed to hormonal imbalances, such as estrogen excess, estrogen-progesterone imbalance, hyperprolactinemia, and effects of gonadal steroids on endogenous opiates. As many as 20%-40% of menstruating women report some symptoms of PMS, which can also occur in postmenopausal women so long as their ovaries are intact.

There is no clear evidence that hormonal treatment(such as progesterone) is effective in this condition, although diuretics and mild analgesics may be of help in relieving physical discomfort.

Physical problems which occur at the time of the menopause are sometimes accompanied by feelings of anxiety and depression. Although hormone replacement therapy is widely used to treat somatic complaints such as "hot flushes" and sweating, its effect on psychological symptoms is uncertain.

6.3.6.2   Puerperal mental disorder

It is well established that there is an increased prevalence of psychiatric disorder amongst women commencing during the puerperium (the 6 weeks period following childbirth), when compared with age – matched, non–puerperal controls. Disorders which occur at this time are puerperal psychosis, postnatal depression and the "maternity blues". ICD–10 does not generally recognise these categories as distinct entities, but their inclusion is justified on clinical grounds.

The incidence of puerperal psychosis is low, with only 1 or 2 women affected in every 1,000 deliveries. It is commoner amongst those having their first baby.

Despite a great deal of research, very little is known about the cause of puerperal psychosis. There is often a family history of mental illness, although a more direct genetic influence has been inferred from the observation that women whose own mothers had a history of puerperal psychosis have a sixfold increased risk of developing the condition themselves. An association with bipolar affective disorder is suggested by a similarity in the clinical presentation of both illnesses, and the high rate of puerperal relapse in women with a history of affective disorder. No clear etiological link has been established with any psychological or environmental factors, although a biological cause might seem likely in view of the dramatic physiological changes which occur at this time. However, no significant endocrine or biochemical abnormality has been detected in these women which distinguishes them from other postpartum females. Non–puerperal episodes of psychosis occur in 50% of these women at some time in the future, which may indicate that many have a life–long tendency to develop major mental ilness.

The onset is often sudden, characteristically between the third and fourteenth day following childbirth, and is usually preceded by 24 – 48 hours of insomnia, restlessness and sometimes confused. Clinically, the condition most frequently resembles an affective disorder, with features of mania (often accompanied by confusion and disorganised speech) or a severe depressive episode with psychotic symptoms (where delusions may focus on the health and well-being of the baby). Less commonly, a schizoaffective or schizophrenic-like disorder develops, with characteristic distortions of thought and perception.

Although hospital admission is frequently required to treat the mother's illness, every effort needs to be made to ensure that she remains with and continues to play a part in the care of her baby. Only if the mother is extremely disturbed should separation be considered, and as soon as her symptoms are under control, she should be reunited with her child. Statistically, the risk of suicide or infanticide is rare. Nevertheless, careful enquiries must always be made to determine if the mother harbours any delusional ideas which might result in harm to her baby or herself.

Many women with puerperal psychosis continue to relate well to their babies during illness, and providing they are carefully supervised by appropriately trained nurses, they can carry out many of the tasks necessary in caring for their infant. This facilitates bonding and allows the mother to feel more competent in coping with her child when she is ready to leave hospital. Where no specialist facility exists, it is common practice to admit both mother and baby onto an acute psychiatric ward. In either case, the continuing involvement of the father and other children should be encouraged. As her mental state improves, supportive individual or group psychotherapy may be of benefit in helping the patient to come to terms with her new role and responsibilities.

The choice of physical treatment will depend upon the clinical presentation of the condition. The possibility of infection should always be borne in mind, and where necessary, treatment with antibiotics started as soon as possible. Severe depressive episodes can be treated with antidepressants (sometimes given in combination with a neuroleptic drug) or ECT. Manic symptoms respond well to lithium and neuroleptics, whilst schizophrenic-like disorders are best treated with neuroleptics alone. However, due attention must be given to the mother's desire to breast feed and the subsequent risk to the infant with certain forms of drug treatment, especially lithium.

6.3.6.3 Involutional psychosis

Involutional psychosis is defined as depressive psychoses appearing during the involutional period(40-55 years for women) in women who have no history of previous mental illness. Based on decrease in the ovaries' production of the hormones estrogen and progesterone, in combination with negetive life events, some women will present severe hot flashes, shivering, sweating, reddening of the skin, and psychiatric symptoms.

Characteristically, such depressions manifest a triad of symptoms, consisting of delusions of sin and guilt or of poverty, an obsession with death, and a delusional fixation on the gastrointestinal tract, all in a setting of agitation and dejection. In some(involutional paranoid state), a fourth major symptom is present in self-referential or persecutory delusions, and this second group with a vivid admixture of paranoid symptoms has a poorer prognosis than the more purely depressive variety. Concern over finances, physical illness, bereavement, enforced retirement, and "loss" of children to marriage or other forms of independence are frequent precipitants. Involutional psychoses account for 5%-10% of first admissions to mental hospitals; their actual incidence is difficult to estimate because many respond favorably to antidepressants administered on an outpatient basis.

Management include psychotherapy, symptomatic drug therapy, and estrogen replacement therapy.

6.4 Mental disorder due to connective tissue disease

Rheumatoid diseases also known as connective tissue disease(CTD), which is a group of autoimmune diseases in which the body's immune system mistakenly attacks healthy tissue of the body. Based on the pathological changes of chronic inflammation of blood vessels and connective tissue, lesions often involve multiple systems and multiple organs.

The three most common CTDs encountered by psychiatrists are rheumatoid arthritis, systemic lupus erythematosus, and fibromyalgia. Although there is no single unifying theory for the development and pathogenesis of these conditions, multidimensional explanations currently aid in integrating them into one category. They involve primarily biological but also psychological and social components.

6.4.1 Systemic lupus erythematosus

Systemic lupus erythematosus(SLE) is the commonest autoimmune disease occurring predominantly in women that causes chronic inflammation of the connective tissue which affects the skin and various internal organs. The skin is red and scaly, joints develop inflammatory arthritis, and the kidneys may be damaged. The brain, heart and lungs may also be affected, with inflamed tissue ultimately becoming scarred. Psychotic symptoms often occur in late stage of the disease with prevalence of 15%-37%, known as Neuropsychiatric Lupus. The psychotic symptoms may be caused by the immune-mediated involvement of autoantibodies in brain vessels, which may affect brain function. In addition, organs such as heart, liver and kidney have been damaged and result in metabolic disorders. Therefore, the secondary psychiatric symptoms occur. Those mental symptoms lack the specificity and varied, easily lead to misdiagnosis.

The neuropsychiatric complications could present as cognitive impairment, psychotic symptoms, and florid delirium with marked behavioral abnormalities. Three symptoms could present: neuroses symptoms such as headache, insomnia, hypomnesis, emotional instability; schizotypal symptoms, e. g. , auditory hallucination, delusions, looseness of thought; manic or depressive symptoms.

Psychiatric treatment is dictated by the predominant clinical picture as it relates to similar primary conditions known to respond to such treatments. Judicious use of antipsychotic agents, mood-stabilizing agents, or both in patients with hallucinations and delusions is reasonable and reportedly effective.

The conflicts of treatment should be put into consideration. The immunosuppressant agents used to modify autoantibody production that seems integral to lupus disease activity can in and of themselves cause psychiatric illness including depression, hypomania, delirium, and various psychotic states. NSAID have been reported to cause delirium as well as mild forms of cognitive dysfunction. Adrenal corticosteroid hormones are notorious for causing psychopathology.

6.4.2   Rheumatoid arthritis

Rheumatoid arthritis(RA) is a systemic, chronic, inflammatory, progressive, and in association with serum rheumatoid factor antibody disease. Patients usually experience a prodromal syndrome that may include vague constitutional symptoms, fleeting musculoskeletal pain, and variable morning stiffness that may last for weeks or months without yielding to diagnosis. Although a few patients experience abrupt onset, most note an insidious beginning followed by gradual involvement of multiple joints in a symmetrical pattern. A few patients have an asymmetrical pattern. It is likely that the problem is of multifactorial origin, and that there is some variation in the genetic and environmental factors involved in individual cases.

Regarding the comorbidity of psychiatric disorders with rheumatoid arthritis, depression is comorbid with rheumatoid arthritis in about 20% of individuals and overlap with somatic neurovegetative signs and symptoms. The incidence of anxiety spectrum disorders is mildly increased in patients with rheumatoid arthritis.

Potential psychiatric side effects of commonly used medications for rheumatoid arthritis are numerous. Cognitive dysfunction and delirium may accompany toxic levels of salicylates. The NSAID cross the blood-brain barrier and contribute to blockade of prostaglandin production, which in turn affects the function of various neurotransmitters. NSAID have been associated with cognitive impairment, frank delirium, depression, mania, and psychotic symptoms. Geriatric patients are especially susceptible to these adverse effects. Mood lability, sleep disruption, delirium, and psychosis are well-recognized potential effects of the glucocorticoids and are often dose sensitive. Patients who require corticosteroids for effective management but tolerate them poorly may benefit from concomitant prophylaxis with lithium. A variety of NSAID increase serum lithium concentrations and require cautious monitoring to avoid lithium intoxication.

Psychotropic agents selected for use in patients with rheumatoid arthritis should minimize the side effects that prove especially problematic for individuals contending with this disease. Sleep, which is often disrupted by pain, can be assisted by the combination of an NSAID and trazodone, with appropriate cautionary advice regarding orthostasis to patients who face decreased mobility. The tricyclic drugs exert mild anti-inflammatory effects independent of their mood-altering benefit. Unfortunately, anticholinergic effects(prominent among the tricyclic drugs and also present with the serotonergic agent paroxetine) can aggravate the significant difficulties with dry oral and ocular membranes in patients whose rheumatoid arthritis is associated with Sjögren's syndrome.

6.5   Mental disorders due to disease of internal organs

Mental disorders caused by diseases of internal organs refer to the mental disorders caused by severe disease of important internal organs(such as heart, liver and kidney). The severity of mental disorders fluctuates with the severity of the primary disease.

6.5.1   Mental disorders due to respiratory diseases

Almost all serious respiratory diseases can cause mental symptoms. There are three pathophysiological factors — hypoxemia, CO_2 retention, and acidosis, which induced by dyspnea on exertion or respiratory failure, synergistically cause dysfunction of cerebral blood vessels and neurons—must be the primary causes of those psychiatric symptoms.

6.5.1.1   Chronic obstructive pulmonary disease

Chronic obstructive pulmonary disease(COPD) is one of the most common respiratory diseases. Psychiatric comorbidity such as anxiety, depression and panic attack frequently present, especially in the severe cases. In patients with COPD, it is necessary to avoid the side effect of respiratory inhibition for anti-anxiety treatment.

The new generation of antidepressants is safer, could be used starting from low doses.

6.5.1.2   Pulmono-encephalopathy

Obstructive lung disease, caused in large part by cigarette smoking, is the most prevalent of the chronic respiratory diseases. Psychiatric complications include acute and chronic encephalopathies related to acute infection or respiratory failure, to sustained hypoxemia and hypercapnia, or to the CNS effects of drugs used in management(oral or inhaled bronchodilators, high-dose prednisone, cough suppressants, or benzodiazepines). Depression is common, as in other chronic medical illnesses, but tend to be characterized by prominent anxiety and paniclike episodes, accounting for frequent prescription of anxiolytics. Psychotic states may occur and are usually related to acute impairment of brain function, which usually manifested as different disturbances of consciousness.

Psychological complications are frequent and include avoidance of therapeutic physical activity because of panic in response to dyspnea, fear of sudden death by asphyxiation, excessive self-blame in patients whose illness is related to smoking, and avoidance of appropriate social activities because of negative body image. Untreated depression in chronic obstructive pulmonary disease increases functional disability. For milder dysphoric states not meeting criteria for a depressive diagnosis, a multidisciplinary rehabilitation and counseling approach improves mood in many patients. For patients with syndromal depressions who do not have severe left ventricular disease or hypercapnia, antidepressant pharmacotherapy with nortriptyline is effective and markedly improves anxiety and severity of somatic symptoms. Important nonpharmacological interventions for anxious depressed patients with chronic obstructive pulmonary disease provide individualized education about the disease and its management, demonstrate to patients how they can modify their own symptoms with appropriate techniques such as breathing retraining, and improve overall physical condition through supervised physical training. Patients with pulmonary disability and those who require home oxygen therapy may benefit from self-help groups.

6.5.2　Mental disorders due to digestive diseases

6.5.2.1　Hepatic encephalopathy

Hepatic encephalopathy, also known as hepatogenic coma, is a prominent syndrome which based on metabolic disturbance of severe liver diseases, excretory clearance, and tend to be characterized by severe somatoform symptoms and encephalopathic states, together with flapping tremor of the outstretched hands, facial grimacing, and fetor hepaticus. It is a significant terminal complication of various liver diseases and the obvious cause of death.

Mental disturbance caused by acute liver diseases include emotional change and abnormal behavior, such as depression, lags in response, wordlessness, decreased activity. Some patients may present anxiety, excited agitation, hypersomnia. The condition may progress to coma, there may be hallucinations and confabulation. Signs of the nervous system may occur as flapping tremor of the outstretched hands, facial grimacing, convulsive seizure, hypermyotonia, pathological reflexes positive. Mental disturbance caused by chronic liver diseases include personality changes and cognitive impairment. Patient may present impatience, grumpiness, irascibility, hypomnesis, impaired concentration, confusion and so on.

Regarding treatment, primary physical disease should be treated first. Due to the liver failure, sedative drugs, psychotroptic drugs will increase the severity of the encephalopathy and should be avoided. In a case of necessity, injection diazepam and low dose of olanzapine tablets could be applicable.

6.5.2.2　Mental disorders due to pancreatic diseases

Acute and chronic pancreatitis, carcinoma of pancreas may result in mental disturbance. As in other acute organic syndromes, there may be hallucinations, confabulation, delirium, depression and disturbance of intelligence. Regarding treatment, symptomatic therapy is the main treatment. Antidepressant, antianxiety agent, psychotroptic drugs could be applicable. If the patient presents disturbance of consciousness, the dosage and mode of the medication should be taken into a careful consideration.

6.5.3　Mental disorders due to renal diseases

6.5.3.1　Renal encephalopathy

Actue or chronic renal disease produce encephalopathic states through their effects on nutrition, metabolism, excretory clearance, and drug disposition. Renal encephalopathy is a mental disorder arised from actue or chronic end-stage renal failure. Symptoms of anxiety, depression, impatience, irascibility, hypomnesis, impaired concentration, confusion occur in about half the patients. There may be hallucinations, confabulation and delirium. There is probably an increased risk of suicide. Impaired capacity to work, reduced physical activity, marital problems, and sexual dysfunction are common. Psychiatric help is mainly sought for mood disorders, difficulties in coming to terms with renal failure or its treatment, and disruptive or uncooperative behaviour. Regarding the treatment, medications with nephrotoxicity should be avoided.

6.5.3.2　Mental disorders due to haemodialysis

Due to uremia, anemia, and other physical complications of the renal failure, some patients with haemodialysis may develop cognitive deficits. When there is dialysis disequilibrium, organic psychiatric syndrome such as lethargy, insomnia, poor concentration, depression and anxiety may occur. The rare occurrence of dialysis dementia is probably due to the aluminium content of the dialysis solutions.

6.6   Mental disorders due to diabetes mellitus

Diabetes mellitus is a chronic condition characterized by a raised concentration of glucose in the blood because of a deficiency in the production and/or action of insulin, a pancreatic hormone made in special celis called the islet cells of Langerhans. It is now generally accepted that good control of blood glucose is the single most important factor in preventing long-term complications.

Diabetes mellitus is requiring prolonged medical supervision and informed self-care. The psychological aspect of treatment should be emphasized because many diabetics show poor self-care and compliance with medical advice, and stressful experience can lead directly to endocrine changes.

Psychological and social problems are more common in diabetics with severe medical complications such as vascular disease, impaired vision, renal failure and sexual dysfunction. They may be caused by restrictions of diet and activity, the need for self-care, and the possibility of serious physical complications. An important minority of those with insulin-dependent and non-insulin-dependent diabetes have difficulties to adapt well to the limitations of their illness. Compliance with blood testing, diet, and insulin use is frequently unsatisfactory, and as a result glycemic control is often less than optimal.

Depression, anxiety and less severe psychological distress are believed to be common psychiatric problems among diabetics. An acute organic syndrome is a prodromal sign of diabetic(hyperglycaemic) coma. It may present as an episode of disturbed behavior (delirium), which may begin either abruptly or insidiously. Other prodromal physical symptoms include thirst, headaches, abdominal pain, nausea, and vomiting. The pulse is rapid and blood pressure is low(dysfunction of autonomic nerve). Dehydration is marked and acetone may be smelt on the breath. Hyperglycemia in diabetics can produce and eventual coma.

Hypoglycemia most commonly occurs in diabetics who use excessive insulin or omit meals, although rarely may be due to an insulinoma. Symptoms of anxiety are often prominent and may be associated with bizarre or aggressive behavior. Prolonged periods of hypoglycemia can lead to irreversible brain damage. The development of cerebral arteriosclerosis may result in a slowly progressive dementia.

Mild cognitive impairment may be caused by recurrent attacks of hypoglycemia or by cerebral arteriosclerosis. Failure to correct blood glucose levels results in progressive impairment of consciousness and eventual coma. Dementia may develop in patients with associated cerebrovascular disease.

With regard to the psychiatric management, specialist psychological intervention such as the treatment of depressive disorder, blood glucose awareness training to improve the ability to recognize and act on fluctuations in blood glucose concentrations, could be usefully supplemented with certain forms.

Apart from the somatic treatment for diabetes mellitus, based on the psychiatric disorders of the diabetics, antidepressant, antianxiety agent, psychotroptic drugs could be applicable in relieving associated psychological and social problems.

Shi Limin

Chapter 7

Mental and Behavioral Disorders Caused by Psychoactive Substance Use

7.1 Introduction

Throughout early history, natives of almost every country have used indigenous psychoactive substances (e. g. , opium, CNS stimulants, cannabis, tobacco) for widely accepted medical, religious, or recreational purposes. In more recent times, based on the development of chemical engineering technology, a wide range of substances(e. g. , central nervous system depressants and stimulants, hallucinogens, and dissociative anesthetics), synthesized denovo or structurally modified from naturally occurring psychoactive compounds, have also become available for self-administration. Psychoactive substance misuse has become a very serious public health problem, which could destroy the society.

Psychoactive substance or drug is defined(by WHO) as any substance that, when taken into a living organism, may modify one or more of its functions, and could result in a maladaptive pattern of substance use. This definition conceptualizes "psychoactive substance" in a very broad concept, including not only the medications but also the other pharmacologically active substances. Common psychoactive substances include opium, alcohol, CNS stimulants, cannabis, tobacco, central nervous system depressants and stimulants, hallucinogens, and dissociative anesthetics. Hard drug is a sociological concept, which pinpoint that it is not only illegal, but addictive as well. After China reopened in 1978, psychoactive substance misuse is getting more and more serious. The control of drug trafficking and the spread of addiction has been virtually considered in the list of society and government agenda.

7.1.1 Classification of psychoactive substances

Based on different pharmacological properties, psychoactive substances could be classified as 7 classes as follows.

(1)CNS depressants, such as alcohol, barbiturates, and benzodiazepines.

(2)CNS stimulants, such as amphetamines, cocaine, and caffeine.

(3)Cannabis(Marijuana). It is a popular recreational drug with biphasic psychoactive effects depending on dosage, frequency and tolerance to the drug. If a small amount is taken orally via a smoking pipe, bong or vaporizer, primary psychoactive effects include a state of relaxation, and to a lesser degree euphoria, sociability and well-being. Secondary psychoactive effects, such as a facility for philosophical thinking, introspection and metacognition. The tertiary psychoactive effects can include an increase in heart rate and hunger.

(4) Hallucinogen. This type of compound, could change the state of consciousness or perception, such as lysergic acid diethylamide(LSD), mescaline, ketamine, and phencyclidine(PCP).

(5) Opioids. This group contains both naturally occurring compounds derived from the opium poppy (opiates) and a number of synthetic derivatives. The fluid or "milk" of the poppy is dried to make opium, the active components of which include morphine and codeine. Heroin(diamorphine) was first synthesised from morphine in an attempt to find a non-addictive substitute for opium. It is approximately twice as potent as the parent compound. Other synthetic derivatives include the analgesics pethidine, dipipanone, methadone and dextropropoxyphene.

(6) Solvent Abuse. This takes the form of the inhalation of chemical fumes from a wide variety of common domestic substances, including glues, plastic cements, paint thinners, petrol, hair lacquer, lighter refills and typewriter correcting fluid, in order to produce an intoxicating effect. Most substances which are used have either toluene or acetone as the main volatile constituent. Fluorinated hydrocarbons contained in aerosol propellants are particularly dangerous, as they may cause spasm of the larynx, although all substances carry the risk of death through inhalation of vomit or asphyxiation.

(7) Tobaccos.

7.1.2　The nomenclature of psychoactive substances abuse

It is helpful to consider some of the terms which are frequently used in association with the problems of substance abuse and dependence.

(1) A drug is any substance that is taken into a living organism and modifies one or more of its functions.

(2) Drug abuse is persistent or occasional excessive illicit use of a drug which is out of keeping with accepted medical practice. After a while tolerance and dependence may develop. The pathological and driven or "compulsive" use of a substance will lead to impaired social or occupational functioning. Abuse is closely related to substance dependence, which also leads to impaired social or occupational functioning, but in addition, includes signs of physiological tolerance or development of a withdrawal syndrome when intake of the drug is reduced or stopped.

(3) Tolerance refers to the way the body adapts to the repeated presence of a drug, so that the user has to increase the dose to achieve the original effect.

For linked to tolerance is the need for increasing dosage to maintain or recapture the desired drug effect; and in general, the more saturated body cells become with any substance, the longer will be the period required to rid them of all traces of the drug. Tolerance of any marked degree also creates serious problems for the drug user in ensuring an adequate supply.

(4) Dependence describes a compulsion to take the drug following its repeated administration. Dependence is of two types, physical and psychological. Physical dependence is present when a specific group of symptoms occur after the individual stops taking the drug. Psychological dependence is present when a craving for the drug exists in order to experience its psychic effects, and sometimes to avoid the discomfort of its absence. This may result in "drug-seeking behavior", such as pressuring doctors for drugs or embarking on a life-style exclusively aimed at obtaining supplies, and at times resorting to criminal behavior to do so.

(5) Withdrawal syndrome is a cluster of time-limited signs and symptoms that develop after abrupt discontinuation, or rapid decrease in dosage, of a psychoactive substance that has been taken repeatedly, usually over a long period of time or in high doses, or both. The syndrome is a manifestation of altered activity of the central nervous system and is often the opposite of the state of acute intoxication induced by the psychoactive substance. It is an indicator of physiologic dependence on the psychoactive substance. Withdrawal syndromes have been described for alcohol, amphetamines, cocaine, nicotine, opioids, and sedative-hypnotic-anxiolytic drugs.

7.1.3　Etiology of psychoactive substances abuse

There is no single cause of drug abuse and dependence. The etiology of psychoactive substances abuse has been involved an integration of bilolgical, psychological, and social factors.

7.1.3.1　Social and environmental factors

In many cultures, the use of certain drugs for social and recreational purposes is widely accepted (e. g., cannabis in the West Indies and opium in the Far East). Consequently, if there are a large number of users, a proportion will inevitably become dependent. Availability and peer group pressure are important factors in the spread of abuse amongst young people who experiment with drugs in societies where they are not condoned.

Cultural factors, social attitudes, peer group attitudes toward, and shared expectations of the benefits of, laws, and drug cost and availability all influence initial experimentation with substances, including alcohol and tobacco. These factors also influence initial use of more socially disapproved drugs such as cocaine and opioids. Drug dependence can be caused iatrogenically by doctors who irresponsibly prescribe potentially addictive medicines to their patients in excessive quantities.

Social and environmental factors also influence continued use(such as enhanced pleasurable activities with drug use; the availability of competing reinforcers in the form of educational, recreational, and occupational alternatives to substance use), although individual vulnerability and psychopathology are probably more important determinants of the development of dependence.

7.1.3.2　Psychological factors

Many younger drug abusers appear to have some degree of personality vulnerability before taking drugs. They often seem to be without resources to cope with the challenges of daily life, inconsistent in their feelings, and critical of society and authority as shown by a poor school record, truancy, or delinquency. Features such as sensation-seeking and impulsivity are also common. Many of those who abuse drugs report depression and anxiety. Some give a history of mental illness or personality disorder in the family. Some may report severe patterns of family dysfunction with high levels of sexual abuse and parental drug use. Such subjects have an increased prevalence of antisocial personality disorder, which is a risk factor for all forms of substance abuse.

Psychological factors — such as the presence of comorbid psychopathology(e. g., depression, anxiety, attention deficit hyperactivity disorder, psychosis); medical illnesses(e. g., chronic pain, essential tremor); or past or present severe stress(e. g., resulting from crime, battle exposure, sexual trauma, or economic difficulties) — have received considerable attention as potential causes for "self-medication". The possibility exists that susceptibility to psychological stressors and substance use disorders may have similar etiologies. For example, some of the etiologic factors that predispose an individual to depression following major losses(e. g., dysregulation of noradrenergic neurotransmission or the hypothalamic-pituitary-adrenal axis) may also contribute to the development of substance use disorders.

7.1.3.3　Biological factors

The fact that not all individuals who self-administer psychoactive agents, during given developmental stages or life circumstances, progress to repeated problematic use, has led to the search for factors that determine individual vulnerability. Biological factors that may contribute to the development of substance use disorders include interindividual differences in the following aspects.

(1) Susceptibility to acute psychopharmacologic effects of a given drug.

(2) Metabolism of the drug.

(3) Cellular adaptation within the CNS to chronic exposure to the drug.

(4) Predisposing personality characteristics (e. g. , sensation seeking or antisocial traits).

(5) Susceptibility to medical and neuropsychiatric complications of chronic drug self-administration.

The fact that individuals often use more than one drug simultaneously, or give a history of having used different drugs sequentially during their lifetime, has led to an emphasis on the similarities rather than the differences among abused substances with respect to the ontogeny of drug use behaviors. Further, the stepwise development of different substance use disorders over time suggests common mechanisms of susceptibility and generalizable diagnostic criteria and treatment strategies.

Neural mechanisms — investigation of the neural pathways that mediate the powerful (positive) reinforcing effects of drugs of abuse have implicated dopamine, opioid, and gamma-amino butyric acid systems within a midbrain-forebrain-extrapyramidal reward circuit with its focus in the nucleus accumbens. The connections of the ventral midbrain and forebrain, commonly called the medial forebrain bundle, are a major conduit for hypothalamic afferents and efferents and also support (more than any other brain region) the repeated self-admin-istration of current through electrodes (an intracranial self-stimulation model of addiction). This system modulates, or filters, signals from the limbic system that mediate basic biological drives and motivational variables, convert emotion intomotivated action and movement via the extrapyramidal system, and may also be the neuronal substrate for the rewarding effects of drugs of abuse. It has been hypothesized that the mesocorticolimbic dopamine system may be critical in motor arousal associated with anticipation of reward, and that all addictive drugs have a psychostimulant (dopaminergic) action as a common underlying mechanism that contributes to reinforcement.

It has been proposed that these dopamine pathways form part of a physiological reward system which has the property of increasing the frequency of behaviors that activate it. Therefore it is of interest that administration of different kinds of drugs of abuse, including alcohol, nicotine, and opiates, to animals increases dopamine release in the nucleus accumbens. This suggests that activation of midbrain dopamine pathways may be a common property of drugs that have a propensity to be abused. While this hypothesis may explain in part the social use of particular drugs, it does not account for the abuse of drugs in some circumstances. Presumably this is a consequence of interactions between the pharmacological properties of the drug, the biological disposition and personality of the user, and the social environment.

Findings from twin and adoption studies demonstrate the relative contributions of genetic and environmental factors in predisposition to drug abuse.

7.2 Mental and behavioral disorders due to use of opioids

7.2.1 Patterns of use

An opioid is any chemical that resembles morphine or other opiates in its pharmacological effects. Opioids work by binding to opioid receptors, which are found principally in the central and peripheral nervous system and the gastrointestinal tract. The receptors in these organ systems mediate the beneficial effects as well as the psychoactive and the side effects of opioids.

Unrefined opium is often smoked using a water pipe. Intravenous use of heroin (mainlining) and morphine is popular because of the short-lived (less than a minute), sudden "rush" produced. Subcutaneous injection is sometimes used, especially if veins have become unusable because of frequent injections. Refined opioids can also be inhaled, a method often preferred by new users. Although the euphoric state of opioid intake is short, the sedative and analgesic effects can continue for hours. Street drugs are frequently "cut" (mixed or combined) with other substances, such as caffeine, powdered milk, quinine, and strychnine, to dilute the concentration of the active ingredient. These other substances can lead to altered clinical effects and medical difficulties beyond those associated with the opioid.

7.2.2 Effects

Opioids are among the world's oldest known drugs; the therapeutic use of the opium poppy predates recorded history. The analgesic (painkiller) effects of opioids are due to decreased perception of pain, decreased reaction to pain as well as increased pain tolerance. The side effects of opioids include sedation, respiratory depression, constipation, and a strong sense of euphoria. Opioids can cause cough suppression, which can be both an indication for opioid administration or an unintended side effect.

The depressant effects of opioids result in bradycardia, suppression of the cough reflex, respiratory depression and constipation. Peripheral vasodilation leads to itching, increased perspiration and a sensation of great warmth with resultant lowering of body temperature. Pupillary constriction occurs and both appetite and sexual ability are diminished, with amenorrhoea a common finding in females who inject opioids intravenously.

Initial use of heroin can be unpleasant due to stimulation of the vomiting centre in the brain stem. With repeated doses this effect disappears and is replaced by "buzz" or "rush", which is intensely pleasurable and has been likened to orgasm. Opioids induce a sense of peace and tranquillity and a relaxed detachment from the outside world. Tolerance and dependence readily develop, so that when the pleasurable effects become less pronounced, drug taking is motivated towards the prevention of withdrawal symptoms. At higher dosages, sedation occurs and can eventually progress to drowsiness, coma and death. Overdosage may be caused by the concurrent use of other depressant drugs, or by addicts who stop taking heroin for a time and then resume at a dosage to which they are no longer tolerant.

The characteristic pharmacologic action of opioids is analgesia. Centrally, opioids are activating at low dosages and sedating at higher dosages. Other major features of intoxication are feelings of euphoria or dysphoria, feelings of warmth, facial flushing, itchy face, dry mouth, and pupil constriction. Intravenous use can cause lower abdominal sensations described as an orgasm-like "rush". This is followed by a feeling of sedation and dreaming. Severe intoxication may cause respiratory suppression, areflexia, hypotension, tachycardia, apnea, cyanosis, and death.

Chronic use of the drug results in general malaise, apathy and a persistent tremor. Signs of poor nutrition, self-neglect and infection may also be evident. Constipation can become so serious that hospitalisation is sometimes necessary to restore bowel function. Not all heroin users become dependent, however, and some limit their experience of the drug to occasional use only.

7.2.3   Withdrawal symptoms

Once dependence is established, sudden cessation of the drug produces a withdrawal syndrome which begins within a few hours of the last dose. Initially, flu-like symptoms develop, including muscle aches, shaking, chills, rhinorrhoea, lacrimation, sweating and yawning. Abdominal cramps, diarrhoea, pupillary dilatation and tachycardia occur later, together with piloerection(goose flesh). This phenomenon gives rise to the term "cold turkey" used in the USA, because it graphically describes the appearance and feel of the skin of addicts who are undergoing withdrawal. The effects are due to autonomic overactivity and reach a peak 8 - 48 hours after the last dose, before subsiding completely within 7-10 days. Withdrawal symptoms could last for several weeks.

7.2.4   Management of opioid withdrawal

Before the management of opioid withdrawal, a correct diagnosis must be made on the basis of history, examination(pin-point pupils during intoxication or withdrawal symptoms) and laboratory tests. These tests include:

(1)Naloxone challenge test(to precipitate the withdrawal symptoms).

(2)Urinary opioids testing: with radio-immunoassay(RIA), free radical assay technique(FRAT), thin layerchromatography (TLC), gasliquid chromatography (GLC), high pressure liquid chromatography (HPLC) or enzyme-multipliedimmuno-assay technique(EMIT).

Based on the clinical fingings, the treatment can be divided into 3 main types: ① treatment of overdose, ② detoxification, ③ maintenance therapy.

The strong physical dependence which opioids induce, combined with a tendency for users to develop serious physical complications, present special problems of management which warrant separate consideration.

Opioid withdrawal and dependence may be treated in several ways. Often a slow taper of methadone(a long-acting opioid that has addiction potential and that currently requires special licensure for use) is given at approved facilities. The main advantage of substituting oral methadone is that, because it is also an opioid, it minimises the development of withdrawal symptoms and yet does not possess the euphoriant properties of heroin. Consequently, the individual is maintained in a "normal" state. Further benefits are that it is effective orally and each dose lasts for relatively long periods. Depending upon the amount of heroin being taken, 20-40 mg of methadone linctus are substituted daily, followed by a gradual reduction over the next 4 weeks.

In other circumstances, a 5 - 10 days taper of the abused opioid or clonidine is used to reduce withdrawal symptoms. Clonidine has the advantage of not being an opioid and not having addicting properties, but it may not provide as smooth a withdrawal. Baseline blood pressure and regular monitoring of blood pressure is advised. Other agents, such as ibuprofen for muscle cramps, loperamide for loose stools, and promethazine for nausea can be helpful adjunctive medications.

Methadone maintenance programs(for 1-2 years or longer) are used in some locations to help reduce the patient's risk of reentering the drug and crime cultures. Some patients on methadone maintenance use other drugs, such as alcohol and cocaine, and may sell the methadone they receive on the streets to support their drug use. A longer-acting opioid called L-alpha-acetylmethadol(LAMM) has also been used for maintenance treatment. Other pharmacologic means of relapse prevention are being investigated and currently include buprenorphine and naltrexone. In the treatment of chronic pain, non-addicting medications(e. g. , carbamazepine and certain antidepressants) and other modalities (e. g. , physical therapy, nerve blocks) should be used in appropriate patients to minimize the likelihood of relapse to opioid use.

Psychological treatment is often provided in the form of group therapy during admission for detoxification. It attempts to help individuals acquire insight into those aspects of their personality and relationships which lead to them abusing drugs, and to find more appropriate ways of dealing with their problems and difficulties. The therapeutic regimen is often strict, and breaking the initial contract by further abuse of drugs results in eviction from the program. In some areas, Narcotics Anonymous groups have been established which adopt a similar philosophy to Alcoholics Anonymous. Help is also provided for relatives(Families Anon), in order to share their problems with other affected families and to learn more about drug abuse from films and lectures.

Long-term rehabilitation may involve the individual residing temporarily in a community with other former addicts. This provides an opportunity to learn new social and living skills, thereby increasing the likelihood of remaining drug-free in the future.

7.2.5   Prevention of drug abuse

Social and political measures to prevent drug-trafficking and dealing have been implemented worldwide, but appear to have had only limited success in restricting supplies. Consequently, the need to educate children and other young people about the dangers of illicit drugs assumes greater importance. Because experimentation with drugs is often facilitated by peer pressure, assertiveness training, which teaches young people how to say "no" when offered them, may prove to be an effective preventive measure.

7.3   Mental and behavioral disorders due to use of alcohol

Ethyl alcohol is a natural product of the breakdown of carbohydrates in plants. Its euphoriant and intoxicating properties have been known from prehistoric times, and almost all cultures have had experience of its use. Ancient Chinese writings made references to alcohol and distinguished its beneficial effects in moderation from the problem of drunkenness. From the 7th century in China(Tang Dynasty), drunkenness was widespread.

Alcohol is still the most widely abused drug in China and worldwide, but because it forms an integral part of the social activities, business life and religious practice of many cultures, it is generally thought of as being far less harmful than other addictive substances which are obtained and used illicitly. Along with rapid economic development in China, alcoholic beverages are readily available at affordable cost with minimal legal restrictions. Accordingly, there is widespread use of alcohol in diverse recreational and work-related circumstances, and traumatic injuries sustained while under the influence of elevated blood alcohol concentrations are among the most common public health problems today. Youngsters with little drinking experience are particularly vulnerable as they first participate in high-risk activities such as sports, sexuality, and driving. Also, heavy drinkers, who often have blood alcohol concentrations that impair judgment and motor skills or who use other drugs in combination with alcohol, are particularly at risk for alcohol-related violence, traumatic injury, and death.

7.3.1   Biochemistry and metabolomics of alcohol

Ethanol(beverage alcohol) is a simple molecule that is well absorbed through the mucosal lining of the digestive tract in the mouth, the esophagus, and the stomach. The most prominent area of absorption, however, is in the proximal small intestine, which is also the site of absorption of many of the vitamin B. Ethanol rapidly enters the bloodstream and, as a result of its high solubility in water, is distributed to almost every body system. As a consequence of its modest fat solubility, alcohol is likely to have effects on body membranes rich in fat, including neurons. The body subsequently metabolizes and excretes approximately one drink(10-12 grams of ethanol) an hour. The rate of alcohol absorption from the digestive tract is likely to be faster on an empty stomach than after a full meal, especially the one rich in fats and carbohydrates.

After absorption into the bloodstream from the small intestine, between 2% and 10% of the alcohol is then excreted unchanged from the lungs or the kidneys or through sweat; the majority is metabolized in the liver. Liver metabolism occurs mostly through four pathways, with each resulting in the production of acetaldehyde.

Most of the process occurs through the actions of alcohol dehydrogenase(ADH) in the cytosol of hepatic cells. Especially at high blood alcohol levels, some of the alcohol is also broken down in the microsomes of the smooth endoplasmic reticulum[the microsomal ethanol oxidizing system (MEOS)system]. The ADH process is the usual rate-limiting metabolic step, occurring relatively slowly because of the liver's need to handle the produced hydrogen ions through use of a co-factor that is in relatively short supply, nicotinamide adenine dinucleotide(NAD).

The acetaldehyde produced by ADH and MEOS is then destroyed by the enzyme aldehyde dehydrogenase(ALDH) in both the liver cell cytosol and mitochondria. This step occurs rapidly, with the result of lower level of this substance; this is fortunate because at high levels acetaldehyde can produce histamine release, which through a variety of mechanisms contribute to low blood pressure, nausea, and vomiting. The ALDH isoenzyme pattern of an individual is related to the risk for developing alcoholism.

7.3.2   Pharmcology of alcohol

Alcohol intoxication proceeds in stages that depend on dosage and time following administration. Apparent CNS stimulation, which occurs early at low dosages of alcohol, results from depression of inhibitory control mechanisms. The most sensitive parts of the brain are the polysynaptic structures of the reticular activating system and the cortex, depression of which causes euphoria and dulling of performance. Excitation resulting from intoxication is characterized by increased activity, verbal communication, and often aggression.

Euphoric feelings or calming effects are typically the expressed reason for drug self-administration. Higher blood concentrations of alcohol cause mild impairment of motor skills and longer reaction time, followed by sedation, decreased motor coordination, impaired judgment, diminished memory and other cognitive deficits, and eventually diminished psychomotor activity and sleep. At still higher concentrations, alcohol can induce stupor, and ultimately coma and death, by progressive depression of midbrain functions and interference with spinal reflexes, temperature regulation, and the medullary centers controlling cardiorespiratory functions.

7.3.3 Psychological impairment due to alcohol abuse

7.3.3.1 Acute alcohol intoxication

The features of alcohol intoxication are well known and the development of inebriation with its variable effects on consciousness, behavior, perception, mood and conversation should be taken into account.

Recent alcohol ingestion result in clinically significant maladaptive behavior or psychological changes (e. g. , inappropriate sexual or aggressive behavior, mood lability, impaired judgment, impaired social or occupational functioning). One (or more) of the following signs, developing during, or shortly after alcohol use: ①slurred speech, ②incoordination, ③unsteady gait, ④nystagmus, ⑤impairment in attention or memory, ⑥stupor or coma.

Those symptoms are not due to a general medical condition and are not better accounted for by another mental disorder.

Pathological intoxication, resulting in highly irrational or aggressive behavior, has been described in certain individuals soon after they have consumed only small amounts of alcohol(which would not produce intoxication in most people).

This may occur in chronic heavy drinkers who have underlying physical damage to the central nerver system. The person was usually amnestic for the episode, and the aggressive behavior was atypical of the person's usual sober comportment.

Alcoholic blackouts consist of a total loss of memory for specific events during heavy bouts of drinking, even though at the time the subject appeared fully conscious, and was behaving and conversing normally. Amnesia also occurs with very high levels of blood alcohol, when consciousness is grossly impaired. Because alcohol lowers the seizure threshold, fits can occur during drinking in those with an epileptic tendency or the established condition.

7.3.3.2 Alcohol dependence

Once dependence is established, a wide spectrum of symptoms can occur when alcohol is withdrawn. These eventually disappear with continued abstinence or if further drinking occurs. They may be conveniently divided into simple withdrawal phenomena, withdrawal fits and delirium tremens.

(1) Simple withdrawal phenomena

These usually commence a few hours after the last drink and reach the peak within the next 24 hours. Symptoms include tremulousness and agitation, sweating, nausea or vomiting, choking or retching (the"dry heaves"), hyperacusis and tinnitus, itching, muscle cramps and early morning wakening. Feelings of panic or guilt may also occur. This syndrome will be relieved by having a drink on the bed in the morning (called "eye opener").

(2) Withdrawal fits

Withdrawal fits happen in about 10% of those dependent on alcohol, and most likely 24–48 hours after the last drink. They are indistinguishable from epileptic seizures and can be prevented by the prophylactic administration of anticonvulsant drugs. Withdrawal fits may occur at any time during the first to the 14th day.

(3) Delirium tremens

Delirium tremens characteristically begins 2–4 days after cessation of drinking in approximately 5% of those with alcohol dependence. It occurs when an individual who is severely dependent on alcohol stops or reduces drinking. This syndrome has a rapid onset, with impairment and fluctuation in the level of consciousness, resulting in profound confusion and disorientation. The patient also experiences perceptual abnormalities in the form of illusions and hallucinations which are commonly visual. Typically, these consist of rapidly moving small animals, such as rodents or snakes. Delusional beliefs develop, particularly with a persecutory content.

Other features of this syndrome include marked tremor of the limbs, body and tongue, marked insomnia, agitation and restlessness. Autonomic disturbance can occur in the form of sweating, tachycardia, dilated pupils and hypertension. Tremor is frequently prominent and ataxia might be evident if the patient attempts to walk. Gastrointestinal disturbances include nausea, vomiting, diarrhoea and anorexia, which may result in dehydration and electrolyte imbalance. Infection and pyrexia can be present from the onset in up to half of all cases, so that prophylactic antibiotic cover is frequently necessary.

Delirium tremens often begins at night and persists for several days, with symptoms worse during the hours of darkness. The episode usually ends with a period of deep prolonged sleep, and on awakening, all symptoms have disappeared, with the subject remembering little of the preceding events.

This syndrome is a disorder of the reticular activating system of the brain, which is responsible for arousal and wakefulness. Because alcohol suppresses rapid eye movement (REM) or dream sleep, when drinking ceases there is a rebound of REM manifested by the perceptual abnormalities seen in this condition.

7.3.3.3   Psychiatric complication of alcohol misuse

(1) Psychotic disorder—alcoholic hallucinosis

In this condition hallucinations occur in clear consciousness. Sometimes these are a continuation of hallucinations first experienced during withdrawal from alcohol. However, halucinations may also commence de novo in a patient who is still drinking.

Usually these experiences are auditory and begin as fragmentary sounds. The sounds gradually become formed and voices are heard, often making unpleasant remarks. The voices may give commands to do things against the subject's will, and persecutory delusions may develop. The experiences may be very compelling and distressing, occasionally resulting in violence or suicide.

(2) Pathological jealousy (othello syndrome)

Firmly held delusions of infidelity may occur in patients who misuse alcohol. They may be precipitated by the patient's feeling of inadequacy stemming from alcohol—induced impotence and further aggravated by the spouse's growing indifference towards a drunken partner. The patient's accusations become repetitive, and aggressive demands for proof may be reinforced by violence. No amount of contrary evidence will dispel the delusion, and cases sometimes end tragically in assault or murder. Alcohol abuse is not the only cause of this syndrome. Treatment is of the underlying condition. Sometimes the only feasible and safe solution is for the couple to separate permanently.

(3) Depression and anxiety

Symptoms of depression are common among excessive drinkers. This is understandable considering the lifestyle of dependent drinkers, who frequently wake with a hangover facing a day overshadowed by the problems caused by drinking.

(4) Cognitive impairment and brain damage

Some 50% – 60% of alcoholics attending specialist clinics perform worse on cognitive testing than would be predicted from their verbal intelligence educational level and age. They commonly show:

1) Impairment of memory, visual more than verbal.

2) Narrowing and rigidity of thought processes, i. e. , difficulty changing from one way of construing and categorising to another.

3) Difficulty learning new material.

4) Impairment of visuospatial and visuoperceptive skills.

A variety of factors may contribute to cognitive impairment among excessive drinkers: the neurotoxic effect of alcohol; thiamine deficiency; repeated head injury; and the consequences of alcohol withdrawal fits.

7.3.3.4　Neurological complication

(1) Alcoholic dementia

Prolonged alcohol intake can lead to a generalised deterioration of mental functioning(evident on psychological testing), which may later progress to a clinically identifiable dementia. The latter bears the hallmark of all dementing illnesses, in that it is an acquired global deterioration of cerebral function involving intellect, memory and personality, in a setting of clear consciousness. The condition tends to have a gradual onset and there is usually a history of heavy drinking for many years. Cognitive impairment may be reversible in the early stages. Computerised axial tomography(CAT scanning) reveals cerebral atrophy and enlargement of the ventricles in about 60% of those subjects dependent on alcohol. However, cognitive impairment does not always parallel the degree of cerebral atrophy seen on a CAT scan, since it may arise from subcortical damage(as in the case of Korsakoff's psychosis.

(2) Wernicke-Korsakoff syndrome

Wernicke's encephalopathy and Korsakoff's psychosis represent different stages of the same disorder. Wernicke's encephalopathy is the acute reaction to severe vitamin B_1(thiamine) deficiency, which is most commonly(but not exclusively) encountered in those who abuse alcohol and therefore have a poor nutritional intake. Other causes of thiamine deficiency are carcinoma of the stomach, malabsorption syndromes, pregnancy, intractable vomiting and malnutrition. Pathological changes are evident in the walls of the third ventricle, floor of the fourth ventricle, thalamus, mamillary bodies, brain stem and cerebellum. The changes consist of cell loss, petechial haemor-rhages and proliferation of blood vessels.

The principal clinical features of Wernicke's encephalopathy are: ① nystagmus, ② ophthalmoplegia (particularly of the lateral rectus muscle), ③ataxia, ④clouding of consciousness and cognitive impairment, ⑤peripheral neuropathy. The onset is frequently sudden and may be missed because it shares several of the features of acute alcohol intoxication. Hypotension, tachycardia and abnormal liver function are sometimes evident. Over 80% of untreated cases progress to the chronic phase of Korsakoff's psychosis, which is classified as the amnesic syndrome in ICD-10.

The onset of the amnesic syndrome can be sudden or insidious. Unlike dementing conditions in which there is global impairment of cerebral function, it involves a specific defect of memory, with preservation of other aspects of intellect and personality. However, it is quite uncommon in its pure form, the clinical picture often being complicated by features of a coexistent global alcoholic dementia.

Although immediate recall, as tested by digit span, is normal, recent memory(e. g. , tested by asking a subject to repeat a name and address after 5 minutes) is defective. The ability to learn new material is therefore severely impaired, and an anterograde amnesia develops. Time sense is invariably defective, with a rearrangement of the chronological sequence of events or telescoping of repeated happenings into one. There may also be a period of retrograde amnesia which extends for weeks, months and occasionally longer before the onset of the illness, although beyond this, more remote memory can be unimpaired.

Confabulation, which is a falsification of memory, is often present, but is not an essential prerequisite for diagnosis. It is best explained in terms of a mind devoid of a store of recent memories, drawing on more distant recollections, and therefore is not a deliberate attempt by the patient to deceive the examiner. For example, a patient who gives an incorrect account of what he had for breakfast that morning may in fact be describing a meal he had some time ago. Some features of Wernicke's encephalopathy, such as nystagmus or peripheral neuropathy, may persist following the development of the amnesic syndrome. The memory disturbance is so incapacitating that the development of this condition is frequently devastating to both the patient and his family. Personality changes, manifesting as apathy, loss of initiative and self−neglect may also be present.

7.3.4   Treatments

Treatments of alcoholism requires a multistage process. Generally patients must go through detoxification, rehabilitation, and then relapse prevention(aftercare). The early recognition of alcohol abuse is of paramount importance in preventing the development of those drink−related problems, as well as the dependence syndrome. Those at risk frequently conceal their drinking behavior, so that the clinician must be aware of the various signs and symptoms which are indicative of alcohol abuse. Careful history−taking, thorough physical examination, laboratory investigations, and the MAST (Michigan alcoholism screening test) or "CAGE" questionnaires will be very helpful for detection of the problems drinker.

7.3.4.1   Physical treatments—detoxification

Medication to minimise withdrawal symptoms makes stopping drinking easier, and in very heavy drinkers, helps prevent seizures and delirium. Hospital admission is only essential when delirium threatens, and/or there is a history of fits or a current medical or psychiatric illness. A long−acting benzodiazepine such as chlordiazepoxide(starting at 60−80 mg/d and reducing to nil over 5−7 days) is usually adequate for community detoxification. Larger doses may be needed in hospital to control agitation and offset the likelihood of confusional states. The final dose should be determined by regular clinical monitoring, but the maximum dose should not exceed 400 mg chlordiazepoxide in 24 hours. It should not be continued for more than 10 days. If there is a history of fits, greater initial doses of the benzodiazepine should be given. In any circumstance the final dose should be determined by regular monitoring. Chlormethiazole effectively controls the withdrawal syndrome, but is not safe for outpatient use, because alcohol/chlormethiazole interactions cause respiratory depression and deaths have occurred. Major tranquillisers are less effective and may increase the risk of withdrawal fits, but are required if psychotic symptoms develop.

The patient should be advised to take time off work, to rest and to drink fruit juices and other soft drinks, but avoid caffeine−containing tea and coffee. In more severe withdrawal it is sensible to check serum urea and electrolytes and aim to maintain an oral fluid intake. In view of the frequency of cognitive impairment in heavy drinkers and its probable relation to vitamin depletion, vitamin supplements should be given to most patients, particularly those who are poorly nourished, and if there is any evidence.

Some medications are used in detoxification to control simple withdrawal symptoms and prevent delirium tremens or fits. Other drugs may also be administered as a form of aversion therapy to prevent a relapse into drinking after abstinence. The limitation of this treatment is that success depends upon the subject's motivation to take the medication regularly. Unfortunately, a few individuals have been known to "drink through" their Antabuse treatment, with disastrous consequences.

Disulfiram inhibits aldehyde dehydrogenase (involved in alcohol metabolism), and its effects in the drinker are largely if not entirely due to accumulation of acetaldehyde. Taken alone, disulfiram causes little or no effects. With alcohol, it causes intense flushing of the face and neck, tachycardia, hypotension, nausea, and vomiting. It has caused death. In treating alcoholism, physicians must use disulfiram with caution and combined with psychosocial treatment modalities.

Disulfiram inhibits other drug-metabolizing enzymes and increases the elimination half-life of several drugs, including phenytoin, warfarin, thiopental, and caffeine. Calcium carbimide, which is available in Canada and other countries, also inhibits aldehyde dehydrogenase and is said by some to be less toxic than disulfiram.

Naltrexone is the only medication approved by the FDA to directly help prevent alcohol relapse. Naltrexone seems to lower alcohol craving and reduce the reinforcing effects of alcohol. It should be used in conjunction with psychosocial forms of therapy. Naltrexone reduces relapse by approximately half that of control subjects over a 2-month to 3-month period(down to a rate of 20% -25%), patients who are unable to remain totally abstinent may obtain more relative benefit from this medication. The type of psychotherapy used with naltrexone appears to influence treatment outcome. Thus lower rates of relapse have been reported in patients using supportive therapy compared to coping skills therapy. For those patients who are unable to maintain total abstinence, the rate of relapse is reduced when naltrexone is combined with coping skills therapy. About 60% of patients on combined naltrexone and supportive therapy remain abstinent over a 2-month to 3-month period, in comparison with about 20% of patients on supportive therapy alone. These results underscore the significant improvements of prognosis that can be obtained with optimal treatment.

Other medications are currently being investigated for alcohol relapse prevention. For example, acamprosate(calcium bisacetylhomotaurinate), a chemical analog of L-glutamic acid, has binding affinity for $GABA_A$, and $GABA_B$ receptor sites. Initial findings suggest that acamprosate increases the mean duration of abstinence over a 200-day period. Without acamprosate treatment, about 20% of alcoholic patients can maintain extended abstinence; with adequate treatment, 65% of typical alcoholic patients maintain abstinence for at least 1 year.

7.3.4.2 Psychological treatments

It is necessary to identify and treat any psychiatric illness, such as depression orschizophrenia, where alcohol may have been used as a self-remedy to alleviate symptoms.

Various forms of psychotherapy are used in the management of alcohol abuse. Brief counselling sessions, group work and individual supportive and dynamic psychotherapy are all advocated. Empathy, warmth and genuineness are important components of all these treatments.

Alcoholics Anonymous is probably the most well-known form of group therapy and was started in Ohio, the USA in 1935 by a stockbroker(Bill W.), and a surgeon(Dr Bob), who was a reformed drinker himself. The philosophy of Alcoholics Anonymous has now spread worldwide and promotes a policy of total abstinence from alcohol, whilst encouraging members to adopt an approach of "one day at a time" in order to overcome their problems. Simple advice and mutual support are offered at group meetings, and although the effectiveness of this form of treatment has not been scientifically evaluated(because few records are kept), Alcoholics Anonymous is probably helpful to many of its large following. Al-Anon provides support for the families of problematic drinkers.

Behavioural techniques have been employed, with limited success, to modify drinking habits by teaching individuals to take smaller sips and drink more slowly. "Drinkwatchers" is an organisation which helps members to control their drinking before they become seriously dependent.

7.3.4.3 Social treatments

It is relatively easy to detoxify patients in hospital, mainly because they are removed from the stressors which induced them to drink in the first place. However, despite effecting changes in life-style and setting realistic goals there remains a high risk of relapse when these individuals are discharged back into the community. For this reason, the involvement of the family should be encouraged, not only to provide information about drinking which the subject does not reveal, but also to support their relatives through the burden of abstinence and possible periods of relapse. Both professional care givers and the family can enhance self-esteem by conveying a sense of hope and encouraging the individual to believe in his ability to control his own destiny.

7.4   Mental and behavioral disorders due to use of barbiturates and benzodiazepines

Barbiturates used to be commonly prescribed as either sedatives to induce relaxation or as hypnotics to help sleep. They have now been largely superseded by the benzodiazepines. Both of them are currently among the most widely prescribed medications and the most commonly misused or abused type of prescription drug. With continuing use, individuals develop tolerance and need larger doses to achieve symptomatic relief. If the physician does not educate the patient and provide careful prescription monitoring, the patient may eventually receive large doses of these medications with attendant side effects such as mood disorders, cognitive dysfunction, social difficulties, impaired work performance, and traumatic injury due to falls or vehicular accidents. In order to maintain symptomatic relief in the face of tighter controls by the prescribing physician, the patient may combine alcohol or other prescribed medications or illicit drugs(e. g. , marijuana, opioids) with the prescribed dose of CNS depressant, seek other physicians to provide additional prescriptions. The combination of alcohol with other CNS depressants greatly increases the risk associated with its use and is the most common clinical cause of severe drug overdoses. Cessation of drug use leads to undesirable, and potentially harmful, withdrawal symptoms(such as seizures). Thus drug-seeking behavior and repeated drug use is often continued in order to prevent these effects. Fulminant withdrawal occasionally results in patients who discontinue CNS depressant use because of illness or other unforeseen circumstances such as hospitalization for a motor vehicle accident.

Small doses of barbiturates induce relaxation, but larger amounts cause sedation in which reaction time is seriously affected, the speech is slurred and body movements become uncoordinated. There is a cumulative effect with alcohol, and overdosage may lead to coma and eventual death.

Prolonged heavy dosages produce an intoxicated state with persistent drowsiness, poor concentration and judgment, motor incoordination, personality changes and lability of mood tending towards depression. Because barbiturates suppress respiration and the cough reflex, heavy users are more prone to the development of chest infections; hypothermia and bradycardia are additional complications.

Long-term barbiturate abuse leads to tolerance(due to hepatic enzyme induction) and the development of both physical and psychological dependence. Withdrawal symptoms are similar to those which occur with alcohol and include anxiety, restlessness, tremor, muscle twitching, marked insomnia and vivid unpleasant dreams. Vomiting may be severe, and sudden withdrawal after high dosages can cause confusion and seizures. Consequently, any attempt to reduce the dosage must be undertaken slowly in hospital to prevent the development of fits. The prophylactic use of an anticonvulsant drug may also be advisable.

Benzodiazepines, including diazepam(Valium), chlordiazepoxide(Librium) and lorazepam(Ativan), are the most commonly prescribed drugs. Also known as minor tranquillisers, they are used as sedatives in the management of anxiety and as hypnotics to induce sleep. In addition to reducing tension, they generally depress mental activity and alertness. Because they produce little euphoria, so they have not become popular for recreational purposes. They are very safe in overdose, but in combination with alcohol can be lethal.

Physical and psychological dependence can develop with benzodiazepines, especially if they have been prescribed for a long time. Withdrawal symptoms, such as anxiety, insomnia, dizziness, palpitations, loss of appetite and hypersensitivity to noise or touch, are often seen following abrupt cessation of medication taken in normal dosage for longer than 3–4 months. Many of them(such as anxiety and insomnia) resemble the original complaints for which the drug was prescribed, thereby encouraging the assumption that medication is still necessary. Convulsions and confusion may occur after sudden withdrawal from high doses. Most symptoms subside within 5–6 weeks, but psychological dependence can persist for much longer.

Planned withdrawal can usually be supervised by the general practitioner or in outpatients over a period of 2–4 months, gradually reducing the dosage at weekly intervals to minimise discomfort. Inpatient care ought to be considered in those withdrawing from very high dosages, or where there is a past history of convulsions. Supportive measures should be offered, such as help in developing alternative means of coping with stress.

7.5   Mental and behavioral disorders due to use of CNS stimulants

Psychostimulants or psychoactive drugs could increase or enhance central nervous system activity, typically manifested as an increase in the level of alertness and/or motivation. Included are analeptics; opiate antagonists; xanthines (such as caffeine); cocaine; amphetamines, methamphetamine, MDMA (ecstasy), ephedrine, methylphenidate, atomoxetine, modafinil, pipradol, phenmetrazine, or similarly acting sympathicomimetics; and other drugs that have been used primarily as anorexiants.

Symptoms of psychostimulant intoxication include increased heart rate and blood pressure, hyperactive reflexes, pupillary dilatation, sweating, chills, nausea, and behavioral changes, such as belligerence, grandiosity, hypervigilance, agitation, impulsivity, and impaired judgment. Chronic use may lead to personality change, and a full-blown delusional(paranoid) psychosis may occur. Withdrawal reactions may occur following prolonged use, with depressed mood, fatigue, and sleep disturbances.

7.5.1   Pharmacological action of amphetamine-type stimulants

The main clinically relevant pharmacologic effect of amphetamine–related stimulants (AST) is the blockade of reuptake of the catecholamine neurotransmitters norepinephrine and dopamine. The sympathomimetics function as direct and indirect agonists at the adrenergic receptor. They block the reuptake of dopamine and norepinephrine into the presynaptic neuron and increase their release into the extraneuronal space. They can act directly at the postsynaptic receptor. The amphetamines produce a feeling of well-being and alertness, decreased need for sleep, and apetite (probably because of their action on the lateral hypothalamic feeding center) leading to weight loss. Side effects include palpitation, sexualexcitement, dizziness, headache, dysphoria, apprehension, and vasomotor disturbances. As a result, many of the signs and symptoms of cocaine and amphetamine intoxication are similar. CNS stimulation and a subjective "high" are accompanied by an increased sense of energy, psychomotor agitation, and autonomic arousal.

The psychoactive effects of most amphetamine-like substances last longer than those of cocaine. Furthermore, because cocaine has local anesthetic actions, the risk of causing severe medical complications such as cardiac arrhythmia and seizures is higher than amphetamine-like stimulants. Amphetamine-related compounds therefore remain popular in stimulant-abusing population.

7.5.2   Clinical feature of ATS abuse

Case report 1:

A woman swallowed two amphetamines at a party and she quickly became disinhibited and euphoric. Afterward, she slaped an acquaintance because she took a kind comment as offense.

Case report 2:

A young woman was dropped on the doorstep of a local emergency room by two men who immediately leave by car. She was agitated and anxious and she kept brushing her arms and legs "to get rid of the bugs". She clutches at her chest, moaning in pain. Her pupils are dialated, her BP is elevated.

Use of amphetamines in the treatment of narcolepsy and attention deficit hyperactivity disorder (ADHD) is rarely associated with abuse. Tolerance may develop if one drug is used for longer than a year.

Smoking, sniffing and inhaling are the most popular methods of ATS use. Oral administration brings self-confidence, exhilaration, an increase in phantasy thoughts, and rapid speech—all described by the user as a feeling of being "turned on". Intravenous administration produces a sudden, generalized, overwhelmingly pleasurable feeling (a "flash" or "rush"), and it is likely to lead to disorganization of thinking and speech, confusing and frightening perceptions and ideas, and perseverative, stereotyped behavior. Some users go on a "run", injecting the drug every 2 hours for 3 or more days, until they "fall out" and sleep for 12–18 hours. They awake lethargic and start a new "run".

Methamphetamine is rapidly absorbed from the lungs and enters into the brain with effects comparable to intravenous administration.

Chronic abuse commonly induces personality and behavior changes such as impulsivity, aggressivity, irritability, and suspiciousness. In some, this progresses to the development of an amphetamine psychosis with persecutory delusions that may be difficult to distinguish from a functional paranoid or schizophrenic episode. The delusions may be accompanied by auditory or tactile hallucinations, lability of mood, hyperactivity, hostility, and violence.

Physical consequences of cocaine and amphetamines abuse include sleep problems, chronic fatigue, severe headaches, nasal sores and bleeding, chronic cough and sore throat, nausea and vomiting. Cocaine abuse can lead to seizures, cerebrovascular accident, cerebrovasculitis, hyperpyrexia and rhabdomyolysis, and dystonias. Possible mechanisms for neuropsychiatric complications include cerebrovascular vasoconstriction, neurotransmitter depletion, and reduced limbic seizure threshold resulting from repeated subconvulsant stimulation. Cocaine abuse is particularly dangerous because of the devastating cardiovascular effects that can occur in healthy and young individuals. These effects include angina pectoris, myocardial infarction, syncope, aortic dissection, pulmonary edema, and sudden arrhythmic death.

7.5.3   Treatment of ATS abuse

The treatment of stimulant intoxication is usually supportive care. Anxiolytics or neuroleptics may be needed for agitation. Psychostimulants can be highly addicting, and chronic users must address causes of relapse and strategies for relapse prevention.

Although pharmacologic agents such as carbamazepine, phenytoin, and tricyclic antidepressants may help prevent relapse, treatment should address the conditions that lead to relapse, that is, reducing the effects of conditioned cues that trigger craving (such as persons with whom, or situations in which, the individual has used cocaine and the availability of cocaine in one's neighborhood). Only if the patient can maintain abstinence beyond the withdrawal period can extinction and ultimate abstinence follow.

If an overdose occurs, further treatment may be needed. In the case of amphetamines, the patient's urine can be acidified with ammonium chloride to increase excretion of the substance. An x−adrenergic antagonist can be used to decrease elevated blood pressure, and antipsychotics, such as Haloperidol, may be needed to diminish CNS overstimulation.

Cocaine overdoses can be more complicated because of the greater potential for cardiac arrhythmia, respiratory failure, and seizures. Haloperidol may be useful in reducing CNS and cardiovascular problems. Artificial respiration or cardiac life support may be needed.

Preliminary studies indicate that cognitive−behavioral therapy may be more effective than interpersonal psychotherapy in prevention of relapse in cocaine−dependent patients. In addition, some preliminary trials suggest that patients with cocaine dependence may benefit from antidepressants such as desipramine and anticonvulsants such as carbamazepine.

7.6   Mental and behavioral disorders and tobacco

Tobacco is a substance commonly used in many countries and across age groups, from early teens to the elderly. Almost 300 million of the Chinese population are using cigarettes at present time. Comparatively high use is found in males, although use in females is increasing. Cigarette smoking is the most common method of use, although cigar smoking, pipe smoking, and smokeless tobacco(snuff) use each have had varying levels of popularity at different times and among different groups. Primarily because of the government policy and educational programs, use of tobacco products has declined over the past 20 years in China, although use increased recently in some subpopulations, such as women and teenagers. The greatest prevalence rate of smoking is in the psychiatric population, especially among patients with schizophrenia or depression.

Nicotine intake has multiple effects. For example, many users report improvedmood, skeletal muscle relaxation, and diminished anxiety and appetite. In addition, cognitive effects including enhanced attention, problem solving, learning, and memory have been reported.

The primary pharmacologic actions of nicotine appear to occur via nicotine binding to acetylcholine receptors in the brain and autonomic ganglia. Several subtypes of nicotinic cholinergic receptors are found in the CNS. Activation of these receptors appears to cause the reinforcing effects and diminished appetite associated with nicotine. Some of the reinforcing actions of nicotine may be due to effects of nicotine on dopamine pathways projecting from the VTA to the dopamine pathways projecting from the VTA to the limbic system and the cerebral cortex. Stimulation of peripheral nicotine receptors causes many of the autonomic effects associated with nicotine use. Short−term use of tobacco appears to increase cerebral blood flow, whereas long−term use has the opposite effect. Aspects of neuroadaptation to nicotine may also be secondary to release of hormones such as β−endor−phin, adrenocorticotropic hormone(ACTH), cortisol, epinephrine, norepinephrine, and vasopressin.

Withdrawal symptoms often occur with abrupt discontinuation of nicotine intake. Symptoms include craving, anxiety, depression, irritability, headaches, poor concentration, sleep disturbances, enhanced blood pressure, and increased heart rate. In some cases, craving may last for years under appropriate circumstances.

The complications of tobacco use are considerable. Much has been written and debated about the adverse effects of tobacco use. It is generally accepted that users have significantly increased risk of many serious illnesses including pulmonary disease(e. g. , emphysema, lung cancer); cardiovascular disease(e. g. , coronary artery disease); peripheral vascular disease, particularly with chronic use; dental disease(e. g. , oral cancer, especially with smokeless tobacco), nicotine stomatitis, and stained teeth; and diminished birth weight in babies of mothers who smoke.

Efforts to stop smoking are nearly always motivated by the associated health risk. The most effective treatment of nicotine addiction is to prevent its occurrence in the first place. Once dependence has been established, however, multiple treatment approaches tend to be used, including external sanctions, hypnosis, self-help groups, family and couples therapy, and behavioral therapies(such as contingency management and cognitive behavior therapy); pharmacological therapies include nicotine replacement therapy(nicotine gum, nicotine, nasal spray, and transdermal nicotine) and bupropion. Varenicline is the first of a new class of partial nicotinic agonists for smoking cessation.

7.7   Prospects

There are 2 classes of pharmacological intervention in drug addiction. First are medications that interfere with the reinforcing effects of drugs of abuse(by interfering with the binding of the drug, with drug-induced dopamine increase, with postsynaptic responses, or with the drug's delivery to the brain, or by triggering aversive responses). Second are medications that decrease the prioritized motivational value of the drug, enhance the saliency value of natural reinforcers, interfere with conditioned responses, interfere with stress-induced relapse, or interfere with physical withdrawal.

Maintenance medications to prevent relapse are most effective in the context of psychotherapy or counseling. Medications in current use include methadone and buprenorphine(for heroin addiction), disulfiram, topiramate, modafinil, propranolol, and baclofen (for cocaine addiction), naltrexone, acamprosate, disulfiram, and topiramate(for alcohol addiction), and bupropion, nicotine replacement(with patch, nasal spray, or gun), and rimonabant(for nicotine addiction). Rimonabant has been reported to be of use in cocaine or alcohol addiction, and odansetron may be of use in alcohol addiction.

Heredity plays a role in all forms of drug addiction, and genes influence the pharmacological effects of the addicting substance and the subject's responsivity to any particular pharmacological agent. Thus no one drug is likely to be equally effective in all who are addicted to a particular drug.

The substance-related mental and behavioural disorders exact an immense toll on the mental and physical well-being of many individuals in our society. Consequently, they jeopardize the integrity of the family and other social institutions. Because of the prevalence of substance-related disorders, and because they can masquerade as diverse medical and other psychiatric disorders, their recognition and initial treatment are relevant to all physicians, in particular, to psychiatrists. Substance-related disorders are heterogeneous in terms of the interactions between the manifest psychopathology of the individual patient and the psychopharmacologic actions of a given drug, within the relevant sociocultural context. This perspective is useful in seeking an etiologic understanding of these disorders, conducting a clinical assessment, planning for the initial treatment of the direct consequences of drug use, and developing and implementing a comprehensive treatment strategy for patients.

Future directions in substance abuse treatment research are likely to focus on understanding issues of comorbid psychiatric conditions, developing new psychopharmacologic treatment options, and combining the use of pharmacotherapy and psychotherapy in the management of these disorders. Agents that can help reduce drug craving and relapse are of particular interest. Overall, considerably more research is needed on the optimal combination of treatment modalities to prevent relapse in substance-dependent patients and improve prognosis.

Shi Limin

Chapter 8

Schizophrenia and Other Psychotic Disorders

8.1 Introduction

Psychosis is a group of mental disorders characterized by abnormal social behavior and failure to understand reality. The predominant clinical features in schizophrenia are hallucinations and delusions, and some patients have persistent impairment. Among these disorders, the most common diseases are schizophrenia, paranoid mental disorders, and acute transient psychosis. In recent years, there have been great breakthroughs in the treatment of schizophrenia, and many patients have been effectively treated.

8.2 Schizophrenia

Schizophrenia is a common mental disorder with unknown etiology. It often occurs in young adults. Common symptoms include false beliefs, unclear or confused thinking, reduced emotional expression and social engagement. People with schizophrenia often have additional mental health problems. Symptoms typically occur gradually, and last a long time. Without active treatment, the disease tends to be chronically inclined or deteriorate.

With the development of biotechnology and brain science in the field of psychiatry, schizophrenia has become the research focus in molecular genetics, neuropathology, neurobiochemistry and neuroimmunology.

8.2.1 Epidemiology

Schizophrenia can be seen in various social cultures and geographical regions. The prevalence of schizophrenia may vary greatly in different regions. Besides the differences of geographical, racial, cultural and other factors, the inconformity in diagnostic criteria is also an important reason. In general, the prevalence of schizophrenia is approximately the same in men and women. Gender differences are mainly reflected in the age of onset and characteristics of disease. The onset age of 90% of schizophrenic patients ranged from 15 to 55 years old. The peak ages of onset are 10−25 years old for males, and 25−35 for females. Unlike men, middle age is the second peak age of onset in women. In female patients, 3% – 10% has been diagnosed after 40 years old. Several follow-up studies supported that the prognosis are better in female than male. In addition, there is an elevated prevalence of substance-use disorders, especially nicotine dependence, among people with schizophrenia. Moreover, schizophrenia patients suffer from somatic disease (especially diabetes, hypertension and heart disease) and accidental injury probability is higher than the general population. Their average life span is shortened by 8–16 years.

The national epidemiological survey in 1993 shows that the lifetime prevalence of schizophrenia is 6.55%, and it is not much different from the result of epidemiological survey of 5.69% in 1982. Most epidemiological data in China indicate that the prevalence of female is slightly higher than men, and the prevalence rate in urban areas is higher than rural areas. Moreover, the prevalence of schizophrenia is negatively correlated with family economic level in both urban and rural areas.

The World Health Organization, with the World Bank and the Public Health School of Harvard University, estimated the total disease burden with disability adjusted life years (DALY). Among the 135 common diseases or health conditions in the 15 – 44 age group, the total disease burden of schizophrenia ranked eighth. In developed countries, direct expenditure due to schizophrenia accounts for 1.4% – 2.8% of all health resources, accounting for about 1/5 of all mental illness expenditures. It is estimated that nearly 7 million people in China suffer from schizophrenia. Therefore, schizophrenia costs huge medical expenses every year, and causes a great loss of productive labor. At present, schizophrenia is still the leading cause of mental disability.

8.2.2　Etiology and pathogenesis

8.2.2.1　Genetic factors

Family surveys have found that the prevalence rate of schizophrenia in those who have a first-degree relative with the disease is 10 times more than in the general population, and the closer the blood relationship is, the higher the expected incidence is. Twin studies have found that the concordance rate of monozygotic twins is 4–6 times of dizygotic twins. Adopt studies have found that the children who had been born by mothers with schizophrenia and brought up in normal families, still have higher prevalence rate. Genetic factors play an important role in the development of schizophrenia. The evidence suggests that schizophrenia is caused by chromosomes and genetic abnormalities. The improvement of molecular biology technology and its application in psychiatric field made many chromosomal abnormalities reported, such as the long arm of 5, 8, 11 and 21 chromosomes, the short arm of chromosome 19, X chromosome, and later 6, 13 and 22 chromosomes. In recent years, molecular genetics research found that schizophrenia might be related to dopamine system (TH gene and MAO gene, $COMT$ gene, $DAT1$ gene, D_1 receptor gene and D_2 receptor gene), 5 – HT system (5 – HT1A receptor gene, 5 – HT2A receptor gene, 5 – HT2C receptor gene and 5 – HT7 receptor gene), the immune system and related gene. A large number of experimental studies suggest that schizophrenia may be a multi gene disease, caused by the superposition of several genes, and its onset is closely related to environmental conditions.

8.2.2.2　Social psychological factors and physical biological factors

As to the etiology research of schizophrenia, besides genetic factors, the influence of psychological stress and somatic disease is also an important aspect.

As for the influence of social psychological factors on schizophrenia, in addition to the social class and economic conditions, many patients can be traced back to the life events, such as family conflicts, love frustration, environmental change unrest in life and insecurity of occupation Occupational instability, especially childhood bereavement(death of parents or permanent separation) effect is more obvious. The domestic investigation found that there is 40% –80% schizophrenia patients' onset related to environmental factors. So far, there is no evidence that the psychological factor is the cause of the disease, but the mental factors may induce the occurrence of schizophrenia. Studies on physical biology factors have found that the incidence of schizophrenia in the people whose mother had a malnutrition or virus infection during the pregnancy is higher. The authors speculate that this is related to the fetal nerve development.

8.2.2.3 Neurobiochemical research

Brain biochemical studies have found that monoamine and other transmitters in the central nervous system play an important role in maintaining and regulating normal mental activity. The therapeutic effects of psychotropic drugs or antipsychotic drugs are closely related to the functions of certain transmitters or receptors.

(1)Dopamine hyperfunction hypothesis

Because antipsychotic drugs can effectively control the symptoms of schizophrenia, its pharmacological effects are related to blocking the function of the dopamine(DA) receptor. In addition, the psychotropic drugs, phenylalanine, can make normal people exhibit symptoms similar to acute schizophrenia. Its pharmacological action is inhibiting the reuptake of DA at the synapse of the central nervous system and increasing the content of dopamine in the receptor site. Many studies have found that the homovanillic acid(the main metabolite of DA or HVA) of schizophrenia patients increased. Autopsy report have found that DA or HVA in the brain tissue is higher than the control group; the PET study found that it is 3 times of the number of striatal D_2 receptor in patients treated with antipsychotics than normal person. Therefore, it is presumed that the hyperactivity of dopamine in the brain is related to psychosis symptoms and supports the hypothesis of hyperfunction of dopamine.

(2)Glutamate hypothesis

The insufficiency of central glutamic acid may be one of the causes of schizophrenia. Glutamic acid is an important excitatory transmitter in cortical neurons studies. Using radioligand binding method and magnetic resonance spectroscopy showed that compared with the normal population, the binding force of the schizophrenic brain glutamate receptor subtypes in some areas has changed significantly. Glutamate receptor antagonist, such as phencyclidine(PCP), could cause hallucinations and delusions and lead to apathy, withdrawal and other negative symptoms. One of the mechanisms of antipsychotic drugs is enhancing the function of central glutamate.

(3)5–hydroxytryptamine hypothesis

The hypothesis that schizophrenia may be associated with 5–hydroxytryptamine(5–HT) metabolic disorders was proposed as early as the Wolley in 1954. In recent 10 years, the widespread application of atypical(antipsychotics) in clinic has focused on 5–HT in the pathophysiology of schizophrenia. It is found that the 5–HT acute schizophrenia patient with obvious emotional and behavioral abnormality is significantly lower than the control group, and it is back to normal with the disappearance of symptoms. In patients with chronic schizophrenia, 5–HIAA in the CSF is slightly decreased. The 5–HT subtype receptors in the frontal lobe of schizophrenia patient is decreased, suggesting that 5–HT may be related to the disease. In recent years, the atypical antipsychotics, such as clozapine, risperidone, and olanzapine, have achieved effective outcomes in the treatment of refractory schizophrenia. The antipsychotic is a strong 5–HT2A receptor antagonist and is relatively weak in binding to the D_2 receptor.

8.2.2.4 Structural brain changes

In the past 30 years, due to the technology development, a large number of subsequent imaging studies have confirmed that 30%–40% of patients with schizophrenia have enlarged ventricles, widened and dysplasia callosum. These changes present in the early episode of schizophrenia, even before onset. It is may be a reflection of the central nervous system disease in the early years of the patient. Autopsy studies have found that the frontal and temporal lobe (hippocampus, olfactory cortex, parahippocampal gyrus) of the patients had brain tissue atrophy. Studies of positron emission imaging (PET) provide a means to study the brain functional activity in vivo. Patients with schizophrenia in test state, such as Wisconsin Card Sorting Test (should be completed by the activities of frontal lobe), do not appear frontal lobe activity enhancement, suggesting that patients had frontal lobe dysfunction.

The histopathology study found that patients have cell structure disorder in hippocampus, frontal cortex, cingulate cortex and olfactory. These changes are not accompanied by glial proliferation. It is presumed to be responsible for the developmental ectopic or differentiation disorder during developing of the brain. The hypothesis of neurodevelopmental abnormalities is put forward.

The study of premorbid function in schizophrenic patients has found that patients have obvious adaptive dysfunction before the onset (speech, exercise, communication, etc.). From the beginning of childhood, the early stage to the late adolescence the adaptive function showed progressive aggravation. This study supports the hypothesis of neurodevelopmental abnormalities in schizophrenia. The authors speculate that genetic factors, viral infection or perinatal injury during pregnancy may play a role in the cause of neuronal migration disorders.

8.2.3 Signs and symptoms

Case report:

Mr. Li, 42 years old, unmarried. He returned to Beijing to stay in his parents' home because of business failure about 1 years ago. Half a year ago, one night, the patient felt a little uneasy when seeing a light coming into his room from the opposite building. Since then, the patient gradually found that neighbors often talk about his privacy, and then he began to suspect that his room was monitored. About 3 months ago, the patient was able to hear a person talking to him in an empty room. The latter came from the National Security Agency and informed him that he had become the top suspect in the country and that the state was monitoring him comprehensively. Later, a woman explained that the patient was a good comrade. These two people often argue which makes patients very annoyed. Half a month ago, patients began to visit various administrative departments, asking for "clarification of facts" and "elution of charges". He plans to write letters to all the world's newspapers to complain about their persecution.

The symptoms of schizophrenia are complex and varied, and the clinical manifestations of different types and stages. The common characteristics are significant alterations in perception, thoughts, mood, and behavior.

8.2.3.1 Early symptoms

The early symptoms of schizophrenia are varied and are generally social withdrawal may occur for example, related to the type of onset. About 2/3 of patients with slow onset, the patient's mental activity becomes dull. They are estranged from others, or taciturn, sat alone; or to wander, don't abide by the rules. Some patients are characterized by abnormal personality, they often lose their temper without self-control, or sensitive and suspicious. Sometimes they will indulge in unrealistic fantasies, talk or laugh to themselves. Some patients may be manifested as symptoms of neurasthenia, impaired performance at work, or compulsive symptoms.

Under the influence of physical infection, poisoning, childbirth and trauma, the disease is often acute onset. The patients could be characterized by sudden excitement, impulsiveness, fear, tension, or disturbance of consciousness.

8.2.3.2　The acute syndrome

During this period, the basic symptoms of schizophrenia become increasingly clear, and the course of disease can present irregular changes, which are manifested as obstacles in thinking, perception, emotion, willpower, behavior and so on.

(1) Disongnaized thinking

This is the most characteristic symptom of schizophrenia. Disorders of the thinking form: in the early stage, there is vagueness in the patient's talk that makes it difficult to grasp their meaning. Thought disorder is reflected in the loosening of association between expressed ideas, and may be detected in illogical thinking. In its severest form, the structure and coherence of thinking are lost, so that utterances are jumbled. Patients with chronic schizophrenia can have poor thinking.

In addition, some patients feel a lot of thinking in their brains. They can't rest at all, and they can hardly control them(Mandatory thinking). Some patients' thinking can be suddenly suppressed without any external causes. At this time, patients feel "my mind is interrupted", but they don't know the reason clearly. Sometimes their logical reasoning is absurd. Some patients use some common words or actions to express some special meanings, no one can understand their meaning(pathological symbolic thinking). Some patients use ordinary words or phrases in unusual ways. All of these are characteristic symptoms of the schizophrenic patients' thinking associative process.

Thinking content obstacle: delusion is one of the most common symptoms of schizophrenia. At the early stages, patients' attitude to their obvious irrational thoughts, is with half believe and half doubt. But as the disease progresses, it is gradually integrated with the morbid faith and firmly believed.

The most common forms of delusion are reference delusion, persecutory delusion, delusion of physical influence and experience of being understood. In addition, there are also pathological jealousy, erotic delusion, delusion of grandeur, hypochondriacal delusions, and delusions of guilt. Patients often begin with doubts, they believe that the behavior of neighbors or colleagues is related to him, and then they felt that all the people around him were aimed at him. Patients feel that the thoughts are being inserted into or withdrawal from one's mind, or "broadcast" to other people(delusion of delusion). Some patients believe that external forces control, interfere and dominate their thinking and behavior(delasion of control). Some patients even think that some special instruments, such as computer, manipulate or control him(delusion of physical influence). Sometimes they are convinced that their inner experience or thinking content has been known to all(experience of being understood). Among these symptoms, feeling of being controlled, delusion of physical influence, and experience of being understood are most valuable in diagnosis. Primary delusion is also a characteristic symptom of schizophrenia. This kind of delusion occurred suddenly, and couldn't be explained by the patient's situation. For example, a schizophrenic patient came to the hospital and suddenly he felt that the outpatient building is about to explode, so he ran out of the building; another example is that a young man saw a girl in the side of the road and shut the door after she entered the house, then he felt that the girl fell in love with him. The delusions of schizophrenia have the characteristics of strange content, logic absurdity, contradiction and generalization.

(2) Disturbances of affective

The earliest symptoms are mainly related to delicate emotions. For example, the thoughtfulness to the colleagues, friends and family, and the emotional response to the environment become dull. With the illness progress, the patient emotional experience becomes more indifferent. Even for events that make people sad or happy, the patient will be insensitive and lose the emotional connection to the environment. For example, the patients may appear indifference when seeing relatives came to see them far away (apathy). The treatment can't arouse the emotional resonance. In addition, it is also visible that the emotional response of the patient is intrinsically wrong, such as he was happy to describe his misfortunes (parathymia). Some patients present discordant with the emotion and the environment.

(3) Disturbances of volitional behavior

The patients gradually become less activity, lack of initiative, living alone or stayed indoors. Their demands for life, study and work are reduced, and behavior gradually becomes withdrawn and isolated from reality (abulia). Some patients can not take care of themselves, or their life is slack, careless about dressing idleness, sitting or completely bedridden. Some other patients can be manifested as parabulia. For example, they will eat something that can not be eaten, such as soap, grass, or suddenly hurt their body. With the influence of hallucinations and delusions, the patients can be manifested as the pathological hyperbulia.

(4) Disturbances of perception

More than half of patients with schizophrenia have the hallucination, and auditory hallucination is the commonest. The content of auditory hallucination is often bizarre, unrealistic and unpleasant to hear. For example, patients hear comments on their speech and behavior (argumental auditory hallucination). The content may also be a threat or command, such as jumping from the building or attack others (command hallucinations); sometimes the patient talks to the sound he has heard; sometimes the voice is accompanied by the patient's behavior. Sometimes the patient's speech was just the content of what he thought (thought hearing). In addition, visual hallucination, gustatory hallucination, olfactory hallucination, tactile hallucination is also very common, and most of them are related to the delusion of victimization.

Disturbance of perceptive synthesis is also common in schizophrenias. For example, the patient feels that headshape changed, eyes are as small as green beans, and the facial features change positions. The patient looked in the mirror repeatedly. Depersonalization is also common, for example, the patient feels that his head separated from body, soul lost, and body left.

(5) Insight disturbance

Most of the patients have no conscious disturbance, hallucinations, delusions, and thinking associative barriers occur in a clear sense of consciousness, with no disturbance of intelligence. However, the patient's insight is partially or completely lost, and it does not admit that he is suffering from mental illness and can not correctly recognize his mental illness.

(6) Cognitive dysfunction

Cognitive function refers to the ability of perception, thinking and learning. It is the basic function of a healthy central nervous system, which generally includes intelligence, advanced planning ability, ability to avoid trouble, and foresight of events that may happen outside. About 85% of the patients with schizophrenia have cognitive impairment. Therefore, it is considered that cognitive dysfunction is one of the core symptoms of schizophrenia.

Intellectual impairment: intelligence tests indicate that there are many aspects of intellectual impairment in schizophrenics, which occur in the first two years after illness or in the first episode. The average intelligence was lower than the normal population, or lower than the patient's own pre-disease level.

Impairment of learning and memory function: there are two kinds of memory, short-term memory and long-term memory. Working memory is one of the main components of short-term memory and is related to the executive function of the central nervous system. Long-term memory consists of explicit and procedural memory. Patients with mild symptoms have only short-term memory impairment, such as word memory impairment, visual memory impairment, speech learning disorders, impairment of digital memory, and so on. Memory impairment in patients with severe symptoms is involved in every aspect of memory. It is believed that memory impairment is associated with some structure changes of the temporal lobe.

Attention impairment: both active attention and passive attention are damaged in patients with schizophrenia. The patients are unable to focus on all kinds of activities, especially brain activity. Therefore, the patient's acceptance of external information is affected, showing a decline in academic achievement and work efficiency.

In addition, there is also movement coordination damage, such as the jumps and irregularities of the eye movement. The patients also have the impairment of language function, such as improper words, poor thinking, breakup of thinking, and neologism, etc.

8.2.3.3　Advanced symptom

In the late stage, due to poor treatment, patients lose work and learning ability, even life needs to be taken care of. The main clinical manifestations are negative symptoms, such as disengagement from reality, indifference, poverty of thought and abulia. Sometimes patients can immerse themselves in hallucinations and delusions, and they behave strangely and eventually develop into a mental recession.

8.2.4　Subtypes of schizophrenia

8.2.4.1　Classification according to clinical symptom group

Schizophrenia is divided into several subtypes, based upon the predominant clinical features. The type is related to the onset, the course of the disease, the response to the treatment and the prognosis. The subtypes are as follows.

(1) Simple schizophrenia

Simple schizophrenia is characterized by the insidious development of odd behavior, social withdrawal, and declining performance at work. Clear schizophrenic symptoms are absent, and there is always the possibility of an earlier acute episode having gone undetected. The early performance is similar to symptoms of neurasthenia, such as dizziness, insomnia, memory loss, attention lax, and the decline of working and learning efficiency. There is a gradual deterioration of functioning with increased amotivation and reduced socialization, impoverished thinking, and abulia. But the hallucinations and delusions are not evident. The changes may be misunderstood as unhappiness or personality problems. They are often diagnosed after years of severe development. Therefore, the effectiveness of treatment is in question.

(2) Adolescence schizophrenia

Adolescence schizophrenia is more common. This type of schizophrenia often onset in adolescence, and abrupt onset, rapid progression. The main manifestations of the patients are the breakdown of thinking, the absurd content of thinking, the illusions and delusions of the patient's delusions and unfixed, so it is difficult to understand. The patient also could be subject to changing moods, change constantly; they look artificial, grimacing, very childish behavior. These patients are often accompanied by incongruous psychomotor excitement and sthenia of instinct (such as sexual desire, appetite). The therapeutic effect is still available.

(3) Catatonic schizophrenia

The type is mostly in young adults onset, and it has the characteristics of rapid onset and rapid development. The patient may appear to be in an early stupor state, the main performance is not food, motionless, mute. In addition, patients do not react to external stimuli (language, cold and heat, pain). For example, their saliva remained in the mouth without swallowing, allowing it to overflow. Patients may also be shown increased muscle tension, such as waxy flexibility, and air pillow. At times the patients may appear to be in a dream-like state. If the patient from the stupor state transition excited for spiritual movement, they may appear impulsive behavior, such as suddenly wake up, to destroy, wounding, impulse. Stuporous and excited catatonia can appear alternately. This type can be self-relieved, and the therapeutic effect is better than other subtypes.

(4) Paranoid schizophrenia

Paranoid schizophrenia is the commonest form. It has a later age of onset, and the onset of disease is slow. The early manifestation of the patient is sensitive and suspicious, gradually forming delusions and further generalization. Common symptoms for paranoid schizophrenia include delusion of reference, delusion of persecution, delusion of jealousy, delusion of physical influence and grandiose delusion. Sometimes it is accompanied by hallucinations and psychosensory disturbance. The patient's emotional and behavior is often subject to hallucinations, delusions, or even self-injury and hurtful behavior. The patients can preserve social functioning and daily work, and emotional reaction is basically normal, but when it comes to delusions, the symptoms are completely unmasked. This type's mental decline is not obvious. It has a better prognosis than the other subtypes.

(5) Undifferentiated schizophrenia

This type refers to patients who do not fit readily into any of the above subtypes, or where there are equally prominent features of more than one of them.

(6) Residual schizophrenia

This type of patient lacks the symptoms of the acute phase. The patients had at least one episode of schizophrenia onset, and they remain 2 or more than 2 positive symptoms or acute symptoms, such as a strange idea, unusual behavior or obvious crankery.

(7) Post-schizophrenia depression

Some patients subsequently experience significant depressive symptomatology after math of a schizophrenic illness. This depression may be an integral part of the schizophrenia, or the psychological reaction, or caused by nerve blocker. This depression is generally not consistent with the severity of depression, but there is a risk of suicide and should be paid attention to.

(8) Degenerated schizophrenia

This type of patient accorded with the symptom standard of schizophrenia. The course of disease was more than 3 years. In the past 1 year, the main symptoms were negative symptoms, and the social function was severely damaged, eventually developing into mental disability.

8.2.4.2 Classification of positive and negative symptom groups

In the early 1980s, Crow described two syndromes of schizophrenia, based on a combination of clinical and neurobiological factors.

(1) Type I schizophrenia

Type I has an acute onset, mainly positive symptoms(hallucinations, delusion, mental form disorder, behavior disorder), no cognitive impairment, and preserved social functioning during remission. The biological basis is dopamine overactivity and structural brain changes. It has a good response to antipsychotic drugs.

(2) Type II schizophrenia

Type II has an insidious onset, mainly negative symptoms(poverty of thought, apathy, abulia, and attention deficit). The patient have cognitive dysfunction with structural brain changes, especially ventricular enlargement and atrophy frontal lobes. There is no evidence of dopamine overactivity. It has a poor response to antipsychotic drugs and outcome.

8.2.5   Diagnosis and differential diagnosis

8.2.5.1   Diagnosis

(1) Key points of diagnosis

1) Course of disease

The age of most patients is from young to middle age, and the course of disease has a slow development.

2) Clinical symptoms

It mainly includes characteristic disturbance of thought, perceptual disturbance, emotional incoordination, indifference and abulia.

3) Signs

There is no special positive sign of this disease. Most patients have a lack of insight, but no disturbance of consciousness and intelligence.

(2) Criteria(ICD-10)

1) Symptoms

The requirement for a diagnosis of schizophrenia is that a minimum of one very clear symptom belonging to any one of the groups listed as 1-4 below, or symptoms from at least two of the groups referred to as 5-9, should have been clearly present for most of the time during a period of a month or more. According to the above requirements, patients with a course of disease less than one month(whether treated or not) should first be diagnosed as schizophrenia-like psychosis. If symptoms persist for a longer time, they will be reclassified as schizophrenia. ①Thought echo, thought insertion or thought withdrawal, and thought broadcasting. ②Delusions of control, influence, or passivity, clearly referred to body or limb movements or specific thoughts, actions, or sensations; delusional perception. ③Hallucinatory voices giving a running commentary on the patient's behavior, or discussing the patient among themselves, or other types of hallucinatory voices coming from some part of the body. ④Persistent delusions that are culturally inappropriate and completely impossible, such as having some religious or political identity or superpower(such as control weather or communicate with alliens). ⑤Persistent hallucinations accompanied by transient or half-formed delusions without clear affective content, or by persistent overvalued ideas, or when occurring every day for weeks or months. ⑥Breaks or interpolations in the train of thought, resulting in incoherence or irrelevant speech, or neologism. ⑦Catatonic behaviors, such as excitement, posturing, or waxy flexibility, negativism, mutism, and stupor. ⑧Negative symptoms, such as marked apathy, paucity of speech, emotional inactivity or incoordination, often cause social withdrawal and social function decline; it must be clear that these symptoms are not due depression or neuroleptic medication. ⑨A significant and consistentchange inpersonal behavior. characterizedas loss of interest, aimlessness, idleness, a self-absorbed attitude, and social withdrawal.

2) Duration

These characteristic symptoms should have been present for most of the time during a period of month or more.

3) Exclusion criteria

Patient with severe depression or manic symptoms should not be diagnosed as schizophrenia without a clear psychotic symptom before the onset of affective disorder. If the psychotic and emotional symptoms present spontaneously and achieve equilibrium, even if the psychotic symptoms are consistent with the diagnostic criteria of schizophrenia, it should be diagnosed as schizoaffective disorder. Patients should not be diagnosed with schizophrenia if they have a clear brain disease or are in drug poisoning or withdrawal.

8.2.5.2 Differential diagnosis

Schizophrenia should be distinguished from a number of other disorders, which are listed below.

(1) Organic syndromes

Organic psychotic disorders include mental disorders caused by brain and body diseases. There is acute encephalopathy syndrome which is acute onset, that is, disturbance of consciousness. There are also chronic encephalopathy syndrome, such as amnesia syndrome, personality change and dementia syndrome, all of which are slow onset. Mental disorders caused by somatic disease often improve with the improvement of physical diseases. If somatic disease is only an inducing factor of schizophrenia, then the symptoms of schizophrenia are becoming more and more clear after the physical disease is better. In addition, we can also identify the disease according to the history, positive signs and laboratory results.

(2) Mania

Schizophrenia patients with acute onset, and excited, many words (hebephrenic type), should be distinguished from mania. Patients with bipolar disorder often show elation and lively, harmony with the environment. Although the patients with schizophrenia have increased speech and movement, they do not go up with elation, action and behavior are naive, divorced from reality and incompatible with the environment.

(3) Depression

The stupor state of schizophrenia (catatonic schizophrenia) should be differentiated from depression. Patients with serious depression show slow thinking and behavior, sometimes up to stupor degree, it is very similar with schizophrenia catatonic type stupor. But through the efforts of doctors, they can get some simple answer. Or the patients' eyes will be in tears because of depression. Schizophrenics have opposite expressions. They often feel indifferent, stiff and difficult to contact. No matter how hard doctors work, they can not arouse emotional resonance or response.

(4) Posttraumatic stress disorder

Posttraumatic stress disorder is closely related to life events. Acute stress reaction often occurs under the influence of severe mental trauma. The main manifestations of patients are psychomotor excitement or psychomotor inhibition. Some patients are accompanied by narrowing of consciousness. The symptoms usually last for a week. The symptoms of delayed stress disorder are mainly manifested in repeated traumatic experiences and reappearance of traumatic situation. The various mental symptoms will gradually reduce with time or changes in the living environment, but schizophrenia has no above characteristics.

(5) Neurosis

Patients with early schizophrenia or simplex type schizophrenia can be characterized by dizziness, insomnia, fatigue, lack of concentration, and low learning efficiency, which is similar to neurasthenia. However, the patients with neurasthenia have complete insight and asked for treatment voluntarily. Patients with schizophrenia had no insight and refused to treat themselves.

Some schizophrenic patients are mainly manifested as obsessive-compulsive symptoms, so they need to be identified with obsessive-compulsive disorder. The content of obsessive-compulsive symptoms in schizophrenic patients is absurd and strange, and the patient's emotional response to compulsive experience is not obvious. In addition, schizophrenic patients lack of self-knowledge and insight, and demand to get rid of compulsive symptoms. These are different from obsessive-compulsive disorder.

Schizophrenia is needed to differentiate with hysterical psychosis. Hysterical attack is often accompanied by strong emotions, the patient's symptoms associated with the trauma, but also with a vent or outward expression tendency, easy to understand, paroxysmal, interictal normal mental state, so it is easy to identify with schizophrenia.

8.2.6   Course and prognosis

The course of disease can be divided into two types: intermittent attack and continuous process. The former can have an incomplete remission period after the sudden onset of mental symptoms and a period of time. The latter has a chronic course of disease and development. Each recurrence can aggravate the mental damage of the patient, make them hard to return to the normal level, so we should maintain the treatment and prevent repetition. Some of the patients showed a persistent course of disease, residual symptoms, or chronic state.

The prognosis of schizophrenia is related to the clinical type and treatment. Generally, the onset of disease is urgent, there are obvious inducements. There is no obvious defect in character before the disease, no family history, and the patient with discontinuous episode is better in prognosis. In contrast, poor outcome in schizophrenia is associated with a slow onset, no external cause, a family history, and younger age of onset. 75% of the first episodes of schizophrenia can be cured with early treatment. In the absence of regular system treatment, 2/3 patients are mentally handicapped. In addition, 10% –15% of the patients died of suicide(Table 8–1).

The continuous progress of modern therapeutics and the widespread use of antipsychotic drugs have prevented many schizophrenic patients from developing to a chronic recession. Domestic data have been reported. After 12 years of follow-up, 48% of the schizophrenic patients with regular treatment have a good prognosis. About 60% of the patients can achieve social remission, that is, a certain social function.

Table 8–1   Factors associated with the prognosis of schizophrenia

Clinical manifestation	Better prognosis	Poor prognosis
Onset form	Acute	Latent
Course of disease	Paroxysmal	Chronic
Past psychiatric history	No	Yes
Affective symptoms	Yes	No
Obsessive thoughts(or compulsive behavior)	No	Yes
Aggressivity	No	Yes
Predisease function	Good	Poor
Marital status	Married	Unmarried
Sexual psychological function	Good	Poor
Soft neurological signs	No	Yes
Abnormality of brain structure	No	Yes
Social position	High	Low
Family history of psychosis	No	Yes

8.2.7   Treatment

The primary treatment of schizophrenia is antipsychotic medications, especially in the acute stage. In the recovery stage, in addition to the maintenance of drugs, it is necessary to combine with psychological rehabilitation. Psychological treatment can improve the social adapt ability of the patients and help them to return to society.

8.2.7.1　Medication

(1) The principle of medication

The drug treatment of schizophrenia should be systematic and standardized, emphasizing the "full course treatment". Drug treatment includes three stages: acute episode, consolidation period treatment and maintenance.

1) Acute episode

The acute phase of schizophrenia refers to the period of very prominent and serious mental symptoms and in the patients with acute exacerbation of the relapse. The objective of acute phase therapy: ①relieve the main symptoms of schizophrenia as soon as possible, including positive symptoms, negative symptoms, agitation, excitement, depression, anxiety and cognitive impairment, and strive for the best prognosis; ②prevent suicide, prevent the occurrence of impulsive. In general, the addition of drugs to the amount of treatment within 1 - 2 weeks can effectively control mental symptoms. The treatment course was at least 6 - 8 weeks at the acute stage.

2) Consolidation episode

After the effective control of the acute mental symptoms, the patient enters a relatively stable period, which is called the consolidation period. The objective of consolidation period therapy: ①prevent the recurrence or fluctuation of the symptoms; ②strengthen the treatment effect; ③it can also control and prevent post schizophrenia depression and obsessive-compulsive symptoms, and can prevent suicide; ④the consolidation period treatment can also promote the recovery of social functions; ⑤consolidation period treatment can also control and prevent common adverse drug reactions caused by long-term medication, such as tardive dyskinesia, amenorrhea, breath overflow, weight gain, abnormal glucose and lipid metabolism, heart, liver and kidney dysfunction. Continue medication uses the same, and the course of treatment generally lasts for 4-6 months.

3) Maintenance episode

The third stage after symptomatic relief and consolidation treatment is the maintenance period. The purpose is to prevent and delay the recurrence of mental symptoms and to improve the functional status of the patients. The dose of the drug can be reduced on the basis of stable curative effect. Reducing the dose of drugs can reduce the adverse reactions of the patients, improve the compliance of medication, which is beneficial to long-term maintenance treatment. The dosage of maintenance therapy should based on patient preference, and drug withdrawal should be gradual, and reduced to 1/3 - 1/2 of the original consolidation dose. It is also possible to reduce the original dose by 20% to the minimum effective dose every 6 months. The maintenance period of treatment can be determined according to the condition of patients, duration of maintenance treatment of first relapse for 2-3 years, second relapse patients took 3-5 years, more than 3 times with recurrent maintenance treatment time should be longer, even lifelong medication. For patients with a history of suicide attempts, violence and aggressive behavior, the maintenance period should be properly extended. The adverse reaction of the patient should be closely moniford.

The dosage of the outpatient should usually be lower than that of inpatients, and the drug should not be stopped suddenly.

(2) Antipsychotic drugs

Antipsychotic drugs, also known as nerve blockers, can effectively control the acute and chronic symptoms of schizophrenia. Antipsychotic drugs can be divided into two types: typical antipsychotics and atypical antipsychotics.

1) Typical antipsychotics

Typical antipsychotics mainly block the D_2 receptor, also known as the dopamine receptor antagonist. The most common atypical antipsychotics include chloropromazine as a representative of phenothiazine, haloperidol as the representative of butylbenzene and chlorprothixene as the representative of sulfur anthracene drugs. The former is represented by chlorpromazine, which main characteristics include strong sedation, anti excitant and anti hallucination, and mild extrapyramidal side effects. The latter is represented by haloperidol and trifluoperazine. These drugs are more effective in anti-hallucination and delusion, but the extrapyramidal side effects are more serious. They have no sedation, no excitatory effects, and less side-effects on visceral function. The commonly used drugs are as follows.

Chlorpromazine: its main functions include obvious sedation, controlling of excitement, anti-hallucination, and delusions. It is suitable for patients with psychomotor excitement and all kinds of acute schizophrenia patients with obvious hallucinations and delusions. The therapeutical dosage is 300-400 mg/d.

Trilafon: the indication of trilafon is almost the same as chlorpromazine, but the former has less sedative effect, and its side-effects on cardiovascular system, liver and hematopoietic system are less than chlorpromazine. It is applicable to elderly patients and patients with poor physical conditions. The therapeutical dose is 40-60 mg/d.

Haloperidol: this medicine can quickly control psychomotor excitement, hallucinations, delusions, and it also has a certain effect on chronic symptoms. The therapeutical dose is 12-30 mg/d.

Sulpiride: in addition to controlling hallucinations, delusions, and logic obstacles in thinking, sulpiride also has a therapeutic effect on improving patients' emotion and affection. The therapeutical dose is 600-800 mg/d.

Long-acting preparation: they are suitable for patients with obvious mental symptoms and refusing to take medicine, as well as for patients need consolidating the efficacy, preventing recurrence, and maintaining treatment. It includes penfluridol, which therapeutical dose and maintenance dose are 40-60 mg per week and 10-30 mg per week, respectively. In addition, fluphenazindecanoate injection is given. The therapeutical dose is 12. 5-50. 0 mg per time, 1 times per 2-3 weeks; the maintenance dose is 12. 5-25. 0 mg per time, 4-6 times per week, 1 times per 4-6 weeks.

2) Atypical antipsychotics (new antipsychotics)

This type of antipsychotic drugs was launched in 1990s. Their mechanism of action is the 5-serotonin and dopamine antagonist, which not only acts on the D_2 receptor, but also on the 5-serotonin receptor. Atypical antipsychotics can treat both positive and negative symptoms. The extra-pyramidal reaction is significantly lower than the typical antipsychotics. At present, the common atypical antipsychotics in China include clozapine, risperidone, olanzapine, quetiapine, and ziprasidone. The main side-effect is metabolic syndrome.

Clozapine: clozapine has antagonistic effect on a variety of neurotransmitters. It has obvious antipsychotic effect, and the extra-pyramidal side effect is very light, and it is better than the typical antipsychotic drug for refractory schizophrenia. The main disadvantage of this medicine is the side effect of granulocytic reduction or even lack, the occurrence rate is about 1% , so it is not used as a first-line drug. The use of clozapine requires regular monitoring of hemogram. Once the granulocytic decline occurs, the drug should be stopped immediately. The therapeutical dose of clozapine is 300-400 mg/d.

Risperidone: risperidone is a 5 - HT2/D_2 receptor balance antagonist, which can improve negative symptoms in addition to positive symptoms such as hallucinations and delusions. The extra-pyramidal side-effects of risperidone were mild, and its therapeutical dose is 3-7 mg/d.

Paliperidone: paliperidone is the active metabolite of risperidone, the mechanism of which is to block the D_2 receptor. It can relieve the positive symptoms of psychosis and stabilize the emotional symptoms. The therapeutical dose of paliperidone is 3–6 mg/d.

Olanzapine: olanzapine mainly acts on D_1, D_2, D_3, D_4 receptor and 5–HT2A receptor. It is effective for both positive and negative symptoms, and there are less adverse reactions in the extrapyramidal system. The therapeutical dose of olanzapine is 5–20 mg/d.

Quetiapine: quetiapine mainly acts on the D_1 receptor, the D_2 receptor, the 5–HT2 receptor and the H_1 receptor. It is effective for both positive and negative symptoms of schizophrenia, with mild sedation and less extrapyramidal reaction. The therapeutical dose of quetiapine is 150–750 mg/d.

Ziprasidone: ziprasidone has strong affinity for D_2 receptor and 5–HT2 receptor, inhibits norepinephrine and 5 – serotonin reuptake, and is suitable for schizophrenia with depression, anxiety and chronic withdrawal. The advantage of ziprasidone is not increasing weight. The therapeutical dose is 80 – 160 mg/d.

Aripiprazole: aripiprazole is a postsynaptic D_2 receptor blocker and a presynaptic receptor agonist, as well as a 5–HT2A receptor antagonist and a partial agonist of 5–HT1A receptor. It has a good effect on the negative symptoms, positive symptoms and cognitive functions of schizophrenia. Its therapeutical dose is 10–30 mg/d.

(3)Combination therapy

In principle, an antipsychotic drug should be used as much as possible in the treatment of schizophrenia. If the effect is not good, the low and high ettisancy nerve blockers can be combined, but one should be the main one. When a schizophrenic has depressive symptoms, an antidepressant can be combined. In the use of antipsychotic drug treatment, if patients have extrapyramidal reactions, they should be combined with the drugs which has the function of anti-extrapyramidal reactions, such as trihexyphenidyl(artane). However, we generally suggest that associated drugs be used only after the side-effects appear.

In addition to antipsychotic drugs in the treatment of schizophrenia, electroconvulsive therapy is an effective treatment, it is mainly applied to acute schizophrenia, catatonic stupor and the patient who is not sensitive to the drug treatment.

8.2.7.2 Modified electroconvulsive therapy

In the treatment of schizophrenia, the indications for modified electroconvulsive therapy(MECT) are excitomania, impulsive symptoms or stupor state. A course of MECT is usually 10–12 times. The frequency of the initial treatment is once a day and twice a week later. Generally, MECT is not the preferred method for the treatment of schizophrenia.

8.2.7.3 Psychotherapy

In the maintenance episode, psychological therapy can improve patients' understanding of ill experience, promote their cognition, attenuation of symptom severity and associated comorbidity, and enhance interpersonal and social functioning. The schizophrenic patients are prone to depression and disappointment after recovery, so psychotherapy is very important in this stage.

8.2.7.4 Psychological and social rehabilitation

The combination of psychosocial intervention and psychotropic drug therapy can improve the course of disease, prevent relapse, improve coping skills, achieve better social and occupational functions. It is not enough for schizophrenic patients to control or eliminate mental symptoms. We should pay attention to the social life of patients, such as entertainment and work therapy. If we want the patient to achieve comprehensive social rehabilitation, we need to restore the energy and physical strength caused by the disease and achieve good health status, restore work or learning ability and rebuild stable interpersonal relationship.

8.2.7.5   Reintegration

For the healed patients, they should be encouraged to participate in social activities. To strengthen the training of the daily life and social ability of the patients with chronic schizophrenia to improve the patient's coping skills. Improve the patient's family environment and interpersonal relationship. Family members should receive psychological education so that they can understand the basic knowledge of schizophrenia, which can increase family members' understanding and support for patients. The above measures have a positive effect on reducing stress in the social life of schizophrenia, reducing recurrence, and promoting psychological and social rehabilitation of the patients.

8.2.8   Prevention

Early detection and early treatment of schizophrenia are very important for the prevention of recurrence. Therefore, we should set up mental prevention institutions in the community, popularize the knowledge of mental disease prevention, eliminate discrimination against psychotic patients, detect and treat the disease early. Through the guidance training and family support of community rehabilitation institutions, the social adaptability of patients can be improved, reduce psychological stress, persist in taking medicine, avoid relapse and reduce disability.

8.3   Paranoid mental disorders

The age of onset of paranoid mental disorders are often after the age of 30. The etiology of this disease is not clear. It is a mental disorder characterized by systematic delusion. It can also exist illusions related to delusional content, but it does not play a prominent role in clinical practice. There is no obvious mental abnormality in the absence of delusion.

Paranoia is rarely seen in clinic and was first named by Kahlbaum in 1863. The protruding characteristics of paranoia are slow progress, persistent, unshakable and highly systematic delusion. The following are the main features of the so-called systematic delusion: delusion can permeate the entire structure and characteristics of the patient's personality; delusions are gradually developed, compact, coordinated and clear, and thus become self-contained; in addition to delusions, the patient's thinking is rational and logical. Their emotions and behavior are consistent with delusions and generally have no hallucinations.

8.3.1   Etiology and pathogenesis

The etiology and pathogenesis of paranoid mental disorder are still unknown. The hereditary factor of the paranoid mental disorder is not obvious, most scholars believe that paranoia is developed by mental stimulation on the basis of personality defects. This kind of patient's character is subjective, stubborn, sensitive, suspicious, strong self-esteem, they are often easily excited and irritable, which constitute the so-called paranoid personality disorders. Because of arrogance and sensitivity, they were mis-interpreted by setbacks and gradually formed delusions. The patient is prone to dissension and conflict with others, which in turn strengthens their delusions.

8.3.2   Clinical features

Case report:

Mr. Xie, male, 46 years old, married, self-employed.

About 5 years ago, the patient began to suspect his wife of having an affair, so he often followed his wife out or checked her cellphone records. When he went out, the patient did not allow his wife to leave home, nor did he allow his wife to go out alone. Each time the patient returned home, he looked around for evidence and asked his son individually about his wife's whereabouts while he was away. If some suspicious phenomena are found, patients will question and even abuse his wife. 2 days ago, because of jealousy and suspicion, the patient beats his wife again. The wife's family takes the patient to the hospital and asks for hospitalization. When talking with doctors, patients communicate smoothly and behave normally when they do not involve wife's derailment. Patients are basically competent at work. However, patients believe that his wife is cheating and do not think he has any mental problems and refuse to be treated.

The incidence of this disease in middle-aged people over 30 years old, more men than women, the higher incidence in mental workers. The disease often begins with the delusion of victimization, and the delusion of delusion occurs later, at last they will intertwine with each other. Patients think someone against himself, thus cause everywhere appeal, or write a letter of complaint, do not give up. Sometimes the patients may think that because of their extraordinary talent, it will make others jealous and persecute them.

The course of this disease is long and may even exist for a lifetime. In the long course of illness, although the mental symptoms can fluctuate because of the influence of environment, the delusions are difficult to disappear once the delusions are formed. However, even if the course of the disease is very long, it does not cause mental failure. The delusion may be mitigated by the weakening of energy after the age of the elderly.

8.3.3   Diagnosis and differential diagnosis

Paranoid mental disorder takes the systemic delusion as the main symptoms, the content of delusion is relatively fixed and related to reality, the main manifestations are victims, jealousy, exaggerated, hypochondriasis or affection. In addition, it can be accompanied by hallucinations. The social function remained good, and there is little mental deterioration. If the course of the disease lasts more than 3 months and other related diseases are excluded, it can be diagnosed as paranoid mental disorder.

Paranoid patients usually remain a perfect emotional state and have no typical symptoms of schizophrenia. Their behaviors, attitude and speech are normal without delusion. They also rarely have a mental deterioration.

8.3.4   Treatments

Antipsychotics can play a role in stabilizing mood and relieving delusions. The main obstacle to the drug treatment of this disease is that the patient is not compliant. This kind of patient can use long effect needle when necessary. Psychotherapy has a poor effect on delusions.

8.4   Acute delusional disorder

Acute delusional disorder is also called transient delusional episode, it is a kind of paroxysmal mental disorders. The onset of the disease is usually not induced. It is often acute onset. There is obvious delusion and other psychopathological symptoms is acute onset or 1 week. The prognosis of this disease is good, and each seizure is completely recovered within 3 months. Acute delusional disorder does not occur in children, and is rarely seen after 50 years old.

8.4.1   Etiology and pathogenesis

The etiology and pathogenesis of acute delusional disorder are still unknown. Some scholars believe that the delusion of this sudden onset is unique to the quality of vulnerability; some people think that this disease is a sudden delusional phenomenon of delusional thinking. Many scholars have pointed out that the emergence of such delusions is "no need for any condition or motivation", that is, the automaticity of delusions. This kind of delusion is not primary, but secondary to the disturbance of consciousness. Electroencephalogram data suggest that during the onset of the disease, the combination of sleep state and wakeup state has been disturbed. The disturbance of morphology and time in these waves suggests that the sensory function of patients is disturbed. This is just like some scholars pointed out according to clinical manifestations, patients are in between "sleep and wake up", which is consistent with the so-called "delusional original state" and "primary delusion experience".

8.4.2   Clinical features

Case report:

Mr. Huang, male, 28 years old, married, casual worker.

Recently, the patient suffered from colds, due to overwork. After symptomatic treatment and rest, his condition improved. One night, the patient suddenly cried out, claiming that the doctor in the outpatient department gave him the wrong medicine. He thought he had taken the poison, and that someone was harming himself. When other workers came to comfort him, the patient thought they were going to send him to the clinic for an injection, with no good intentions. So he hurt his colleagues with tools. The patient was immediately sent to a psychiatric hospital for emergency treatment, and he fell asleep after injection. The patient's mental state returned to normal after two days. Afterwards, patients could basically recall the scene of onset. He felt sorry for what he had done, and hoped his colleagues could forgive him.

The patient was previously healthy. He denied that he had a history of mental illness and no drinking history.

Patients of this disease often have a sudden onset, and their delusions are suddenly erupted. The content of delusions is varied and changeable, often characterized by delusions, exaggeration and physical influence, and the delusions of some patients are full of fantasy. These delusions may be accompanied by vivid hallucinations, especially in the phonism, the patients could have a strong emotional experience and can be behaved for excitement or anxiety, depression, emotional fluctuations. From the appearance of the patients, their consciousness seems clear. Patients often have good orientation and ability to adapt to the life. Although patients speak clearly and fluently, in fact, their state of consciousness is often characterized by slight obstacles, such as attentional laxation, absence and coldness, reflecting or listening, and indulging in vivid delusion. Once the symptoms are relieved, the patient feels as if it is free from a nightmare or unthinkable confusion. Individual cases may turn to paranoia or schizophrenia after repeated episodes.

8.4.3   Diagnosis

(1) The patient suddenly produces a variety of loosely structured and indeterminate delusions, such as

victimization, exaggeration, jealousy, or religious delusion. It can be accompanied by trance, illusion, transient hallucination, disintegration of personality, increased or reduced exercise.

(2) The course of this disease is short, but some cases can be up to 3 months.

(3) The following diseases are excluded: reactive psychosis, mental disorders caused by psychoactive substances and non-addictive substances, or schizophrenia like disorders with persistent hallucinations and characteristic disturbance of thought.

8.4.4　Treatments

The outcome of antipsychotic drugs is generally good. Patients recover in a few days or weeks, and individual cases will recover in a few months. No residual symptoms are left after treatment.

Psychological therapy is based on reasoning education and should be repeated and continued. Some patients can help to improve their condition by adjusting work or living environment.

8.5　Acute transient psychosis

Acute transient psychosis includes a group of mental disorders with the following common characteristics. ①Abrupt onset. ②The disease mainly manifested as symptoms of mental illness, including fragments of hallucination, disorder ofspeech or catatonia. ③Most patients can be completely or mostly remission.

Some patients can show schizophrenia-like symptoms, and if the duration is less than one month, it can be diagnosed as schizophreniform psychosis. Some patients get sick on the journey, they often have comprehensive factors such as overexertion, mental stress and lack of sleep before onset. The main symptoms are sudden disturbance of consciousness, fragmented delusion, hallucination, disorder of language, etc. , which can be relieved after a full rest.

Li Youhui, Lian Nan

Chapter 9

Mood Disorders

9.1 Introduction

The term "mood" denotes an emotional state that may affect all aspects of the individual's life. The syndromes are characterized by pathologically depressed mood and should be regarded as existing on a continuum with normal mood. A diagnosis is appropriate when the mood disturbance is "primary" and central to the illness and not secondary to some other physical or psychological state. The ICD-10 includes the following categories of mood disorders: ①major depressive episode; ②bipolar disorder; ③mania episode; ④recurrent depressive disorder; ⑤persistent mood disorder; ⑥other mood disorders (dysthymic disorder; cyclothymic disorder); ⑦unspecified mood disorder.

9.2 Overview

9.2.1 Major depression and bipolar disorder

Mood can be defined as a pervasive and sustained emotion or feeling tone that influences a person's behavior and colors his or her perception of being in the world. Disorders of mood — sometimes called affective disorders — make up an important category of psychiatric illness consisting of depressive disorder, bipolar disorder, and other disorders.

A variety of adjectives are used to describe mood: depressed, sad, empty, melancholic, distressed, irritable, disconsolate, elated, euphoric, manic, gleeful, all descriptive in nature. Some can be observed by the clinician, and others are subjective (e. g. , hopelessness). Mood can be labile, fluctuating, or alternate rapidly. Other signs and symptoms of mood disorders include changes in activity level, cognitive abilities, speech, and vegetative functions.

These disorders virtually always result in impaired interpersonal, social, and occupational functioning. It is tempting to consider mood disorders on a continuum with normal variations in mood. Patients with mood disorders, however, often report an ineffable, but distinct, quality to their pathological state. The concept of a continuum, therefore, may represent the clinician's over-dentification with the pathology, thus possibly distorting his or her approach to patients with mood disorder.

Patients with only major depressive episodes have major depressive disorder or unipolar depression. Patients with both manic and depressive episodes or only manic episodes are known to have bipolar disorder. The terms "unipolar mania" and "pure mania" are used for patients who are bipolar but do not have depressive episodes. Three additional categories of mood disorders are hypomania, cyclothymia, and dysthymia. Hypomania is an episode of manic symptoms that does not meet the criteria for manic episode. Cyclothymia and dysthymia as disorders represent less severe forms of bipolar disorder and major depression, respectively.

In the past 20 years, major depression and bipolar disorder have been considered to be two separate disorders. Bipolar disorder is actually a more severe expression of major depression has been reconsidered recently, however. Many patients given a diagnosis of a major depressive disorder reveal, on careful examination, past episodes of manic or hypomanic behavior that have gone undetected.

9.2.1.1 Depression

A major depressive disorder occurs without a history of a manic, mixed, or hypomanic episode. A major depressive episode must last at least 2 weeks, and typically a person with a diagnosis of a major depressive episode also experiences at least four symptoms from a list that includes changes in appetite and weight, changes in sleep and activity, reduced energy, feelings of guilt, problems thinking and making decisions, and recurring thoughts of death or suicide.

9.2.1.2 Mania

A manic episode is a distinct period of an abnormally and persistently elevated, expansive, or irritable mood lasting for at least 1 week or less if a patient must be hospitalized. A hypomanic episode lasts at least 4 days. It is similar to a manic episode except that it is not sufficiently severe to cause impairment in social or occupational functioning, and no psychotic features are present. Both mania and hypomania are associated with self-important ideas, a decreased need for sleep, distractibility, over physical and mental activity, and over-involvement in pleasurable behavior.

9.2.1.3 Dysthymia and cyclothymia

Dysthymic disorder and cyclothymic disorder are characterized by the presence of symptoms that are less severe than those of major depressive disorder and bipolar I disorder, respectively. Dysthymic disorder is characterized by at least 2 years of depressed mood that is not sufficiently severe to fit the diagnosis of major depressive episode. Cyclothymic disorder is characterized by at least 2 years of frequently occurring hypomanic symptoms that can not fit the diagnosis of manic episode and of depressive symptoms that can not fit the diagnosis of major depressive episode.

9.2.2 Epidemiology

The prevalence of mood disorders are common. Most recent surveys, show that major depressive disorder has the highest lifetime prevalence(almost 17%) of psychiatric disorders. Which is 5%-17%. The annual incidence of bipolar disorder is less than 1%, but it is difficult to estimate because milder forms of bipolar disorder are difficult to identify.

9.2.2.1 Sex

An almost universal observation, independent of country or culture, is the two fold greater prevalence of major depressive disorder in women than in men. The reasons for the difference are hypothesized to involve hormonal differences, the effects of childbirth, differing psychosocial stressors for women and for men, and behavioral models of learned helplessness. Manic episodes are more common in men, and depressive episodes are more common in women. When manic episodes occur in women, they are more likely than men to present a mixed picture (e. g., mania and depression). Women also have a higher rate of being rapid cyclers, defined as having four or more manic episodes in a one-year period.

9.2.2.2　Age

The onset of bipolar disorder is earlier than major depressive disorder. The age of onset for bipolar disorder ranges from childhood (as early as 5 or 6 years old) to 50 years or even older in rare cases, with a mean age of 30. The mean age of onset for major depressive disorder is about 40 years, with 50% patients having an onset between 20 and 50 years of age. Major depressive disorder can begin in either childhood or in old age. Recent epidemiological data suggest that the incidence of major depressive disorder may be increasing among people younger than 20 years. This may be related to alcohol and drugs of abuse in this age group.

9.2.2.3　Marital status

Major depressive disorder occurs most often in persons without close interpersonal relationships and in those who are divorced or separated. Bipolar disorder is more common in divorced and single persons than married persons, but this difference may reflect the early onset and the resulting marital discord characteristic of the disorder.

9.2.2.4　Socioeconomic and cultural factors

No correlation has been found between socioeconomic status and major depressive disorder. A higher than average incidence of bipolar disorder is found among the upper socioeconomic groups. Bipolar disorder is more common in persons who did not graduate from college than in college graduates, however, which may also reflect the relatively early age of onset for the disorder. Depression is more common in rural areas than in urban areas. The prevalence of mood disorder does not differ among races.

9.2.3　Comorbidity

Individuals with major mood disorders are at an increased risk of comorbid disorders. The most common disorders are alcohol abuse or dependence, panic disorder, obsessive-compulsive disorder (OCD), and social anxiety. Conversely, individuals with substance use disorders and anxiety also have an elevated risk of lifetime or current comorbid mood disorder. In both unipolar and bipolar disorder, whereas men more frequently present substance use disorders, women more frequently present comorbid anxiety and eating disorders. In general, patients with bipolar show more comorbidity of substance use and anxiety disorders than patients with unipolar major depression. In the Epidemiological Catchment Area (ECA) study, the lifetime history of substance use disorders, panic disorder, and OCD was approximately twice as high as patients with bipolar disorder (61%, 21% and 21%, respectively) than patients with unipolar major depression (27%, 10% and 12%, respectively). Comorbid substance use disorders and anxiety disorders worsen the prognosis of the illness and markedly increase the risk of suicide among patients with unipolar major depressive and bipolar.

9.3 Etiology

9.3.1 Biological factors

Many studies have reported biological abnormalities in patients with mood disorders. Until recently, the monoamine neurotransmitters — norepinephrine(NE), dopamine, serotonin, and histamine—were the main focus of theories and research about the etiology of these disorders. A progressive shift has occurred from focusing on disturbances of single neurotransmitter systems in favor of studying neurobehavioral systems, neural circuits, and more intricate neuroregulatory mechanisms. The monoaminergic systems, thus, are now viewed as broader, neuromodulatory systems, and disturbances are as likely to be secondary or epiphenomenal effects as they are directly or causally related to etiology and pathogenesis.

9.3.1.1 Biogenic amines

Of the biogenic amines, NE and serotonin are thetwo neurotransmitters most implicated in the pathophysiology of mood disorders.

(1)Norepinephrine

Evidences have shown that decreased regulation of β-adrenergic receptors are associated with depression evidence. Activation of β_2 receptors results in a decrease of the amount of NE released also implied its involvement in depression. Presynaptic β_2-receptors are also located on serotonergic neurons and regulate the amount of serotonin released. The clinical effectiveness of antidepressant drugs with noradrenergic effects—for example, venlafaxine(Effexor)—further supports a role for NE in the pathophysiology of at least some of the symptoms of depression.

(2)Serotonin

With the effect of the selective serotonin reuptake inhibitors (SSRIs)— for example, fluoxetine (Prozac)—serotonin has become the biogenic amine neurotransmitter most commonly associated with depression. The identification of multiple serotonin receptor subtypes has also increased the excitement within the research community about the development of even more specific treatments for depression. Besides that SSRIs and other serotonergic antidepressants are effective in the treatment of depression, serotonin is involved in the pathophysiology of depression. Depletion of serotonin may precipitate depression, and some patients with suicidal impulses have low cerebrospinal fluid(CSF) concentrations of serotonin metabolites and serotonin uptake sites on platelets.

(3)Dopamine

Although NE and serotonin are the biogenic amines most often associated with the pathophysiology of depression, dopamine may be involved in the pathophysiology. It is suggested that dopamine activity may be reduced in depression and increased in mania. The discovery of new subtypes of the dopamine receptors and an increased understanding of the presynaptic and postsynaptic regulation have enriched research. Drugs that reduce dopamine concentrations — for example, reserpine(Serpasil) — and diseases that reduce dopamine(e. g. , Parkinson disease) are associated with depressive symptoms. In contrast, drugs that increase dopamine concentrations, such as tyrosine, amphetamine, and bupropion(Wellbutrin), reduce the symptoms of depression. Two recent theories about dopamine and depression are that the mesolimbic dopamine pathway may be dysfunctional in depression and that the dopamine D_1 receptor may be hypoactive in depression.

9.3.1.2   Other neurotransmitter

Acetylcholine (ACh) is found in neurons that are distributed diffusely throughout the cerebral cortex. Cholinergic neurons have reciprocal or interactive relationships with all three monoamine systems. Abnormal levels of choline, which is a precursor to ACh, have been found at autopsy in the brains of depressed patients, reflecting abnormalities in cell phospholipid composition. Cholinergic agonist and antagonist drugs have different clinical effects on depression and mania. Agonists can produce lethargy, anergia, and psychomotor retardation in healthy subjects, can exacerbate symptoms in depression, and can reduce symptoms in mania. These effects generally are not sufficiently robust to have clinical applications, and adverse effects are problematic. In an animal model of depression, strains of mice that are super−or sub−sensitive to cholinergic agonists have been found susceptible or more resistant to developing learned helplessness (discussed later). Cholinergic agonists can induce changes in hypothalamic − pituitary adrenal (HPA) activity and sleep that mimic those associated with severe depression. Some patients with mood disorders in remission, as well as their never−ill first−degree relatives, have a trait−like increase in sensitivity to cholinergic agonists.

γ−aminobutyric acid(GABA) has an inhibitory effect on ascending monoamine pathways, particularly the mesocortical and mesolimbic systems. Reductions of GABA have been observed in plasma, CSF, and brain GABA levels in depression. Animal studies have also found that chronic stress can reduce and eventually deplete GABA levels. By contrast, GABA receptors are upregulated by antidepressants, and some GABAergic medications have weak antidepressant effects.

The amino acids glutamate and glycine are the major excitatory and inhibitory neurotransmitters in the CNS. Glutamate and glycine bind to sites associated with the N−methyl−D−aspartate(NMDA) receptor, and an excess of glutamatergic stimulation can cause neurotoxic effects. Importantly, a high concentration of NMDA receptors exists in the hippocampus. Glutamate, thus, may work in conjunction with hypercortisolemia to mediate the deleterious neurocognitive effects of severe recurrent depression. Emerging evidence suggests that drugs that antagonize NMDA receptors have antidepressant effect.

9.3.1.3   Second messengers and intracellular cascades

The binding of a neurotransmitter and a postsynaptic receptor triggers a cascade of membrane−bound and intracellular processes mediated by second messenger systems. Receptors on cell membranes interact with the intracellular environment via guanine nucleotide−binding proteins(G proteins). The G proteins, in turn, connect to various intracellular enzymes(e. g. , adenylate cyclase, phospholipase C and phosphodiesterase) that regulate utilization of energy and formation of second messengers, such as cyclic nucleotide[e. g. , cyclic adenosine monophosphate(cAMP) and cyclic guanosine monophosphate(cGMP)], as well as phosphatidylinositols(e. g. , inositol triphosphate and diacylglycerol) and calcium−calmodulin. Second messengers regulate the function of neuronal membrane ion channels. Increasing evidence also indicates that mood−stabilizing drugs act on G proteins or other second messengers.

9.3.1.4   Alterations of hormonal regulation

Lasting alterations in neuroendocrine and behavioral responses can result from severe early stress. Animal studies indicate that even transient periods of maternal deprivation can alter subsequent responses to stress. Activity of the gene coding for the neurokinin brain−derived neurotrophic growth factor(BDNF) is decreased after chronic stress, as is the process of neurogenesis. Protracted stress thus can induce changes in the functional status of neurons and, eventually, cell death. Recent studies in depressed humans indicate that a history of early trauma is associated with increased HPA activity accompanied by structural changes

(i. e. , atrophy or decreased volume) in the cerebral cortex.

Elevated HPA activity is a hallmark of mammalian stress responses and one of the clearest links between depression and the biology of chronic stress. Hypercortisolema in depression suggests one or more of the following central disturbances: decreased inhibitory serotonin tone; increased drive from NE, ACh, or corticotropin-releasing hormone(CRH); or decreased feedback inhibition from thehippocampus.

Evidence of increased HPA activity is apparent in 20%–40% of depressed outpatients and 40%–60% of depressed inpatients.

Elevated HPA activity in depression has been documented via excretion of urinary-free cortisol (UFC),24-hour(or shorter time segments) intravenous collections of plasma cortisol levels, salivary cortisol levels, and tests of the integrity of feedback inhibition. A disturbance of feedback inhibition is tested by administration of dexamethasone(Decadron,0.5–2.0 mg), a potent synthetic glucocorticoid, which normally suppresses HPA axis activity for 24 hours. Nonsuppression of cortisol secretion at 8:00 A. M. the following morning or subsequent escape from suppression at 4:00 P. M. or 11:00 P. M. is indicative of impaired feedback inhibition. Hypersecretion of cortisol and dexamethasone nonsuppression are imperfectly correlated (approximately 60% concordance). A more recent development to improve the sensitivity of the test involvesinfusion of a test dose of CRH after dexamethasone suppression.

These tests of feedback inhibition are not used as diagnostic tests because adrenocortical hyperactivity (albeit usually less prevalent) is observed in mania, schizophrenia, dementia, and other psychiatric disorders.

(1) Thyroid axis activity

Approximately 5%–10% of people evaluated for depression have previously undetected thyroid dysfunction, as reflected by an elevated basal thyroid-stimulating hormone(TSH) level or an increased TSH response to a 500 mg infusion of the hypothalamic neuropeptide thyroid-releasing hormone(TRH). Such abnormalities are often associated with elevated antithyroid antibody levels and, unless corrected with hormone replacement therapy, can compromise response to treatment. An even larger subgroup of depressed patients(e. g. ,20%–30%) shows a blunted TSH response to TRH challenge. To date, the major therapeutic implication of a blunted TSH response is evidence of an increased risk of relapse despite preventive antidepressant therapy. Of note, unlike the dexamethasone-suppression test(DST), blunted TSH response to TRH does not usually normalize with effective treatment.

(2) Growth hormone

Growth hormone (GH) is secreted from the anterior pituitary after stimulation by NE and dopamine. Secretion is inhibited by somatostatin, a hypothalamic neuropeptide, and CRH. Decreased CSF somatostatin level have been reported in depression, and increased level have been observed in mania.

(3) Prolactin

Prolactin is released from the pituitary by serotoninstimulation and inhibited by dopamine. Most studies have not found significant abnormalities of basal or circadian prolactin secretion in depression, although a blunted prolactin response to various serotonin agonists has been described. This response is uncommon among premenopausal women, suggesting that estrogen has a moderating effect.

Alterations of sleep neurophysiology. Depression is associated with a premature loss of deep (slow-wave) sleep and an increase in nocturnal arousal. The latter is reflected by 4 types of disturbance: ①an increase in nocturnal awakening, ②a reduction in total sleep time, ③increased phasic rapid eye movement (REM) sleep, ④increased core body temperature. The combination of increased REM drive and decreased slow-wave sleep results in a significant reduction in the first period of non-REM(NREM) sleep, a phenomenon referred to as reduced REM latency. Reduced REM latency and deficits of slow−wave sleep typically persist after recovery of a depressive episode. Blunted secretion of GH after sleep is associated with decreased slow−wave sleep and shows similar state−independent or trait−like behavior. The combination of reduced REM latency, increased REM density, and decreased sleep maintenance identifies approximately 40% of depressed outpatients and 80% of depressed inpatients. False−negative findings are commonly seen in younger, hypersomnolent patients, who may actually experience an increase in slow−wave sleep during episodes of depression. Approximately 10% of healthy individuals have abnormal sleep profiles, and, as with dexamethasone non-suppression, false−positive cases are not uncommonly seen in other psychiatric disorders.

Patients manifesting a characteristically abnormal sleep profile have been found to be less responsive to psychotherapy and have a greater risk of relapse or recurrence and may benefit preferentially from pharmacotherapy.

9.3.1.5   Immunological disturbance

Depressive disorders are associated with several immunological abnormalities, including decreased lymphocyte proliferation in response to mitogens and other forms of impaired cellular immunity. These lymphocytes produce neuromodulators, such as corticotropin−releasing factor (CRF), and cytokines, peptides known as interleukins. There appears to be an association with clinical severity, hypercortisolism, and immune dysfunction, and the cytokine interleukin−1 may induce gene activity for glucocorticoid synthesis.

9.3.1.6   Structural and functional brain imaging

Computed tomography (CT) and magnetic resonance imaging (MRI) scans have permitted sensitive, non-invasive methods to assess brain, including cortical and subcortical tracts, as well as white matter lesions. The most consistent abnormality observed in the depressive disorder is increased frequency of abnormal hyperintensities in subcortical regions, such as periventricular regions, the basal ganglia, and the thalamus. More common in bipolar I disorder and among elderly adults, these hyperintensities appear to reflect the deleterious neurodegenerative effects of recurrent affective episodes. Ventricular enlargement, cortical atrophy, and sulcal widening have also been reported in some studies. Some depressed patients may also have reduced hippocampal or caudate nucleus volumes, or both, suggesting more focal defects in relevant neurobehavioral systems. Diffuse and focal areas of atrophy have been associated with increased illness severity, bipolarity, and increased cortisol levels.

The most widely replicated positron emission tomography (PET) finding in depression is decreased anterior brain metabolism, which is generally more pronounced on the left side. From a different vantage point, depression may be associated with a relative increase in nondominant hemispheric activity. Furthermore, a reversal of hypofrontality occurs after shifting from depression into hypomania, such that greater left hemisphere reductions are seen in depression compared with greater right hemisphere reductions in mania. Other studies have observed reduced cerebral blood flow or metabolism, or both, in the dopaminergically innervated tracts of the mesocortical and mesolimbic systems in depression. Again, evidence suggests that antidepressants at least partially normalize these changes.

In addition to a global reduction of anterior cerebral metabolism, increased glucose metabolism has been observed in several limbic regions, particularly among patients with relatively severe recurrent depression and a family history of mood disorder. During episodes of depression, increased glucose metabolism is correlated with intrusive ruminations.

9.3.1.7   Neuroanatomical considerations

Both the symptoms of mood disorders and biological research findings support the hypothesis that mood disorders involve pathology of the brain. Modern affective neuroscience focuses on four brain regions in the regulation of normal emotions: the prefrontal cortex(PFC), the anterior cingulate, the hippocampus, and the amygdala. The PFC holds representations of goals and appropriate responses to obtain these goals. Such activities are particularly important when multiple, conflicting behavioral responses are possible or when it is necessary to override affective arousal. Evidence indicates some hemispherical specialization in PFC function. For example, whereas left-sided activation of regions of the PFC is more involved in goal-directed or appetitive behaviors, regions of the right PFC are implicated in avoidance behaviors and inhibition of appetitive pursuits. Subregions of the PFC appear to localize representations of behaviors related to reward and punishment.

The anterior cingulate cortex(ACC) is thought to serve as the point of integration of attentional and emotional inputs. Two subdivisions have been identified: an affective subdivision in the rostral and ventral regions of the ACC and a cognitive subdivision involving the dorsal ACC. The former subdivision shares extensive connections with other limbic regions, and the latter interacts more with the PFC and other cortical regions. It is proposed that activation of the ACC facilitates control of emotional arousal, particularly when goal attainment has been thwarted or encountered new problems .

The hippocampus is most clearly involved in various forms of learning and memory, including fear conditioning, as well as inhibitory regulation of the HPA axis activity. Emotional or contextual learning appears to involve a direct connection between the hippocampus and the amygdala.

The amygdala appears to be a crucial way station for processing novel stimuli of emotional significance and coordinating or organizing cortical responses. Located just above the hippocampus, the amygdala has long been viewed as the core of the limbic system. Although most research has focused on the role of the amygdala in responding to fear or pain, it may be ambiguity or novelty, rather than the aversive nature of the stimulus per se, that brings the amygdala on line.

9.3.2　Genetic factors

Family, adoption, and twin studies have long documented the heritability of mood disorders. Recently, the primary focus of genetic studies has been to identify specific susceptibility genes using molecular genetic methods.

9.3.2.1　Family studies

Family studies address the question of whether a disorder is familial. More specifically, is the rate of illness in the family members of someone with the disorder greater than that of the general population? Family data indicate that if one parent has a mood disorder, a child will take a risk of between 10% and 25% for mood disorder. If both parents are affected, this risk roughly doubles. The more members of the family who are affected, the greater the risk is to a child. The risk is greater if the affected family members are first-degree relatives rather than more distant relatives. A family history of bipolar disorder indicates a greater risk for mood disorders in general and, specifically, bipolar disorder. Unipolar disorder is typically the most common form of mood disorder in families of bipolar probands. The familial overlap suggests some degree of common genetic underpinnings between these two forms of mood disorder. The presence of more severe illness in the family also indicates a greater risk.

9.3.2.2　Adoption studies

Adoption studies provide an alternative approachto separating genetic and environmental factors in familial transmission. Only a limited number of such studies have been reported, and their results have been mixed. One large study found a three-fold increase at the rate of bipolar disorder and a two-fold increase in unipolar disorder in the biological relatives of bipolar probands. Similarly, in a Danish sample, a three-fold increase in the rate of unipolar disorder and a six-fold increase in the rate of completed suicide in the biological relatives of affectively ill probands were reported. Other studies, however, have been less convincing and have found no difference in the rates of mood disorders.

9.3.2.3 Twin studies

Twin studies have provided the most powerful approach to separating genetic from environmental factors, or "nature" from "nurture." The twin studies provide compelling evidence that genes explain only 50% -70% of the etiology of mood disorders. Environment or other non-heritable factors must explain the remainder. Therefore, it is a predisposition or susceptibility to disease that is inherited. Considering unipolar and bipolar disorders together, these studies find a concordance rate for mood disorder in themonozygotic (MZ) twins of 70% -90% compared with the same-sex dizygotic (DZ) twins of 16% -35%. This is the most compelling data for the role of genetic factors in mood disorders.

9.3.2.4 Linkage studies

DNA markers are segments of DNA of known chromosomal location, which are highly variable among individuals. They are used to track the segregation of specific chromosomal regions within families affected with a disorder. When a marker is identified with disease in families, the disease is said to be genetically linked. Chromosomes 18 q and 22 q are the two regions with strongest evidence for linkage to bipolar disorder. Several linkage studies have found evidence for the involvement of specific genes in clinical subtypes. For example, the linkage evidence on 18 q has been shown to be derived largely from bipolar I — bipolar II sibling pairs and from families in which the probands had panic symptoms.

Gene-mapping studies of unipolar depression have found very strong evidence of linkage to the locus for cAMP response element-binding protein (CREB1) on chromosome 2. Eighteen other genomic regions were found to be linked; some of these displayed interactions with the CREB1 locus. Another study has reported evidence for a gene-environment interaction in the development of major depression. Subjects who underwent adverse life events were shown, in general, to be at an increased risk for depression. Of such subjects, however, those with a variant in the serotonin transporter gene showed the greatest increase in risk. This is one of the first reports of a specific gene-environment interaction in a psychiatric disorder.

9.3.3 Psychosocial factors

9.3.3.1 Life events and environmental stress

A long-standing clinical observation is that stressful life events more often precede first, ratherthan subsequent, episodes of mood disorders. This association has been reported for both patients with major depressive disorder and bipolar I disorder. One possible explaination is that the stress accompanying the first episode results in long-lasting changes in the brain's biology. These long-lasting changes may alter the functional states of various neurotransmitter and intraneuronal signaling systems, changes that may even include the loss of neurons and an excessive reduction in synaptic contacts. As a result, a person has a high risk of undergoing subsequent episodes of a mood disorder, even without an external stressor.

Some clinicians believe that life events play a principal role in depression; others suggest that life events have only a limited role in the onset and timing of depression. The most compelling data indicate that the life event most often associated with development of depression is losing a parent before the age of 11. The environmental stressor most often associated with the onset of an episode of depression is the loss of a spouse. Another risk factor is unemployment; persons out of work are three times more likely to report symptoms of an episode of major depression than those who are employed. Guilt may also play a role.

9.3.3.2 Personality factors

No single personality trait or type uniquely predisposes a person to depression; all humans, of whatever personality pattern, can and do become depressed under appropriate circumstances. Persons with certain personality disorders — OCD, histrionic, and borderline — may be at greater risk for depression than persons with antisocial or paranoid personality disorder. The latter can use projection and other externalizing defense mechanisms to protect themselves from their inner rage. No evidence has indicated that any particular personality disorder is associated with later development of bipolar I disorder; however, patients with dysthymic disorder and cyclothymic disorder are at risk of later developing major depression or bipolar disorder.

Recent stressful events are the most powerful predictors of a depressive episode onset. From a psychodynamic perspective, the clinician is always interested in the meaning of the stressor. Research has demonstrated that stressors that the patient experience as reflecting negatively on his or her self−esteem are more likely to produce depression. Moreover, what may seem to be a relatively mild stressor to outsiders may be devastating to the patient because of particular idiosyncratic meanings attached to the event.

9.3.3.3 Psychodynamic factors in depression

The psychodynamic understanding of depression defined by Sigmund Freud and expanded by Karl Abraham is known as the classic view of depression. That theory involves four key points: ①disturbances in the infant−mother relationship during the oral phase(the first 10−18 months) predispose to subsequent vulnerability to depression; ②depression can be linked to real or imagined object loss; ③introjection of the departed objects is a defense mechanism invoked to deal with the distress connected with the object's loss; ④because the lost object is regarded with a mixture of love and hate, feelings of anger are directed inward at the self.

Melanie Klein understood depression as involving the expression of aggression toward loved ones, much as Freud did. Edward Bibring regarded depression as a phenomenon that sets in when a person becomes aware of the discrepancy between extraordinarily high ideals and the inability to meet those goals. Edith Jacobson saw the state of depression as similar to a powerless, helpless child victimized by a tormenting parent. Silvano Arieti observed that many depressed people have lived their lives for someone else rather than for themselves. He referred to the person for whom depressed patients live as the dominant other, which may be a principle, an ideal, or an institution, as well as an individual. Depression sets in when patients realize that the person or ideal for which they have been living is never going to respond in a manner that will meet their expectations. Heinz Kohut's conceptualization of depression, derived from his self−psychological theory, rests on the assumption that the developing self has specific needs that must be met by parents to give the child a positive sense of self−esteem and self−cohesion. When others do not meet these needs, there is a massive loss of self−esteem that presents as depression. John Bowlby believed that damaged early attachments and traumatic separation in childhood predispose to depression. Adult losses are said to revive the traumatic childhood loss and so precipitate adult depressive episodes.

9.3.3.4 Psychodynamic factors in mania

Most theories of mania view manic episodes as a defense against underlying depression. Abraham, for example, believed that the manic episodes may reflect an inability to tolerate a developmental tragedy, such as the loss of a parent. The manic state may also result from a tyrannical superego, which produces intolerable self−criticism that is then replaced by euphoric self−satisfaction. Bertram Lewin regarded the manic patient's ego as overwhelmed by pleasurable impulses, such as sex, or by feared impulses, such as aggression. Klein also viewed mania as a defensive reaction to depression, such as omnipotence, in which the person develops delusions of grandeur.

9.3.4　Other formulations of depression

9.3.4.1　Cognitive theory

According to cognitive theory, depression results from specific cognitive distortions present in persons susceptible to depression. These distortions, referred to as depressogenicschemata, are cognitive templates that perceive both internal and external in ways that are altered by early experiences. Aaron Beck postulated a cognitive triad of depression that consists of: ①views about the self—negative and self—precept, ②about the environment—atendency to experience the world as hostile and demanding, ③about the future — the expectation of suffering and failure. Therapy consists of modifying these distortions.

9.3.4.2　Learned helplessness

The learned helplessness theory of depression connects depressive phenomena to the experience of uncontrollable evens. For example, when dogs in a laboratory were exposed to electrical shocks from which they could not escape, they showed behaviors that differentiated them from dogs that had not been exposed to such uncontrollable events. The dogs exposed to the shocks would not cross a barrier to stop the flow of electric shock when put in a new learning situation. They remained passive and did not move. According to the learned helplessness theory, the shocked dogs learned that outcomes were independent of responses, so they had both cognitive motivational deficit(i. e. , they would not attempt to escape the shock) and emotional deficit(indicating decreased reactivity to the shock). In the reformulated view of learned helplessness as applied to human depression, internal causal explanations are thought to produce a loss of self—esteem after adverse external events. Behaviorists who subscribe to the theory stress that improvement of depression is contingent on the patient's learning a sense of control and mastery of the environment.

9.4　Clinical features

Case report:

Female, 29 years old. 2 years ago, due to work stress, she began to feel unhappy, want to cry all day, lose interest in everything. She didn't want to do anything. She felt the reaction speed and the working efficiency was decreased. She blamed herself and regreted for what she has done with low self evaluation. She felt too tired to live. She thought if she dies, she and her family would be reliefed. She lost her appetite, sleepless at night, woke up at 4 in the morning and couldn't fall asleep again. Her family found out that she was in a bad mood. Her family made her stop working for about 1 months. Her mood improved gradually, and so did her diet and sleep. After resting, she returned to normal work. About 3 weeks ago, for no reason, she appeared to be in a good mood. She felt her brain reacted faster. She was confident that she was stronger than others and can achieve great goal. She thought she can be a department leader. She often spends money to buy things for others. She likes to talk to others. She only slept 3 hours a day, and it would be enough. She was still energetic and busy during the day. She lost her temper when she was stopped by her family or colleagues. Her family found her abnormality unusual and sent her to the hospital. She thought she was not sick and refused treatment.

The two basic symptom patterns in mood disorders are depression and mania. Depressive episodes can occur in both major depressive disorder and bipolar disorder. Researchers have attempted to find reliable differences between bipolar disorder depressive episodes and episodes of major depressive disorder, but the differences are elusive. In a clinical situation, only the patient's history, family history, and future course can help differentiate the two conditions. Some patients with bipolar disorder have both manic and depressive features, and some seem to experience brief — a few minutes to a few hours — episodes of depression during manic episodes.

9.4.1 Depressive episodes

A depressed mood and a loss of interest or pleasure are the key symptoms of depression. Patients may say that they feel blue, hopeless, in the dumps, or worthless. For a patient, the depressed mood often has a distinct quality that differentiates it from the normal emotion of sadness or grief. Patients often describe the symptom of depression as one of agonizing emotional pain and sometimes complain about being unable to cry, a symptom that resolves as they improve.

About two–thirds of all depressed patients contemplate suicide, and 10% –15% commit suicide. Those recently hospitalized with a suicide attempt or suicidal ideation have a higher lifetime risk of successful suicide than those never hospitalized for suicidal ideation. Some depressed patients sometimes seem unaware of their depression and do not complain of a mood disturbance even though they exhibit withdrawal from family, friends, and activities that previously interested them. Almost all depressed patients (97%) complain about reduced energy; they have difficulty finishing tasks, are impaired at school and work, and have less motivation to undertake new projects. About 80% of patients complain of trouble sleeping, especially early morning awakening(i. e. , terminal insomnia) and multiple awakenings at night, during which they ruminate about their problems. Many patients have decreased appetite and weight loss, but others experience increased appetite and gain weight and sleep longer than usual. These patients are classified as having atypical features.

Anxiety, a common symptom of depression, affects as many as 90% of all depressed patients. The variouschanges in food intake and rest can aggravate coexisting medical illnesses such as diabetes, hypertension, chronic obstructive lung disease, and heart disease. Other vegetative symptoms include abnormal menses and decreased interest and performance in sexual activities. Sexual problems can sometimes lead to inappropriate referrals, such as to marital counseling and sex therapy, when clinicians fail to recognize the underlying depressive disorder. Anxiety (including panic attacks), alcohol abuse, and somatic complaints (e. g. , constipation and headaches) often complicate the treatment of depression. About 50% of all patients describe a diurnal variation in their symptoms, with increased severity in the morning and lessening of symptoms by evening. Cognitive symptoms include subjective reports of an inability to concentrate (84% of patients in one study) and impairments in thinking(67% of patients in another study).

9.4.1.1 Depression in children and adolescents

School phobia and excessive clinging to parents may be symptoms of depression in children. Poor academic performance, substance abuse, antisocial behavior, sexual promiscuity, truancy, and running away may be symptoms of depression in adolescents.

9.4.1.2 Depression in older people

Depression is more common in older persons than it is in the general population. Various studies have reported prevalence rates ranging from 25% to almost 50% . Several studies indicate that depression in older persons may be correlated with low socio–economic status, the loss of a spouse, a concurrent physical illness, and socialisolation. Other studies have indicated that depression in older persons is underdiagnosed and undertreated, perhaps particularly by general practitioners. The underrecognition of depression in older persons may occur because the disorder appears more often with somatic complaints in older, than in younger groups. Further, ageism may influence and cause clinicians to accept depressive symptoms as normal in older patients.

9.4.2   Manic episodes

An elevated, expansive, or irritable mood is the hallmark of a manic episode. The elevated mood is euphoric and often infectious and can even cause a counter transferential denial of illness by an inexperienced clinician. Although uninvolved persons may not recognize the unusual nature of a patient's mood, those who know thepatient recognize it as abnormal. Alternatively, the mood may be irritable, especially when a patient's overtly ambitious plans are thwarted. Patients often exhibit changes of predominant mood from euphoria early in the course of the illness to later irritability.

The treatment of manic patients in an inpatient ward can be complicated by their testing of the limits of ward rules, tendency to shift responsibility for their acts onto others, exploitation of the weaknesses of others, and propensity to create conflicts among staff members. Outside the hospital, manic patients often drink alcohol excessively, perhaps in an attempt to self-medicate. Their disinhibited nature is reflected in excessive use of the telephone, especially in making long-distance calls during the early morning hours.

Pathological gambling, a tendency to disrobe in public places, wearing clothing and jewelry of bright colors in unusual or outlandish combinations, and inattention to small details(e. g. , forgetting to hang up the telephone) are also symptomatic of the disorder. Patients act impulsively and at the same time with a sense of conviction and purpose. They are often preoccupied by religious, political, financial, sexual, or persecutory ideas that can evolve into complex delusional systems. Occasionally, manic patients become regressed and play with their urine and feces.

Mania in adolescents: Mania in adolescents is often misdiagnosed as antisocial personality disorder or schizophrenia. Symptoms of mania in adolescents may include psychosis, alcohol or other substance abuse, suicide attempts, academic problems, philosophical brooding, OCD symptoms, multiple somatic complaints, marked irritability resulting in fights, and other antisocial behaviors. Although many of these symptoms are seen in normal adolescents, severe or persistent symptoms should cause clinicians to consider bipolar I disorder in the differential diagnosis.

9.4.3   Coexisting disorders

9.4.3.1   Anxiety

In the anxiety disorders, symptoms of anxiety can coexist with significant symptoms of depression. Whether patients who exhibit significant symptoms of both anxiety and depression are affected by two distinct disease processes or by a single disease process that produces both sets of symptoms is not yet resolved. Patients of both types may constitute the group of patients with mixed anxiety – depressive disorder.

9.4.3.2   Alcohol dependence

Alcohol dependence frequently coexists with mood disorders. Both patients with major depressive disorder and those with bipolar I disorder are likely to meet the diagnostic criteria for an alcohol use disorder. The available data indicate that alcohol dependence is more strongly associated with a coexisting diagnosis of depression in women than in men. In contrast, the genetic and family data about men who have both mood disorder and alcohol dependence indicate that they are likely to have two genetically distinct disease processes.

9.4.3.3 Other substance—related disorders

Substance—related disorders other than alcohol dependence are also commonly associated with mood disorders. The abuse of substances may be involved in precipitating an episode of illness or, conversely, may represent patients' attempts to treat their own illnesses. Although manic patients seldom use sedatives to dampen their euphoria, depressed patients often use stimulants, such as cocaine and amphetamines, to relieve their depression.

9.4.3.4 Medical conditions

Depression commonly coexists with medicalconditions, especially in older persons. When depression and medical conditions coexist, clinicians must try to determine whether the underlying medical condition is pathophysiologically related to the depression or whether any drugs that the patient is taking for the medical condition are causing the depression. Many studies indicate that treatment of a coexisting major depressive disorder can improve the course of the underlying medical disorder, including cancer.

9.5 Diagnosis and differential diagnosis

9.5.1 Diagnosis

9.5.1.1 Major depressive disorder, single episode

Depression may occur as a single episode or may be recurrent. Differentiation between these patients and those who have two or more episodes of major depressive disorder is justified because of the uncertain course of the former patients' disorder. Several studies have reported data consistent with the notion that major depression covers a heterogeneous population of disorders. Some studies assessed the stability of a diagnosis of major depression in a patient over time, and found that 25% –50% of the patients were later reclassified as having a different psychiatric condition or a nonpsychiatric medical condition with psychiatric symptoms. Some studies evaluated first—degree relatives of affectively ill patients to determine the presence and types of psychiatric diagnoses for these relatives over time. These studies found that depressed patients with more depressive symptoms are more likely to have stable diagnoses over time and are more likely to have affectively ill relatives than are depressed patients with fewer depressive symptoms. Also, patients with bipolar Ⅰ disorder and bipolar Ⅱ disorder(recurrent major depressive episodes with hypomania) are likely to have stable diagnoses over time.

9.5.1.2 Major depressive disorder and recurrent

Patients who are experiencing at least a second episode of depression are classified as having major depressive disorder, recurrent. The essential problem with diagnosing recurrent episodes of major depressive disorder is choosing the criteria to designate the resolution of each period. Two variables are the degree of resolution of the symptoms and the length of the resolution. DSM—5 requires that distinct episodes of depression be separated by at least 2 months during which a patient has no significant symptoms of depression.

9.5.1.3 Bipolar disorder

The ICD—10 criteria for a bipolar disorder requires the presence of a distinct period of abnormal mood lasting at least 1 week and includes separate bipolar I disorder diagnoses for a single manic episode and a recurrent episode based on the symptoms of the most recent episode. The designation bipolar disorder is synonymous with what was formerly known as bipolar disorder — a syndrome in which a complete set of mania symptoms occurs during the course of the disorder.

9.5.2   Differential diagnosis

9.5.2.1   Major depressive disorder

(1) Medical disorders

The diagnosis of mood disorder due to a general medical condition must be considered. Failure to obtain a good clinical history or to consider the context of a patient's current life situation can lead to diagnostic errors. Clinicians should have depressed adolescents tested for mononucleosis, and patients who are markedly overweight or underweight should be tested for adrenal and thyroid dysfunctions. Homosexuals, bisexual men, prostitutes, and persons who abuse a substance intravenously should be tested for acquired immune deficiency syndrome (AIDS). Older patients should be evaluated for viral pneumonia and other medical conditions.

Many neurological and medical disorders and pharmacological agents can produce symptoms of depression. Patients with depressive disorders often first visit their general practitioners with somatic complaints. Most medical causes of depressive disorders can be detected with a comprehensive medical history, a complete physical and neurological examination, and blood and urine tests. The thyroid and adrenal functions should be tested because disorders of both of these endocrine systems can appear as depressive disorders. In substance-induced mood disorder, any drug a depressed patient is taking should be considered a potential factor in the mood disorder. Cardiac drugs, antihypertensives, sedatives, hypnotics, antipsychotics, antiepileptics, antiparkinsonian drugs, analgesics, antibacterials, and antineoplastics are all commonly associated with depressivesymptoms.

1) Neurological conditions

The most common neurological problems that manifest depressive symptoms are Parkinson's disease, dementing illnesses (including dementia of the Alzheimer's type), epilepsy, cerebro-vascular diseases, and tumors. About 50% –75% of the patients with Parkinson disease have marked symptoms of depressive disorder that do not correlate with the patient's physical disability, age, or duration of illness but do correlate with the abnormalities found on neuropsychological tests. The symptoms of depressive disorder can be masked by the almost identical motor symptoms of Parkinson's disease. Depressive symptoms often respond to antidepressant drugs or ECT. The interictal changes associated with temporal lobe epilepsy can mimic a depressive disorder, especially if the epileptic focus is on the right side. Depression is a common complicating feature of cerebrovascular diseases, particularly in the 2 years after the episode. Depression is more common in anterior brain lesions than in posterior brain lesions and, in both cases, often responds to antidepressant medications. Tumors of the diencephalic and temporal regions are particularly likely to be associated with depressive disorder symptoms.

2) Pseudodementia

Clinicians can differentiate the pseudodementia of major depressive disorder from the dementia of a disease, such as dementia of the Alzheimer's type. The cognitive symptoms in major depressive disorder have a sudden onset, and other symptoms of the disorder, such as self-reproach, are also present. A diurnal variation in the cognitive problems, which is not seen in primary dementias, may occur. Whereas depressed patients with cognitive difficulties often do not try to answer questions ("I don't know"), patients with dementia may confabulate. During an interview, depressed patients can sometimes be coached and encouraged into remembering, an ability that demented patients lack.

(2) Mental disorders

Depression can be a feature of virtually any mental disorder, but the mental disorders particular consideration in the differential diagnosis.

(3) Other mood disorders

Clinicians must consider a range of diagnostic categories before making at a final diagnosis. Mood disorder caused by a general medical condition and substance induced mood disorder must be ruled out. Clinicians must also determine whether a patient has had episodes of mania—like symptoms, indicating bipolar Ⅰ disorder(complete manic and depressive syndromes), bipolar Ⅱ disorder(recurrent major depressive episodes with hypomania), or cyclothymic disorder(incomplete depressive andmanic syndromes). If a patient's symptoms are limited to those of depression, clinicians must assess the severity and duration of the symptoms to differentiate among major depressive disorder(complete depressive syndrome for 2 weeks), minor depressive disorder(incomplete but episodic depressive syndrome), recurrent brief depressive disorder(complete depressive syndrome but for less than 2 weeks per episode), and dysthymic disorder(incomplete depressive syndrome without clear episodes).

(4) Other mental disorders

Substance—related disorders, psychotic disorders, eating disorders, adjustment disorders, somatoform disorders, and anxiety disorders are all commonly associated with depressive symptoms and should be considered in the differential diagnosis of a patient with depressive symptoms. Perhaps the most difficult differential is that between anxiety disorders with depression and depressive disorders with marked anxiety. An abnormal result on the dexamethasone—suppression test, the presence of shortened REM latency on a sleep electroencephalogram(EEG), and a negative lactate infusion test result support a diagnosis of major depressive disorder in particularly ambiguous cases.

(5) Uncomplicated bereavement

Uncomplicated bereavementis not considered a mental disorder even though about one—third of all bereaved spouses for a time meet the diagnostic criteria for major depressive disorder. Some patients with uncomplicated bereavement do develop major depressive disorder, but the diagnosis is not made unless no resolution of the grief occurs. The differentiation is based on the symptoms' severity and length. In major depressive disorder, common symptoms that evolve from unresolved bereavement are a morbid preoccupation with worthlessness; suicidal ideation; feelings that the person has committed an act(not just an omission) that caused the spouse's death; mummification(keeping the deceased's belongings exactly as they were); and a particularly severe reaction, which sometimes includes a suicide attempt. In severe bereavement depression, the patient simply pines away, unable to live without the departed person, usually a spouse. These patients do have a serious medical condition. Their immune function is often depressed, and their cardiovascular status is precarious. Death can ensue within a few months of that of a spouse, especially among elderly men. Such considerations suggest that itwould be clinically unwise to withhold antidepressants from many persons experiencing such an intense mourning.

(6) Schizophrenia

It is difficult to distinguish a manic episode from schizophrenia. Although difficult, a differential diagnosis is possible. Merriment, elation, and infectiousness of mood are much more common in manic episodes than in schizophrenia. The combination of a manic mood, rapid or pressured speech, and hyperactivity weighs heavily toward a diagnosis of a manic episode. The onset in a manic episode is often rapid and is perceived as a marked change from a patient's previous behavior. Half of all patients with bipolar I disorder have a family history of mood disorder. Catatonic features may be part of a depressive phase of bipolar I disorder. When evaluating patients with catatonia, clinicians should look carefully for a past history of manic or depressive episodes and for a family history of mood disorders. Manic symptoms in persons from minority groups(particularly blacks and Hispanics) are often misdiagnosed as schizophrenic symptoms.

(7) Medical conditions

In contrast to depressive symptoms, which are present in many psychiatric disorders, manic symptoms are more distinctive, although they can be caused by a wide range of medical and neurological conditions and substances. Antidepressant treatment can also be associated with the precipitation of mania in some patients.

9.5.2.2   Bipolar disorder

When a patient with bipolar disorder has a depressive episode, the differential diagnosis is the same as that for a patient being considered for a diagnosis of major depressive disorder. When a patient is manic, however, the differential diagnosis includes bipolar disorder, cyclothymic disorder, mood disorder caused by a general medical condition, and substance-induced mood disorder. For manic symptoms, borderline, narcissistic, histrionic, and antisocial personality disorders need special consideration.

9.5.2.3   Major depressive disorder versus bipolar disorder

To decide whether a patient has major depressive disorder or bipolar disorder is a major challenge in clinical practice. Numerous studies have shown that bipolar disorder is not only confused with personality, substance use, and schizophrenic disorders but also with depressive and anxiety disorders. Certain features especially in combinationare predictive of bipolar disorder(Table 9-1).

Table 9-1   Clinical features predictive of bipolar disorder

(1) Early age at onset
(2) Psychotic depression before 25 years of age
(3) Postpartum depression, especially one with psychotic features
(4) Rapid onset and offset of depressive episodes of short duration(<3 months)
(5) Recurrent depression(more than five episodes)
(6) Depression with marked psychomotor retardation
(7) Atypical features(reverse vegetative signs)
(8) Seasonality
(9) Bipolar family history
(10) High-density, three-generation pedigrees
(11) Trait mood lability(cyclothymia)
(12) Hyperthymic temperament
(13) Hypomania associated with antidepressants
(14) Repeated(at least three times) loss of efficacy of antidepressants after initial response
(15) Depressive mixed state(with psychomotor excitement, irritable hostility, racing thoughts, and sexual arousal duringmajordepression)

More broad indicators of bipolarity include the following conditions, none of which, by itself, confirms a bipolar diagnosis, but should raise clinical suspicion in that direction: agitated depression, cyclical depression, episodic sleep dysregulation, or a combination of these; refractory depression (failed antidepressants from three differentclasses); depression in someone with an extroverted profession, periodic impulsivity, such as gambling, sexual misconduct, andwanderlust, or periodic irritability, suicidal risks, or both; and depression with erratic personality disorders.

9.5.3 Mental status examination

9.5.3.1 Major depressive episodes

(1) General description

Generalized psychomotor retardation is the most common symptom of depression, although psychomotor agitation is also seen, especially in older patients. Hand wringing and hair pulling are the most common symptoms of agitation. Typically, a depressed patient has a stooped posture, no spontaneous movements, and a downcast, averted gaze. On clinical examination, depressed patients exhibiting gross symptoms of psychomotor retardation may appear identical to patients with catatonic schizophrenia.

(2) Mood, affect, and feelings

Depression is the key symptom, although about 50% of patients deny depressive feelings and do not appear to be particularly depressed. Family members or employers often bring or send these patients for treatment because of social withdrawal and generally decreased activity.

(3) Speech

Many depressed patients have decreased rates and volume of speech; they respond to questions with single words and exhibit delayed responses to questions. The physician may literally have to wait 2 or 3 minutes for a response to a question.

(4) Perceptual disturbances

Depressed patients with delusions or hallucinations are said to have a major depressive episode with psychotic features. Even in the absence of delusions or hallucinations, some clinicians use the term psychotic depression for grossly regressed depressed patients — mute, not bathing, soiling. Such patients are probably better described as having catatonic features.

Delusions and hallucinations that are consistent with a depressed mood are said to be mood congruent. Mood-congruent delusions in a depressed person include those of guilt, sinfulness, worthlessness, poverty, failure, persecution, and terminal somatic illnesses (such as cancer and a " rotting" brain). The content of mood-incongruent delusions or hallucinations is not consistent with a depressed mood. For example, a mood-incongruent delusion in a depressed person might involve grandiose themes of exaggerated power, knowledge, and value. When that occurs, a schizophrenic disorder should be considered.

(5) Thought

Depressed patients customarily have negative views of the world and of themselves. Their thought content often includesnon-delusional ruminations about loss, guilt, suicide, and death. About 10% of all depressed patients have marked symptoms of a thought disorder, usually thought blocking and profound poverty of content.

(6) Sensorium and cognition

①Orientation. Most depressed patients are oriented to person, place, and time, although some may not have sufficient energy or interest to answer questions about these subjects during an interview. ②Memory. About 50% –75% of all depressed patients have a cognitive impairment, sometimes referred to as depressive pseudodementia. Such patients commonly complain of impaired concentration and forgetfulness.

(7) Impulse control

10% –15% of all depressed patients commit suicide, and about two-thirds have suicidal ideation. Depressed patients with psychotic features occasionally consider killing a person as a result of their delusional systems, but the most severely depressed patients often lack the motivation or the energy to act in an impulsive or violent way. Patients with depressive disorders are at increased risk of suicide as they begin to improve and regain the energy needed to plan and carry out a suicide(paradoxical suicide). It is usually clinically unwise to give a depressed patient a large prescription for a large number of antidepressants, especially tricyclic drugs, at the time of their discharge from the hospital. Similarly, drugs that may be activating, such as fluoxetine, may be prescribed in such a way that the energizing qualities are minimized(e. g. , be given a benzodiazepine at the same time).

(8) Judgment and insight

Judgment is assessed by patients' actions in the recent past and their behavior during the interview. Depressed patients' descriptions of their disorder are often hyperbolic; they overemphasize their symptoms, and life problems. It is difficult to convince such patients that improvement is possible.

(9) Reliability

In interviews and conversations, depressed patients overemphasize the bad and minimize the good. A common clinical mistake is to unquestioningly believe a depressed patient who states that a previous trial of antidepressant medications did not work. Such statements may be false, and they require confirmation from another source. Psychiatrists should not view patients' misinformation as an intentional fabrication; the admission of any hopeful information may be impossible for a person in a depressed state of mind.

(10) Rating scales for depression

Rating scales for depression can be useful in clinical practice for documenting the depressed patient's clinical state.

1) Zung self-rating depression scale

The Zung self-rating depression scale is a 20-item report scale. A normal score is 34 or less; a depressed score is 50 or more. The scale provides a global index of the intensity of a patient's depressive symptoms, including the affective expression of depression.

2) Raskin depression scale

The Raskin depression scale is a clinician-rated scale that measures the severity of a patient's depression, as reported by the patient and as observed by the physician, on a 5-point scale of three dimensions: verbal report, displayed behavior, and secondary symptoms. The scale has a range of 3-13; a normal score is 3, the out off of depression is 7.

3) Hamilton rating scale for depression

The Hamilton rating scale for depression(HAMD) is a widely used depression scale consisted of 24 items, each of which is rated 0-4 or 0-2, with a total score of 0-76. The clinician evaluates the patient's answers to questions about feelings of guilt, thoughts of suicide, sleep habits, and other symptoms of depression, and the ratings are derived from the clinical interview.

9.5.3.2 Manic episodes

Manic patients are excited, talkative, sometimes amusing, and frequently hyperactive. At times, they are grossly psychotic and disorganized and require physical restraints and the intramuscular injection of sedating drugs.

(1) Mood, affect, and feelings

Manic patients classically are euphoric, but they can also be irritable, especially when mania has been present for some time. They also have a low frustration tolerance, which can lead to feelings of anger and hostility. Manic patients may be emotionally labile, switching from laughter to irritability to depression in minutes or hours.

（2）Speech

Manic patients can not be interrupted while they are speaking, and they are often intrusive nuisances to those around them. Their speech is often disturbed. As the mania gets more intense, speech becomes louder, more rapid, and difficult to interpret. As the activated state increases, their speech is filled with puns, jokes, rhymes, plays on words, and irrelevancies. At a still greater activity level, associations become loosened, the ability to concentrate fades, and flight of ideas, clanging, and neologisms appear. In acute manic episode, speech can be totally incoherent and indistinguishable from that of a person with schizophrenia.

（3）Perceptual disturbances

Delusions occur in 75% manic patients. Mood-congruent manic delusions are often concerned with great wealth, extraordinary abilities, or power. Bizarre and mood-incongruent delusions and hallucinations also appear in mania.

（4）Thought

The manic patient's thought content includes themes of self-confidence and self-aggrandizement. Manic patients are often easily distracted, and their cognitive functioning in the manic state is characterized by an unrestrained and accelerated flow of ideas.

（5）Sensorium and cognition

Although the cognitive deficits of patients with schizophrenia have been fully discussed, less has been reported about similar deficits in patients with bipolar disorder. These deficits can be interpreted as reflecting diffuse cortical dysfunction; subsequent work may localize the abnormal areas. Grossly, orientation and memory are intact, although some manic patients may be so euphoric that they answer questions testing orientation incorrectly. Emil Kraepelin named the symptom "delirious mania."

（6）Impulse control

About 75% manic patients are assaultive or threatening. Manic patients do attempt suicide and homicide, but the incidence of these behaviors is unknown.

（7）Judgment and insight

Impaired judgment is a hallmark of manic patients. They may break laws about credit cards, sexual activities, and finances and sometimes involve their families in financial ruin. Manic patients also have little insight into their disorder.

（8）Reliability

Manic patients are notoriously unreliable in their information. Because lying and deceit are common in mania, inexperienced clinicians may treat manic patients with inappropriate disdain.

9.6   Course and prognosis

Studies of the course and prognosis of mood disorders have generally concluded that mood disorders tend to have long courses and patients tend to have relapses. Although mood disorders are often considered benign in contrast to schizophrenia, they exact a profound toll on affected patients.

9.6.1 Major depressive disorder

9.6.1.1 Course

（1）Onset

About 50% of patients having their first episode of major depressive disorder exhibited significant depressive symptoms before the first identified episode. Therefore, early identification and treatment of symptoms may prevent the development of a full depressive episode. Although symptoms may have been present, patients with major depressive disorder usually have not had a premorbid personality disorder. The first depressive episode occurs before the age of 40 years in about 50% of patients. A later onset is associated with the absence of a family history, antisocial personality disorder, and alcohol abuse.

(2) Duration

An untreated depressive episode lasts 6 – 13 months; most treated episodes last about 3 months. The withdrawal of antidepressants before 3 months has elapsed almost always results in the return of the symptoms. As the course of the disorder progresses, patients tend to have more frequent episodes that last longer. Over a 20-year period, the mean number of episodes is five or six.

(3) Development of manic episodes

5% – 10% of patients with an initial diagnosis of major depressive disorder have a manic episode 6–10 years after the first depressive episode. The mean age for this switch is 32 years, and it often occurs after two to four depressive episodes. Although the data are inconsistent and controversial, some clinicians report that the depression of patients who are later classified as having bipolar I disorder is often characterized by hypersomnia, psychomotor retardation, psychotic symptoms, a history of postpartum episodes, a family history of bipolar disorder, and a history of antidepressant-induced hypomania.

9.6.1.2 Prognosis

Major depressive disorder is not a benign disorder. It tends to be chronic, and patients tend to relapse. Patients who have been hospitalized for a first episode of major depressive disorder have about a 50% chance of recovering in the first year. The percentage of patients recovering after repeated hospitalization decreases with passing time. Many unrecovered patients remain affected with dysthymic disorder. About 25% of patients experience a recurrence of major depressive disorder in the first 6 months after release from a hospital, about 30% – 50% in the following 2 years, and about 50% – 75% in 5 years. The incidence of relapse is lower than these figures in patients who continue prophylactic psychopharmacological treatment and in patients who have had only one or two depressive episodes. Generally, as a patient experiences more depressive episodes, the shorter time between the episodes, and the heavier severity of each episode.

Prognostic indicators: many studies have focused on identifying both good and bad prognostic indicators in the course of major depressive disorder. Mild episodes, the absence of psychotic symptoms, and a short hospital stay are good prognostic indicators. Psychosocial indicators of a good course include a history of solid friendships during adolescence, stable family functioning, and generally sound social functioning for the 5 years preceding the illness. Additional good prognostic signs are the absence of a comorbid psychiatric disorder and of a personality disorder, no more than one previous hospitalization for major depressive disorder, and an advanced age of onset. The possibility of a poor prognosis is increased by coexisting dysthymic disorder, abuse of alcohol and other substances, anxiety disorder symptoms, and a history of more than one previous depressive episode. Men are more likely than women to experience a chronically impaired course.

9.6.2 Bipolar disorder

9.6.2.1 Course

The natural history of bipolar disorder is such that it is often useful to make a graph of a patient's disorder and to keep it up to date as treatment progresses. Although cyclothymic disorder is sometimes diagnosed retrospectively in patients with bipolar disorder, no identified personality traits are specifically associated with bipolar disorder.

Bipolar disorder most often starts with depression(75% of the time in women,67% in men) and is a recurring disorder. Most patients experience both depressive and manic episodes,although 10%–20% experience only manic episodes. The manic episodes typically have a rapid onset(hours or days) but may evolve over a few weeks. An untreated manic episode lasts about 3 months;therefore,clinicians should not discontinue giving drugs before that time. Of persons who have a single manic episode,90% are likely to have another. As the disorder progresses,the time between episodes often decreases. After about 5 episodes,however,the interepisode interval often stabilizes at 6–9 months. Of persons with bipolar disorder,5%–15% have four or more episodes per year and can be classified as rapid cyclers.

Bipolar disorder in children and older persons:Bipolar disorder can affect both the very young and older persons. The incidence of bipolar disorder in children and adolescents is about 1%,and the onset can be as early as age 8 years old. Common misdiagnoses are schizophrenia and oppositional defiant disorder. Bipolar disorder with such an early onset is associated with a poor prognosis. Manic symptoms are common in older persons,although causes is broad and includes nonpsychiatric medical conditions,dementia,and delirium,as well as bipolar disorder. The onset of bipolar disorder in older persons is relatively uncommon.

9.6.2.2 Prognosis

Patients with bipolar disorder have a poorer prognosis than patients with major depressive disorder. 40%–50% of patients with bipolar disorder may have a second manic episode within 2 years of the first episode. Although lithium prophylaxis improves the course and prognosis of bipolar disorder,probably only 50%–60% of patients achieve significant control of their symptoms with lithium. One 4–year follow–up study of patients with bipolar disorder found a premorbid poor occupational status,alcohol dependence,psychotic features,depressive features,inter episode depressive features,and male gender were all factors that contributed to a poor prognosis. Short duration of manic episodes,advanced age of onset,few suicidal thoughts,and few coexisting psychiatric or medical problems predict a better outcome.

About 7% of patients with bipolar disorder do not have a recurrence of symptoms;45% have more than one episode,and 40% have a chronic disorder. Patients may have from 2 to 30 manic episodes,although the mean number is about nine. About 40% of all patients have more than ten episodes. On long–term follow–up,15% of all patients with bipolar disorder are well,45% are well but have multiple relapses,30% are in partial remission,and 10% are chronically ill. One–third of all patientswith bipolar disorder have chronic symptoms and evidence of significant social decline.

9.7 Treatments

Treatments of patients with mood disorders should be directed toward several goals. First,the patient's safety must be guaranteed. Second,a complete diagnostic evaluation is necessary. Third,a treatment plan that addresses not only the immediate symptoms but also the patient's prospective well–being should be initiated. Although current treatment emphasizes pharmacotherapy and psychotherapy addressed to the individual patient,stressful life events are also associated with increases in relapse rates. Thus,treatment should address the number and severity of stressors in patients' lives.

Overall,the treatment of mood disorders is rewarding for psychiatrists. Specific treatments are now available for both manic and depressive episodes,and data indicate that prophylactic treatment is also effective. Because the prognosis for each episode is good,optimism is always warranted and is welcomed by both the patient and the patient's family. Mood disorders are chronic, however, and the psychiatrist must educate the patient and the family about future treatment strategies.

9.7.1　Hospitalization

The most critical decision a physician must make is whether a patient should hospitalize or recive outpatient treatment. Indications for hospitalization are the risk of suicide or homicide, a patient's grossly reduced ability to get food and shelter, and the need for diagnostic procedures. A history of rapidly progressing symptoms and the rupture of a patient's usual support systems are also indications for hospitalization.

A physician may safely treat mild depression or hypomania in the office if he or she evaluates the patient frequently. Clinical signs of impaired judgment, weight loss, or insomnia should be minimal. The patient's support system should be strong, neither over involved nor withdrawing from the patient. Any adverse changes in the patient's symptoms or behavior or the attitude of the patient's support systemmay suffice to warrant hospitalization.

Patients with mood disorders are often unwilling to enter a hospital voluntarily and may have to be involuntarily committed. These patients often can not make decisions because of their slowed thinking, negative weltanschauung, and hopelessness. Patients who are manic often have such a complete lack of insight into their disorder that hospitalization seems absolutely absurd to them.

9.7.2　Psychosocial therapy

Although most studies indicate — and most clinicians and researchers believe — that a combination of psychotherapy and pharmacotherapy is the most effective treatment for major depressive disorder, some other studies suggest that: either pharmacotherapy or psychotherapy alone is effective, at least in patients with mild major depressive episodes, and the regular use of combined therapy adds to the cost of treatment and exposes patients to unnecessary adverse effects.

Three types of short-term psychotherapies — cognitive therapy, interpersonal therapy, and behavior therapy—have been studied to determine their efficacy in the treatment of major depressive disorder. Although its efficacy in treating major depressive disorder is not as well researched as these three therapies, psychoanalytically oriented psychotherapy has long been used for depressive disorders, and many clinicians use the technique as their primary method. What differentiates the three short-term psychotherapy methods from the psychoanalytically oriented approach are the active and directive roles of the therapist, the directly recognizable goals, and the end points for short-term therapy.

Accumulating evidence is encouraging about the efficacy of dynamictherapy. In a randomized, controlled trial comparing psychodynamic therapy with cognitive behavior therapy, the outcome of the depressed patients was the same in the two treatments.

The National Institute of Mental Health(NIMH) treatment of depression collaborative research program found the following predictors of response to various treatments: low social dysfunction suggested a good response to interpersonal therapy, low cognitive dysfunction suggested a good response to cognitive–behavioral therapy and pharmacotherapy, high work dysfunction suggested a good response to pharmacotherapy, and high depression severity suggested a good response to interpersonal therapy and pharmacotherapy.

9.7.2.1　Cognitive therapy

Cognitive therapy, originally developed by Aaron Beck, focuses on the cognitive distortions postulated to be present in major depressive disorder. Such distortions include selective attention to the negative aspects of circumstances and unrealistically morbid inferences about consequences. For example, apathy and low energy result from a patient's expectation of failure in all areas. The goal of cognitive therapy is to alleviate depressive episodes and prevent recurrence by helping patients identify and test negative cognitions; develop alternative, flexible, and positive ways of thinking; and rehearse new cognitive and behavioral responses.

Studies have shown that cognitive therapy is effective in the treatment of major depressive disorder. Most studies found that cognitive therapy is equal in efficacy to pharmacotherapy and is associated with fewer adverse effects and better follow-up than pharmacotherapy. Some studies have indicated that the combination of cognitive therapy and pharmacotherapy is more efficacious than either therapy alone, although other studies have not found that additive effect. At least one study, the NIMH treatment of depression collaborative research program, found that pharmacotherapy, either alone or with psychotherapy, may be the treatment of choice for patients with severe major depressive episodes.

9.7.2.2　Interpersonal therapy

Interpersonal therapy, developed by Gerald Klerman, focuses on one or two of a patient's current interpersonal problems. This therapy is based on two theories. First, current interpersonal problems are likely to have their roots in early dysfunctional relationships. Second, current interpersonal problems are likely to be involved in precipitating or perpetuating the current depressive symptoms. Controlled trials have indicated that interpersonal therapy is effective in the treatment of major depressive disorder and, not surprisingly, may be specifically helpful in addressing interpersonal problems. Some studies indicate that interpersonal therapy may be the most effective method for severe major depressive episodes when the treatment choice is psychotherapy alone.

The interpersonal therapy program usually consists of 12-16 weekly sessions and is characterized byan active therapeutic approach. Intrapsychic phenomena, such as defense mechanisms and internal conflicts, are not addressed. Discrete behaviors — such as lack of assertiveness, impaired social skills, and distorted thinking — may be addressed but only in the context of interpersonal relationships.

9.7.2.3　Behavior therapy

Behavior therapy is based on the hypothesis that maladaptive behavioral patterns result in a person's receiving little positive feedback and perhaps outright rejection from society. By addressing maladaptive behaviors in therapy, patients learn to function in the world in such a way that they receive positive reinforcement. Behavior therapy for major depressive disorder has not yet been the subject of many controlled studies. The limited data indicate that it is an effective treatment for major depressive disorder.

9.7.2.4　Psychoanalytically oriented therapy

The psychoanalytic approach to mood disorders is based on psychoanalytic theories about depression and mania. The goal of psychoanalytic psychotherapy is to effect a change in a patient's personality structure or character, not simply to alleviate symptoms. Improvements in interpersonal trust, capacity for intimacy, coping mechanisms, the capacity to grieve, and the ability to experience a wide range of emotions are the aim of psychoanalytic therapy. Treatment often requires the patient to experience periods of anxiety and distress during the course of therapy, which may last for several years.

9.7.2.5　Family therapy

Family therapy is not generally viewed as a primary therapy for the treatment of major depressive disorder, but increasing evidence indicates that helping a patient with a mood disorder to reduce and cope with stress can lessen the chance of a relapse. Family therapy is indicated if the disorder jeopardizes a patient's marriage or family functioning or if the mood disorder is promoted or maintained by the family situation. Family therapy examines the role of the mood-disordered member in the overall psychological well-being of the whole family. It also examines the role of the entire family in the maintenance of the patient's symptoms. Patients with mood disorders have a high divorce rate, and about 50% of spouses report that they would not have married or had children if they had known that the patient was going to develop a mood disorder.

9.7.3 Vagal nerve stimulation

Experimental stimulation of the vagus nerve in several studies designed for the treatment of epilepsy found that patients showed improved mood. This observation led to the use of left vagal nerve stimulation (VNS) using an electronic device implanted in the skin, similar to a cardiac pacemaker. Preliminary studies have shown that a number of patients with chronic, recurrent major depressive disorder went into remission when treated with VNS. The mechanism of action of VNS to account for improvement is unknown. The vagus nerve connects to the enteric nervous system and, when stimulated, may cause release of peptides that act as neurotransmitters. Extensive clinical trials are being conducted to determine the efficacy of VNS.

9.7.4 Transcranial magnetic stimulation

Transcranial magnetic stimulation(TMS) shows promise as a treatment for depression. It involves the use of short pulses of magnetic energy to stimulate neurons in the brain. It is specifically indicated for the treatment of depression in adults who have failed to achieve satisfactory improvement from one prior antidepressant medication at or above the minimal effective dose and duration in the current episode.

Repetitive transcranial magnetic stimulation(rTMS) produces focal secondary electrical stimulation of targeted cortical regions. It is nonconvulsive, requires no anesthesia, has a safe side-effect profile, and is not associated with cognitive side-effects.

The patients do not require anesthesia or sedation and remain awake and alert. It is a 40-minute outpatient procedure that is prescribed by a psychiatrist and performed in a psychiatrist's office. The treatment is typically administered daily for 4-6 weeks. The most common adverse event related to treatment was scalp pain or discomfort.

TMS therapy is contraindicated in patients with implanted metallic devices or nonremovable metallic objects in or around the head.

9.7.5 Sleep deprivation

Mood disorders are characterized by sleep disturbance. Mania tends to be characterized by a decreased need for sleep, but depression can be associated with either hypersomnia or insomnia. Sleep deprivation may precipitate mania in patients with bipolar I disorder and temporarily relieve depression in those who have unipolar depression. Approximately 60% of patients with depressive disorders exhibit significant but transient benefits from total sleep deprivation. The positive results are typically reversed by the next night of sleep. Several strategies have been used in an attempt to achieve a more sustained response to sleep deprivation. One method used serial total sleep deprivation with a day or two of normal sleep in between. This method does not achieve a sustained antidepressant response because the depression tends to return with normal sleep cycles. Another approach used phase delay in the time patients go to sleep each night, or partial sleep deprivation. In this method, patients may stay awake from 2 A. M. to 10 P. M. daily. Up to 50% of patients get same-day antidepressant effects from partial sleep deprivation, but this benefit also tends to wear off in time. In some cases, however, serial partial sleep deprivation has been used successfully to treat insomnia associated with depression. The third, and probably most effective, strategy combines sleep deprivation with pharmacological treatment of depression. A number of studies have suggested that total and partial sleep deprivation followed by immediate treatment with an antidepressant or lithium (Eskalith) sustains the antidepressant effects of sleep deprivation. Likewise, several reports have suggested that sleep deprivation accelerates the response to antidepressants, including fluoxetine (Prozac) and nortriptyline (Aventyl, Pamelor). Sleep deprivation has also been noted to improve premenstrual dysphoria.

9.7.6　Phototherapy

Phototherapy was introduced in 1984 as a treatment for SAD (mood disorder with seasonal pattern). Patients typically experience depression as the photoperiod of the day decreases in winter. Women consist of at least 75% of all patients with seasonal depression, and the mean age of presentation is 40 years. Patients rarely present older than the age of 55 years with seasonal affective disorder.

Phototherapy typically involves exposing the affected patient to bright light in the range of 1,500 – 10,000 lux or more, typically with a light box that sits on a table or desk. Patients sit in front of the box for approximately 1–2 hours before dawn each day, although some patients may also benefit from exposure after dusk. Alternatively, some manufacturers have developed light visors, with a light source built into the brim of the hat. These light visors allow mobility, but recent controlled studies have questioned the use of this type of light exposure. Trials have typically lasted 1 week, but longer treatment durations may be associated with greater response.

Phototherapy is well-tolerated. New light sources tend to use lower light intensities and come equipped with filters; patients are instructed not to look directly at the light source. As with any effective antidepressant, phototherapy, on rare occasions, has been implicated in switching some depressed patients into mania or hypomania.

In addition to seasonal depression, the other major indication for phototherapy may be in sleep disorders. Phototherapy has been used to decrease the irritability and diminished functioning associated with shift work. Sleep disorders in geriatric patients have reportedly improved with exposure to bright light during the day. Likewise, some evidence suggests that jet lag might respond to light therapy. Preliminary data indicate that phototherapy may benefit some patients with OCD that has a seasonal variation.

9.7.7　Pharmacotherapy

After a diagnosis has been established, a pharmacological treatment strategy can be formulated. Accurate diagnosis is crucial because unipolar and bipolar spectrum disorders require different treatment regimens.

The objective of pharmacologic treatment is symptom remission, not just symptom reduction. Patients with residual symptoms, as opposed to full remission, are more likely to experience a relapse or recurrence of mood episodes and to experience ongoing impairment of daily functioning.

9.7.7.1　Major depressive disorder

The use of specific pharmacotherapy approximately doubles the chances that a depressed patient will recover in 1 month. All currently available antidepressants may take up to 3–4 weeks to exert significant therapeutic effects, although they may begin to show the effects earlier. Choice of antidepressants is determined by the side effect profile least objectionable to a given patient's physical status, temperament, and lifestyle. That numerous classes of antidepressants (Table 9–2) are available, many with different mechanisms of action, represents indirect evidence for heterogeneity of putative biochemical lesions. Although the first antidepressant drugs, the monoamine oxidase inhibitors(MAOIs) and tricyclic antidepressants(TCAs), are still in use, new compounds have made the treatment of depression more clinician and patient friendly.

Table 9-2　Antidepressant medications

Generic(brand) name	Usual daily dose/mg	Common side effects	Clinical caveats
(1)NE reuptake inhibitors			
Desipramine(Norpramin, Pertofrane)	75-300	Drowsiness, insomnia, OSH, agitation, CA, weight ↑, anticholinergic[a]	Overdose may be fatal. Dose titration is needed
Protriptyline(Vivactil)	20-60	Drowsiness, insomnia, OSH, agitation, CA, anticholinergic[a]	Overdose may be fatal. Dose titration is needed
Nortriptyline(Aventyl, Pamelor)	40-200	Drowsiness, OSH, CA, weight ↑, anticholinergic[a]	Overdose may be fatal. Dose titration is needed
Maprotiline(Ludiomil)	100-225	Drowsiness, CA, weight ↑, anticholinergic[a]	Overdose may be fatal. Dose titration is needed
(2)5-HT reuptake inhibitors			
Citalopram(Celexa)	20-60		Many SSRIs inhibit various cytochrome P450 isoen-zymes. They are better tolerated than tricyclics and have high safety in overdose. Shorter half-life SSRIs may be associated with discontinuation symptoms when abruptly stopped
Escitalopram(Lexapro)	10-20		
Fluoxetine(Prozac)	10-40		
Fluvoxamine(Luvox)[b]	100-300	All SSRIs may cause insomnia, agitation, sedation, GI distress, and sexual dysfunction	
Paroxetine(Paxil)	20-50		
Sertraline(Zoloft)	50-150		
Vortioxetine(Brintellix)	10-20		
(3)NE and 5-HT reuptake inhibitors			
Amitriptyline(Elavil, Endep)	75-300	Drowsiness, OSH, CA, weight ↑, anticholinergic[a]	Overdose may be fatal. Dose titration is needed
Doxepin(Triadapin, Sinequan)	75-300	Drowsiness, OSH, CA, weight ↑, anticholinergic[a]	Overdose may be fatal
Imipramine(Tofranil)	75-300	Drowsiness, insomnia and agitation, OSH, CA, GI distress, weight ↑, anticholinergic[a]	Overdose may be fatal. Dose titration needed
Trimipramine(Surmontil)	75-300	Drowsiness, OSH, CA, weight ↑, anticholinergic[a]	—
Venlafaxine(Effexor)	150-375	Sleep changes, GI distress, discontinuation syndrome	Higher doses may cause hypertension. Dose titration is needed. Abrupt discontinuation may result in discontinuation symptoms
Duloxetine(Cymbalta)	30-60	GI distress, discontinuation syndrome	—
(4)Pre-and postsynaptic active Agents			
Nefazodone	300-600	Sedation	Dose titration is needed. No sexual dysfunction
Mirtazapine(Remeron)	15-30	Sedation, weight ↑	No sexual dysfunction

Continue to Table 9-2

Generic(brand) name	Usual daily dose/mg	Common side effects	Clinical caveats
(5)Dopamine Reuptake Inhibitor			
Bupropion(Wellbutrin)	200-400	Insomnia or agitation, GI distress	Twice-a-day dosing with sustained release. No sexual dysfunction or weight gain
(6)Mixed Action Agents			
Amoxapine(Asendin)	100-600	Drowsiness, insomnia or agitation, CA, weight ↑, OSH, anticholinergic[a]	Movement disorders may occur. Dose titration is needed
Clomipramine(Anafranil)	75-300	Drowsiness, weight ↑	Dose titration is needed
Trazodone(Desyrel)	150-600	Drowsiness, OSH, CA, GI distress, weight ↑	Priapism is possible

Note; dose ranges are for adults in good general medical health, taking noother medications, and age 18-60 years. Doses vary depending on theagent, concomitant medications, the presence of general medical orsurgical conditions, age, genetic constitution, and other factors. Brandnames are those used in the United States.

CA, cardiac arrhythmia; 5-HT, serotonin; GI, gastrointestinal; NE, norepinephrine; OSH, orthostatic hypotension; SSRIs, selective serotonin-reuptake inhibitor.

[a] Dry mouth, blurred vision, urinary hesitancy, and constipation.

[b] Not approved as an antidepressant in the United States by the US Food and Drug Administration.

(1)General clinical guidelines

The most common clinical mistake leading to an unsuccessful trial of an antidepressant drug is the use of low a dosage for a short time. Unless adverse events prevent it, the dosage of an antidepressant should be raised to the maximum recommended level and maintained at that level for at least 4 or 5 weeks before a drug trial is considered unsuccessful. Alternatively, if a patient is improving clinically on a low dosage of the drug, this dosage should not be raised unless clinical improvement stops before maximal benefit is obtained. When a patient does not begin to respond to appropriate dosages of a drug after 2 or 3 weeks, clinicians may decide to obtain a plasma concentration of the drug if the test is available for the particular drug being used. The test may indicate either noncompliance or particularly unusual pharmacokinetic disposition of the drug and may thereby suggest an alternative dosage.

(2)Duration and prophylaxis

Antidepressant treatment should be maintained for at least 6 months or the length of a previous episode, whichever is greater. Prophylactic treatment with antidepressants is effective in reducing the number and severity of recurrences. One study concluded that when episodes are less than 2.5 years, prophylactic treatment for 5 years is probably indicated. Another factor suggesting prophylactic treatment is the seriousness of previous depressive episodes. Episodes that have involved significant suicidal ideation or impairment of psychosocial functioning may indicate that clinicians should consider prophylactic treatment. When antidepressant treatment is stopped, the drug dose should be tapered gradually over 1-2 weeks, depending on the half-life of the particular compound. Several studies indicate that maintenance antidepressant medication appears to be safe and effective for the treatment of chronic depression.

Prevention of new mood episodes (i.e., recurrences) is the aim of the maintenance phase of treatment. Only patients with recurrent or chronic depressions are candidates for maintenance treatment.

(3)Initial medication selection

The available antidepressantsdo not differ in overall efficacy, speed of response, or long-term effectiveness. Antidepressants, however, do differ in their pharmacology, drug interactions, short-term and long-term side effects, likelihood of discontinuation symptoms, and ease of dose adjustment. Failure to tolerate or to respond to one medication does not imply that other medications will also fail. Selection of the initial treatment depends on the chronicity of the condition, course of illness(a recurrent or chronic course is associated with increased likelihood of subsequent depressive symptoms without treatment), family history of illness and treatment response, symptom severity, concurrent general medical or other psychiatric conditions, prior treatment responses to other acute phase treatments, potential drug interactions, and patient preference. In general, approximately 45% -60% of outpatients with uncomplicated(i. e. , minimal psychiatric and general medical comorbidity), nonchronic, nonpsychotic major depressive disorder who begin treatment with medication respond(i. e. , achieve at least a 50% reduction in baseline symptoms). However, only 35% -50% achieve the standard of remission(i. e. , the virtual absence of depressive symptoms).

(4)Treatment of depressive subtypes

Clinical types of major depressive episodes may have varying responses to particular antidepressants or to drugs other than antidepressants. Patients with major depressive disorder with atypical features may preferentially respond to treatment with MAOIs or SSRIs. Antidepressants with dual action on both serotonergic and noradrenergic receptors demonstrate greater efficacy in melancholic depressions. Patients with seasonal depression can be treated with light therapy. Treatment of major depressive episodes with psychotic features may require a combination of an antidepressant and an atypical antipsychotic. Several studies have also shown that ECT is effective for this indication — perhaps more effective than pharmacotherapy. For those with atypical symptom features, strong evidence exists for the effectiveness of MAOIs. SSRIs and bupropion (Wellbutrin) are also of use in atypical depression.

(5)Comorbid disorders

The concurrent presence of another disorder can affect initial treatment selection. For example, the successful treatment of OCD associated with depressive symptoms usually results in remission of the depression. Similarly, when panic disorder occurs with major depression, medications with demonstrated efficacy in both conditions are preferred(e. g. , tricyclics and SSRIs). In general, the non-mood disorder dictates the choice of treatment in comorbid states.

Concurrent substance abuse raises the possibility of a substance-induced mood disorder, which must be evaluated by history or by requiring abstinence for several weeks. Abstinence often results inremission of depressive symptoms in substance-induced mood disorders. For those with continuing significant depressive symptoms, even with abstinence, an independent mood disorder is diagnosed and treated.

General medical conditions are established risk factors in the development of depression. The presence of a major depressive episode is associated with increased morbidity or mortality of many general medical conditions(e. g. , cardiovascular disease, diabetes, cerebrovascular disease, and cancer).

(6)Therapeutic use of side-effects

Choosing more sedating antidepressants[e. g. , amitriptyline (Elavil, Endep)] for more anxious, depressed patients or more activating agents(e. g. , desipramine) formore psychomotor-retarded patients is not generally helpful. For example, any short-term benefits with paroxetine, mirtazapine, oramitriptyline(more sedating drugs) on symptoms of anxiety orinsomnia may become liabilities over time. These drugs often continueto be sedating in the longer run, which can lead to patients prematurely discontinuing medication and increase the risk of relapseor recurrence. Some practitioners use adjunctive medications(e. g. , sleeping pills or anxiolytics) combined with antidepressants to providemore immediate symptom relief or to cover those side effects to whichmost patients ultimately adapt.

A patient's prior treatment history is important because an earlierresponse typically predicts current response. A documented failure on a properly conducted trial of a particular antidepressant class(e. g. ,SSRIs,tricyclics,or MAOIs) suggests choosing an agent from analternative class. The history of a first-degree relative responding to a particular drug is associated with a good response to the same class ofagents in the patient.

(7)Acute treatment failures

Patients may not respond to amedication,because:①they can not tolerate the side effects,even in the face of a good clinical response;②an idiosyncratic adverse event may occur;③the clinical response is not adequate;④wrong diagnosis has been made. Acute phase medication trials should last 4-6 weeks to determine if meaningful symptom reduction is attained. Most(but not all) patients who ultimately respond fully show at leasta partial response(i. e. ,at least a 20%-25% reduction inpretreatment depressive symptom severity) by week 4 if the dose is adequate during the initial weeks of treatment. Lack of a partial response by 4 to 6 weeks indicates that a treatment change is needed. Longer time periods — 8-12 weeks or longer — are needed to define the ultimate degree of symptom reduction achievable with amedication. Approximately half of patients require a second medication treatment trial because the initial treatment is poorly tolerated or ineffective.

(8)Selecting second treatment options

When the initialtreatment is unsuccessful,switching to an alternative treatment oraugmenting the current treatment is a common option. The choice between switching from the initial single treatment to a new single treatment(as opposed to adding a second treatment to the first one)rests on the patient's prior treatment history,the degree of benefit achieved with the initial treatment,and patient preference. As a rule, switching rather than augmenting is preferred after an initial medication failure. On the other hand,augmentation strategies are helpful with patients who have gained some benefit from the initial treatment but who have not achieved remission. The best-documented augmentation strategies involve lithium(Eskalith) or thyroidhormone. A combination of an SSRIs and bupropion(Wellbutrin) is also widely used. In fact,no combination strategy has been conclusively shown to be more effective than another. ECT is effectivein psychotic and nonpsychotic forms of depression but is recommended generally only for repeatedly nonresponsive cases or inpatients with very severe disorders.

A new therapy involves the use of the anesthetic agent ketamine,which has been shown to be effective in treatment resistant depression. It has a mechanism of action that inhibits the postsynaptic glutamate binding protein NDMA receptor. Because abnormalities inglutamatergic signaling have been implicated in major depressive disorder,this may account for its efficacy. Patients usually receive a single infusion of ketamine over a 30-minute period at a concentration of 0. 5 mg/kg. A positive response is usually seen within 24 hours,andimproved mood lasts for 2-7 days. The most common side-effects are dizziness,headache,and poor coordination,which are transitory. Dissociative symptoms,including hallucinations,may also occur.

(9)Combined trectment

Medication and formal psychotherapy are often combined in practice. If physicians view mood disorders as fundamentally evolving from psychodynamic issues,their ambivalence about the use of drugs may result in a poor response,non-compliance and probably inadequate dosages for a short treatment period. Alternatively,if physicians ignore the psychosocial needs of a patient,the outcome of pharmacotherapy may becompromised. Several trials of a combination of pharmacotherapy and psychotherapy for chronically depressed outpatients have shown a higher response and higher remission rates for the combination than for either treatment used alone.

9.7.7.2　Bipolar disorders

The pharmacological treatment of bipolar disorders is divided into both acute and maintenance phases. Bipolar treatment, however, also involves the formulation of different strategies for the patient who is experiencing mania, hypomania or depression. Lithium and its augmentation by antidepressants, antipsychotics, and benzodiazepines has been the major approach to the illness, but three anticonvulsant mood stabilizers — carbamazepine(Tegretol), valproate(Depakene), and lamotrigine(Lamictal) — have been added more recently, as well as a series of atypical antipsychotics, most of which are approved for the treatment of acute mania, for monotherapy of acute depression, and for prophylactic treatment. Each of these medications is associated with a unique side effect and safety profile, and no one drug is predictably effective for all patients. Often, it is necessary to try different medications before an optimal treatment is found.

(1)Treatment of acute mania

The treatment of acute mania, or hypomania, usually is the easiest phases of bipolar disorders to treat. Agents can be used alone or in combination to bring the patient down from a high. Patients with severe mania are best treated in the hospital where aggressive dosing is possible and an adequate response can be achieved within days or weeks. Adherence to treatment, however, is often a problem because patients with mania frequently lack insight of their illness and refuse medication. Because of the impaired judgment, impulsivity, and aggressiveness combine to put the patient or others at risk, many patients in the manic phase are medicated to protect themselves and others from harm.

1)Lithium carbonate

Lithium carbonate is considered the prototypical "mood stabilizer". Because the onset of antimanic action with lithium can be slow, it usually is supplemented in the early phases of treatment by atypical antipsychotics, mood-stabilizing anticonvulsants, or high-potency benzodiazepines. Therapeutic lithium levels are between 0.6 and 1.2 mEq/L. The introduction of newer drugs with more favorable side-effects, lower toxicity, and less need for frequent laboratory testing has resulted in adecline in lithium use. For many patients, however, its clinical benefits can be remarkable.

2)Valproate

Valproate[valproic acid (Depakene) or divalproex sodium (Depakote)]has surpassed lithium in use for acute mania. Unlike lithium, valproate is only indicated for acute mania, although most experts agree it also has prophylactic effects. Typical dose levels of valproic acid are 750–2,500 mg/d, achieving blood levels between 50 and 120 μg/mL. Rapid oral loading with 15–20 mg/kg of divalproex sodium from day 1 of treatment has been well to lerated and associated with a rapid onset of response. A number of laboratory testsare required during valproate treatment.

3)Carbamazepine and oxcarbazepine

Carbamazepine has been used as a first-line treatment for acute mania worldwide for decades but hadn't gained approval in the United States until 2004. Typical doses of carbamazepine to treat acute mania range between 600 and 1,800 mg/d associated with blood levels of between 4 and 12 μg/mL. The keto congener of carbamazepine, oxcarbazepine, may possess similar antimanic properties. Higher doses than those of carbamazepine arerequired because 1,500 mg of oxcarbazepine approximates 1,000 mg of carbamazepine.

4)Clonazepam and lorazepam

The high-potency benzodiazepine anticonvulsants used in acute mania include clonazepam(Klonopin) and lorazepam(Ativan). Both may be effective and are widely used for adjunctive treatment of acute manic agitation, insomnia, aggression, dysphoria, as well as panic. The safety and the benign side effect profile of these agents render them ideal adjuncts to lithium, carbamazepine, or valproate.

5) Atypical and typical antipsychotics

All of the atypical antipsychoticshave demonstrated antimanic efficacy and are approved by the Food and Drug Administration for this indication. Compared with olderagents, such as haloperidol(Haldol) and chlorpromazine(Thorazine), atypical antipsychotics have a lesser liability for excitatory postsynaptic potential and tardive dyskinesia; many do not increase prolactin. However, they have a wide range of substantial to no risk for weight gain with its associated problems of insulin resistance, diabetes, hyperlipidemia, hypercholesterolemia, and cardiovascular impairment. Some patients, however, require maintenance treatment with an antipsychotic medication.

(2) Treatment of acute bipolar depression

The relative usefulness of standard antidepressants in bipolar illness, in general, and in rapid cycling and mixed states, in particular, remains controversial because of their propensity to induce cycling, mania, or hypomania. Accordingly, antidepressants are often enhanced by a mood stabilizer in the first-line treatment for a first or isolated episode of bipolar depression. A fixed combination of olanzapine andfluoxetine(Symbyax) has been shown to be effective in treating acute bipolar depression for an 8-week period without inducing a switch tomania or hypomania.

Paradoxically, many patients with bipolar in the depressed phase do not respond to treatment with standard antidepressants. In these instances, lamotrigine or low-dose ziprasidone(20-80 mg per day) may be effective. Quetiapine or lurasidone may also be used.

Electroconvulsive therapy may also be useful for patients with bipolar depression who do not respond to lithium or other mood stabilizers and their adjuncts, particularly in cases in which intense suicidal tendency presents as a medical emergency.

Other agents: when standard treatments fail, other types of compounds may be applied. The calcium channel antagonistverapamil(Calan, Isoptin) has acute antimanic efficacy. Gabapentin, topiramate, zonisamide, levetiracetam, and tiagabine have not been shown to have acute antimania effects, although some patients may benefit from a trial of these agents when standard therapies have failed. Lamotrigine does not possess acute antimanic properties but does help prevent recurrence of manic episodes. Small studies suggest the potential acute antimanic and prophylactic efficacy of phenytoin. ECT is effective in acute mania. Bilateral treatments are required because unilateral, nondominant treatments have been reported to beineffective or even to exacerbate manic symptoms. ECT is reserved for patients with rare refractory mania and for patients with medical complications, as well as extreme exhaustion(malignant hyperthermia or lethal catatonia).

(3) Maintenance treatment of bipolar disorder

Preventing recurrences of mood episodes is the greatest challenge facing clinicians. Not only must the chosen regimen achieveits primary goal—sustained euthymia—but the medications should not produce unwanted side-effects that affect functioning. Sedation, cognitive impairment, tremor, weight gain, and rash are some side-effects that lead to treatment discontinuation.

Lithium, carbamazepine, and valproic acid, alone or in combination, are the most widely used agents in the long-term treatment of patients with bipolar disorder. Lamotrigine has prophylactic antidepressant, potentially, mood-stabilizing properties. Patients with bipolar disorder depression taking lamotrigine exhibit a rate of switch intomania that is the same as the rate with placebo. Lamotrigine appearsto have superior acute and prophylactic antidepressant properties compared with antimanic properties. Given that breakthrough depressions are a difficult problem during prophylaxis, lamotriginehas a unique therapeutic role. Very slow increases of lamotrigine help avoid the rare side effect of lethal rash. A dose of 200 mg/d appears to be the average in many studies. The incidence of severe rash(i. e. , Stevens-Johnson syndrome, a toxic epidermal necrolysis) is now thought to be approximately two in 10,000 adults and four in 10,000 children.

Thyroid supplementation is frequently necessary during long-termtreatment. Many patients treated with lithium develop hypothyroidism, and many patients with bipolar disorder haveidiopathic thyroid dysfunction. T3(25-50 μg/d), because of its short half-life, is often recommended for acute augmentation strategies, but T4 is frequently used for long-term maintenance. In some centers, hypermetabolic doses of thyroid hormone are used. Data indicate improvement in both manic and depressive phases with hypermetabolic T4-augmenting strategies. Table 9-3 summarizes the principles of treatment of bipolar disorders.

Table 9-3   Principles in the treatment of bipolar disorders

(1) Maintain dual treatment focus: acute short term and prophylaxis

(2) Chart illness retrospectively and prospectively

(3) Mania as medical emergency: treat first; chemistries later

(4) Load valproate and lithium(Eskalith); titrate lamotrigine(Lamictal) slowly

(5) Careful combination treatment can decrease adverse effects

(6) Augment rather than substitute in treatment-resistant patient

(7) Retain lithium in regimen for its antisuicide and neuroprotective effects

(8) Taper lithium slowly, if at all

(9) Educate patient and family about illness and risk-to-benefit ratios of acute and prophylactic treatments

(10) Give statistics(i. e. ,50% relapse in first 5 months off lithium)

(11) Assess compliance and suicidality regularly

(12) Develop an early warning system for identification and treatment of emergent symptoms

(13) Contract with patient as needed for suicide and substance use avoidance

(14) Use regular visits; monitor course and adverse effects

(15) Arrange for interval phone contact when needed

(16) Develop fire drill for mania re-emergence

(17) Inquire about and address comorbid alcohol and substance abuse

(18) Targeted psychotherapy; use medicalization of illness

(19) Treat patient as a coinvestigator in the development of effective clinical approaches to the illness

(20) If treatment is successful, be conservative in making changes, maintain the course, and continue full-dose pharmacoprophylaxis in absence of side effects

(21) If treatment response is inadequate, be aggressive in searching for more effective alternatives

Chen Ce

Chapter 10

Neurosis

10.1　Introduction

Neurosis is a group of mental disorders which common features are as follows. ①Onset of neuroses often associated with psychological and social factors. ②There are certain quality and personality features before the disease onset. ③Main symptoms include mood symptoms, obsessive–compulsive symptoms, hypochondriac symptoms, a variety of physical discomfort and so on. These symptoms, which often are mixed in different types of neuroses patients, affect the psychological function and social function to varying degrees although no evidence of organic disease and these symptoms are not commensurate with the reality. ④Patients without psychotic symptoms, the pain is obvious, and patients have a insight of disease and desire to seek treatment. ⑤Patients social function is relatively complete and their behavior is usually maintained within the scope of social norms. ⑥The course is more persistent.

The total prevalence of neuroses is about 5% worldwide. The prevalence of China in 1993 was 2.1%, and women(2.7%) were higher than men(2.67%). Neuroses always begin in the 16−35 age. This period is the most important period of life and career development stage which will have important and decisive impact on life.

10.2　Pathogenesis of neurosis

The etiology of neurosis is unknown. Its onset is often closely related to the individual genetic factors, life experiences, and psychological conflicts. It is generally agreed that external psychological factors combined with intrinsic quality factors are main causes of neurose and the two factors are causal.

10.2.1　Mental stress factors

For a long time, neuroses are considered to be a major mental disorder associated with psychosocial stress factors. Many studies have shown that patients with neuroses suffered more negative events than others such as poor interpersonal relationships, unharmonious marital and sexual relations, economic distress, family conflicts, job-related stress. On the one hand, individuals who suffer from mental events may be more susceptible to neuroses. On the other hand, the personality of neurosis patients may be more likely to feel "dissatisfied with life", more sensitive to life events or more likely to damage interpersonal communication resulting in more conflict and stress in life.

Stress events that cause neurosis have the following characteristics. ①The stress events is often not very strong, but repeated and durative. Although catastrophic intense stress events can also cause neuroses, daily trivia is more important factor. This is different characteristics from reactive mental disorders. ②Chronic stress events often have a special significance for the onset of neurosis. These life stress events may seem insignificant from the perspective of healthy people, but some neurosis are particularly sensitive to these. The key is not the positive and negative nature of the events but whether they cause individual inner conflicts. ③Patients with stress events caused by psychological difficulties or conflicts have a certain understanding and also efforts to adapt these events to eliminate the psychological impact from these events. However, the idea of patients always can not be changed into action to save themselves from the plight of the conflict and contradictions so that long-term persistence of stress. Ultimately, the stress is more than the protection provided by self-adaptability or social support leading to disease. ④Stress events of neurosis patients not only from the outside but also more from the psychological need. Neurosis patients are often rational, ethical, and traditional. They always ignore and suppress their own needs to adapt to environment, feel dissatisfied with others and their behavior, live with regret and inner contradictions. Therefore, the pain comes from the personality of patients.

10.2.2 Personality factors

Most researchers believe that personality traits or individual susceptibility are more important for the onset of neuroses compared psychosomatic events. Even biological etiology (such as genetics) also suggests that genetic effects of the parent were characterized by personality of susceptible. Generally, the personality characteristics of patients determine the degree of sensitivity to neuroses in the first. Pavlov believes that people whose nerve is weak, strong and uneven are susceptible to neuroses. Eysenck and others believe that people whose personality is old-fashioned, serious, sentimental, anxiety, pessimistic, conservative, sensitive, eccentric issusceptible to neurological disorders. Secondly, different personality characteristics determine the tendency to develop a particular type of neurological disorder. Pavlov also believes that people who are the weak type belonging to the art type (the first signal system is stronger than the second signal system) are susceptible to neurosis, belonging to thinking type (the first signal system is weaker than the second signal system) are susceptible to obsessive-compulsive disorder and belonging to the middle type (two signal systems are balanced) are susceptible to neurasthenia. Even some special personality types are same as those neuroses subtypes such as compulsive personality and obsessive-compulsive disorder.

10.2.3 Biological factors

Neuroses are a group of mental disorders that are unexplained. Biological studies have shown that some changes in the structure or function of the central nervous system may be related to the occurrence of neuroses. The enhancement of central norepinephrine and serotonin activity and the lack of function of inhibitory amino acids (such as γ-aminobutyric acid) may be associated with anxiety disorders. The reduction of central serotonin may be associated with obsessive-compulsive disorder and depression disorder. Some obsessive-compulsive disorder patients be found bilateral caudate nucleus volume reduction by brain CT and MRI. However, the study results of different scholars are inconsistent. It is inconclusive that these changes are the cause or the results. The pathogenesis of neuroses has a long history and different psycho-genres have different interpretations about that, and these theories have different curative effects on neuroses.

10.3 Clinical features, diagnosis and treatments of neurosis

10.3.1 Clinical features

The clinical manifestations of neurosis are complex. Different symptoms have different levels of severity and are mixed in different subtypes. Common symptoms are as follows.

10.3.1.1 Brain disorders symptoms

(1) Excitable spirit

It has three main characteristics. ①Association and memories increased. The patients are easy to cause mental excitement in daily life, including work, study or rest, manifesting as the memory and association increased but messy, repeated thinking. The patients know that woolgather do not make sense, want to control, but can not control causing psychological conflict and feel pain. ②Diversion of attention. The patients can easily be attracted by subtle changes in environment so that they are difficult to focus. On the other hand, the patients can not focus on a particular topic so that associations and memories continually lead thinking to the astray way. ③Enhanced feeling. The patients are particularly sensitive to sound and light. The general noise is unbearable for them. Them may have photophobia and like working or learning in a darker place, also like putting down the curtainsin daylight. The patients feel more about their own body. They feel a tight sense in chest when breathing, feel tachycardia and asthma when moving. These symptoms often appear in neurasthenia, anxiety disorder and so on.

(2) Mental fatigue

The patients mainly manifest as decreased energy and fatigue after a short period of work. Serious patients have thinking difficulties, inattention, confusion, poor memory and low efficiency in work and learning. However, this fatigue is not accompanied by motivation diminished. These symptoms often appear in neurasthenia and so on.

10.3.1.2 Emotional symptoms

(1) Anxious

The most common symptoms in neurosis. It is extremely disturbing status without reason, a kind of endless anxiety. The clinical manifestations are tension, anxiety and panic, accompanied by autonomic nervous system dysfunction and exercise anxiety. Forms of clinical manifestations are continuity and intermittent. The latter also known as panic attack that is an extreme anxiety accompanied by suffocation, dying and self-uncontrol. It can attack in the context of chronic anxiety or attack single. Some patients have a normal emotion in the interval. Some patients will anxiety persistently worry about the next attack.

(2) Irritability

A state which easy to provoke an emotion. The patients feel anger, rage, and quarrel with another because of a small thing but regrets later. They are often self-repressed, but erupt again after suppressed a certain time. It is so-called "trilogy".

（3）Depression

Depression in neuropathy always is less severe. The patients often showed lack of confidence, interest decrease, hopeless, loss of libido, appetite and fatigue, feeling weakness, chronic pain and so on. These symptoms are not serious but always fluctuate and persistent.

（4）Fear

It is a normal protective emotional response. It can remind individuals to make a decision to escape or duel as soon as possible in danger. Fear symptom refers to an unreasonable fear of normal objective stimulus. The patients know that the mood is absurd and unnecessary, but can not escape. Fear symptom is the main clinical manifestation of phobia, accompanied by a series of autonomic nervous symptoms, such as flushing or pale, breathing and heart rate faster, fluctuation of blood pressure and so on.

10.3.1.3   Obsession and compulsion

Obsession and compulsion refers to concept, impulse or behavior appeared over and over again. The patients are very painful, as they know it is unnecessary but can not get rid of it. The symptoms include the following three categories.

（1）Obsessive idea

The patients repeatedly think about the same concept, they know it is unnecessary but can not get rid of it, such as "Which came first, the chicken or the egg?" or repeatedly doubt and recall about what they have done.

（2）Obsessive intention

It is a compulsive impulse which not yet put into action. The patients feel a strong driving force drive themself do something which violate their own wishes such as there is "jumping" impulse when they stand on the high building.

（3）Compulsive behavior

The common behaviors include compulsive washing, compulsive counting, compulsive examination and compulsive ritual such as patients wash their hands more than ten times a day and tens of minutes every time. They know it is unnecessary and too much but can not get rid of it. They will get upset if they not wash their hands. Obsession and compulsion often appear inobsessive—compulsive disorder or other neuroses.

10.3.1.4   Hypochondriac symptoms

The patients are overly concerned with their health or certain body functions and suspect that they have some kind of physical or mental illness. The repeatedly explain of doctor and repeated medical examination can not eliminate the hypochondria. They see a doctor and make medical examination repeatedly. Hypochondriac symptoms often appear in hypochondria or other neuroses.

10.3.1.5   Physical symptoms

Neuroses patients have many physical symptoms and seek medical attention in various clinical departments. Main symptoms are chronic pain, system symptoms caused by autonomic nervous system dysfunction.

（1）Chronic pain

It is a clinically common symptom. It may indicate a potential organic damage, a tense mental state, even a waywhich contact others' attention, emotion and interpersonal relationships. Pain often appears in head and neck. Secondly, pain appears in the lower back, limbs. The pain always is persistent or fluctuant.

（2）Dizziness

It is one of the common complaints in neurosis. The patients describe as "giddy" "brain is unclear". Dizziness is accompanied by headache and head swelling. Meanwhile, the patients have unclear mind, memory loss, analysis of comprehensive ability reduced. Dizziness is actually a comprehensive description of a variety of symptoms.

（3）Autonomic nervous system symptoms

Function of nerve is regulate the activities of internal organs to body and environmental change. The autonomic nervous system of neuroses patients dysfunction showing a lot of physical symptoms such as anxiety patients have sympathetic hyperfunction symptoms including palpitation, tachycardia or bradycardia, frequent urination, urgent urination, sweating, dry mouth, abdominal pain, and diarrhea.

10.3.1.6   Somnipathy

Somnipathy is the common symptom of neurosis, especially insomnia. Insomnia is mainly manifested as short sleep time or poorsleep quality, or lack of self-satisfaction sleep. Insomnia is generally divided into three forms: difficulty falling asleep, easy waking up, waking up in early. Patients with neuroses are more likely to have difficulty falling asleep. The patients mostly are psychogenic somnipathy. They often worry about "may not sleep tonight" "how is work tomorrow" before go to bed. They are very nervous. They are trying to fall asleep, such as numbering in heart, excluding distractions and so on. Inversely, the more nervous they became, the more they can not sleep. This is expectancy anxiety and affects sleep badly. The patients prolong the latency of sleep because of complicated thinking, anxiety and muscle tension. Even if they barely fall asleep, they also think they are hard to sleep, easy to wake up, short sleep time, shallow sleep and more dreams. They feel sleepy, drowsy and hard during the day. The study also showed that some patients with neuroses had short sleep time in reality.

Other somnipathy are rare in neuroses including nightmare, night terror, sleep-walking and so on.

10.3.2   Diagnosis

The diagnosis of neurosis is based on the diagnostic criteria of international psychiatric classification. The diagnostic criteria include the general criteria and sub-standard criteria. Any sub-standard criteria must meet the general criteria. The following Table 10-1 shows the coding of diagnosis of neuroses in ICD-10.

Table 10-1   The comparison of diagnosis of neurosis in ICD-10 and the textbook

ICD-10	The textbook
F40 Phobic	10.3 Phobic
F41 Other anxiety disorders	
F41.0 Panic disorder	10.4 Panic disorder
F41.1 General anxiety disorder	10.5 General anxiety disorder
F42 Obsessive-compulsive disorder	10.6 Obsessive-compulsive disorder
F45 Somatoform disorder	10.7 Somatoform disorder
F48 Other neuroses	
F48.0 Neurasthenia	10.8 Neurasthenia

Neuroses are a group of mental disorders characterized primarily as anxiety, depression, fear, compulsion, hypochondriasis or neurasthenia. The symptoms have a certain personality basis and often affected by social environment. The symptoms are not based on verifiable organic disease and are not commensurate with the real situation of patient. However, the patients are painful and incompetent to the symptoms. Insight of the patients are integrity or basic integrity. The course is procrastinated.

10.3.2.1   Symptom criteria

At least one of the following: fear, obsession and compulsion, panic attack, anxiety, somatoform, somatization, hypochondriac symptoms, neurasthenie symptoms.

10.3.2.2   Severity criteria

Social function of the patients are damaged. They can not get rid of the psychic pain. The symptoms can promote them to seek medical treatment initiatively.

10.3.2.3   Time criteria

The symptoms persist for 3 months at least. Panic has other criteria.

10.3.2.4   Exclusion criteria

Organic mental disorders, mental disorders which caused by psychoactive substances and non-addictive substances, various mental disorders(such as schizophrenia and paranoid mental disorders), mood disorders should be excluded.

On the other hand, various neuroses or their combinations can be found in infections, poisoning, visceral diseases, endocrine diseases, metabolic diseases and brain organic diseases. These are called neurological disorder syndrome.

10.3.3   Treatment

Treatments of neurosis includes drug therapy and psychotherapy. In general, drug therapy is effective in controlling symptoms. But psychological treatment is equally important because occurrence of neurosis are closely related to psychosocial factors and personality traits. Psychiatric treatment of neuroses should be based on the specific treatment purpose.

10.3.3.1   Psychotherapy

(1)The purpose of psychotherapy is to reduce the burden and pain on patients and provide general support for the consolidating treatment. The main methods of psychotherapy include psychological conversation, psychological counseling, long-term guidance, supportive psychotherapy and relaxation therapy.

(2)The purpose of psychotherapy is to change behavior of the patients, relieve symptoms, change the conditions and thinking. It includes a variety of behavioral therapy and some operational treatment.

(3)The purpose of psychotherapy is to enhance judgments of the patient ability to resolve conflicts, change attitudes and promote mental maturity. The basic treatment is psychodynamic psychotherapy. It paves the way for further psychological treatment by eliminating symptoms and stabilizing personality.

(4)Effective treatment be determined and adjusted in work according to the type and severity of the mental disorder of patients, the personality structure, the living condition, the motivation and experience in past treatment, the level and experience of the psychological training of the psychotherapist. It can also be worked in the form of group therapy, twin therapy and family therapy.

10.3.3.2   Drug treatment

In addition to psychological treatment, we also consider the applicability of physical and drug treatment. It is important to carefully assess the severity, type, and psychiatric use of patients with neuroses. For neuroses patients with fear, depression, anxiety and compulsion, antidepressants and benzodiazepine drugs should be used in time to relieve symptoms. There are many types of drugs to treat neurological disorders, such as anxiolytic drugs, antidepressants and brain metabolism promoting drugs. Drugs should be selected by symptoms of the patients. The advantage of drug treatment is to control the target symptoms rapidly. It combines with psychological therapy having aid in relieving symptoms, improving confidence, promoting psychological treatment effect and patient compliance behavior. Medication and the possible side effects must be explained to the patient before the treatment so that the patients have fully psychological prepared. The aim is to increase patient compliance and avoid patients giving up treatment or frequent changes in treatment programs due to diligence sensitive, anxiety and hypochondriacal in treatment programs. It is not conducive to rehabilitation of patients.

10.4 Phobia

A phobia is a type of disorder defined by a persistent and excessive fear of an object or situation. Those affected will go to great lengths to avoid the situation or object, to a degree greater than the actual danger posed. Phobia affects their normal activities. In 1982, a epidemiological survey of neurosess ackess 12 regions showed that the prevalence of phobia was 0.59‰ and the prevalence of urban and rural areas was similar. In 1996, Magee et al reported that the lifetime prevalence of three subtypes of phobia in the United States was 6.7% (square phobia), 13.3% (social phobia) and 11.3% (special phobia). Women are more likely to be affected by phobia than men. The highest prevalence of the crowd is 25-44 age. The most age of onset is about 20 years old. Phobia patients account for about 5% in neuroses specialist clinics.

Most of course of phobia patients is delay. There is a trend to chronic development. The longer the course, the worse the prognosis. Children and single phobia patients have better prognosis. The phobia patients who fear several objects have worse prognosis.

10.4.1 Etiology and pathogenesis

10.4.1.1 Genetic factors

Square phobia has a family genetic predisposition. In particular, it affects female more than male. The reason is unclear. The twin study also suggested that square phobia may be related to inheritance. There is a certain connection with panic disorder. Some specific phobia have obvious genetic predisposition such as blood and injection phobia. About 2/3 biological relatives of the patients have the same disease. The response of average person to terrifying stimuli is different from the response of phobia patients. Phobia patients show bradycardia rather than tachycardia and prone to syncope.

10.4.1.2 Neurobiology

Some studies found that plasma epinephrine of patients with social phobia increased when they suffered from fear. Through the experiment which clonidine caused growth hormone unresponsive, the social phobia patients accompanied by norepinephrine dysfunction are determined.

10.4.1.3 Psychosocial factors

In the early 19th century, the United States psychologists explained the mechanism of phobia by the conditional reflex. They thought that the expansion and persistence of the symptoms of phobia is caused by the recurrence of symptoms make anxiety conditionalization and avoidance behaviors hinder the subsidence of anxiety conditionalization. This is also the theoretical basis of behavioral therapy. Freud viewed fear as a result of a sexual conflict that originated in childhood. In his view, fear comes from the self-dangerous response and the level of response is due to the initial attribution. Thus, the evocation of this dangerous experience is due to the influence of the external context, the internal drive, the frustration and rejection of the self. Fear as a signal that the self in trying to prevent that the subconscious drive causes the frustration experience of consciousness to allowing the self effectively monitor and manage the instinct that caused the frustration experience. Phobia also is known as "anxiety hysteria" in theory of freud. That is due to the oedipus conflict in early childhood. In adulthood, the internal drive continues to show a strong oedipus or erosconflict which provoke a castrated anxiety. Poor social environment, poor family and school education can become the cause of phobia. The inappropriate behavior of parents and educational methods, especially the parents of spoil, scare and threat are mainly cause. In addition, the disharmony the between family members will also bring panic and anxiety to the child.

10.4.2　Clinical features

Case report:

Linda is a 23 year old girl. She is nervous in daily interactions with others and does not dare to look directly at others. When she communicates with strangers, she is flustered, red-faced, short of breath, and trembling. Knowing that it is a psychological problem, but it is difficult to control, seriously affecting daily work and life, and nothing happens when she is alone. Her parents said, "she was introverted, unsociable, unsocial and sensitive to things. Their excessive love makes her more pampered. She was ranked among the best in primary grades, and people around her praised her, which gradually formed her self-centered personality. She thought she was perfect, stronger than other peers, and should be praised and favored. However, once she spoke, she made a mistake and caused the classmates laughing. After returning home, she became dumb and lasted for a long time. Since then, her academic performance begun to decline, and she has been afraid to go out, do not dare to associate with others."

Hundreds of phobia objects are found in the literature. Usually, they can be classfied into three categories.

10.4.2.1　Agoraphobia

It also known as square phobia, wilderness phobia, party phobia. It is the most common kind of phobia, about 60%. The disease occurs in about 25 years old and about 35 years old is another peak age. Women are more likely to have agoraphobia than men. Mainly manifestation of phobia is fear of specific circumstances such as height, open spaces, closed environment and crowded public places. The patients fear for entering the store, theater, station or public transport. Patients are worried that they feel fear in these places, can't get help and can't escape lead them to try to avoid these environments. Phobia often accompanied by depression, obsession and compulsion, personality disintegration and other symptoms.

10.4.2.2　Social phobia

Social phobia mostly occurs at the age of 17 – 30. It often have no obvious cause and suddenly happen. It often have no obvious incentive and onset suddenly. The main performance is the patients avoid social as they feel shy, cramped, embarrassed and clumsy. They are afraid to be ridiculed in front of others in social activities or work. They feel tension, fear and blush before the social contact. Once they have socializing with others, they immediately appear uncontrollable blush, palpitation, embarrassed and want to immediately leave the situations. The patients have a strong desire to interact with others but they are afraid of interacting with others. The patients form psychological conflict and feel miserable. Some patients are afraid of look at each other. They think that others know their inner misconduct and despise as long as eye contact. Some patients think they have malicious eyesight that will hurt each other and not dare to face with others(red face fear). Some patients are afraid to interact with people because they think they can not control the behavior of secretly observing people will be found by others and the people think they are not serious(eye fear). Some patients not want to go to public places for fear of eating or urinating in public.

The object of social phobia can be acquaintances, relatives or people who do not know. The more common fear of the object is the same age of the opposite sex, severe boss, parents of fiancee and so on. When a patient is forced into a social occasion, he or she will be anxious seriously.

10.4.2.3 Specific phobia

It also known as a simple phobia. It refers to patients have an unreasonable fear of a specific object or animal. The most common fear object is animal or insect, such as snakes, dogs, cats, rats, spiders, worms, caterpillars and so on. Some patients are afraid of blood or sharp items. Some patients are fear of natural phenomena, such as darkness, wind, thunder, lightening. The symptoms of a specific phobia are constant. It limits to a particular object. It is neither change nor generalization. Some patients may have eliminated the fear of an object but emerge a new fear object. Specific phobia often begins in childhood. Women are more likely to have specific phobia.

10.4.3 Diagnosis and differential diagnosis

Characters of phobia are unreasonable fear of particular object or scenario and the patients avoid fear object actively.

10.4.3.1 Diagnostic criteria

(1)Meeting the diagnostic criteria of neuroses.

(2)The main feature are as follow. ①There are strong fear of a certain object or situation. The degree of fear and the actual risk are not commensurate. ②There are anxiety and autonomic nerve symptoms and continuous avoidance behavior. ③Fear is unreasonable and unnecessary, but uncontrol.

(3)The avoidance of fear scenes and things must be or have been prominent symptoms.

(4)Exclusion of anxiety disorders, schizophrenia and hypochondria.

10.4.3.2 Differential diagnosis

Phobia should be identified with the following diseases.

(1)Anxiety disorder

Main symptoms of phobia and anxiety disorder are anxiety. But the anxiety in phobia caused by a specific object or situation is situationality and paroxysmal. To reduce the anxiety, the phobia patients have reduplicative avoidance behavior. The anxiety patients have no obvious object of anxiety and anxiety is persistent.

(2)Obsessive-compulsive disorder

Fear of obsessive-compulsive disorder stems from some thoughts or ideas in the heart. The patients are fear of losing self-control, not fear of the environment.

(3)Hypochondriasis

Phobia patients who is fear of disease may be similar to hypochondriasis patients. But the fear of hypochondriasis patients is not prominent and they think that their concerns are reasonable. The fear object of anxiety disorder patients is external. They think that their fear are unreasonable and can not get rid of it.

10.4.4   Treatments

10.4.4.1   Psychotherapy

It is one of the important treatments in this disease. The common treatments include system desensitization, exposure or shock therapy and muscle relaxation training.

10.4.4.2   Pharmacotherapy

Anxiolytics and antidepressants can be used to treat phobia. Their mainly effect is to relieve anxiety and depression. One good effect on social phobia patients is to give 20–40 mg a day of paroxetine or 50–150 mg a day of sertraline. To alleviate anxiety symptoms, benzodiazepine drugs such as alprazolam or lorazepam can be added. Pharmacotherapy combined with psychotherapy is good for shortening the course of treatment, improving treatment confidence, reducing recurrence.

10.5   Panic disorder

Panic disorder is also known as acute anxiety disorder. Panic disorder patients repeatedly appear significant palpitations, sweating, tremor and other autonomic symptoms accompanied by a strong sense of nearness or uncontrollability. Panic disorder characterized by unpredictability and uncontrollability. The patients have a strong response such as anxiety, tension and fear for worried catastrophic end but often stop quickly.

The lifelong prevalence of panic disorder is about 2%–4%. In the 1980s, a epidemiological survey of adults found that the lifetime prevalence of panic attacks was 3.6% and the lifetime prevalence of panic disorder was about 1.5% in the United States. The data showed that 9%–10% of people have experienced of panic attack. Most of the patients rehabilitate without treatment. A few patients developed into panic disorder. In the 1990s, another survey showed that the lifetime prevalence of panic disorder was 3.5% in the United States. Women are more likely to have panic disorder. The ratio of female to male was 5 : 2 (Kessler, et al. 1994). Panic disorder often begins in the late adolescence or early adulthood. The age range is 15–40 years. The average age of onset is 25 years.

10.5.1   Etiology and pathogenesis

10.5.1.1   Genetic factors

The genetic research of the disease has involved in many content. In the family survey, Crowe, Harris, Crow, et al. (1983) respectively found that the risk of the disease of first–degree relatives of the patient were 24.7%, 20% and 17.3% and the risk of the disease of first–degree relatives of the normal were 2.3%, 4.8% and 1.8%. The results showed that panic disorder had familial aggregation. Torgersen(1983) reported that a twin study on panic disorder with MZ than DZ rate of with 5 times but the rate of panic disorder with MZ only is 31%. This suggested that non–genetic factors on the occurrence of the disease play an important role.

10.5.1.2   Neurobiological factors

Sodium lactate and yohimbine is easy to induce panic attacks. During panic attacks, patients show palpitations, trembling, sweating and other symptoms of a large number β–adrenergic receptor excitement. β–adrenergic receptor blockers such as propranolol have the effect of reducing panic attacks and anxiety. The

5-HT system plays an important role in panic disorder evidenced by the efficacy of antidepressants in panic disorder.

10.5.1.3 Psychosocial factors

Traumatic or negative life events and the formation of childhood and adulthood are significantly related to panic disorder. Patients with panic disorder are more sensitive to post-traumatic stress, especially involving the separation and attachment relationship rupture. It suggests that the parental attachment rupture of childhood is related to panic disorder of adulthood. Recent traumatic stress can play a role in panic attacks. The interaction of life events and genetic susceptibility are the underlying cause of panic disorder of adulthood.

10.5.2 Clinical features

Case report:

Helen is a 42-year-old woman. Two years ago, she had episodes of palpitation, chest tightness, and shortness of breath due to family conflicts. It lasted for a few minutes to 10 minutes and self-reliefed. This situation is closely related to emotions, with nervousness, worry, fear, and trembling. These symptoms were recurrent. Her physical examination showed no obvious abnormalities. During the episode, she was worried about the next symptom recurrence. Three days ago, she had no obvious cause of the above symptoms, feeling flustered, chest tightness, difficulty breathing, cold back, limbs shaking, numbness, stiffness, sudden death, accompanied by nervousness, worry, fear. The attack lasted a long time, ranging from a few minutes to an hour, and improved after oxygen inhalation and rehydration therapy in emergency department.

A strong panic experience suddenly emerge in the daily living environment without special fear accompanied by the feel of dying, losing control and serious autonomic nervous system symptoms. The patients often scream, cry or run as extremely nervous, fear, unbearable and feel of choking death while a strong heart palpitations, chest pain and tightness, precordial sense of oppression, breathing difficult and throat obstruction. Someone have over-ventilated, headache, dizziness, sweating, pale or flushing, gait instability, hand and foot tremor, numbness and other autonomic symptoms. The onset of panic attacks usually is acute. The process takes about 5-20 minutes and more than 1 hour rarely. After panic attacks, the patients take a few days to recover. In interrupted interval, 60% patients have evasive behavior such as not alone to go out and not to go many places for the expected anxiety which fear of panic attacks relapse but with help.

In addition to the aforementioned symptoms, panic attacks at least 3 times in 1 month or the anxiety of fear of recurrence for 1 month after the first episode. The long-term prognosis of panic disorder is good. 40% patients comorbid depression which lead to a worse prognosis of panic disorder. Substance abuse, especially alcohol abuse, increases in patients with panic disorder. About 7% patients may have suicidal behavior.

10.5.3 Diagnosis and differential diagnosis

10.5.3.1 Diagnostic criteria

According to the diagnostic criteria of ICD-10, the diagnostic basis of panic disorder is the attack has at least 3 times in 1 month and every time no more than 2 hours. The attack impacts daily activities. The intermittent period between the two attacks not have obvious other symptoms except for fear of recurrence. In addition to this, panic disorder has the following characteristics.

(1) There is no real danger in the episode of attacks.

(2) The attack is not limited to known or predictable circumstances.

(3)There are almost no anxiety symptoms in the intermittent period of panic attacks.

(4)The attack is not the result of physical fatigue physical disease(such as hyperthyroidism) or substance abuse.

10.5.3.2 Differential diagnosis

(1)Panic attacks can not be caused by physical diseases, such as heart disease, hyperthyroidism, epilepsy, transient ischemic attack, pheochromocytoma or hypoglycemia. EEG and myocardial enzymes are necessary for patients who are suspected of being heart attack.

(2)Panic attacks may occur in phobia, such as agoraphobia, social phobia and specific phobia. We do not make the diagnosis of panic disorder under the circumstances. Only unpredictable panic attacks make the diagnosis of panic disorder.

(3)Panic disorder can be secondary to depression, especially men. If the patients meet the diagnostic criteria for depression at the same time, panic disorder should not as the main diagnosis.

10.5.4 Treatments

The goal of treatment for panic disorder is to reduce or eliminate panic attacks, improve anxiety and avoidance behavior and improve quality of life. At the beginning of treatment, we should tell the patient panic attacks are the result of physiological and psychological disorders. The physical symptoms usually do not lead to life-threatening. Pharmacotherapy and psychotherapy are effective.

10.5.4.1 Pharmacotherapy

Benzodiazepine drugs(BZD) take effect rapidly. Alprazolam or clonazepam also can be used to treat panic disorderbut long – term use easily lead to substance dependence. The conventional drug is alprazolam. itspotency at treatment dose than diazepam and its sedative effect is weaker. It takes 2–3 weeks to increase the amount of medicine. Withdrawal medication needs to be slow. It generally takes more than 6 weeks.

Tricyclic antidepressants(TCAs)are also used to treat panic disorders. Daily dose of imipramine is 50–300 mg. The dose begins to a small dose with 10 mg or 25 mg and gradually be increased. It often works at 150 mg/d. Chlorpheniramine can also be used to treat panic disorder with 25–200 mg/d. However, the dose need to begin to a small dose due to tricyclic antidepressants have more adverse reactions. The excessive dose is easy to lead to poison.

Serotonin reuptake inhibitors(SSRIs), serotonin and norepinephrine reuptake inhibitors(SNRIs), norepinephrine and specific serotonin reuptake inhibitors(NaRIs) are effective with the treatment for panic disorder. As a result of broad spectrum of them, their roles are more appropriate when panic disorder comorbid depression, social anxiety disorder, generalized anxiety disorder, post-traumatic stress disorder or substance abuse. The common drugs include paroxetine(20–60 mg/d) fluoxetine(5–20 mg/d), sertraline(50–150 mg/d), fluvoxamine(150 mg/d), venlafaxine and its sustained-release tablet and mirtazapine(taking in morning) to take control of panic attacks. It usually takes 2–3 weeks to work and no havesubstance abuse and dependence. Long-term use of SSRIs can significantly reduce resuscitation rate of the patients.

Clinically, BZD combined with SSRIs is used to improve patients with panic disorder faster than SSRIs alone but BZD can be reduced after 5–6 weeks to avoid short comings of the long-term use of BZD and the early effects of SSRIs.

10.5.4.2 Cognitive behavior therapy

The first thing for therapies is helping the patients to understand the process of panic attacks and the intermittent situation. The patient exposure to panic attacks by meditation to eliminate the response of various autonomic nervous of patients. The method of situational therapy is takes on-site exposure to make patients to gradually adapting fear to alleviate avoidance behavior and subsequent agoraphobia. In accordance with the order from top to bottom to shrink and relax the muscles of head and face, upper limb, chest, abdomen and lower limbs to reduce anxiety. The other methods are instruct patients some knowledge about breathing exercise, relaxing body muscles, regulating breathing, omphaloskepsis, eliminating distractions and so on. Cognitive reorganization: reasonable explanation of the physical sensation and emotional experience of patients can make them realize their feeling and experience are advantageous and will not cause serious damage to health.

10.6   Generalized anxiety disorder

General anxiety disorder(GAD) is a generalized and persistent anxiety and not limited to a specific external environment. The symptoms is changeable. The patients always feel nerves and muscle tension, trembling, exercise anxiety, sweating, top-heavy, palpitations, dizziness and epigastric discomfort. Patients often feel that they or their loved ones will suffer from serious illness or catastrophe. The anxiety often associated with psychological and social stress. Disease fluctuations of the disease is chronic.

In 12 districts across the country, the epidemiological survey(1982) of neuroses showed that the prevalence of generalized anxiety disorder was 0.148%. Women are more likely to have GAD than men. The ratio of female to male was about 2 : 1. GAD mostly beginsat 20-40 age. The prognosis of GAD is largely related to individual quality. In general, the patients who have short course of disease, mild symptoms, good social adaptability before the disease and no obvious defects of indications have better prognosis.

10.6.1   Etiology and pathogenesis

10.6.1.1   Genetic factors

Heredity plays an important role in the occurrence of anxiety disorder. The comorbidity rate of anxiety disorder is 15% in the blood relatives much higher than the normal residents. The comorbidity rate of anxiety disorderis 2.5% in dizygotic twins. The comorbidity rate of anxiety disorderis 50% in monozygotic twins. Someone think that anxiety disorder result in environmental factors and susceptible factors. The susceptible factors are determined by heredity.

10.6.1.2   Pre-morbid personality

Pre-morbid personality includes low self-esteem and self-confidence, cowardice, prudence and tension for slight frustration or physical discomfort, anxiety, mood swings.

10.6.1.3   Mental factors

Mental factors such as slight setback and dissatisfaction can induce anxiety disorder.

10.6.1.4   Biological factors

The physiological basis of anxiety response is sympathetic and parasympathetic nervous system often activation accompanied by adrenaline and norepinephrine excessive release. Somatic symptom is determined by the balance between sympathetic and parasympathetic nervous. There are different views on the pathogenesis of anxiety disorder. Some scholars emphasized the connection between emotional centers (such as amygdala hypothalamus) and anxiety disorder. It supported by a discovery which benzodiazepine receptor be found in the limbic system and neocortex. Some scholars suggested that β−adrenergic blockers can effectively improve physical symptoms and relieve anxiety. The psychoanalysis school suggested that anxiety disorder is due to the threat from excessive self−conflict. Based on the theory of learning, some scholars believed that anxiety is a habitual behavior which the connection between anxiety stimulation and neutral stimulation lead to generalization of the stimulation and formation of general anxiety. Lader suggested that heredity is the important physiology and psychology basis of this disease. Once strong anxiety response arisen, the environment strengthening or self−strengthening formed anxiety disorder.

10.6.2   Clinical features

Case report：

Melody is a 45−year−old woman. After her husband died year ago, she was in a bad mood, upset, fidgety and nervous panic. She became irritable, angry, worried about bad things, and tried to reliet herself by banging her head against a wall. Her sleep is of poor quality. There was no obvious abnormality in the physical examination.

GAD also known as chronic anxiety disorder. It is the most common anxiety disorder. It has a slow onset. Frequent or persistent anxiety is its main clinical features. The patient is always too worried, nervous and afraid accompanied by autonomic nervous disorders and exercise anxiety(such as dry mouth, sweating, palpitation, shortness, frequent urination, urgent urination, pacing back and forth, tremor, restless) but no threat, danger, negative outcome in fact. In addition, the patients often have difficulties in sleeping, more dreams. Sometimes, they may have night terror, nightmare and other sleep disorders.

10.6.3   Diagnosis and differential diagnosis

10.6.3.1   Diagnosis

The diagnosis is made according to the clinical features of anxiety. GAD is based on persistent primary anxiety accompanied by autonomic nerve symptoms and exercise anxiety but no clear object, fixed content or fear. The course lasts more than 6 months. The patient is suffered from impaired social function.

10.6.3.2   Differential diagnosis

(1)Anxiety caused by physical disease

Many physical diseases have anxiety symptoms such as thyroid disease, heart disease, certain neurological diseases(encephalitis, cerebrovascular disease, brain degeneration disease, systemic lupus erythematosus and so on). Anxiety in elder patients, have no psychological stress factors, have pre−illness good personality may be secondary to physical disease. Inquiring the history of disease detailedly, physical examination, mental status examination and appropriate laboratory examination are necessary to avoid misdiagnosis.

(2)Drug−induced anxiety

Some drugs can cause anxiety disorders such as some quasi−sympathetic drugs amphetamines cocaine, some hallucinogens such as LSD and opioids, long−term use of hormones, sedative hypnotics, antipsychotic drugs caused by anxiety disorder can be identified, according to the history of medication.

(3)Anxiety caused by mental disorder

Schizophrenia, depression, hypochondria, obsessive−compulsive disorder, phobia, post−traumatic stress disorder are often associated with anxiety or panic attack. Depression is more associated with anxiety. Other neuroses also associated with anxiety, but anxiety symptoms in these diseases are often not the main clinical feature.

10.6.4 Treatments

10.6.4.1 Psychotherapy

Psychotherapy of anxiety disorder includes cognitive therapy, behavioral therapy or cognitive-behavioral therapy. The personality characteristics of anxiety patients often manifest as demanding reality, too high life expectations, unclear perception to disease, pessimism, long-term high alert state. It leads to some distortion know and it is one of the causes of anxiety disorder in delay. At the same time, anxiety often cause muscle tension, autonomic nervous system dysfunction, cardiovascular system and digestive system symptoms. Therefore, cognitive therapy can change unreasonable and distorted perception to the disease, the behavioral therapy such as relaxation training, and system desensitization can alleviate physical symptoms. It often can receive good results. Specific treatment methods see this book psychological treatment chapter.

10.6.4.2 Pharmacotherapy

(1) Benzodiazepine drugs

They have strong anti-anxiety effect, take effect quickly and safety. The basic pharmacological effect on γ-aminobutyric acid to relieving anxiety, relaxant muscle, sedation, analgesia and hypnosis. According to the different half-life, Benzodiazepine drugs can be divided into long-range effect drugs, medium-range effect drugs and short-range effect drugs. Long-range effect drugs include diazepam, nitrazepam, clonazepam and so on. Mid-range drugs inculde alprazolam, nordazepam, chlorine hydroxyl diazepam and so on. Short-term effect drugs include triazolam and midazolam. Short-term effect drugs are used in paroxysmal anxiety. Long-term effect drugs are used in persistent anxiety.

Application of drugs should start from the small dose and gradually increased to the best effective dose. The drugs maintain 2-6 weeks before the gradual withdrawal. Withdrawal process of drugs can not shorter than 2 weeks to prevent symptoms rebound.

At present, benzodiazepine drugs be used in the early stage and combine with selective serotonin reuptake inhibitors and then gradually disable benzodiazepine drugs to selective serotonin reuptake inhibitors such as paroxetine, sertraline, fluvoxamine and other antidepressants have a good effecton anxietyand no addiction.

(2) β-adrenergic receptor blockers

The most commonly used β-adrenergic receptor blockers is propranolol. It has good effect on physical symptoms such as palpitations, tachycardia, tremor, sweating, short of breath and suffocation caused by autonomic nervous system hyperfunction. Generally, it often combined with other anxiolytic drugs. The common dose is 10-30 mg, 2-3 times a day. The patients who have asthma bradycardia ban β-adrenergic receptor blockers.

(3) Other drugs

Antidepressants and aromatic piperazine anxiolytic drugs such as buspirone have a good effect on anti-anxiety. They be widely used in the treatment of anxiety disorders due to no dependence, no sleep effect, no-prolonging. The dose is 5-10 mg, 3 times a day. But they work after 7-14 days. So, the treatment can be combined with benzodiazepine drugs in early. SSRIs (such as fluvoxamine, sertraline) also have a good effect. Deanxit and venlafaxine, also have a significant effect.

10.7   Obsessive-compulsive disorder

Obsessive-compulsive disorderis a type of neurological disorder with obsessive-compulsive symptoms as the main clinical feature. The neuroses epidemiological survey data shown that prevalence of obsessive-compulsive disorder was 0.3 ‰ at 12 regions of China in 1982. Foreign data shown that prevalence of obsessive-compulsive disorder was 0.5‰ in the general population. The prevalence is similar between male and female.

10.7.1   Etiology and pathogenesis

Etiology is unclear. Genetic factors, compulsive personality traits and psychosocial factors play a role in the onset of obsessive-compulsive disorder.

10.7.1.1   Genetic factors

Comorbidity rate of obsessive-compulsive disorderin the blood relatives is higher than the normal residents. The disease prevalence in parents of the patients is 5%-7%. The twins study also supported that obsessive-compulsive disorder related to inheritance.

10.7.1.2   Personality characteristics

1/3 of obsessive-compulsive disorder patients have pre-morbid compulsive personality. Their parents and children may have compulsive personality. The personality characteristics include cautiousness, hesitation, thrift, caution, attention to detail, enjoying think, pursuing perfection, strictnessbut lack of flexibility.

10.7.1.3   Mental factors

The survey data shown that 35% of patients had pre-morbid mental factors in Shanghai. The factors such as social psychological factors and heavy mental injury accidents which can cause long-term mental stress and anxiety cancause obsessive-compulsive disorder.

10.7.2   Clinical features

Case report :

Jane works in a hospital. Six months ago, her father died of illness, and she was very sad. Since then, Jane has always feared that she could get cancer as working in a hospital and always wash her hands more than 10 times after work. When she got home, she changed all her clothes and shoes to avoid bringing cancer home. Although doctors told her that cancer is not contagious, Jane is not convinced. Later on, she became too afraid to sit in a chair that someone else had sat in. When someone touched her, she would wash her hands until she thought they were clean. It took her a lot of time to "clean" each day, and it made her tired and seriously affected her work. Although she knew it was not necessary and tried not to think about it, the idea persisted and came up again and again. Jane felt very miserable, but she just couldn't control herself.

The disease usually occurs in adolescence or childhood and mostly slow onset. Tension or psychological stress often is inducement. The basic symptoms are compulsive idea, compulsive intention and compulsive behavior. Someone just have one main symptom. Someone have several symptoms. The most common symptom compulsive idea includes compulsive suspicion(the patients repeated doubts about the correctness of his words and deeds), compulsive rumination(the patients repeated thinking about natural things or natural phenomena), compulsive association(an idea appear in brain of patients and the patients involuntarily associate with another idea), compulsive recollection (the things which patient has experienced involuntarily re-peated emergence) and compulsive opposing thinking (the patients involuntarily think of opposite things or ideas when they meet a thing or idea). Patients know that these ideas are meaningless but can not be got rid of them. Compulsive behavior is that has to be taken to all eviate the anxiety caused by compulsive idea. Common compulsive behaviors include compulsive exam, compulsive interrogation, compulsive washing and so on. Some patients heard the advised of doctor "less think, brain cells will dead if you think too much", then this concept repeated in brain of the patients and they visit the famous doctors repeatedly to asked and confirmed "will brain cells dead?" They repeatedly ask the question in the outpatient to relax themselves but soon rejuvenate after returning home. Compulsive intention refers to the patient repeated ex-perience a strong inner impulse which they want to make action which violates their own wishes and they know that is absurd but can not get rid of the inner impulse. The characteristic of obsessive-compulsive dis-order is self-compulsive and self-opposing-compulsive consciousness appears at the same time. The sharp conflict makes the patients anxious and painful. Impulses of patients come from themselves inner and they recognize obsessive-compulsive symptom is abnormal but can not get rid of it. The main symptom in pa-tients with prolonged disease course is ritualized action and mental pain to reduce. Their social function is significantly damaged at this time.

The patients with obsessive-compulsive disorder often accompany depression, anxiety and other symp-toms of neuroses. But they are not main clinical features just secondary to obsessive – compulsive symptoms.

10.7.3   Diagnosis and differential diagnosis

Diagnosisis not difficult for the patients with symptoms in line with clinical feature, typical compulsive symptoms and asking for treatment. However, some patients who fail to try to get rid of obsessive-compul-sive symptoms easy to form behavior of adapt to the disease. At this time, treatment becomes not necessary. This should be noted. Obsessive-compulsive disorder need to be identified with the following dis-eases in clinical practice.

10.7.3.1   Schizophrenia

Schizophrenia patients also have obsessive-compulsive symptoms. However, the patients don't feel pain for the symptoms, don't desire to get rid of compulsive and don't take the initiative to require treatment. Ob-sessive-compulsive symptoms of schizophrenia patients are more bizarre. They have no self-conciousness but have schizophrenia symptoms.

10.7.3.2   Depressive disorder

Patients with depression can accompany obsessive-compulsive symptoms and patients with obsessive-compulsive disorder can also accompany depressive symptoms. The key of identification is what symptom is primary.

10.7.3.3   Phobia

The fear in phobia cause by objective while the fear of patients with obsessive-compulsive disorder cause by the subjective experience. The avoidance behavior of patients with obsessive-compulsive disorder is related to compulsive suspicion and compulsive worry.

10.7.3.4   Mental disorders caused by brain organic diseases

Organic lesions of the central nervous system, especially the basal ganglia lesions, may lead to obsess-ive-compulsive symptoms. At this time, the key of identification is whether the patients have neurological history, sign and related auxiliary examination.

10.7.4   Treatments

Pharmacotherapy combines with psychotherapy to favourable effect.

10.7.4.1   Psychotherapy

The purpose of psychotherapy is to make the patients have a correct understanding for own personality characteristics and illnesses and have a correct judge for surrounding environment and situation to remove spiritual burden and insecurity. The purpose of psychotherapy also is to learn how enhance self-confidence to reduce the sense of uncertainty but not to pursue perfection to remove the sense of imperfection. At the same time, their relatives mobilize to help patients actively engaged in literature, sport or social activities so that the patients gradually free from obsessive rumination.

Behavioral therapy, cognitive therapy and psychoanalytic therapy can be used for treating obsessive-compulsive disorder. The specific treatments are in psychotherapy section.

10.7.4.2   Pharmacotherapy

Clomipramine is more commonly used and has good effect. The treatment dose is 150-300 mg, 2-3 times a day. Usually, it works after 2-3 weeks. The dose starts with small and gradually adds to the amount of treatment. If it no work after 4-6 weeks, switching drug or combining with other drugs can be considered. The treatment time is 3-6 months. However, it is non-preferred due to its strong anti-cholinergic side effects. Selective serotonin reuptake inhibitors (fluvoxamine, fluoxetine, paroxetine and so on) and clomipramine have similar effect on treating obsessive-compulsive disorder. Selective serotonin reuptake inhibitors are easy more to be accepted due to mild side effects. Therefore, serotonin reuptake inhibitors have become the main drug for treating obsessive-compulsive disorder. For refractory obsessive-compulsive disorder, selective serotonin reuptake inhibitors combined with mood stabilizers (such as sodium valproate, carbamazepine) may have certain effect. They combined with risperidone or aripiprazole are also effective. In addition, clonazepam has a certain effect on the patients with obsessive-compulsive disorder accompanied by anxiety for clonazepam can act on γ-aminobutyric acid and serotonin at the same time. Clonazepamcan combine with serotonin reuptake inhibitors as one of the measures which enhance the efficacy of serotonin reuptake inhibitors.

10.8   Somatoform disorders

Somatoform disorders belong toneuroses characterized by the dominant idea which persistently worrying or belief various somatic symptoms. Patients are repeatedly hospitalized for these symptoms. Repeated negative result of medical examination and the explanation of doctor can not dispel their doubts. Even if there is sometimes a physical disorder, it can not explain the nature and extent of symptoms, the pain and the dominant idea. The patients are often accompanied by anxiety or depression. Although the occurrence and persistence of symptoms are closely related to unpleasant life events, difficulties and conflicts, patients often deny the presence of psychological factors. The prevalence of this disease is not very different between men and women. The course is fluctuant and chronic.

Somatoform disorders include somatization disorder, undifferentiated somatoform disorder, hypochondriasis, somatoform autonomic dysfunction and somatoform pain disorder.

10.8.1 Etiology and pathogenesis

10.8.1.1 Genetic factors

Some studies suggested that somatoform disorders associated with genetic susceptibility. Foster study (Clongdengde) suggested that genetic factors may were associated with the functional somatic symptoms.

10.8.1.2 Personality characteristics

Some studies found that the patients often were neurotic personality which is sensitive, suspicious, stubborn and excessive concern for health. They focus on their own discomfort and related events with resulting in sensitivity threshold decreased and sensitivity of the body sensation increased. This is easy to produce a variety of physical discomfort.

10.8.1.3 Neurophysiology

Someone suggested that patients with somatoform disorders had filtration dysfunction in brain stem network structure. Generally, individuals do not feel the normal activity of organs as the feel are filtered out in the integration mechanism of the mesh or the edge system to ensure that the individuals are pointing to the outside and not be interfered by various inner physiological activities. Once the filtration function is disordered and the inner feel of patients enhance, the patients continue accepting a variety of physiological changes which maybe deemed to physical symptoms.

10.8.1.4 Psychological and social factors

Attitude of parents toward disease and patients live with who have chronic diseases in early life are susceptible factors of somatization disorders. Their symptom model often is the symptoms of their relatives which they see in childhood. The patients who were over-cared or lack care in early childhood are easy to have somatization disorders in adulthood. Psychoanalysis theory suggests that somatic symptoms are a substitute for fear of the internal or external environment of the individual and emotional release. Parsons put forward secondary gain concept that emphasize the social role and privilege of patients. The patients can avoid the responsibility they don't want to take and get the care of others because of the disorder.

10.8.2 Clinical features

Case report:

Peter is a 29-year-old man. More than 5 years ago, there was no obvious cause for headache, mainly on the left side, with different duration, sometimes accompanied by nausea. He repeatedly visited various hospitals, no obvious abnormalities were found in electroencephalogram, head CT and MRI. The medication effect was not good. For this reason, he felt irritable, incompetent, less interested and less confident. The pain and emotion are closely related. In the past four months, his sleep guality was poor, a tendency to wake up in dreams, sometimes difficulty sleeping, and a worse headache the next day.

10.8.2.1 Somatization disorder

It is also known as Briquet syndrome. The clinical features is recurring and changing physical symptoms. The symptoms may involve any part of the body but various medical examinations can not confirm that any organic disease to explain its somatic symptoms sufficiently. This often leads to repeated medical attention, obvious social dysfunction, anxiety and depression. The onset always is before the age of 30 years old. Women are more likely to have somatization disorder. The course is at least 2 years. Common symptoms can be grouped into the following.

(1) Pain

This are a group of frequent symptoms. The parts of pain often are very wide such as head, neck, abdomen, back, joints, limbs, chest and rectum and soon. The parts are not fixed and the pain can occur in menstrual period, sexual intercourse or urination.

(2) Gastrointestinal symptoms

The symptoms is also common such as belching, acid reflux, nausea, vomiting, bloating, diarrhea or some special discomfort caused by food. Gastrointestinal examinations just have superficial gastritis or intestinal irritation syndrome which is difficult to explain the serious symptoms.

(3) Genitourinary symptoms

The common symptoms include frequent urination, urgency urination, dysuria, genital discomfort, frigidity, erection and ejaculation disorders, menstrual disorders, excessive menstrual blood, vaginal secretions abnormality.

(4) Pseudo-neurological symptoms

The symptoms imply nervous system diseases but physical examination can not find evidence of neurological damage. The common symptoms include ataxia, limb paralysis, weakness, dysphagia or pharyngeal obstruction, aphonia, urinary retention, hallucinations, loss of tactile or pain, diplopia, blindness, deafness, convulsions and other symptoms.

10.8.2.2   Undifferentiated somatoform disorder

The patients complain one or more somatic symptoms and feel painful. However, medical examinations can not find evidence of any organic disease. The course is more than 6 months. The patients have significant social dysfunction. Common symptoms include fatigue, lack of appetite, gastrointestinal or urinary system discomfort. The clinical type can be seen as atypical somatization disorder. The symptoms involved are not as extensive as somatization disorder. The course is not necessarily up to 2 years.

10.8.2.3   Hypochondriasis

Hypochondriasis is a type of somatoform disorder characterized by hypochondriac symptoms. The patients are overly concerned about their health or illness. They fear or believe that they are suffering from a serious illness which is disproportionate to the actual. The patients are particularly alert to changes in their body. Any slight changes of body function(such as heart beat, abdominal distension and so on) will cause attention of the patients. These changes are insignificant for the normal people but the patients give them special attention. The patients unconsciously exaggerate or distort these changes and think they have serious illness. On the basis of an increased alertness, the slight sensation also can cause unwell, seriously disturbed and unbearable feel so that the patient convince that they are suffering from serious illness. Although the results of the various tests do not support the speculation and the doctor also patiently explained and repeatedly ensure that they not have serious illness, the patients are often skeptical about the reliability of the test results, disappointed with the explanation of doctors and still adhere to their own hypochondriac concept leading they repeatedly asked for check or treatment. Because the all or most attention of patients focus on health, learning, work, daily life and interpersonal communication often are affected obviously.

The above symptoms are not consistent in different patients. Someone have obvious hypochondriac discomfort associated with anxiety or depression(sensory hypochondriac disorder). Someone just have hypochondriac concept but physical discomfort and mood changes are not significant(conceptual hypochondriac disorder). Someone have vague or broader hypochondriac symptoms. Someone have single and clear hypochondriac symptoms but never reach absurd and delusion(single hypochondriac disorder). Most patients know that their evidence is not sufficient and yearn for further confirm the diagnosis by repeated examination and require treatment.

10.8.2.4　Somatoform autonomic dysfunction

Somatoform autonomic dysfunctionis a kind of syndrome of organ controlled by the autonomic nervous system(such as cardiovascular, gastrointestinal and respiratory system) which caused by neurological disorder. Patients with autonomic nervous excitement symptoms(such as palpitations, sweating, flushed and tremor) have nonspecific but individual and subjective symptoms(such as pain, burning, heaviness, the tight feeling and swelling in uncertainty area). There results of examinations can not prove that there are somatic disorders in the organs and systems. The characteristics of somatoform autonomic dysfunction are significant autonomic involvement, non-specific symptoms, subjective complaints and adherence to the symptoms due to particular organ or system.

10.8.2.5　Somatoform pain disorder

It is sustained and severe pain which can not be explained by physiological process or physical disorder. The patients feel pain and their social function are damaged. Medical examination can not find any corresponding somatopathy in the pain site. Common pains include headache, atypical facial pain, low back pain, chronic pelvic pain. Pain can occur anywhere else in the body such as surface, deep tissue or internal organs. The natures of pain include dull pain, swelling pain, acheor sharp pain. There is evidence in the clinic indicate that psychological factors or emotional conflicts play an important role in the pain occurrence, aggravation, persistence and severity.

The peak incidence of age is between 30 to 50 years old. Women are twice as likely as men. Labourers are more likely to have an somatoform pain disorder. There is a tendency to family gather. The patients have chronic pain as a main symptom lead to doctor repeatedly. They often used a variety of drug, physical therapy, even surgical treatmentwhich not have exact effect often but result in sedative and analgesic drug dependence. The patients accompany anxiety, depression and insomnia.

Onset age of somatoform pain disorder is earlier. Women are more likely to have somatoform pain disorder than men. The course is chronic with acute onset. The patients treated in early have a good prognosis. Someone have delayed course.

10.8.3　Diagnosis and differential diagnosis

Common feature of these diseases are a variety of physical symptoms. Different clinical types have their own outstanding performance but medical examination can not find evidence of organic diseaseor the symptoms of the continued and the severity is not commensurate with physical examination. Patients are deeply concerned about the physical illness and pain. Their social functions are damaged. There is evidence that the occurrence, persistence and exacerbation of somatic symptoms are closely related to psychological factors. But somatoform disorders need to be identified with the following diseases.

10.8.3.1　Physical disease

Some diseases may not be able to find objective medical evidence in early. Therefore, the diagnosis of various somatoform disorders requires 6 months of course at least. When the age of onset is 10 years of age, physical symptoms are single, fixed, and continued to increase, physical disease should be considered at first and close observation. It is not appropriate to hastily make diagnosis of somatoform disorder. Clinical practice shows that diagnosing somatoform disorders just according to mental incentives, no positive signs at the initial examination and patients are easy to accept the implied may lead to misdiagnosis.

10.8.3.2　Depression and anxiety disorder

Depression and anxiety in varying degrees often occur in somatoform disorders but light. Patients with depression have "triad depression" accompanied by fewer physical symptoms which mainly concentrate in the gastrointestinal system. ICD – 10 noted that physical symptoms appear after 40 years of age, especially male likely to be an early manifestation of primary depression. Anxiety symptoms are more obvious and physical symptoms are not lasting in anxiety disorder.

10.8.4　Treatments

10.8.4.1　Psychotherapy

Establishing good doctor–patient relationship is the key to the success of psychotherapy. In addition to complaining physical symptoms, the patients have a long and no effect of treatment experience, emotional tension and anxiety. Doctors should be patient listening to patients and make patients have confidence to doctors and treatments.

In the course of treatment, doctors contact skills are essential. Patients often show dependent, performing and injury behavior. They always complain or feel wronged. Someone indulge in pain and is accustomed to dependence on drugs. Someone even have hostility and threats so that doctors are in a passive position or lack patience. Doctors should not only understand the pain of the patients but also guide the patient to focus on the established treatment goals and the results obtained such as sleep improvement, pain relief and so on. Doctors should encourage patients to peaceful coexistence with slight physical discomfort regarding as normal perception. The patients should gradually increase activity. The purpose of treatment is to make patients understand their own bad behavior. The treatments include analysising the relevant factors of the disease, finding a solution together, and establishing the correct attitude of life events and physical illness. At the same time, adjusting the environment of patients is essential to adjust disease behavior and develop healthy behavior. Doctors should help patients to enhance social environment and family adaptability and encourage patients to learn to self–regulation as soon as possible to get rid of dependence. Their spouses, relatives and friends should understand and sympathy the patient suffered and change negative, indifferent and discriminatory attitude to establish positive, and caring family atmosphere. Studies have shown that short–term or long–term family therapy is very effective on improving patient relationships.

10.8.4.2　Pharmacotherapy

The patients with somatoform disorders often accompany anxiety, depression, insomnia and other symptoms. Psychological symptoms and physical symptoms are each other cause and form vicious cycle. Psychotherapy works slow. Anti–anxiety drugs and antidepressants should be used as soon as possible.

Common antidepressants include tricyclic antidepressants(amitriptyline and the treatment dose is 50 – 100 mg per day for 2 times), serotonin reuptake inhibitors(such as paroxetine, fluvoxamine, sertraline) which has become the first choice for good effect and few side effects, serotonin and norepinephrine reuptake inhibitors(such as venlafaxine, duloxetine) which also have good effects especially on pain.

Doctors should emphasize that the treatment of this disease have treatment stage and the consolidation stage and the drug reduction process should be slow. The patients can not stop the medicine by themselves to avoid recurrence. The length of treatments time depends on the course, personality, environment and other factors. Once the symptoms have been alleviated, the psychological, family and social rehabilitation measures should be strengthened.

10.9 Neurasthenia

Neurasthenia was proposed in 1869 by G. Beard who is the American neurologist. He was thought that neurasthenia is an unexplained organic disorder. The mainly clinical features of neurasthenia are more than 70 kinds of various physical and psychosomatic symptoms such as fatigue, headache, poor appetite and so on. The main symptoms are fatigue. However, neurasthenia was deleted in DSM–Ⅲ in 1978 due to its ambiguity concept. For some disease which the main clinical feature is fatigue can not be classified, there is a diagnosis of "chronic fatigue syndrome" (CFS). Someone think that is a replica of neurasthenia. At present, most scholars in china believe that neurasthenia is still a disease entity and not going to disappear for canceled in DSM–Ⅲ. Therefore, ICD–10 still retains the diagnostic category of neurasthenia based on the view of oriental scholars.

The survey (1982) shown the prevalence of neurasthenia was 13.03‰ in China. The WHO multicenter epidemiological survey (In 1995, Sartorius et al.) found that the prevalence of neurasthenia was 5.4% and 2/3 of the patients accompanied anxiety or depression symptoms.

The neurasthenia is usually slow onset. The symptoms are chronic and volatility. The decline of the symptomsis relates to psychological conflict. Therefore, neurasthenia is tends to fluctuate and delay in the patients who have susceptible quality and life stress events.

10.9.1 Etiology and pathogenesis

10.9.1.1 Psychological factors

It is important causes of neurasthenia. Those which can cause long–term nervous activity overweight and negative emotions may be the risk factors of neurasthenia such as the death of their kinsfolk, inharmonious family, career failure, relationship strain, life rhythm reversed and long–term psychological contradiction.

10.9.1.2 Personality characteristics

Patients who have sensitive, suspicious, timid, subjective and poor self–control personality are susceptible to neurasthenia due to general mental stimulation and disease. Patients whose personality traits were not to be strong have neurasthenia foe more lasting mental stimulation.

10.9.1.3 Physical factors

Various of weaken the body function of various factors can contribute to the occurrence of this disease. All kinds of physical and functional weaken can contribute to the occurrence of neurasthenia.

10.9.2 Clinical features

Case report:

Julie is a 43–year–old woman. 6 months ago, she had no obvious cause of dizziness, dark mask and nausea, and each attack lasted about 5 minutes. Rest and self–administered drugs to improve the microcirculation could be relieved (details are not clear). She felt weak limbs, slightly anxious mood, not clear mind, poor sleep at night. During the relief period, she felt dizzy. Over the past 6 months, the symptoms are often repeated, paroxysmal, emotional anxiety. No positive signs were found in the neurological examination.

10.9.2.1 Brain dysfunction symptoms

Brain dysfunction symptoms include easy excitement and fatigue. The excitement is mainly manifested in the growth of associations and memories and confusion. The content is always repeated, messy, meaningless. The patients know these are meaningless but can not get out. The patients can not control but want to try to control these causing psychological conflict and pain. Their attention can not focus on one subject and feel chaos and is easy to be transferred by external stimuli. At the same time, their sense is enhanced. They have photophobia and like working and learning in a darker place. During the day, they also like putting down the curtain. They are afraid of noise, like silence and can't stand the noise. As their sense enhance, they always feel chest tight when breathing, abdomen and chest skin uncomfortable when clothing is closing to abdomen and chest, heart beat fast and shortness breath when moving. In short, the patient is unbearable for the normal stimulation.

Spiritual fatigue as the core symptoms of neurasthenia presented by G. Beard is still the main feature of neurasthenia. Fatigue in neurasthenia patients is a brain function regulation system dysfunction often accompanied by emotional symptoms. It is also known as emotional fatigue. It has the following features. ①The fatigue often accompanied by negative mood(such as tension, depression). Rest can not relieve fatigue but it can be improved by emotional symptoms reducing or disappearing. ②Fatigue is situational. When engaged in not interested things, the patients are particularly fatigue. When engaged in interested things, the patients are not fatigue. ③Fatigue often is diffuse. Neurasthenia patients are fatigue doing everything unless they do work which they like or can do. ④Fatigue is not associated with the decline of desire and motivation. The patients fatigue and have a lot of desire suffering from the "lack of ability" or "ability not equal to their ambition". They feel pain for not realizing their ambition. ⑤Mental fatigue is core symptom and physical fatigue is not necessarily.

10.9.2.2　Emotional symptoms

Emotional symptoms of neurasthenia mainly include trouble, irritability and tension. Generally, it has the following 3 features. ① The patients seek help for pain. ② The patients are difficult to control themselves. ③ The intensity and duration of emotions are not commensurate with life events or situations. The patients worry about trivial matters all day long. Irritability is means to easy to be angry, can not control quarreling with others and regret and self-repression after quarreling. After a period of time, they also can not control quarreling with others. They repeat the "trilogy". Irritability would damage interpersonal relationship and poor interpersonal relationship also intensify irritability. Patients feel that life is full of burden, work and study are stressful and their moods often are in a state of tension.

10.9.2.3　Psychological and physiological symptoms

Neurasthenia patients often have some physical symptoms but a variety of examinations can not find evidence of pathological changes. These symptoms are actually a physiological dysfunction and closely relate to the mental state of patients. The most common symptoms include sleep disorders, tension headaches and physical discomfort. Sleep disorders in neurasthenia patients are characterized by difficulty falling asleep, shallow sleep, dreaminess, fatigue after waking up. Tension headache is characterized by inconstant pain, tight grip on the head, a feeling of stress, dizziness, distension, head swelling and unsharpness as being in cloud. Increased fatigue can be reduced by mood improvement. Physical discomfort mainly manifested as autonomic nervous system dysfunction such as dyspepsia, loss of appetite, abdominal distension, diarrhea, impotence, spermatorrhea, premature ejaculation, irregular menstruation, panic, shortness of breath, chest tightness and so on.

10.9.2.4　Hypochondriac concept, anxiety and depression

The patients always suspect that they may suffer from a serious illness which can not be diagnosed by the current medical technology, because they have many discomfort symptoms. However, multiple medical examination can not discover the organic disease. The patients are worried and repeatedly seeking the doctor but the treatments are not effective. They worry that their disease no improve and affect their health, work and study so that they are in a state of anxiety and depression. However, these symptoms of anxiety and depression don't last long. Once the situation improves, the symptoms will disappear.

10.9.3　Diagnosis and differential diagnosis

Neurasthenia can be found in almost all mental disorders and many somatic diseases due to its unspecific clinical symptoms. So diagnostic of neurasthenia must be based on hierarchy. If the clinical features are consistent with the diagnostic criteria for neurasthenia and the criteria for another disease at same time, the first diagnosis is the other disease. In this way, other physical and mental diseases can be excluded.

In addition to the clinical symptoms, the diagnosis requires the course more than 3 months. The severity standard requires neurasthenia affect social function of the patients or the patients feel pain leading to seeking treatment initiatively.

Symptoms of neurasthenia are common in other brain organic diseases and somatic diseases. At this time, the diagnosed should is neurasthenic syndrome.

Neurasthenia often needs to identify with the following diseases.

10.9.3.1　Dysthymia

Dysthymia is a type of depressive disorders. It is characterized by persistent(at least 2 years) low mood state duo to depressed personality and negative life events. The patients are not interested in anything, no confidence, no hope, no sense of life and low self-evaluation. But they still have responsibility on the family. They tend to ascribe bad status to objectivity. Depression in neurasthenia is not persistent and mild.

10.9.3.2　Anxiety disorder

Prominent symptom of anxiety disorder is anxiety experience without clear objects and specific content. Anxiety in neurasthenia has the reality of the specific reasons and content in reality.

10.9.4　Treatments

10.9.4.1　Psychotherapy

Cognitive therapy, morita therapy and relaxation therapy can be applied. In the begining, detailed medical history and comprehensive physical examination to possess rich information is available for the diagnosis. At the same time, trust between doctors and patients is good for psychological treatment. Psychotherapy helps patients understand the nature of the disease, relieves the anxiety and mental stress, improves confidence, stabilizes the mood and helps the patient to find psychosocial factors that cause symptoms to linger. The etiology is related not only to external factors, but also to susceptibility of patients.

The patients always are introverted, sensitive, suspicious, high self-esteem and inferiority. They pay special attention to their own situation and body changes and evaluation of other people to themselves. The failure is common in life. Once getting frustrated, they will feel more disappointed and helpless. So, promoting cognitive change of the patients helping patients adjust their expectations of life to reduce their mental stress can achieve good results. To help patients analyze individual weaknesses and help them to correct and enhance their ability to adapt is also an important psychological treatment purposes and that has an important role in promoting disease recovery and avoiding recurrence. In addition, this is necessary to properly arrange life, not perfectionism, appropriate self-relaxation, self-liberation without affecting the interests of others as much as possible. Physical exercise has a good effect on enhancing physical fitness, promoting physical sleep and reducing the physical discomfort.

10.9.4.2　Pharmacotherapy

First choice drugs are antianxiety agents. Benzodiazepines(such as alprazolam, lorazepam) have a certain effect on improving tension, reducing the level of irritability, relaxing muscle and eliminating physical discomfort. Buspirone is a type of anxiolytic drugs without abirritative and hypnotic effect which also have effect on symptoms of neurasthenia but it work after 7-14 day. so can be combined with benzodiazepines in early. After the buspirone is work, benzodiazepine drugs could be reduced and gradually stop in order to avoid drug resistance and dependence as using benzodiazepines for a long time. The dose of buspirone is 5-10 mg, 3 times a day. Deanxit, neurostan and some exciting drugs also have good effect on anxiety and weakness symptoms. The patients with obvious depression symptoms also canused SSRIs such as fluvoxamine, sertraline, citalopram, paroxetine and so on.

Autonomic dysfunction can be added with puerolol(2-3 times a day, long at a time).

10.10　Neuroses rehabilitation

With the change of medical science from biological model to biological-psychological-sociological model, the role of psychosocial factors(such as environment, emergency events, personality traits and so on) should be emphasized in the progression of neuroses. Bad mood, type and severity of the patients have great effect on the disease course and prognosis.

Psychological rehabilitation is also known as mental rehabilitation. It can also be understood as making mental activity and psychological behavior being adjusted and recovery as far as possible with limited conditions and measures. The psychological rehabilitation not only include the application of drugs or other clinical treatment to control psychotic symptoms but also help patients to eliminate the psychological burden and bad mood which is more importantly. At same time, training patients to adapt to surrounding environment and restoring social function is to achieve medical rehabilitation.

Conventional treatment of neuroses includes pharmacotherapy and psychotherapy. On the basis of conventional psychotherapy and pharmacotherapy, rehabilitation treatment for additional family therapy has great influence on the recovery of social function of patients. Patients with neuroses always have psychological vulnerability, interpersonal sensitivity, emotional instability and evident social function defects. The treatment can not be limited to the treatment of physical and psychological symptoms, which improving society function is more important for really achieve psychological rehabilitation. Therefore, it is necessary to strengthen family therapy and social support in rehabilitation period.

10.10.1　Family therapy

Family is the basic unit of society. Pathogenic factorsin some mental illness come from the family. Different people play a different family rolein different families and bear different family responsibilities. Family plays an important role in the occurrence, development and fate of mental illness. Paying attention to family therapy is the best way to get patients to achieve psychological rehabilitation. At present, the families of patients with mental illness exist ignorance, incomprehension, prejudice even discrimination. The families lack confidence and patience for the treatment and lack care, understood and psychological support for patients. This directly affects treatment and psychological rehabilitation so that it is difficult for patients to return to society. Family therapy is an important way to promote the psychological rehabilitation and return to society as soon as possible. Family members understand the relationship between the occurrence, development and mechanism of the disease and the family and society by interviewing with family members to correct understanding of family to the disease and full support treatment. At the same time, family members should get along with the patients to stabilize the emotions of patients, relieve the psychological pressure of the patients and make patients adapting to society and family. The position of the patient in the family and the psychological contradiction can bring about the family conflict. On the contrary, the family conflict can aggravate the occurrence and development of the mental disease. Therefore, strong family therapy is helpful for understanding and support between family members, resolving family conflicts and psychological rehabilitation. It makes the patients returning to society to reshape his status and image in their family.

10.10.2 Social support

Social support refers to the individual obtain material and spiritual support from the family, friends and colleagues in the stress. Coping style is cognitive behavioral effort of individual in stress. The mental health level of patients with neurosis is relatively low. The incidence is susceptible to external social support system and coping style. Strong social support system and positive coping style can reduce the recurrence of neurosis. Patients should actively try or brave acceptance social support and should not reject the care and help of others. This is the key to improving social support. Learning and mastering positive coping skills is very favorable for maintaining a good emotional experience, relieving psychological stress and promoting their mental health.

Wang Yiming

Chapter 11

Dissociative Disorders

11.1　Introduction

Dissociative disorders are characterized by a disconnection between thoughts, identity, consciousness and memory. Dissociative disorder, formerly known as hysteria, is redefined in ICD-10, due to significant psychological factors such as life events, inner conflicts or strong emotional experiences, suggestion or self-hints that act on susceptible individuals that cause a group of illnesses, no basis of organic disease. The morbidity rate of dissociative disorder is reported differently. Epidemiological survey showed that the prevalence rate of ordinary people was 3.55 ‰ in China in 1982. Foreign data showed that prevalence of female among the residents was 3‰–6‰ and more women than men. The incidence in backward areas of culture is higher, most starting age is 20–30 years old, there is the mass phenomenon on young students in part of our country and has the recurrent tendency. It onset acutely more based on the promotion of psychological factors and develop rapidly meanwhile the prognosis is better, 60%–80% of patients can be self-mitigation within a year.

11.2　Etiology and pathogenesis

The occurrence of dissociative disorder relate to genetic factors and personality characteristics which summarized as based on a certain character, it occurs due to coping with trauma which most often form in children exposed to long-term physical, sexual, emotional abuse, nature disasters or combat. Common causes of dissociative disorders are as follows.

11.2.1　Genetic factors

Neurosis is generally considered to be a group of heterogeneous diseases. Various factors (such as heredity, environment and personality type) play different roles in different types of neurosis and different individuals. They can affect the onset of neurosis at different stages. The formation and development of patients with bad personality are not only affected by environmental factors but also by genetic factors. Foreign data showed that the incidence of dissociative disorder in the close relatives of patients with dissociative disorders was 1.7%–7.3%, which was higher than general population. The incidence of female relatives was 20%. It reported that patients with positive family history accounted for 24% in Fu Jian. Shields had studied the symptoms of neurosis in 62 twins(12–15 years old) of the same sex(27 males and 35 females), their symptoms properties of neurosis depended genetic factors to a large extent. This suggests that genetic factors are more important than psychiatric factors for some patients.

11.2.2 Morbid personality

It refers to the patient's performance of emotion and personality, this morbid personality appears more prominently after the disease.

11.2.2.1 Highly emotional

The ordinary mood is naive, easy to move, squeamish, capricious, irritable, sensitive, suspicious, losing temper or cry for trifles, grumpy, small–minded, eager to be praised and pitied, not afford criticism. The expression is exaggerated, contrived and to attract the attention of others. The emotional reaction is too strong, from one extreme to the other extreme, with exaggerated and dramatic color, acts impetuously.

11.2.2.2 Ideas of reference

It refers to the hint when patients that are susceptible to the surrounding people's words, actions, attitudes, and produce the corresponding association and reaction. It refers to the self–talk when some of their own feelings are not unfit for producing the corresponding association and reaction. The hint depends on patients emotional tendencies of patients, if patients produce emotional tendencies on something or some person, are easily hinted.

11.2.2.3 High degree display of self

It refers to the self–centered tendency which brag and show themselves too much. The patients like to become the center of attention. After the disease, exaggerating symptom and praying for sympathy is main expression.

11.2.2.4 Excessive fantasy

Fantasy content is vivid, which is easy to confuse reality and fantasy giving the impression of lying under the influence of strong emotions giving the impression of lying. The patients have rich emotion. Their reaction is very volatile and they are emotionalism.

11.2.3 Psychodynamic theory

It holds that the pathogenesis of dissociative disorder originated in the negative emotions of repression. The repressed concepts form a strong psychological conflict. One solution is to separate part of the consciousness from the subject consciousness separation, which produces dissociation symptoms. The other solution is to translate the psychological conflict into physical symptom through complex psychological defense mechanism, which produces conversion symptoms. But the explanation of psychodynamics can not be scientifically demonstrated.

11.2.4 Reflection theory

It holds that dissociative disorder is essentially a class of instinctive reaction originally of the nervous system, people under a strong stimulation are likely to produce such reactions, the reactions are the symptoms.

11.3 Clinical features

Case report :

Lily is a 25-year-old girl. 3 days ago, Lily was suddenly fired. After hearing the news, Lily was silent and looking blank. Then she stopped suddenly, lifted the quilt, threw down her baby, jumped out of bed, screamed wildly, and rushed out the door. Her family stopped her, and the crowd held her and locked her in the house. In the room, she hit the door against the window, hit her head against the wall, and cried loudly. After several twists and turns, Lily fell into bed and cried, gradually exhausted and fainted. The next day, she work up as usual and recalled the process of the onset.

The main clinical features are dissociation symptoms and conversion symptoms. Dissociation refers to complete or partial inconformity to the past experience, current environment and self-identity. Conversion refers to the emotional response caused by mental stimulation followed by physical symptoms. Once the physical symptoms come, emotional reactions will fade or disappear. The physical symptoms are called conversion symptoms. The sensory disturbance, cinesipathy or altered state of consciousness manifested by dissociative disorder lacks the corresponding organic basis. Common symptoms have the characteristics of affectation, exaggeration, full of emotion and so on. Sometimes, the symptoms are induced by hint but also disappeared forhint. The symptoms have recurrent tendency. Psychiatric symptoms are outstanding performances including disorders of consciousness and emotion majorly such as psychogenic amnesia, psychogenic fugue, multiple personality, depersonalization and so on. Conscious disturbance is mainly the narrowing of consciousness, twilight state, oneirismand so on. This accompany by a strong emotional experience. The behavior is explosive and performance including laughing and crying together, beating breast and shouting loudly. Most of the dissociative disorder come on acutely under the stimulation of spiritual factors and develop to a critical stage rapidly. The clinical manifestations are complex and diverse. In summary, it can be divided into the following three types.

11.3.1 Dissociative disorders

Main features of dissociative disorders refer to disruptions or breakdowns of memory, awareness, identity, or perception. The performances include forgetting, roaming, personality changing and others. The symptoms are paroxysmal. The psychological factors are often obvious before it occurs. the onset of the disease often help patients out of the woods, vent depression mood, getting attention and sympathy from others, getting support and compensation but the patient himself may deny it. Symptoms are recurrent and appearfor recalling and associating events or situations which associate with previous traumatic experiences. In suitable environment or the therapy of hypnosis or psychoanalysis, the separation of the mental world can be restored. Sometimes, it can be restored quickly.

11.3.1.1 Dissociative amnesia

The main symptom is the temporary less of recall memory, specifically episodic memory, due to a traumatic or stressful event. But, there is always a fixed core content in the state of awakening which always can not be remembered. Forgetting is not caused by organic reason. The forgetting can not be explained by the general forgetfulness or fatigue.

11.3.1.2 Dissociative fugue

The manifests unplanned travel or wandering. The patients often leave an intolerable environment to a place which may be familiar or have emotional significance in the past.

At the moment, the scope of awareness of patients become narrow at the moment, but the daily basic living(such as eating and living) ability and simple social contact(such as buying tickets, travelling, asking way) still maintain lasting for several minutes to a few days. After they sober from the course of the disease, theycan not recall completely.

11.3.1.3 Dissociative stupor

It is often triggered by traumatic experience and psychic trauma. Patients have complete suppression of mental activity, maintaining a fixed position in long time, completely or almost have no words and spontaneous movement. The behavior is in line with the standard of catalepsy, whichcan not find the evidence of physical illness by checking. Usually, the patients wake up on after a few minutes.

11.3.1.4 Trance and possession disorders

The performance is the temporary loss of personal identity and full awareness of the surrounding environment and to forget the process in whole or in part. In some cases, behaviors of the patientsare like being replaced by another personality, elves, gods, or "forces" and attention of the patients are limited or focus on the one or two sides of the environment often along with a series of sports, posture, pronunciation which are limited and repeated. The trance state refers to involuntary state. A person thinks that he or she is replaced by a god, a ghost, other people, or a person who has died and claims himself is a supernatural or a person who has died, which is disorders trance state. Trance and possession disorders are the pathological process of involuntary and selfless.

11.3.2 Conversion disorder

Clinical manifestations of dissociative motor and sense disorders are complex such as motor and sense dysfunction. Physical examination, neurological examination and laboratory tests can not found organic lesion in internal organ and nervous system. The symptoms and signs do not meet the physiology and anatomy characteristics of nervous system. The symptoms are often more serious when observed and the symptoms tend to be worse when anxiety increases.

11.3.2.1 Dissociative motor disorders

The performances of limbs paralysis are monoplegia, paraplegia or hemiplegia accompanied by the strengthen and relaxation of muscular tension. The patients whose muscular tension increase are often fixed in a certain position and appears obvious resistance when active passively. Chronic cases may have limb contracture or muscle disuse atrophy. Examination can not find the evidence of neurological damage.

The performances of limbs tremor, twitch and myoclonusare limbs tremble, twitch irregularly and a group of muscle twitch rapidly similar to dance-like action. The symptoms will be worse when anxiety.

The performances of Astasia-Abasia are upper limbs may have severe tremor and violent shaking. The both lower limbs can be active but can not stand. The patients need support or dump to one side. But they usually not fall off. The patients can not walk, put their feet together when walking or appear swinging gait. They may dance with the music under the hint.

Amusia refer to the patient who wants to speak but can not make a sound or only can talk through whisper or hoarse voice. Checking the nervous system finds not organic pronunciation disease or other psychiatric symptoms.

11.3.2.2 Convulsions

It also known as pseudoseizures. It is similar to the state of epileptic seizures but no clinical features of epileptic seizures and the corresponding electrophysiological changes. It often break out when the patients rage or be hinted such as the doctor or family come into the ward. When seizures occurs, the patients slowly fell to the ground or lie in bed, no reaction when someone calls him, their whole body is rigid, there is limb jitter. They roll on the bed, show opisthotonos posture or breath urgent or stop. They also pull clothes or hair, beat their breast, and bite. Some patients grimace and eyes wet with tears. But they are not biting their tongue and on have incontinence. Most symptoms will relief in ten minutes. There is not sluggish spirit or sleepiness after the outbreak. There is no corresponding change in EEG.

11.3.2.3 Dysociate anaesthesia and sensory loss

It can be expressed as numbness, loss, allergy, abnormality of the body, or having special sensory disturbance. Numbness skin area of the patients is close to concept of somatic disease. It unlike neuroanatomy and is inconsistent with objective examination.

The performances of anaesthesia are the lack of local or systemic skin feeling, the missing of half-body pain or feel of appearing gloves and socks. Lack feelings can be pain, touch and temperature.

The performances of algesia are that the skin is particularly sensitive to the touch and a slight touch can cause severe pain.

The patients with paresthesia feel that pharynx has foreign body feeling or obstruction feeling and pharynx examination can not detect abnormality. It was called globushysterieus. But it should be identified with styloid process syndrome caused by the styloid process is too long. The latter can be confirmed by pharyngeal touch or X-ray.

The performances of defective vision are amblyopia, blindness, tunnel vision, contraction of visual field, monocular diplopia. It often occurs suddenly and returned to normal suddenly after be treated. Although the patients complaint visual deprivation, they surprisingly retain the ability to move. Normal visual evoked potential was which can is standard for normal vision.

The performance of hearing disorder is sudden hearing loss, but electrical audiometry and auditory evoked potentials are normal.

11.3.3 Special form of expression

11.3.3.1 Dissociative identity disorder

Dissociative identity disorder is a mental disorder characterized by the maintenance of at least two distinct and relatively enduring personality states. The disorder is accompanied by memory gaps. He or she conducts daily social activities in a different way. And presents into two or more distinct personality, which each has respective memory, hobbies and behavior, completely independent, alternately appearing, no contact. In first onset, the change of the personality is sudden and often relate closely to mental trauma. Afterwards, the transformation of personality can be triggered by association or special events. At some point, only one personality be showed. Each identity is not aware of the existence of other identities, when another identity appears. This identity seems to have lost for some time. The patients with two personalities are called double personality or alternating personality, one personality is dominant.

11.3.3.2 Ganser syndrome

It is a group of psychiatric symptoms described by Ganser as a special type of dissociative disorder. The patient has a mild sense of confusion, the question can be understood, but often give an approximate answer such as 2 +2 = 3, cattle have five legs. If you ask the patient to struck a match, he or she turns the match stem upside down and wipe the matchbox using the end without gunpowder. Telling him to use the key to open the door, he or she back the key to insert the keyhole. The patients leave others the impression of affectation accompany by odd behaviors or excitement and stupor attacking alternately.

11.3.3.3 Emotional outburst

It often occurs suddenly after someone suffer from serious mental trauma such as quarreling with people or emotion excite. The disturbance of consciousness of patients is lighter. The performances are crying, shouting, rolling on the ground, beating chest and stamping feet, tearing clothes, pulling hair or banging head against the wall. The speech and act has the character of venting the inner feelings. In the group, it is particularly intense. Generally, it needs to last for several minutes to quiet down, some may be forgotten afterwards.

11.3.3.4 Mass hysteria

It often occurs in the groups that live together such as school, churches, monastery or public places. It usually get epidemic in the environment which the economic status, and the educational level of the group are not high, feudal superstition activities more popular. Most of the patients are mostly young women. The patients under mental stress, fatigue, lack of sleep, menstrual period and having the personality of performance are more susceptible to get the sick. Some special scene and atmosphere like praying in the church, practicing certain qigong collectively often provide conditions for the prevalence of the disease. Recently reported that the disease occur mostlyin primary and secondary students after vaccination or collective meal. At beginning, one person develops symptoms and the witnesses are affected developing similar symptoms in succession. Due to unknown the disease in this circumstance, it often causes widespread tension and fear in this group. Under the influence of mutual hints and autosuggestion, the disease outbreak in short order. Most of the episodes are short-lived and similar in form. Isolating patients, especially the first patient, and giving symptomatic treatment, the epidemic can be controlled quickly.

11.4   Diagnosis and differential diagnosis

11.4.1 Diagnostic criterias

The diagnosis must have the following points.

(1) Possessing various clinical features of dissociative disorder.

(2) No evidence of physical disorders which can explain the symptoms.

(3) Evidence of mental illness clearly related to time and stressful events, problems or disorganized relationship(even if the patient denies it).

11.4.2 Differential diagnosis

11.4.2.1 Epileptic graviton

Convulsions in dissociative disorders should be distinguished from epileptic graviton. The consciousness lost totally and the pupils mostly dilate and the light reactions disappear when epileptic graviton attacks. Epileptic graviton occurs at night. It have three stages of tetanus, spasm and recovery. The limbs twitch regularly when in spasm accompanied by biting tongue and lip, falling and incontinence. The patients can not recall anything after the attack and EEG examination has characteristic changes of sharp and slow wave, spike and ware wave and others.

11.4.2.2 Acute stress disorder

The occurrence and development of acute stress response are closely related to mental stimulation factors. The illness immediately occurs after a severely catastrophic stress. The course is short generally lasting no more than 3 days. There is no recurrent history. The prognosis is good.

11.4.2.3 Malinger

Imitating forgetting with intent often associates with some obvious problems. Deliberate imitation of action and feel losing is generally difficult to identify with dissociative disorder. The identification depends on careful observation and a comprehensive understanding patient. Examination of the corresponding indicators in laboratory is an important criterion for identification.

11.4.2.4 Stupor

It can be divided into schizophrenia stupor, drug-induced stupor and depressive stupor based on medical history.

11.4.2.5 Organic sensation and movement disorder

Some progressive diseases, especially multiple sclerosis and systemic lupus erythematosus, can be confused with dissociative sensation and movement disorder in the early. In order to clarify the diagnosis, it needs to take a relatively long time to observe and evaluate. Other neurological disorders also need to be considered identified in the early such as myasthenia gravis, periodic paralysis, brain tumor, optic neuritis, part of vocal cord paralysis, Guillain-barre syndrome, Parkinson disease switch syndrome, basal ganglia and peripheral nerve degeneration, subdural hematoma, acquired, or genetic dystonia, Creutzfeldt-Jacob disease and AIDS. Dissociative convulsion should be distinguished from it comorbidity with epileptic seizure.

11.4.2.6 Other

Trance and possession disorders should be differential with schizophrenia, multiple personality, temporal lobe epilepsy, head trauma, psychoactive substances and others.

11.5 Treatments

Dissociative disorders are functional. Therefore, psychological treatment plays an important role. Medication treatment is mainly taking anxiolytic drugs appropriately to enhance the effect of psychological treatment.

11.5.1 Psychotherapy

The patients are apprehensive because they convince that their suffering from a serious disease. Their family are also very nervous. The patients pay special attention to words and actions of doctor, even an eye of doctor will cause their emotional response. So, doctors need to care for and sympathy patients, detailed examine the history, take physical examination carefully. Examination can exclude organic disease and obtain the trust of patients and their families. It is conducive to get success of psychological treatment. When the patients talk about the cause of disease, let the patient abandon vent and pour discontent. Doctors give understanding and comfort. The specific psychological treatments are as follows.

11.5.1.1 Suggestive therapy

It is a classical method of treating dissociative disorder. In the past the treatment is intravenous injection aether 0.5 mL, with verbal suggestion that the disease will attack after a particular smell, they do not worry about anything and will recovery completely. After the peak of its attack, doctors inject proper amount distilled water into the skin of chest with verbal suggestion that the disease can be cured after the injection. This suggestive therapy with inducing the symptoms at first and then terminating the symptoms is more effective than only injecting distilled water. Induction therapy takes full advantage of the clinical characteristics that diseases are easy to come on under the suggested. It makes patients believe that doctors can "call it" and "play it". People who have had a history of general anesthesia should not use this therapy because patient has an experience of using ether, which go against suggestion. In addition, pregnant women contraindicate it and menstrual period with caution, because ether can cause uterine contractions. Suggestive therapy is suitable for acute and higher suggestibility patient. Witty suggestive therapy often can receive dramatic effects. Currently, injecting 10% calciumgluconate 10 mL slowly with verbal suggestion has good effect on the treatment of dissociative physical disorder.

11.5.1.2 Hypnotherapy

In the hypnotic state, it can reappear traumatic experience what has been forgotten and release depressed emotion to reach the goal of eliminating symptoms. It is suitable for treating amnestic disorder, multiple personality, silent disorder, stuporous state, emotional injury and depression in dissociative disorder.

11.5.1.3 Behavioral therapy

It is suitable for patients with chronic limb dysfunction or speech training patients with system desensitization stepwise.

11.5.1.4 Other psychotherapy

Such as interpretive psychotherapy. The main purpose is to guide patients to assess psychological stimulation factor correctly and understand the nature of the disease fully to help patients overcoming personality defects, learning to deal with stress correctly, strengthening self – exercise and promoting psychosomatic health.

11.5.2 Physiotherapy

Acupuncture and electro-stimulation have good effect on paralysis, deafness, blindness, anaudia, body twitch and other dysfunction in dissociative disorders. They are used in different symptoms.

It is important to note thattreatment procedures must is complete and thorough before implementing any kind of psychotherapy and estimate for possible situation is full in order to take effective measures in time to ensure the success of treatment. Once the treatment fails, that will increase the difficulty of the next treatment, and even may cause the condition aggravation. Therefore, psychotherapy must be implemented by therapists with experience and should not be abused.

11.5.3 Pharmacotherapy

Psychotic seizure, passion, excitatory and convulsion in dissociative disorder need emergency treatment such as intravenous injection of diazepam 10−20 mg changing to oral medicine after patients quiet. Generally, the preferred drug is a weak stabilizer such as alprazolam(0.4 mg, 2−3 times a day). Some patients with significant anxiety and depression can also use antidepressant drugs such as Deanxit, Neurostan, Maprotiline. The patients who have obvious psychotic symptoms or minor tranquilizer is invalid to them can use antipsychotic drugs such as chlorpromazine. Once the disease recover, it should be stop and not need to maintain treatment in generally.

11.6   Prevention and healthcare of dissociative disorders

Developing a healthy personality has great significance to reduce the incidence of this disease for a child. The adverse factors about the environment play an important role in the development of children personality disorder and behavior disorder such as the trauma in childhood, improper parenting, divorced family environment, skip-generation raising and so on. That has far-reaching influence on the development of abnormal personality and mental abnormality in child. So, mental health must be educated to children. Family education should be paid the primary attention. Family is the main place where children live. Parents are enlightenment teacher and example of children. Child like a piece of white paper and is good at imitating and accepting everything around him or her. All this play an important role in the development of personality and sound in body and mind of children. The school education is also very important which focus on developing good character of children such as honesty and integrity. So, the school and the family should cooperate closely to discover and correct the neuropsychiatric disorders which appear possibly in the childhood. Confirming and handling cases in time can correct and cure the disease.

Wang Yiming

Chapter 12

Stress Related Disorders

12.1 Introduction

Stress related disorders, which used to be referred to as reactive mental disorders or psychogenic mental disorders, refer to the severity and persistence of the group of mental disorders closely related to social psychological factors. It mainly includes: acute stress disorder (ASD), post – traumatic stress disorder (PTSD) and adjustment disorder. Acute stress disorder refers to the transient mental disorder that occurs immediately after a sudden and significant mental stimulation; stress related disorder is a relatively persistent mental disorder that occurs after the individual suffers intense mental stimulation; adjustment disorder refers to the individual in a milder and more persistent mental disorder caused by a more prolonged psychological event. The common features of these disorders are that mental factors constitute a key factor in promoting the diseases. If there is no corresponding psychological factor, these people would not become ill. Moreover, the symptoms and prognosis of these disorders are related to mental inducements. PTSD is the most common disorder in this kind of disorders; there are many studies related to PTSD, in which of them indicate certain brain damage.

12.1.1 Etiology and pathogenesis

The occurrence of stress related disorders involves two key factors, stressful events and individual's susceptibility to the disorder. The eventually leads to stress related disorders. However, the interaction between these two factors is still a complex issue that needs further study. For example, how severe mental stress can lead to disease? How is the degree of mental stress assessed quantitatively? Why individuals sometimes suffer from the same mental stress, some people do not get sick and the manifestations of the disease are also different?

Stressful events refer to the kinds of events encountered by individuals in their living environment. According to the difference between the speed and intensity of stress events, mental stress can be acute and severe. For example, the natural and man–made disasters that threaten the safety of life or position can also be chronic and lasting, such as long–term environmental pressure or internal conflict. Generally speaking, ASD or PTSD is often associated with strong and acute mental stressors. According to the different nature of the stress events, the stress events can be the irresistible natural events, such as earthquake, tsunami, nonhuman factors, etc. , and can also be caused by human−related, such as the injury caused by beating, rape, killing and dereliction of duty. Generally speaking, stressful events cause more intense mental trauma to individuals. It should be noted that after a stressful event, most individuals produce a variety of psychological reactions, such as sleep disorder, uneasiness, subjective pain, fear, and anger, but these reactions don't have significant impact on the normal function, these reactions will gradually fade away, which is the psychological response of normal people after stressful events. Only when the mental and psychological reactions of the individual appear more symptoms, severe to the individual's obvious pain, the individual work learning and other living functions, the individual mental disorders such as ASD or PTSD are considered. It can lead to strong stressful events that can cause ASD or PTSD to susceptible individuals, such as earthquake, tsunami and other major natural disasters, war, terrorist incidents, accidents such as traffic accidents, production accidents, or sudden death of relatives, loss of freedom and other loss of events, which constitute spiritual traumatic events.

In the face of traumatic events, whether an individual is sick is also related to the individual's susceptibility. Individuals are susceptible to stress related disorders, both internal and external. The intrinsic predisposing factors mainly include individual genetic background, age, gender, personality characteristics and physical condition. The individual's genetic background will affect the susceptibility of individuals to stress related disorders through the characteristics of the HPA axis, the prefrontal lobes, the hippocampus and the amygdala. However, the external vulnerability includes the lack of necessary social support system, childhood trauma experience and negative life events. In order to be more beneficial to clinical intervention and research, some scholars also distinguish the predisposing factors according to the time of occurrence, that is, before the traumatic event, the peri traumatic period and after the traumatic event. Pretraumatic factors include the individual background or family history of anxiety or affective disorder, low IQ, mild nervous system development disorder. The factors of peri trauma include three aspects: the severity of individual's response to traumatic events, individual's cognition of traumatic events, and social support. Posttraumatic factors are related to the timely and effective intervention of the post−traumatic intervention, whether the traumatic event is overlapped, and the individual endocrine and other biological characteristics after the trauma.

In the study of the mechanism of various types of stress−related disorders, the current research mainly focuses on PTSD research. The main reason is that the course of PTSD is long, the symptoms seriously affect the life, and the relative course of ASD is shorter, and the adjustment disorder involves many environmental and psychological factors, and the degree is relatively milder. The research on the pathogenesis of PTSD mainly involves three main aspects: neurophysiology, neuroendocrine and neuroimaging.

(1) Neurophysiological event related potential(event−related potentials, ERPs) is a record of electrical activity recorded from the scalp after receiving a specific stimulus, after cognitive processing. This long latency evoked potential mainly reflects the cognitive process of brain activity. The P300 wave is related to the functions of the temporal lobe, the parietal lobe, the frontal region and the hippocampus. In the study of PTSD, it was found that in the non traumatic interference stimulus, the patient had the neutral target stimulation, the amplitude of P3b decreased and the latency delayed, which reflected the reduction of the processing resource allocation ability of the non−threatening information. In the trauma related stimuli, the amplitude of P3b increased and the degree was related to the task difficulty, reflecting the patient's interference. The response amplification indicated that patients' anxiety and alertness were increased. Compared with non−patients who also have traumatic exposure, the amplitude of P3b increased, suggesting that patients pay more attention to trauma related stimuli. In summary, the results of the P300 study in patients with PTSD suggest that the patient is separated from the information processing of situational dependence, excessively weakening the neutral stimulus and excessively enhancing the processing of trauma related stimuli.

(2) When neuroendocrine in the face of traumatic events, neuroendocrine changes are the precursor of the changes of all organs, and the basis of the plasticity of the function of the nervous system. The changes of neuroendocrine system are very complicated under stress. It involves a variety of transmitters, tempering and receptor systems, such as the excitatory amino acid system, GABA suppressor system, serotonin system, dopamine system, cholinergic system, neurosteroid system, pituitrin, endorphin, neuropeptide, cholecystokinin, and substance P. But the stress related processes are renin angiotensin system and HPA axis system, also known as stress system. A large number of studies suggest that there is chronic dysfunction of HPA axis during PTSD. This feature is different from that seen in other mental disorders. The results include elevated corticotropin releasing hormone in CSF, lower urinary cortisol, and elevated urine norepinephrine/cortisol, and response reduced in regulating factor of adrenocorticotropin with adrenocorticotropic hormone, cortisol inhibition after dexamethasone administration, and decreased number of lymphocyte glucocorticoid receptors. These results suggest that the high response of stress to cortisol is consistent with the high sensitivity of HPA axis.

(3) Neuroimaging in recent years has been widely studied in the aspects of PTSD's brain function and structure. Most of the results suggest that there are abnormal in the hippocampus, the parahippocampal gyrus, the amygdala and the prefrontal lobes. The prefrontal lobe regulates the reaction of amygdale to fear. When the function of the frontal lobe is diminished, the regulation of the amygdala is weakened and overreacted, which leads to a series of clinical manifestations, such as repeated trauma experience, heighten alertness, and anxiety. Whether these changes in brain structure and function are the results or causes of traumatic stress disorder need to be further explored and demonstrated.

12.1.2　Epidemiology

Epidemiological studies on stress related disorders are mostly focused on PTSD. The prevalence of PTSD reported varies widely from a few percent to more than 50%. This is mainly determined by the difference of research objects and the standards adopted. According to the American Psychiatric Association, the prevalence of PTSD in the United States was 1%–14%, an average of 8%, and the lifetime risk was 3%–58%, while the total risk was 1.3% in the German population and 37.4% in Algeria. The risk of suicide in PTSD group is higher than that in general group, up to 19%. Studies on the PTSD of different groups after the Wenchuan earthquake suggest that the prevalence rate is above 10%–30%. The risk of PTSD after traumatic events is related to the intensity and nature of traumatic events. A general human–made traumatic event was significantly higher than a nonhuman violent event, for example: a survey from the United States showed that 50% of the people after rape, capture, torture or kidnapping got PTSD, and 9.2% after the general community trauma experience. Studies have also found that PTSD is not the same age among different sexes. For example, Kessler reported that the age of high incidence of male PTSD was 45–54 years, while that of women was 25–34 years. In general, the incidence of female PTSD is higher than that of men, about two times that of men. The phenomenon is attributed to more traumatic events that women face, such as rape, sex invasion, and the fear of traumatic events in women's psychological characteristics. Epidemiological studies on ASD focus on different groups after major disasters or mass trauma events. Some reports suggest that the incidence of ASD in traffic accident survivors is 13%–14%, the victims of violent crime are 19% , and the massacre witnesses are 33% . The investigation and study of some affected groups after the Wenchuan earthquake found that the incidence of ASD was 30% –60% . Adjustment disorders are always accompanied by acute or chronic stressful events, and there is still no authoritative mass data. The only survey of people aged 18 – 64 , including the five European countries, showed that the prevalence of adjustment disorders was less than 1% . Another report indicates that patients with adjustment disorders account for 5% –20% in psychiatric outpatient department.

12.1.3   prognosis

The prognosis of stress related disorders varies with specific circumstances. In general , ASD recovered within 1 month and partially developed into PTSD , while about 1/3 of PTSD patients developed chronic disease or significantly impaired labor force. The problem of comorbidity of PTSD is also prominent. About 50% of them will be associated with substance abuse , depression and anxiety. The risk of suicide rate in PTSD patients is higher. The occurrence of PTSD is often associated with public emergencies , and the prevention and intervention may affect the use and deployment of a large number of social resources , and also constitute one of the mental diseases that seriously affect the labor force. The prognosis of adults with adjustment disorders is relatively good , most patients can be alleviated by self adjustment or medical treatment. Symptoms may worsen if some stress factors persist. Sometimes , after the removal of stress factors , patients may still turn into severe depression. For the 5 year follow–up study of patients with adjustment disorders , about 71% of adult patients recovered completely , and about 21% of them converted to severe depression or alcohol abuse. The prognosis of adolescent adjustment disorders was poor , and about 43% turned into severe mental disorders , including schizophrenia , schizoaffective disorders , major depressive disorder , substance abuse or personality disorder. Unlike adults , behavioral disorders or adjustment disorders in adolescents will be a predictor of mental disorders in the future.

12.2   Acute stress disorder

Acute stress disorder(ASD) is a kind of transient disorder , which refers to a serious physical or psychological response under a strong stressor to an individual with no obvious mental disorder , usually relieved for hours or days. A stressor can be an extraordinarily traumatic experience , such as a serious threat to the safety or physical integrity of a person or person he loves(such as natural disasters , accidents , wars , violent attacks or rapes) , or a dramatic threat to the personal social status or social network (such as the loss of many relatives or fire in home). The risk of developing the disease increased if individual hasphysical exhaustion or organic factors , such as the elderly. The clinical data of ASD are as follows.

12.2.1   Clinical features

Case report:

Hua Li , Male , 32 years old , Married , Production line worker. Five days before admission , Li's wife and 6 months' son died due to Wenchuan earthquake. Li cried when he heard the news. After a while , he couldn't recognize his families and shouted , "My lovely wife and baby , you can't die…where is this…" with incoherent language. He can sleep only after taking sleeping pills at night. The next day he was quiet , but his face was blank , his eyes looked straight , and he had no emotional reaction. He needed help in life.

12.2.1.1   PTSD similar symptoms

The main symptom of ASD is a group of symptoms similar to PTSD , including the flash back of traumatic experience, numbness and avoidance, and high alertness. Flash back refers to the repeated recurrence of traumatic events in consciousness and the reappearance in dreams. Numbness and avoidance are manifested as active avoidance or emotional numbness in traumatic experience.

12.2.1.2 Dissociative symptoms

It is also one of the common symptoms of ASD, such as blankness, trouble, slow reaction, decreased consciousness, feeling of unreality, dissociative amnesia, personality or reality dissociation. Dissociation symptoms usually occur within minutes or hours after strong mental stressor, most of which are sustained for 2-3 days, and in a few cases the symptoms can last for 1 month. After the symptom is relieved, the patient partially or completely forgets the attack process.

12.2.1.3 General symptoms

In addition to the characteristics of the above two types of symptoms, ASD patients can also show some general symptoms, including anxiety, depression, fear, and autonomicnervous symptoms (such as palpitation, sweating, muscle tension, movement uneasiness).

12.2.1.4 Psychosis

Some ASD patients may show psychiatric symptoms associated with stressful events, such as fragmental hallucinations and delusions, and associated severe anxiety and depression reactions.

12.2.2 Diagnosis and differential diagnosis

12.2.2.1 Diagnosis

The diagnosis of ASD relies mainly on clinical characteristics. Laboratory and other auxiliary examinations are usually used as the basis for excluding other diseases.

The occurrence of ASD must be stressed from minutes to hours after intense mental stress, lasting more than 2 days, generally within 1 week, and the longest not more than 1 month. If the symptoms of ASD persist for more than 1 month, it is diagnosed as PTSD.

The clinical diagnosis of ASD has two main characteristics: first, three symptoms similar to PTSD, that is, flash back, avoidance of numbness and over alertness. The second is the dissociative of symptoms, manifested as limited consciousness, attention narrowing, numbness, and orientation disorder.

The diagnosis of acute stress disorder was diagnosed in three main diagnostic criteria of mental illness in ICD-10, DSM-5 and CCMD-3. The diagnostic essentials of acute stress disorder (DSM-5) are as follows.

The diagnostic criteria 308.3 (F43.0) of acute stress disorder are as follows.

(1) Exposure to actual or threatened death, serious injury, or sexual violation in one (or more) of the following ways.

1) Directly experiencing the traumatic event(s).

2) Witnessing, in person, the event(s) as it occurred to others.

3) Learning that the event(s) occurred to a close family member or close friend.

Note: in cases of actual or threatened death of a family member or friend, the event(s) must have been violent or accidental.

4) Experiencing repeated or extreme exposure to aversive details of the traumatic event(s) (e. g. , first – aid responders collecting human remains, police officers repeatedly exposed to details of child abuse).

Note: this does not apply to exposure through electronic media, television, movies, or pictures, unless this exposure is work related.

(2)Presence of nine(or more) of the following symptoms from any of the five categories of intrusion, negative mood, dissociation, avoidance, and arousal, beginning or worsening after the traumatic event(s) occurred.

1)Intrusion symptoms

①Recurrent, involuntary, and intrusive distressing memories of the traumatic event(s). Note: in children, repetitive play may occur in which themes or aspects of the traumatic event(s) are expressed. ②Recurrent distressing dreams in which the content and/or affect of the dream are related to the event(s). Note: In children, there may be nightmares without recognizable content. ③Dissociative reactions(e. g., flashbacks) in which the individual feels or acts as if the traumatic event(s) were recurring. Such reactions may occur on a continuum, with the most extreme expression being a complete loss of awareness of present surroundings. Note: In children, trauma–specific reenactment may occur in play. ④Intense or prolonged psychological distress or marked physiological reactions in response to internal or external cues that symbolize or resemble an aspect of the traumatic event(s).

2)Negative mood

Persistent inability to experience positive emotions(e. g., inability to experience happiness, satisfaction, or loving feelings).

3)Dissociative symptoms

①An altered sense of the reality of one's surroundings or oneself(e. g., seeing oneself from another's perspective, being in a daze, time slowing). ②Inability to remember an important aspect of the traumatic event(s) (typically due to dissociative amnesia and not to other factors such as head injury, alcohol, or drugs).

4)Avoidance symptoms

①Efforts to avoid distressing memories, thoughts, or feelings about or closely associated with the traumatic event(s). ②Efforts to avoid external reminders(people, places, conversations, activities, objects, situations) that arouse distressing memories, thoughts, or feelings about or closely associated with the traumatic event(s).

5)Arousal symptoms

①Sleep disturbance(e. g., difficulty falling or staying asleep, restless sleep). ②Irritable behavior and angry outbursts(with little or no provocation), typically expressed as verbal or physical aggression toward people or objects. ③Hypervigilance. ④Problems with concentration. ⑤Exaggerated startle response.

(3) Duration of the disturbance (symptoms in Criterion B) is 3 days to 1 month after trauma exposure.

Note: symptoms typically begin immediately after the trauma, but persistence for at least 3 days and up to a month is needed to meet disorder criteria.

(4)The disturbance causes clinically significant distress or impairment in social, occupational, or other important areas of functioning.

(5)The disturbance is not attributable to the physiological effects of a substance(e. g., medication or alcohol) or another medical condition(e. g., mild traumatic brain injury) and is not better explained by brief psychotic disorder.

12. 2. 2. 2 Differential diagnosis

(1)Acute psychotic disorder

The severity of the mental stressor in ASD is obviously strong, the appearance time of the disease is closely related to the mental factors, the symptoms are relatively short, the change of the symptoms is closely related to the mental stress factors, that is, the symptoms are relieved quickly after the release of mental stress factors. Symptomatic features are also different. Symptoms of ASD are recurrent, avoiding numbness, heighten alertness, and separating symptoms.

(2)Affective disorder

Affective disorder may be caused by some stressful events before, but the intensity of stressful events and the relationship between time and the development of symptoms are often not as close as stress disorders. In terms of the content of the symptoms, the emotional coordination of affective disorder is high or low, and the symptoms are longer and repeated.

(3)Dissociative disorder

The dissociative disorder has various manifestations of hysteria with hyperbole, performance and affectation, and the patient has hysteria personality traits, such as high emotion, high suggestive, fantasies and self center.

(4)Organic mental disorders

Some physical diseases, such as the infection of the central nervous system, poisoning, can appear acute mental disorders, which can be shown as delirium, psychomotor excitement, fear, and consciousness disorder. However, organic mental disorders are often unlike acute stress disorders that have direct and strong psychological incentives, and a history of disease, physical examination and laboratory examination can detect the corresponding qualitative basis. The symptoms do not have the main characteristics of stress disorder, namely: reappearance, avoidance of numbness and heighten alertness.

12.2.3 Treatments

Because ASD affects the system of individual belief and meaning, interpersonal relationship, occupational function and physical health, treatment often requires the integration of multiple treatment model.

12.2.3.1 Medicine treatment

Medication is limited to the treatment of symptoms. Clonidine can be used in the treatment of increased alertness. Propranolol, clonazepam and alprazolam are used to treat anxiety and panic reaction. SSRIs, such as fluoxetine, are used for the treatment of avoidance symptoms. Trazodone or topiramate is used for insomnia or nightmares. When ASD develops to PTSD, antidepressants can be used. These antidepressants include SSRIs, MAOIs and tricyclic.

12.2.3.2 Psychotherapy

Studies have shown that cognitive behavioral therapy, exposure therapy, therapeutic writing and supportive treatment are effective for ASD. Psychological education therapy is also a single variable cognitive behavior therapy, which is 3−4 times stronger than supportive therapy in preventing ASD from developing into PTSD. Psychological education therapy combined with cognitive construction of catastrophic events can be used to deal with anxiety by intentional technology, and also to help patients identify and strengthen the positive aspects of emotions and feelings. For example, some people can discover their abilities and talents in crisis time. Group and family therapy can help ASD patients enhancing the effectiveness of coping strategies and reduce social isolation caused by trauma. These treatments give the patient a chance to describe their experiences, to allow the patient to accept the care of the listener, to help the memory conditioning of the event.

(1)Critical incident stress debriefing(CISD) is a therapeutic intervention technique given to individuals who suffer from mental traumatic events(within 48 hours). The aim of the therapy is to weaken the acute symptoms of mental trauma and prevent patients from developing towards comprehensive PTSD. CISD usually contains four steps: ①the description of traumatic events; ②sharing the emotional responses of the survivors to the event; ③open discussion of the symptoms caused by the events; ④explaining that these symptoms are the normal response to the trauma, and then discussing the various coping strategies.

(2) Critical incident stress management(CISM) is an integrated intervention system, which refers to a specially trained professional team that goes to the site of a disaster trauma event to provide a number of different forms of service, such as one to one risk support, and 45−75 minutes for brief collective crisis management briefings, emotional discussions to traumatic events(group discussions on events) against the affected group. CISM is particularly helpful in preventing ASD rescue personnel's exhaustion, such as police, ambulance crews, and health−care workers. In short, immediate crisis intervention after natural disasters and major trauma can help victims express feelings, thereby reducing potential ASD as PTSD develops.

12.2.3.3　Other therapies

Many mainstream professionals also recommend some traditional natural therapies, such as proper nutrition and regular exercise. In addition, yoga and other traditional fitness methods can resist ASD related anxiety and insomnia through muscle contraction and relaxation. Hydrotherapy can be used to treat post−traumatic muscle pain and spasm. Certain herbs can be used to treat functional symptoms of the digestive tract. In addition, prayer, meditation, or talks with spiritual tutors can help or treat individuals who are affected by traumatic events in the belief system.

12.2.4　Prognosis

In social life, trauma such as natural disasters or accidents, can not be completely avoided. But human beings have the responsibility to reduce the degree or frequency of disasters and accidents, and to establish and improve health support social networks. The prevention of ASD mainly includes public mental health education and crisis intervention.

12.2.4.1　Public mental health education

The aim of psychological health and positive psychology education is not only to increase the public's mental health knowledge, but also to cultivate positive psychological quality, including positive values and attitude to life, independent initiative, emotional pressure management ability, active solution and strategy to the problem, sense of humor, communication and collaboration skills, etc. These are all preventive interventions for emergency related barriers. It is necessary to improve the psychological endurance and resilience of individuals after traumatic stress, and to prevent the occurrence of ASD, or to develop ASD to PTSD.

12.2.4.2　Crisis intervention after trauma

Crisis intervention should be carried out as soon as possible after the traumatic events. Interventions include getting out from the crisis environment of traumatic events, giving material support for food, water, and adequate sleep conditions, providing environmental conditions to discuss traumatic events or emotional catharsis, strengthening social support, moderately promoting the normalization of life, and reducing excessive responsibility requirements.

12.3　Post traumatic stress disorder

Posttraumatic stress disorder(PTSD) is a complex disorder involving memory, emotional response, intelligent process, and nervous system damage after one or more traumatic experiences. PTSD is a normal response after abnormal events. In the DSM-5 diagnostic system, PTSD is classified into the category of anxiety disorders.

12.3.1 Clinical features

Case report:

Bingbing, 11 years old, Male, 5th grade primary school. One months ago, a magnitude 6.7 earthquake happened when the patient was in the classroom. When the students ran away, there was stampede and his friend died. The patient's memory repeatedly appeared before. In the evening, the patient woke up with a nightmare. He did not want to go to school and was afraid of noise at home. The patient appeared to be in a trance, slow speech and poor appetite.

12.3.1.1 Symptoms of recurrence

(1) Flashbacks repeatedly recreate traumatic experiences, including palpitations, sweating and other physiological symptoms.

(2) Recurrent distressing dreams.

(3) Intense intrusive imagery.

Reproducing symptoms may cause difficulties in daily life. It can be induced by personal thoughts or feelings. Speech, objects or situations that can cause memories of events can be a contributing factor.

12.3.1.2 Avoidance and numbness

(1) Avoidance of reminders of the events.

(2) Inability to feel emotion.

(3) Strong self reproach, depression or worry.

(4) Diminished interest in activities.

(5) Difficulty in recalling stressful events at will.

Events that remind individuals of traumatic events can ignite evasive symptoms. These symptoms can cause daily life to change. For example, after a serious traffic accident, a person who used to drive may avoid driving or taking a bus.

12.3.1.3 Hyperarousal

(1) Is easy to be frightened.

(2) Feel nervous or uneasy.

(3) Insomnia and/or irritability.

Hyperarousal is often persistent, not only irritated by the inducements of traumatic events, but also irritated by other irrelevant things. High alert symptoms make a person feel irritation and anger. These symptoms make people's daily life difficult, such as sleep, diet, or concentration.

12.3.1.4 Other symptoms

In addition to the above three typical symptoms, PTSD patients also show an increased risk of substance abuse, aggressive behavior or suicidal risk. At the same time, it will also be accompanied by depression, anxiety symptoms and/or coucentration, memory, decreased and other cognitive impairment.

12.3.1.5 The clinical characteristics of PTSD in children

The clinical manifestation of PTSD in children also covers the symptom of adult group, but with different characteristics. For example, children's recurrent symptoms are characterized by repeated nightmares, related to traumatic events. Sometimes they go through trauma related scenes or play games related to trauma, recurring daydreams or flashbacks. They will feel sad and be emotional when they are in a scene. Avoidance symptoms are characterized by efforts to avoid trauma related scenes, activities or associations, thus showing anxiety, withdrawal, sticky and unwilling to fall asleep. Heightening alertness is characterized by excessive panic reaction, lack of concentration, irritability, cowardice, fear of darkness, and fear of nightmares. At the same time, there will be symptoms of cognitive impairment such as school weariness and poor academic performance. Similar to adults, children's PTSD also experience behavioral problems such as impulsive attack, self injurious suicide and addictive behavior.

12.3.2 Diagnosis and differential diagnosis

12.3.2.1 Diagnosis

In the three major diagnostic classification systems of DSM−5, ICD−10 and CCMD−3, the corresponding diagnostic categories of "post traumatic stress disorder(PTSD)" have their respective attribution. In the DSM−5 diagnosis system, PTSD is classified as the major category of "anxiety disorder", and in ICD−10, it is classified as "serious stress response", and in CCMD−3, PTSD is classified as a major stress related disorder. In these three diagnostic systems, there is a similar train of thought for defining the symptom characteristics and duration of the disease. That is, the main symptoms can be diagnosed for more than 1 month. The diagnostic criteria of DSM−5 defines acute as symptoms within 3 months, while chronic diseases are more than 3 months.

ICD−10 introduces the definition and characteristics of PTSD, which makes diagnosis more flexible and requires that the diagnoser has high clinical recognition ability. ICD−10's clinical description of the PTSD classification criteria is as follows.

This is a delayed and/or prolonged response to unusually threatening or catastrophic events or situations, and such events can produce almost everyone's sufferings(such as natural and man−made disasters, wars, serious accidents, witnessing the death of others, being subjected to torture, being a victim of terrorist activity, rape, or other criminal activity). Personality traits(such as compulsion, weakness) or the history of a past neurotic disease can reduce the threshold of the syndrome or make it more serious, but it is unnecessary and inadequate to explain the occurrence of the symptoms with these susceptibility factors.

Typical symptoms include the constant backdrop of "numbness" and emotional delay, repeated recollection of trauma in intruding memories("flashbacks") or dreams, estranged from others, unresponsive to the surrounding environment, lack of pleasure, and avoidance of activities and situations that are easily associated with trauma. In general, it is possible that the patient's original clue to trauma is the object of fear and avoidance. Occasionally dramatic acute outbreaks of fear, panic, or attack are seen, which are triggered by memories and/or reacting stimuli to the trauma or the original response.

Usually there is a hyperexcitability of the autonomic nervous system, characterized by excessive alertness, startle reaction and insomnia. Anxiety and depression often coexist with the above symptoms and signs. The idea of suicide is not uncommon. Another factor that complicate matters is excessive drinking and drug abuse.

After trauma, the incubation period varies from weeks to months(but rarely exceeds 6 months). The course of the disease is fluctuating, and most of the patients can be recovered. A few cases are characterized by chronic disease which has not been cured for many years or transformed into enduring personality changes.

ICD−10's diagnostic points for the PTSD classification criteria are as follows.

The diagnosis of this obstacle should not be too wide. There must be evidence that it occurred within

6 months after severe trauma. However, if the clinical manifestation is typical, and no other suitable diagnosis (such as anxiety, compulsion, depression) can be chosen, even if the event and the onset interval are more than 6 months, it is possible to give a "possible" diagnosis. In addition to the evidence of trauma, there must be repeated, intrusive recollections or recurring in daytime imagination or sleep. There are obvious feelings of alienation, numbness, and avoidance that may evoke traumatic memories. But these are not necessary for diagnosis. Autonomic disorders, mood disorders and behavioral abnormalities are helpful in diagnosis, but they are not essential.

12.3.2.2 Differential diagnosis

(1) Acute stress disorder

The clinical characteristics of acute stress disorder and PTSD are similar. The main point of identification is onset time and course of disease. Acute stress disorder(ASD) quickly became ill within hours after a traumatic event, most of which resumed within 1 week. The symptoms are more characteristic by dissociation symptoms.

(2) Generalized anxiety disorder

The precondition personality of the patients with generalized anxiety disorder is often characterized by anxiety, such as lack of sense of security, tension and anxiety, easy worry, and excessive attention to the physical state of the body. Its onset is not like PTSD's strong and time related traumatic events as a cause, and its symptom characteristics also lack the recurrence of PTSD's trauma experience.

(3) Panic disorder

The onset of panic disorder is not the cause of PTSD, which has strong and time related traumatic stress events. The symptoms are episodic tension, fear, and nervous tension symptoms of autonomic nerve, but not PTSD's flashback and avoidance.

(4) Adaptive disorder

The occurrence of adaptive disorder is related to the relatively light and persistent stress factors, often the changes in the living environment, such as the obvious changes in the situation of immigrant and living. Clinical manifestations were mainly emotional disorders such as anxiety and depression, or maladjustment.

12.3.3 Treatments

PTSD can be applied to all kinds of psychotherapy, and can also be treated with the corresponding drug therapy or the combination of the two methods. Research shows that PTSD can be treated by a variety of psychotherapy, drug treatment can alleviate the various symptoms, and also help to promote the consolidation of psychotherapy. The combination of drug therapy and psychotherapy is the best way. Therefore, the treatment of PTSD needs the cooperation of psychiatrists and psychotherapists. The situation of each PTSD patient is different, so the treatment strategy adopted for each patient is different. It is important that PTSD therapy is performed by a professional psychiatrist or psychotherapist who is professionally trained of PTSD. There are also differences in the types of symptoms treated by different treatments.

12.3.3.1 psychotherapy

A series of different psychotherapy methods, including cognitive behavioral therapy(CBT), hypnotic therapy, eye movement desensitization reprocessing(EMDR) and psychoanalysis, are used in the treatment of the disease. The ways and functions of all kinds of psychotherapy are as follows.

(1) Cognitive behavioral therapy

A number of comparative studies on CBT treatment of PTSD showed that CBT therapy has a good effect on the treatment of PTSD's core symptoms and related symptoms. There are two main approaches to CBT treatment for PTSD. One is exposure therapy. The principle is to induce patients to desensitization to traumatic memories. Another training for anxiety management is to teach patients to reduce anxiety. These include relaxation training, biofeedback, social skills training, decentralization, or cognitive reconstruction.

(2) Kinetic psychotherapy

This method will help the patient recover the feeling of self while learning new coping strategies and methods, so as to deal with the intense emotion related to the trauma. Usually, the treatment process consists of three stages: ①establishing a sense of security for the patient; ②deep exploration of the trauma; ③helping the patient to reestablish the link between the family, the friends, the wider society, and the resources of all other meanings.

(3) The establishment of discussion groups or peer groups

These groups are usually supervised by experts specializing in different trauma problems, such as different types of trauma experts for war, rape/incest, or natural disasters. They help patients recognize other survivors, share similar experiences and emotional reactions. This approach is very helpful for patients who feel guilty and feel guilty about traumatic events. For example, some patients compromise to keep their lives, or they are killed in some disasters, but they survive themselves.

(4) Family therapy

Family therapy should be recommended for patients whose family life is affected by PTSD symptoms.

12.3.3.2　Medication

For patients with severe symptoms of PTSD, medication is often needed. Drug therapy can not only treat the core symptoms of PTSD, that is, the recurrence of traumatic experience, numbness, the increase of alertness, and the treatment of symptoms, anxiety and depression. At present, there are many kinds of drugs used to treat symptoms of PTSD, usually involving the following species.

(1) Selective serotonin reuptake inhibitors(SSRIs): SSRIs has been used as a first-line drug for the treatment of PTSD. The study showed that sertraline, 50-200 mg/d, was effective in treating increased alertness and numbness, effective over 50%, and effective for prevention of recurrence, which was officially approved by the US Food and Drug Administration(FDA). In addition, other kinds of SSRIs, such as paroxetine, fluoxetine and citalopram, etc., are also used clinically in the treatment and prevention of PTSD recurrence.

(2) Other updated serotonin antidepressant: evidence showed that venlafaxine (average dose 225 mg/d) or mirtazapine(average dose 34 mg/d) could significantly improve the symptoms of PTSD.

(3) Tricyclic antidepressant drugs including imipramine, Doxepin and amitriptyline are effective in improving the symptoms of depression and anxiety in PTSD patients, but the effect of PTSD's main symptoms such as recurrence and avoidance of symptoms is not obvious.

(4) Monoamine oxidase inhibitor(MAOIs), phenylhydrazine(45-75 mg/d), is used for the treatment of traumatic dreams, flashback, panic response and sudden violence, and is effective for intrusive trauma symptoms, and is better than imipramine.

(5) Adrenergic blocker beta blocker, propranolol, 120-160 mg/d, is effective in treating temper irritability, nightmare, sleep disorders, intruder symptoms, hyperarousal, and phobia . Norepinephrine α_2 receptor antagonist clonidine, 0.2-0.4 mg/d for 6 months of emotion self-control, relieving temper irritable to improve sleep, relieving panic, hyperarousal and intruding symptoms, and improving psychosocial function. The α_1 adrenergic antagonist, prazosin, is an antihypertensive drug, but it has been proved that 1-4 mg/d prazosin is effective in treating the nightmare symptoms of PTSD, and is also effective for daytime symptoms, such

as relieving pain.

(6) Mood stabilizers and anticonvulsant drugs lithium carbonate, carbamazepine and sodium valproate are effective in the treatment of PTSD's irritability and anger symptoms and heighten alertness. About three fourth of topiramate 50 mg/d was effective after 4 weeks of treatment.

(7) Atypical antipsychotics also have symptomatic effects on PTSD. Quetiapine can be used to improve disease related sleep problems. Risperidone 2-4 mg/d changed the symptoms of flashback, high alertness, anxiety and psychotic symptoms in PTSD patients.

12.4 Adjustment disorder

Adjustment disorder is a stressful or difficult situation for a long time, and the patient has certain personality defects, resulting in emotional disorders such as annoyance and depression, as well as behavior disorder or physiological dysfunction, and impaired social function. The course of disease is long, but generally not more than 6 months. It usually starts within 1 month after stressful events or changes in life. With time passing, by the elimination of stimulus or adjustment to emergency, mental disorders will ease. The disorder may occur in all ages due to the causes: the death of the loved one, the divorce or the relationship problems, the changing of the habitual life, the physical or health problems of the person or the lover, the new family or the new city, the unforeseen disaster, worry about the economy problem. The common sources of stress for adolescents are family problems or conflicts, school problems or related sexual problems.

12.4.1 Clinical features

Case report:

Lili, 22 years old, female, college student. 6 months ago, Lili went to the United States to study. Lili feel pressure, and gradually appear insomnia, lack of concentration, memory decline. She felt depressed and tired. She also complained about dizziness and headache.

The clinical manifestations of adaptive disorders are varied. Depressive symptoms, anxiety symptoms, trauma stress behavior symptoms, or the combination of the three.

12.4.1.1 Depressive symptoms

Patients with general adjustment disorder have mild depressive symptoms, including loss of interest, disappointment, crying, nervousness and cowardice.

12.4.1.2 Anxiety symptoms

Anxiety, worry, despair, sleep disorder, concentration less, collapse and suicide.

12.4.1.3 Behavioral disorders

Irritability, fighting, reckless and indiscreet, forgetting important tasks (such as paying bills, homework), avoiding family and friends, lowering academic performance, playing truant, destroying property and so on.

12.4.2 Diagnosis and differential diagnosis

12.4.2.1 Diagnosis

In the three main diagnostic classification systems of DSM-5, ICD-10 and CCMD-3, there are indications for diagnosis. The description of adjustment disorders in ICD-10 is that a state of subjective pain and emotional disorder usually hinders social function and behavior, and occurs during adaptation to the consequences of obvious changes in life or stressful the events. The stessor may affect the integrity of the individual social network(bereavement or separation experience), or the broader social support system and value system(immigrant or refugee state). Stressors can involve individuals themselves, or influence groups or communities. Compared with other disorders, individual susceptibility plays a more important role in the occurrence of adjustment disorders and in the form of expression. But we are still asseme that if there is no stressor, this will not happen. Various clinical manifestations, including depression, anxiety, annoyance (or the mixture of the various symptoms mentioned above), feel that the current situation can not be dealt with, the plan is impossible, it is difficult to continue. In addition, there is a certain degree of function defect in daily affairs. Patients may feel prone to unexpected behavior or sudden violence, but this rarely happens. However, conduct disorders, such as aggression or non social behavior, can be accompanied by characteristics, especially adolescents. Any individual symptom is insufficient in severity and prominence to meet a more specific diagnosis. In children, bed – wetting, childish voice and sucking fingers can be repeated. These degenerative phenomena are usually part of the whole symptom.

Adjustment disorders usually occur within 1 month after stress events or changes in life. The duration of symptoms is generally not more than 6 months.

Diagnostic points: the diagnosis of adjustment disorders depends on conscientiously evaluating the following relationship.

(1)The form, content and severity of symptoms.

(2)Past medical history and personality.

(3)Stressful events, situations or life crises.

The existence of these third factors must be clearly identified and there should be evidence(although presumably) of no disorder without stress. If the stress is weak or does not confirm the time connection(less than 3 months), it should be classified in other disorders according to the characteristics presented.

12.4.2.2　Differential diagnosis

(1)Depression

Adjustment disorders often show depressive symptoms and need to be differentiated from depression. Depression is characterized by more severe depressive symptoms, often accompanied by negative suicidal thoughts or behaviors. Severe depression has a day and night light change. The inducement of depression is often less obvious than that of adjustment disorder. At the same time, depression may have a history of depressive episode or bipolar disorder in the past, and is more likely to have family history.

(2)Personality disorders

The emotional state and behavior characteristics of personality disorder are consistent, without obvious and specific stressors, often accompanied by many years of interpersonal maladjustment. The discomfort of personality disorder can be aggravated by stressor, but stress is not the dominant factor of the formation of personality disorder. If people with personality disorders have new symptoms in the role of stress sources and meet the diagnostic criteria for adjustment disorders, they can be diagnosed with dual disorders of adjustment disorders and personality disorders.

12.4.3　Treatments

12.4.3.1　Solving the source of stress

Most of the patients with adjustment disorder will relieve their symptoms after removing the stress factors or changing the uncomfortable environment. Therefore, it has a direct therapeutic effect on patients with adjustment disorders to solve stressors reasonably.

12.4.3.2 Psychotherapy

Although the source of stress has a direct therapeutic effect on adjustment disorders, many stressors are unavoidable or difficult to solve in real life. Therefore, it will play an important role in the treatment of adjustment disorders by reducing the psychological stress level of the stressor by psychotherapy and improving the adaptability and resilience of individual stress.

Treatment modalities for adjustment disorders can be individual therapy, group therapy, crisis intervention, and family therapy. The goal of the treatment is to encourage negative emotional expression, to reduce the degree of pain caused by negative emotions, to promote cognition, understanding and learning problems/coping styles, to establish connections and supportive networks and to adjust positive emotions.

(1) Cognitive behavioral therapy(CBT) is mainly to help patients deal with their feelings: ①first, therapists should help patients understand negative emotions and thoughts; ②then the therapist helps the patient enter the helpful mental state and healthy action.

(2) Other treatment. ①Long course therapy: in the course of long course treatment, the individuals who have adjustment disorder can used for months to explore their own thoughts and feelings and to clarify the significance of stress, and then actively comprehend and construct. ②Family therapy: therapists work with family members, clarify problems, build connections and support. ③Self-help group: help patients get different perspectives on adversity and build contacts and support with people who share problems.

12.4.3.3 Medicine treatment

For patients with severe symptoms, medication can be considered, such as serious anxiety, serious sleep disorders, or excessive sadness. Drug therapy can not only relieve the symptoms of patients, but also increase the effect of psychotherapy. Drug therapy is usually based on the specific circumstances of the patient to select relatively short-term anxiolytic drugs and/or antidepressant drugs.

Deng Hong

Chapter 13

Physiological Disorders Related to Psychological Factors

13.1 Introduction

Physiological disorders related to psychological factors are a group of mental disorders characterized by physical dysfunctions related to psychosocial factors. The disorders covered in this chapter include eating disorders, sleep disorders and sexual dysfunctions.

The concept of psycho-physiological disorder first developed in the United States since the 1960s. Now, in DSM-5, physiological disorders related to psychological factors are described in different chapters, respectively, as selected sleep-wake disorders, eating disorders and sexual dysfunctions. In ICD-10, it is also known as behavioral syndrome with physiological dysfunction and somatic factors.

Physiological disorders related to psychological factors and psychosomatic diseases belong to psychosomatic medicine that is a branch of studying the relationship between mind and body. Psychosomatic medicine promotes the transformation of medical model from biomedical model to bio-psycho-social medical model.

13.2 Eating disorders

Eating disorders(ED) are persistent disturbance related to eating or eating-related behaviors, combined with an intense preoccupation with body weight and shape. Eating disorders can cause physical symptoms (e. g. ,heart and kidney problems) and even death.

Eating disorders are also common with mental disorders(e. g. ,anxiety disorders,depression,and substance abuse).

The cause of eating disorders is not clear but involves biological,psychological,and socio-cultural factors. Socio-cultural and interpersonal elements can trigger onset,and changes in neural networks can sustain the illness.

The present lifetime prevalence of all eating disorders is about 5% and common, especially in young adults and adolescents. Eating disorders are more common in women than in men, usually start in adolescence. Treatment involves monitoring, nutritional counseling, psychotherapy and sometimes medicines.

According to ICD-10, the code classification of eating disorders(F50) is behavioral syndromes associated with physiological disturbances and physical factors(F50-F59). The categories of eating disorders by ICD-10 areanorexia nervosa(AN, F50. 0), atypical anorexia nervosa(F50. 1), bulimia nervosa(BN, F50. 2), atypical bulimia nervosa(F50. 3), overeating(binge-eating) associated with other psychological disturbances(F50. 4), vomiting associated with other psychological disturbances(F50. 5), other eating disorders(F50. 8), and eating disorders, unspecific(F50. 9). The disorders focused in this section are anorexia nervosa, bulimia nervosa and psychogenic or nervous vomiting.

13.2.1 Anorexia nervosa

13.2.1.1 Overview

Anorexia nervosa is a chronic eating disorder characterized by very low body weight, an extreme concern about weight and shape . characterized by an intense fear of gaining weight and becoming fat. Some people with anorexia may also engage in binge-eating. Anorexia can cause malnutrition, amenorrhea, osteoporosis, loss of skin integrity, heart problems and suicide. It is a fatal disorder.

13.2.1.2 Epidemiology

Anorexia nervosa is a life-threatening eating disorder. Anorexia nervosa has been reported more frequently over the past several decades. Most patients are young women. It usually begins in adolescence or young adulthood, although childhood-onset and older-onset cases and encountered. It is estimated a lifetime prevalence of 0.9%-4.3% among women and 0.2%-0.3% in men in Western countries. The male-female ratio is about 1 : 10. The range of onset is between 10 and 30 years old although it typically begins in adolescence. The most common age of onset is between 14 and 18 years old. 5% of anorectic patients have the onset in their early 20s. There is a secondary peak of individuals their 40s. Rates of anorexia nervosa have increased significantly over the last few decades. The risk of developing an anorexia nervosa is higher in models, actors, dancers and athletes such as gymnasts and figure skaters.

13.2.1.3 Etiology and pathogenesis

The exact etiology is not known. Genetic, biological, psychological, socio-cultural and personal factors are implicated in the causes of anorexia nervosa.

(1) Genetic factors

Numerous studies have shown a possible genetic predisposition toward anorexia nervosa. There is an increased risk for the disorder in biological siblings of patients with anorexia nervosa. Twin studies have shown a heritability rate of between 28% and 58%. In addition, epigenetic mechanisms mean by which environmental effects alter gene expression, such as DNA methylation, may contribute to the development or maintenance of anorexia nervosa.

(2) Biological factors

Neurobiological factors: some evidences have shown that anorexia nervosa is linked to abnormal neurotransmitter activity in the part of rain that controls pleasure and appetite. Evidences from physiology, pharmacology and neuroimaging imply serotonin may play a role in anorexia. Serotonin dysregulation such as alterations in 5-HT1A and 5-HT2A receptors and the 5-HT transporter may affect mood, impulse control and feeding behavior. Serotonin dysregulation is also involved in other mental disorders such as depression and anxiety disorders. Research in these areas are relatively new and the mechanisms are unclear.

Brain imaging: brain CT studies have shown that patients with anorexia nervosa have increased CSF clearance (brain drain and ventricular enlargement) after long periods of starvation. Resting state fMRI has identified the insular cortex and corticolimbic circuitry as likely brain areas responsible for the symptomology of anorexia nervosa. Positron emission tomographic scan studies have shown that the metabolism of caudate nucleus is higher in the anorectic state than after realimentation.

(3) Psychological factors

The cause of anorexia linked are to childhood sexual abuse or troubled relationships. Psychological issues related to feelings of helplessness and difficulty in establishing autonomy have also been suggested as contributing to the development of anorexia nervosa. Studies have shown family dynamics can play a part in the cause of anorexia. Some patients of anorexia nervosa resist parental control by dieting in order to resolve family conflicts. In addition, patients with anorexia nervosa might have a history of being teased about their size or weight. Other psychological causes include feelings of inadequacy, anger, anxiety, depression and loneliness.

Psychoanalysis agrees that young anorectic patients have been unable to separate psychologically from their mothers and have greedy and unacceptable oral desires. Therefore, these desires are projectively disavowed.

(4) Personal factors

Certain personality traits appear to more vulnerable to developing anorexia nervosa. Anorectics tend to be perfectionists who have a right-or-wrong, black-or-white, all-or-nothing way of seeing situations. Some anorectics lack a strong sense of identity and have low self-worth or low self-esteem.

(5) Socio-cultural factors

Socio-cultural factors are associated with the development of anorexia nervosa. Rates of this disorder appear to vary among different cultures and change across time as cultures evolve. Social stress and values are also the reasons of anorexia nervosa. Vocational and avocational interests interact with other vulnerability factors to increase the probability of developing anorexia nervosa. For example, people of certain occupation (such as models, dancers, actress, jockeys and wrestlers) requiring to be thin are more likely to develop anorexia. Those with anorexia have much higher contact with cultural sources that promote weight loss. When there is a constant pressure from people to be thin, teasing, bullying can cause psychological symptoms. In addition, different culture can have very different expectations related to appearance and weight. In cultures where being thin is idealized, the individual may try to maintain an unhealthy and unrealistic weight. Modern western and eastern culture emphasizes that the thinner, the more beautiful, so that women tend to gain social recognition and appreciation through their pursuit of slim bodies.

13.2.1.4   Clinical features

Case report:

The patient, female, 13 years old, 165 cm, junior high school student. Three year ago, her friend said: "you play piano wonderfully, but you look a little fat." After that, the patient began to control her diet and paid more attention to the body shape and weight. She only ate vegetables, and took various methods to avoid weight gaining, such as taking weight-loss drugs and self-induced vomiting. Her weight decreased gradually from 48 kg to 30 kg. Her hair fell out, and her menstruation was irregular. Four months ago, amenorrhea appeared. But she still considered herself too fat and refused eating.

The symptoms of anorexia include extreme weight loss, fear of gaining weight, body image disturbance, physical symptoms and psychiatric symptoms.

(1) Weight loss

Patients of anorexia nervosa are not really anorexic, but normal appetite.

Patients attempt to lose weight and stay slim by limiting energy intake and consuming energy, vomiting, misusing laxatives, exercising excessively, etc. Firstly, patients may be preoccupied with dieting. They usually eat very little despite being underweight or at a healthy weight. Some cut food into tiny pieces, refusing to eat around others and hiding or discarding of food. Patterns of obsessively measuring caloric intake or weight may be prominent. Many patients restrict themselves from eating more than 1,000 calories each day, stay away from fattening foods, and completely eliminate meats from their diets. Secondly, some may repeat self-induced vomiting or catharsis by using laxatives, enemas, diet pills, ipecac syrups, diuretics, and water pills. Lastly, patients lose weight by excessively physical exercise including running, dancing, jumping, micro-exercising such as making small persistent movements of fingers or toes.

Some odd behavior directed toward losing weight occurs. For example, patients usually refuse to eat with their families or in public places.

(2) Fear of gaining weight and body image disturbance

No matter how weight loss is achieved, even is underweight, starved or malnourished, an intense fear of gaining weight and becoming overweight is present in all patients with the disorder. Patients are so fear of even the slightest weight gain that they take all precautionary measures to avoid gaining weight or becoming obese. Patients are addicted to an obsession with counting calories and monitoring fat contents of food. The fear of weight gain is a persistent criterion for anorexia nervosa.

Body image disturbance: body image disturbance is at least two components. Firstly, there is adistorted perception of body size, weight and shape so that either the whole body or specific body parts appear larger or "fatter" to the individual. Patients believe themselves to be too fat while in reality they are dangerously and severely underweight. The overvalued ideas about body shape and weight are the central psychological features of anorexia nervosa. This belief explains why most patients do not want to be helped to gain weight. Secondly, it is body image disparagement, where the body is viewed as repulsive or loathsome. Body image disparagement can also be generalized or focused on specific parts of the body and is often accompanied by body shape avoidance(i. e., the avoidance of situations that places a focus on shape and weight, such as looking in a mirror).

(3) Physical symptoms

Patients usually come to medical attention when their weight loss becomes apparent. As the weight loss grows profound, physical signs and symptoms appear, patients show a variety of metabolic changes(Table 13-1).

(4) Psychiatric symptoms

It is important to identify that just how many of psychiatric symptoms are a result of anorexia nervosa rather than a cause of it. Insomnia, obsessive-compulsive behavior, social phobia, depression, anxiety, solitude, and irritability are most frequently psychiatric symptoms of anorexia nervosa noted clinically. Anorexia nervosa also have high rates of comorbidity(about 50%) with major depressive disorders. The suicide rate is high in persons with anorexia nervosa. Some patients may keep away from friends and families, and become more social withdraw.

Table 13-1   Physical symptoms of anorexia nervosa

Item	Physical symptoms of anorexia nervosa
Vital sign	Bradycardia
General condition	Dry hair and skin, lanugo, edema, muscle atrophy, loss of body fat, malnutrition, looking pale, sunken eyes, halitosis, low weight, hypothermia(as low as 35 ℃)
Cardiovascular system	Hypotension, bradycardia
Nervous system	Paralysis, fainting or dizziness, headaches, heightened sensitivity to cold
Digestive system	Constipation, nausea, vomiting, fullness after eating, bloating, epigastric discomfort
Endocrine system	Spanomenorrhea, amenorrhea, asexuality, infertility, delayed psychosocial sexual development
Hematologic system	Anemia, leukopenia
Urinary system	Prerenal azotemia
Mental problems	Chronic fatigue, suicide

13.2.1.5   Diagnosis and differential diagnosis

(1)Diagnosis

In ICD-10 and DSM-5, it is defined by different criteria. According to ICD-10, for a definite diagnosis of anorexia nervosa, all the following are required.

Symptoms criteria: low body weight, body weight is maintained at least 15% below that expected(either lost or never achieved), or body mass index(BMI) is less than 17.5 kg/m^2, or under 85% of weight expected for height, age and sex. Prepubertal patients may show failure to make the expected weight gain during the period of growth. Self-induced behaviour, the weight loss is self-induced by avoidance of "fattening foods". One or more of the following may also be present, self-induced vomiting; self-induced purging; excessive exercise; use of appetite suppressants and/or diuretics. Distorted body image, body image distortion with a dread of fatness: an extreme concern about weight and shape characterized by an intense fear of gaining weight and becoming fat, a strong desire to be thin. Endocrine disorder, a widespread endocrine disorder involving the hypothalamic-pituitary-gonadal axis; manifesting in women as amenorrhoea and in men as a loss of sexual interest and potency. Pubertal delayed or arrested, if onset is prepubertal, the sequence of pubertal events is delayed or even arrested(growth ceases; in girls the breasts do not develop and there is a primary; in boys the genitals remain juvenile). With recovery, puberty is often completed normally, but the menarche is late.

Course criteria: symptoms last at least three months.

Severity criteria: the symptoms cause clinically significant distress or affect social and vocational function.

exclusion criteria: exclusion of symptoms caused by other physical diseases(e.g., liver cirrhosis, hypothyroidism, cancer); exclusion of symptoms caused by other mental disorders(e.g., depression, anxiety disorder, schizophrenia) and medications.

(2)Differential diagnoses

The medical disease: weight loss, vomiting, and peculiar food handling may occur in medical disorder such as tuberculosis, brain tumor or cancer. Clinicians should do the relevant examination to eliminate the medical disease. Endocrine disorder is common in the individual of anorexia nervosa so it should be eliminated somatic disorder through related examinations.

Depressive disorder: both depressive disorder and anorexia nervosa have several features in common, such as loss weight, sadness, depression, anxiety, obsessive idea, and occasional suicidal thoughts. The two disorders, however, have some distinguishing features. Generally, patient with a depressive disorder has decreased appetite, whereas patient with anorexia nervosa claims to have normal appetite and to have hungry feel; only in the severe stages of anorexia nervosa do patients actually have decreased appetite. Intense fear of obesity, disturbance of body image, purging behaviour or hyperactivity is typical of patients with anorexia nervosa but is absent in patients with a depressive disorder.

Schizophrenia: patients with schizophrenia pay more attention to the food to be poisoned and are seldom concerned with caloric(calorie) of food, and are rarely preoccupied with a fear of gaining weight.

13.2.1.6 Course and prognosis

The course of anorexia nervosa varies greatly. The outcome of anorexia nervosa varies from spontaneous recovery to a waxing and waning course to death. Some are spontaneous recovery without treatment, some recover after a variety of treatments, some deteriorate course result in death caused by complications of starvation.

After a series of comprehensive treatment of anorexia nervosa, about 45% of patients have better prognosis without any problems. About 30% of patients have a moderate prognosis with many symptoms and weight problems. About 25% of patients have poor prognosis, with chronic underweight condition, recurrent attacks, and repeated inpatient treatment. 5%–15% of patients die of multiple organ failure, cardiac complications, secondary infection, and suicide. The prognosis of patients with short course are better than that with long course.

13.2.1.7 Treatments

According to the complicated psychological and medical implications of anorexia nervosa, a comprehensive treatment, including nutrition therapy, somatic support therapy, pharmacotherapy, and psychotherapy is recommended. Effective treatment also requires close cooperation among multidisciplinary professionals, including nutritionist, physician, pediatrician, psychiatrist, therapist, social worker, patients and their families. Early intervention and treatment are more effective. Treatment for anorexia nervosa tries to address three main areas: restoring the patients to a healthy weight; treating the psychological problems related to this disorder; reducing or eliminating behavior or thought that originally led to this disorder.

(1)Nutrition and somatic support therapy

The priority of anorexic treatment is addressing and stabilizing any serious health issues. Hospitalization may be necessary if patients are with dangerously low weight, comorbidity(e. g. , depression), dangerous and fatal complications, suicide or suicide risk, outpatient care treatments failed.

Somatic support therapy: the purpose is to save lives and maintain the stability of vital signs. It mainly includes correcting disorders of water and electrolyte metabolism, balancing acid and alkaline, providing enough energy to sustain life, eliminating edema and removing the threat of life. Nutrition therapy: the goal is to regain normal weight. Nutrition is the most essential factor to patients, and must be tailored to each person's condition. Dietary intake should start from small amount and increase gradually. Food variety is important according to different needs, for which fluid, semi-liquid or soft food can be selected; adequate energy, protein, vitamins, and inorganic salts must be ensured as well to help the body recovery, regaining the normal weight.

(2)Psychotherapy

Psychotherapy has been clinically proven to reduce the severity, shorten the duration of anorexia nervosa. Cognitive and behavioral therapy(CBT) has been found effective for inducing weight gain and reducing relapse rates in anorexia nervosa. It is important to make a specific dietary plan, monitor food intake and binging and/or purging behaviors. While emphasizing that weight control is only one aspect of the problem, help should be offered with cognitive restructuring to identify automatic thoughts, challenge their core beliefs, and resolve their problems in interpersonal relationships. Family therapy has been advocated, reflecting the belief that family factors are important in the origins of anorexia nervosa. Systematic reviews suggest family therapy is successful for adolescents with anorexia nervosa. In addition, Guidelines also suggest cognitive analytic therapy(CAT) and interpersonal therapy(IPT) for anorexia nervosa, but the evidence is limited.

　(3)Pharmacotherapy

Pharmaceuticals can be used as adjuvant therapy although they have limited benefit for anorexia itself. Antidepressants(specifically selective serotonin re-uptake inhibitors; e. g. , SSRIs), anti-anxiety or antipsychotics can also be used to treat anorexia nervosa. Medication should not be used as the sole or primary treatment for anorexia nervosa, rather, it should be used in conjunction with therapy. Patients have significant symptoms of depression, antidepressants such as SSRIs are sometimes used for this indication. Antipsychotics such as olanzapine may aid initial weight gain.

13.2.2　Bulimia nervosa

13.2.2.1　Overview

Bulimia nervosa(BN) is a chroniceating disorder characterized by binge eating(uncontrolled excessive eating)followed by purging. Bulimia was first described by Russell(1979)as a variant of anorexia, and soon was accepted as a separate diagnosis. The main features of bulimia are binge eating and purging behaviors in order to preventing weight gain. Three essential criteria of bulimia are recurrent binge eating, recurrent compensatory behaviour, and preoccupation with own body weight or shape. Bulimia may have symptoms that overlap anorexia. This disease is a gluttony caused not by organic disease, nor by epilepsy, schizophrenia and other psychiatric disorders.

13.2.2.2　Epidemiology

Bulimia nervosa is more prevalent than anorexia nervosa and has been reported dramatic increased over the past several decades. Bulimia nervosa occurs more frequently in developed countries and occurs more in cities than in rural areas. Bulimia nervosa is more common in women than in men, and more common in late adolescence and early adulthood. The lifetime prevalence is 1. 0% (about 1. 5% in women and 0. 5% in men). The prevalence of bulimia is around 1% among women aged between 16 and 40 years in western societies. Generally, bulimia has its first onset in adolescence or young adulthood, which is often later in adolescence than that of anorexia. Although bulimia is often present in normal-weight young women, sometimes they have a history of obesity.

13.2.2.3　Etiology and pathogenesis

The causes of neurobiology, genetics, psychology, and socio-culture are similar to those described above for anorexia(see 13.2.1.3 Etiology and pathogenesis).

　(1)Genetic factors

Family studies of bulimia have consistently found a higher lifetime prevalence of bulimia among their relatives. Further, numerous twin studies suggest that liability to bulimia is significantly influenced by additive genetic factors. Increased frequency of bulimia is found in first-degree relatives of patients with the disorder. Although many molecular genetic studies have been conducted, they do not yield an unanimous finding.

　(2)Biological factors

Some studies have attempted to associate the symptom of binging and purging with various neurotransmitters. Because antidepressants often benefit patients with bulimia. Some studies have shown serotonin affects binging behavior in bulimics. Research has also focused on abnormalities in the structure or activity of hypothalamus. Studies suggest that the hypothalamus of bulimics may be lack of initiation of a normal satiation(feeling full or finished) response. MRI studies suggest that overeating in bulimia nervosa may result from an exaggerated perception of hunger signals related to sweet taste mediated by the right anterior insula area of the brain.

(3)Psychological factors

Psychological factors are precipitating factors of bulimia. Patients with bulimia are outgoing, angry, and impulsive. Object—relations theory insists patients with bulimia are difficult to separate from caretakers, as manifested by the absence of transitional objects during their early childhood. Psychoanalysis views that bulimia nervosa is imbalance between superego and ego(lack superego control and the ego strength). Studies show psychiatric disorder, including a family history of psychiatric disorder, especially depression, substance misuse and emotional lability(including suicide attempts) are associated with bulimia. Certain family attitudes or dynamics may contribute to the risk of a child or teenager developing an eating disorder. Sexual abuse may be a risk factor for the development of bulimia.

(4)Socio—cultural factors

Bulimia occurs most often in industrialized cultures where there is an emphasis on thinness and slim figure, especially if thinness is linked to success. Media have created an unrealistic thin image of the perfect, successful person. The stress to be thinner and higher achievers can lead to bulimia, even in very young children.

(5)Others

Bulimia nervosa occurs in persons with high rates of mood disorders and impulse control disorders, substance—related disorders and personality disorders. 25% of patients with bulimia have a history of a previous episode of anorexia nervosa. Professions and sports such as ballet dancer, model, swimmer may respond to societal pressures to be slender which indirectly encourageeating disorders.

13.2.2.4 Clinical features

Case report:

The patient, female, 20 years old, 160 cm, 52 kg before illness, a college student. Two years ago, after breaking up with her boyfriend, She felt upset. One day after shopping, she found it was very pleasant to eat too much. After that, there is an irresistible desire to eat, and need to eat a lot of food immediately (the amount of food is several times than usual. She can eat 1 kg rice, 10 steamed buns, etc.). Gluttony almost happen every day. After binge eating, she fears of weight gain so much that she often use a variety of means to avoid gaining weight such as increasing excretion, reducing absorption or doing excessive exercise. Now, she weights 53 kg and has normal menstruation.

Bulimia nervosa is a serious and potentially life—threatening eating disorder characterized by the three central features, physical symptoms and psychiatric symptoms.

(1)The three central features

The main features of bulimia nervosa are recurrent binge eating, recurrent compensatory behaviour, andbody image disturbance(overvalued ideas concerning shape and weight). This cycle may be repeated several times a week, or in more serious cases, several times a day.

Recurrent binge eating: an episode of binge eating is characterized by the following: eating much faster than normal during a binge perhaps in a short space of time; eating a large amount when not hungry that is definitely larger than most people would eat during a similar period of time and circumstances; eating until feeling uncomfortably full; eating alone or secretly; a sense of lack of control over eating during the episode; binges may be planned in advance; feelings of guilty, shame or disgust following a food binge.

Recurrent compensatory behaviour: recurrent inappropriate compensatory behaviour are practiced after binge eating to prevent weight gain primarily by self-induced vomiting, abusing laxatives or diuretics, using enemas, or exercising obsessively (see 13. 2. 1. 4 Clinical features). Some use a combination of all these forms of purging. Vomiting is common and is usually induced by sticking a finger down the throat. Some patients are able to vomit at will. Vomiting can decrease the abdominal pain and the feeling of being bloated and allows patients to continue eating without gaining weight. Individuals with bulimia "binge and purge" can maintain normal or above normal body weight.

Fear of gaining weight and body image disturbance (overvalued ideas concerning shape and weight, see 13. 2. 1. 4 Clinical features).

Both bulimia nervosa and anorexia nervosa have body image disturbance. However, their core psychopathologies are different. In contrast to anorexia nervosa, symptoms of bulimia nervosa are more ego-dystonic, dysphoria, guilt, self-loathing and overwhelming "loss of control".

(2) Physical consequences

Bulimia nervosa have less physical consequences than anorexia nervosa. However, there are some physical complications worthy of further discussion. Electrolyte imbalance such as hypokalaemia, caused by repeated vomiting, can lead to weakness, cardiac arrhythmias, cardiac arrest, and even death. Esophagitis, metabolic alkalosis, abdominal pain or nausea may occur. The teeth become pitted and erosion of dental enamel by the acidic vomitus, and patients often complain of dental pain and sensitivity. Rarely, urinary infections, tetany, and epileptic fits may occur. Unlike patients with anorexia nervosa, those with bulimia nervosa may maintain a normal or above body weight.

(3) Psychiatric symptoms

As in anorexia nervosa, general psychiatric symptoms are prominent in bulimia nervosa. Depressive symptoms are more prominent in bulimia nervosa than in anorexia nervosa, and are probably secondary to the eating disorder. In addition, patients with bulimia nervosa also have increased rates of anxiety disorders, bipolar disorder, dissociative disorders and obsessive-compulsive features. Patients with bulimia nervosa engage in maladaptive behaviours such as self-harm, alcohol and drug misuse, shoplifting and sexual abuse. However, different from those with anorexia nervosa, women with bulimia nervosa are generally more sexually active than general population.

13. 2. 2. 5   Diagnosis and differential diagnosis

(1) Diagnosis

Many individuals with bulimia "binge and purge" are in secret and maintain normal or above normal body weight, so they can often successfully hide their problem from others for years.

Symptoms criteria: the preoccupation with eating and food, and irresistible desire of food, eating a large amount of food in a short time and an uncontrollable binges; recurrent inappropriate compensatory behaviour in order to prevent weight gaining, such as self-induced vomiting, misuse of laxatives, enemas, diuretics, or other medication (e. g. , appetite suppressant, thyroxine agent), fasting and excessive exercise; psychopathology including the morbid fear of obesity and strict weight limit that is far below the standard. Some patients (but not all) have a history of anorexia nervosa. The interval between bulimia nervosa and anorexia nervosa ranges from months to years.

Course criteria: the binge eating and inappropriate compensatory behaviour both occur, on average, at least twice a week for 3 months.

Severity criteria: the symptoms cause clinically significant distress or affect social and vocational function.

Exclusion criteria: exclusion of symptoms caused by other physical diseases (e. g. , liver cirrhosis, hypothyroidism, cancer); exclusion of symptoms caused by other mental disorders (e. g. , depression, anxiety disorder, schizophrenia, anorexia nervosa) and medications.

(2) Differential diagnoses

Binge eating disorder: both binge eating disorder and bulimia nervosa are characterized by episodic bouts of the intake of excessive amounts of food. The two disorders, however, have some distinguishing features. Binge eating disorder has nopurging or compensatory behavior, however, bulimia nervosa has.

Kleine-Levin syndrome: both Kleine-Levin syndrome and bulimia nervosa have hyperphagia. Kleine-Levin syndrome is a sleep disorder characterized by persistent episodic hypersomnia (lasting for 2-3 weeks) and cognitive or mood changes. Many patients also experience episodic hypersomnia, disorientation, manic impulse, hypersexuality, and other symptoms besides hyperphagia. Patients with Kleine-Levin syndrome have not overvalued ideas concerning shape and weight, and purging or compensatory behavior.

13.2.2.6   Course and prognosis

Compared with anorexia nervosa, bulimia nervosa has better prognosis. Those treated cases are much better than those untreated cases. Patients untreated tend to remain chronic or small improvement with time. A longer duration of the disorder, childhood obesity and low self-esteem may be associated with a worse prognosis and outcome.

13.2.2.7   Treatment

There are two main types of treatment: pharmacological and psychosocial treatments.

(1) Psychotherapy

There are several supported psychosocial treatments for bulimia. CBT should be considered the benchmark, first-line treatment for bulimia nervosa. The data supporting the efficacy of CBT are based on strict adherence to rigorously implemented, highly detailed, manual-guided treatments that include about 18-20 sessions over 5-6 months. CBT is quite effective for treating bulimia nervosa in adults. Family-Based Treatment (FBT) might be more helpful to younger adolescents who need more support and guidance from their families. Psychodynamic treatment of patients with bulimia nervosa has been of limited studied. Some researchers have also claimed positive outcomes in hypnotherapy.

(2) Pharmacotherapy

Antidepressant medications such as SSRIs have been shown to be helpful in treating bulimia. This may be based on elevating central 5-hydroxytryptamine levels. Antidepressant medications can reduce binge eating and purging independent of the presence of a mood disorder. Fluoxetine (Prozac) is approved by FDA for the treatment of bulimia, and other antidepressants such as sertraline may also be effective for treating bulimia.

13.2.3   Psychogenic vomiting

13.2.3.1   Overview

Psychogenic vomiting is a group of mental disorders that spontaneous or self-induced vomiting. According to ICD-10, psychogenic vomiting is called vomiting associated with other psychological disturbances (F50.5)

13.2.3.2   Etiology and pathogenesis

Psychogenic vomiting is often related to psychosocial factors such as distress, emotional upset, tension. Patients with psychogenic vomiting are usually self-centered, easy to be implied, exaggerated, artificial, etc. Psychogenic vomiting is more common in women than in men, and usually presents in early or middle adult life.

13.2.3.3　Clinical features

Case report:

The patient, female, 15 years old. One year ago, after being criticized by her teacher, the patient vomited after eating. The vomited substance was stomach contents. She vomited more than 10 times a day without obvious nausea or other discomfort. Later, she suffered repeated attacks under similar circumstances. The patient denied that she wanted to lose weight. In the past year her weight is not significant reduction, and menstruation is normal.

Psychogenic vomiting is chronic and episodic vomiting without an organic cause, which commonly occurs after meals without nausea, endocrine disorder and other discomfort. Recurrent vomiting is spontaneous or self-induced after eating, with just eaten food, and does not affect appetite. More than 80% of patients are normal weight. Psychogenic vomiting can be accompanied by the clinical symptoms of dissociative disorders such as exaggeration, affectation, sudden onset, and strong suggestibility.

13.2.3.4　Diagnosis and differential diagnosis

(1) Diagnosis

Symptoms criteria: spontaneous or self-induced of recurrent vomiting is freshly eaten food; usually more than 80% of patients are normal weight (weight loss of patients is not obvious) and some of patients even gain weight.

Course criteria: vomiting occurs almost every day, at least for 3 months.

Severity criteria: the symptoms cause significant distress or affect social and vocational function.

Exclusion criteria: exclusion of symptoms caused by other physical diseases (e. g. , cancer); exclusion of symptoms caused by other mental disorders (e. g. , bulimia nervosa, hypochondriacal disorder, dissociative disorders) and medications. Exclusion of excessive vomiting caused by pregnancy.

(2) Differential diagnoses

Bulimia nervosa: it should be distinguished from bulimia nervosa, in which self-induced vomiting follows episodes of binge eating (uncontrolled overeating).

13.2.3.5　Course and prognosis

The prognosis of psychogenic vomiting is good.

13.2.3.6　Treatments

Treatments are differed according to the various factors considered. For patients who principally present psychological problems such as stress, psychotherapy are suggested (see 13.2.1.7 Treatments). It is reported that psychotherapy can be helpful in psychogenic vomiting. In addition, sometimes pharmacotherapy is needed. Nutrition and somatic support therapy may be necessary according to the condition. Antidepressant medications such as SSRIs and anxiolytic drug are helpful in psychogenic vomiting.

13.3　Sleep disorders

Sleep disorders are the general terms for various functional disorders associated with specific stages of sleep, which include disorders of initiating and maintaining sleep, disorders of excessive somnolence and disorders of sleep-wake schedule. In many cases, sleep disorders are one of the symptoms of another mental or physical disorder. Even if a particular sleep disorder appears to be clinically independent, there are may mental and/or somatic factors that may be associated with it. Sleep disorders are independent, or simple feature of other disorders, should be determined to its reason, course, clinical feature and lab examination. In any case, the diagnosis of sleep disorders can be made by the patient's main complaint.

The ICD-10 classification of sleep disorders is rather different from DSM-5 and ICSD-3 classification of sleep disorders. The ICD-10 system sets aside two areas for sleep disorders: organic(ICD-10 code: G47) and nonorganic(ICD-10 code: F51), but it only includes a few actual sleep disorder diagnoses. This chapter mainly discuss nonorganic sleep disorders. The nonorganic sleep disorders' classifications in accordance with the ICD-10 include the following: nonorganic insomnia, nonorganic hypersomnia, nonorganic sleep-wake schedule disorders, sleep-walking disorder, sleep terror, nightmare disorder, other nonorganic sleep disorders and nonorganic sleep disorder(not specific).

13.3.1 Nonorganic insomnia/insomnia

13.3.1.1 Overview

Nonorganic insomnia/Insomnia is the most common sleep disorder characterized by unsatisfactory quality and/or quantity of sleep. The predominant complaint in insomnia is difficulty with sleep initiation, sleep maintenance, or early awakening despite adequate opportunity, time and circumstance for sleep or quality associated with daytime functional impairment. Insomnia can occur independently or as a result of another problem. Insomnia can cause anxiety, depression, irritability, impairment in social, occupational, or other important areas of function. In the case of children or cognitively impaired adults, often the parent or caregiver who reports the problem.

13.3.1.2 Epidemiology

Insomnia is very common. Approximately one-third has several serious bouts of insomnia yearly. Ninety percent of the general population has experienced acute insomnia at least once. Approximately 10% of the population may suffer from chronic insomnia. The prevalence of insomnia in the general population is 10% – 20%. Insomnia affects people of all ages including children, although it is more common in adults and its frequency increases with age. Population surveys show a 1 – year prevalence rate of 30% – 45% in adults. Between 15% –30% of adults and 10% –23% of adolescents have insomnia. The prevalence rates of male and female is not significantly. Different approximately half of insomnia is related to a psychiatric disorder.

13.3.1.3 Etiology and pathogenesis

Insomnia can be caused by a variety of causes. The main causes are:

(1) Environmental factors

Poor sleeping environment, e. g. , ambient noise, light, air pollution, over-crowding, or sudden changes of the sleep environment.

(2) Psychological factors

Many life changes can trigger insomnia. Situational stress(e. g. , relationships, academic stress, job-related stress, financial problems, noise stress, medical worries) and unhappiness life or work event can lead to insomnia. In addition, high health requirement and excessive attention of sleep is also easy to lose sleep.

(3)Sleep rhythm changes

Travel or other factors, such as work schedules that disrupt sleep routine, also may trigger insomnia. Frequent shifts in day and night can change circadian rhythms and cause insomnia.

(4)Physiological factors

Physiological factors such as hunger, fatigue, sexual excitement, daytime naps, stimulation before bedtime, etc.

(5)Medication, substance abuse and food factors

Medication, substance abuse and food factors such as alcohol, caffeine, tea, nicotine, benzodiazepine misuse, antidepressants[selective serotonin reuptake inhibitors(SSRIs) and monoamine-oxidase inhibitors (MAOIs)], sympathomimetics(salbutamol, pseudoephedrine), anti-hypertensives(beta-blockers, calcium-channel blocker), non-steroidal anti-inflammatory drugs, corticosteroids(agitation), recreational drugs, drug withdrawal(hypnotics), etc.

(6)Mental disorders

Insomnia can occur as a result of a coexisting mental disorder. Many mental disorders(e. g. , anxiety disorder, depression, bipolar disorder, post-traumatic stress disorder, schizophrenia) are associated with sleep disorders, and insomnia is often part of mental symptoms. Insomnia may also manifest as a clinical feature of a more predominant mental disorder.

(7)Medical condition

Insomnia can occur as a result of medical condition such aschronic obstructivepulmonary disease, renal disease, Parkinson's disease, fibromyalgia, arthritis, cancer, pain, etc.

13.3.1.4　Clinical features

Case report:

The patient, female, 32 years old. 2 years ago, She had difficulty in falling asleep, maintaining sleep and had many nightmares. She felt daytime sleepiness. Her memory, attention and ability to work were impaired. She felt tension, headaches, increased errors and mistakes. She became worried about sleep more. Sometimes she was unhappy, anxious and irritable. One month ago, these symptoms worsen so that she couldn't go to work.

(1)Sleep problems

The main symptom of insomnia is trouble falling or maintaining asleep, which leads to lack of sleep. Symptoms include as follows. Sleep-onset insomnia: lying awake for a long time before you fall asleep (difficulty in initiating sleep). Sleep-maintenance insomnia: sleeping for only short periods(difficulty in maintaining sleep with frequent awakenings or problems returning to sleep; being easy to wake up because of sound or light). Early-morning awakening: wake up too early. Feeling as if you haven't slept at all.

In adolescents and young adults, the main concerns are generally noted in trying to fall asleep; in older adults, just the opposite is true, and older adults often report trouble maintaining sleep.

(2)Impairment of daytime function

Impairment of daytime function is the defining and the most common symptom of insomnia. The daytime functional impairment in insomnia include daytime sleepiness, daytime fatigue, poor attention or concentration, impaired memory, reduced motivation or lack of energy, tension, headaches, increased errors and mistakes, gastrointestinal symptoms, as well as concerns and worries about sleep. Insomnia has an increased risk of depression, anxiety and irritability. In adults, insomnia is also associated with cognitive impairment, increased job absenteeism, increased accident risks, higher health care costs, lower values of quality of life and impaired social and vocational function. In children insomnia is associated with poor school performance.

13.3.1.5 Diagnosis and differential diagnosis

(1)Diagnosis(diagnostic criteria,ICD-10)

Doctor will diagnose insomnia based on medical and sleep histories and some physical exams[e. g. , polysomnography(PSG)].

Symptoms criteria: difficulty in falling asleep, or difficulty in maintaining sleep, or poor quality of sleep; the preoccupation with insomnia and the consequences of insomnia; the excessive attention to sleep; impairment of daytime function.

In assessing symptoms, be sure to examine bedtime behaviors and sleep-wake schedules, especially in children and adolescents, where diagnosing this condition is rare.

Course criteria: insomnia occurs at least three times a week and lasts more than one month.

Severity criteria: the length of sleep and/or unsatisfactory quality of sleep have caused obvious distress or affect social and vocational function.

Exclusion criteria: exclusion of insomnia caused by other physical diseases(e. g. , hypertensive, peripheral neuritis, cancer); exclusion of insomnia caused by other mental disorders(e. g. , depression, anxiety disorder, schizophrenia).

(2)Differential diagnoses

Short duration sleep: it's important to make a distinction between insomnia and short duration sleep. Short duration sleep may be normal in some patients who may require less time for sleep without feeling daytime impairment.

Sleep deprivation: in insomnia, adequate time and opportunity for sleep is available, whereas in sleep deprivation, lack of sleep is due to lack of opportunity or time to sleep because of intentional avoidance of sleep.

Narcolepsy: both insomnia and narcolepsy have the trouble of sleeping. Narcolepsy is usually one or more of the additional symptoms such as falls, sleep paralysis, and pre-sleep hallucinations. However, there are certain clinical and EEG features that can help in differentiating insomnia from narcolepsy.

13.3.1.6 Course and prognosis

Insomnia has a good prognosis, but the treatment of refractory insomnia is highly demanding for patients.

13.3.1.7 Treatments

(1)Cognitive-behavior therapy for Insomnia

Cognitive-behavior therapy for Insomnia(CBT-I) includes stimuli control therapy(SCT), sleep restriction therapy(SRT), sleep hygiene education, relaxation training and cognitive reconstruction. Among these, SRT, SCT and sleep hygiene education are three primary treatments. Interestingly, despite the "C" in CBT-I, it is not the case that formal cognitive therapy but a routine part of CBT-I interventions. There is clear evidence that CBT-I is an efficacious evidence-based treatment that produces clinical gains. Adult chronic insomnia disorder management guide recommends CBT-I as a first-line treatment for insomnia (ACP,2016).

Sleep hygiene education: as a treatment, the intervention requires the clinician and patient review a set of instructions which are geared toward maintaining good sleep habits. It is useful for all patients with insomnia and can be applied in primary care. Sleep hygiene is the recommended behavioral and environmental practice that is aimed to promote better quality sleep. This recommendation was developed in the late 1970s as a method to help people with mild to moderate insomnia. These include keeping regular bedtime and arousal, limited maps, release worry, and having a peaceful, comfortable, quiet and dark sleep environment. In addition, it is important to reduce preoccupation with stressors that disturb sleep-wake schedule and thinking of unnecessary events or factors. Avoid overexcitement before going to bed, late-evening exercise, large late meals, alcohol, nicotine, caffeine, and other stimulants before bedtime, excessive alcohol and smoking, excessive daytime sleep, too much time in bed lying awake.

Sleep restriction therapy(SRT): this intervention requires patients to limit the length they spend in bed and evaluated by a sleep diary. In order to accomplish this, the clinician works with the patient to establish a fixed wake time and decrease sleep opportunity by prescribing a later bedtime.

Stimulus control therapy: the goal of this intervention is to bring sleep under better stimulus control. Typical instructions include the following: sleep only in the bedroom(not on the chair or couch); do not stay in bed except for sleep and sex; engage in a distracting, but not too stimulating, activity that provides a focus of attention other than sleep; leave the bedroom when awake for approximately 15-20 minutes and stop trying to sleep.

(2) Pharmacotherapy

Both pharmacological and non-pharmacological approaches can be used to treat insomnia. Drugs were widely used in the past, but non-pharmacological approaches are now recommended as first-line treatment.

Insomnia is commonly treated with benzodiazepine hypnotics(temazepam, alprazolam, clonazepam) or non-benzodiazepine hypnotics [zolpidem, eszopiclone (Lunesta), zaleplon (Sonata)], and other hypnotics. Hypnotic drugs should be used with care. In general, sleep medications should not be prescribed for more than 2 weeks because tolerance and withdrawal may result. Patients with obvious anxiety and depression can be used anti-anxiety or antidepressant medications.

13.3.2   Nonorganic hypersomnia

13.3.2.1   Overview

Nonorganichypersomnia/hypersomnia, the new diagnosis of hypersomnolence disorder(HD) or hypersomnolence in DSM-5, is a sleep disorder of excessive sleepiness by prolonged sleep episodes or daytime sleep episodes occurring almost daily. People with a hypersomnia may fall asleep at times that is inconvenient, debilitating, dangerous or even potentially life-threatening such as at work, during a meal, in the middle of a conversation or while driving. Hypersomnia may also have other sleep-related difficulties such as a lack of energy and trouble thinking clearly and cause distress or impairment in social, occupational, or other important areas of functioning.

13.3.2.2   Epidemiology

Hypersomnia affects approximately 5% of the general population, with a higher prevalence for men due to the sleep apnea syndromes. This disorder becomes most apparent in late adolescence and early adulthood (age 17-24).

13.3.2.3   Etiology and pathogenesis

The etiology is not clear. It rarely occus in children, but it is related to psychological factors. Partly lethal and familial hypersomnia have familial agglomeration, which may be associated with genetic factors.

13.3.2.4   Clinical features

Case report:

The patient, male, 18 years old. He had excessive sleepiness (usually more than 9 hours sleep) and still report nonrestorative and disturbed sleep. He had excessive and sudden bursts of daytime sleep. Once he suddenly fall in sleepiness when he was walking. He got bruise and broken his right calf. He had lost recent memory, and his thinking and learning ability was decline.

The symptoms of hypersomnia are excessive daytime sleepiness (EDS) , prolonged nighttimesleep or nonrestorative sleep(sleep can not relieve fatigue). Among these, the most common characterization of hypersomnia by self-reported is excessive sleepiness.

Excessive sleepiness: the average individual sleep between 6 and 9 hours a night. Hypersomnia has an abnormal increase of 25% or more in time spent sleeping. The sleep cycle of hypersomnia often exceeds 9-hour period, and the individual may have trouble waking up, staying awake or repeated daytime naps that usually provide no relief from symptoms.

Nonrestorative sleep: it occurs with poor sleep quality, and individuals report they are exhausted after what would be considered an adequate amount of sleep. Although it is a common symptom related to hypersomnia disorder, if it occurs alone without the other related symptoms, it is not considered hypersomnia, and another disorder that captures this specific symptom should be considered.

Some may lead to severe physical and cognitive impairment manifested as loss of recent memory, decrease of thinking and learning ability. Some may lead to physical impairment such as bruise, fracture and, eventually death.

Excessive sleep causes significant stress, impairment of social function or decline in quality of life.

13.3.2.5　Diagnosis and differential diagnosis

(1) Diagnosis(diagnostic point, ICD-10)

Symptoms criteria: excessive daytime sleep or sleep onset may not be accounted for by an inadequate amount of sleep; recurrent episodes of sleep or lapses in sleep within the same day(i. e. , may need to take repeated naps, can develop dangerous automatic behavioral routines); sleep more than 9 hours and still report nonrestorative and disturbed sleep. (i. e. , always feels tired and reports sleep is not restful); prolonged nighttime sleep; difficulty waking up after an abrupt wakening(i. e. , can not seem to get moving to complete important tasks; sluggish, resulting in frustration and distress for the individual).

Course criteria: symptoms occurs for at least 1 month.

Severity criteria: symptoms has caused obvious distress or affect social and vocational function.

Exclusion criteria: the excessive sleep is not better accounted for by insomnia, does not occur exclusively during the course of another sleep disorder, and can not be accounted for by an inadequate amount of sleep. The disturbance is not caused by physiological effects of a substance, mental disorders(e. g. , depression, anxiety disorder, schizophrenia), or a general medical condition.

(2) Differential diagnoses

Narcolepsy: the identification of hypersomnia and narcolepsy is critical. Both of them have excessive sleepiness. Narcolepsy is usually one or more of the additional or auxiliary symptoms such as falls, sleep paralysis, and pre-sleep hallucinations. The sleep episodes of narcolepsy are irresistible and invigorating. Nighttime sleep of narcolepsy is short. In contrast, hypersomnia has fewer episodes during the day and lasted longer. Patients can prevent it from happening; nighttime sleep of hypersomnia is usually prolonged and it is difficult to achieve full arousal when waking up. However, there are certain clinical and EEG features that can help in differentiating hypersomnia from narcolepsy.

Sleep apnea syndrome: most patients with sleep apnea syndrome has apnea at night, typical intermittent rhonchi, obesity, high blood pressure, impotence, cognitive impairment, hyperactivity and sweat at night, morning headaches and bad fraternal movement except signs of excessive daytime sleep.

13.3.2.6   Treatments

(1)Etiological treatment

Finding the causes as much as possible. For example, hypersomnia arises from medical conditions, drug or substance use.

(2)Sleep hygiene and CBT

The regular lifestyle: drinking more coffee, tea and other beverages during the day, going to bed at night on time, arranging a relatively fixed and moderate amount of physical activity such as walking, exercise, running, and tai chi(see 13.2.1.7 Treatments).

(3)Pharmacotherapy

The main goal is to control symptoms and improve the quality of life. The ideal treatment for hypersomnia is based on the symptoms. There is cure for these conditions, but symptoms are managed with either the wake promoting substance modafinil(Provigil; first−line treatment) or traditional psycho−stimulants such as amphetamines and their derivatives(if modafinil fails). Central stimulants(e. g. , Methylphenidate/Ritalin, Pemoline) can improve excessive daytime sleepiness. But it needs to be used with caution because of the dependence. Other drugs used to treat hypersomnia include clonidine, levodopa, bromocriptine, activating antidepressants, and monoamine oxidase inhibitors.

13.3.3   Non−organic sleep−wake schedule disorders/nonorganic sleep−wake rhythm disorders

13.3.3.1   Overview

The sleep−wake cycle is one of the most prominent circadian rhythms, and is regulated by a complex interaction between the homeostatic process(a drive for sleep which builds up during wakefulness and declines during sleep) and the circadian process(a sleep−wake independent 24−hour oscillatory rhythm that modulates sleep and wake propensity). For optimal sleep, the required sleep and wake times should be in synchrony with the timing of the intrinsic circadian rhythm of sleep and wake propensity. The normal sleep−wake rhythm for most people is sleeping at night and waking up during the day.

Nonorganic sleep−wake schedule disorders(nonorganic sleep−wake rhythm disorders) arecaused by a mismatch between circadian rhythms and required sleep−wake cycle. These disorders are persistent or recurrent patterns of sleep disruption due to an alteration of the circadian system or misalignment between the endogenous circadian rhythm and sleep − wake schedule required by an individual's environment or schedule. In other words, a person's natural biological clock for sleep is at odds with times required for them to go to sleep and wake up. This disease is common in adults, rare in children or adolescents.

13.3.3.2   Etiology and pathogenesis

The basic underlying etiology is a desynchrony between an individual's internal circadian biological clock and the desired or conventional sleep−wake cycle. Under normal circumstances the internal circadian pacemaker is reset each day by bright light, social cues, stimulants, and activity. In cases such as circadian dysrhythmia(working at night, irregular life, jet lag, etc.) and stress(anxiety caused by stress can lead to delay sleep, wake up early and disrupt the whole rhythm structure) in which these factors fail to reset the circadian rhythm, Nonorganic sleep−wake schedule disorders occur. Some studies have shown it is associated with genetic factors.

13.3.3.3　Clinical features

Case report:

Mike, male, 32 years old, writer, late sleep for 4 years. 4 years ago, Mike began to sleep late because of difficulty in falling asleep. He fell asleep during 1 o'clock to 3 o'clock, and got up at noon. After getting up, he felt dizzy and could not focus on work. But he was energetic at night, active in thinking and effective in work. So he worked at night and postponed his sleep time. He felt upset because he couldn't participate in social activities due to his work schedule. So he came to the hospital for treatment.

Nonorganic sleep-wake schedule disorders include conditions in which the sleep times are out of alignment. Patients with the disorders does not follow the normal sleep times at night and are accompanied by worry, fear, mental activity disability and social functional impairment. The main symptoms:

The sleep rhythm is reversed: the symptoms are the daytime sleep and the nighttime awake.

Delayed sleep phase disorder: this disorder is a sleep pattern that is delayed by two or more hours so that patients go to sleep later at night and sleeps later in the morning. These patients, are commonly referred to as night owls, are more alert in the evening and early nighttime, stay up later, and are more tired in the morning.

Advanced sleep-wake phase disorder: this disorder is characterised by falling asleep several hours before normal bedtime and wake up earlier than normal. These patients, are sometimes called early birds or larks, are drowsy in the evening, want to sleep earlier, awaken earlier, and are more alert in the early morning.

Irregular sleep-wake rhythm disorder: this disorder is patients' circadian rhythms to be so disorganized that there is no clear sleep or wake pattern. People with this sleep disorder may sleep off and on in a series of naps over a 24-hour period. The sleep-wake pattern is temporally disorganized, and the timing of sleep and awake is unpredictable.

Shift work disorder: a non-traditional work(e. g. , transportation, health care) schedule involving night shifts can cause shift work disorder. The patients sleep quality is poor and consistent feelings of fatigue or exhaustion.

13.3.3.4　Diagnosis

Symptoms criteria: it is a misalignment between the individual's sleep wake pattern and normal sleep-wake pattern of his culture or environment; insomnia during the main sleep phase, but drowsiness when sober.

Course criteria: these symptoms occur almost every day for more than 1 month or recurrent over a short period of time.

Severity criteria: the unsatisfactory of quality or quantity and/or disturbance of circadian rhythm of sleep lead to clinically significant distress or impairment in social, occupational, or other important areas of function.

Exclusion criteria: these disorders do not occur exclusively during the course of another sleep disorder or other mental disorder. These disorders are not due to the direct physiological effects of a substance (e. g. , a drug of abuse, a medication) or a general medical condition.

13.3.3.5　Treatments

(1)Sleep hygieneand CBT

The prerequisite step in any case is to follow "sleep hygiene", although for people with nonorganic sleep-wake schedule disorders it is generally not sufficient to normalize their schedule (see 13. 3. 1. 7 Treatments).

(2) Chronotherapy

Chronotherapy, also called chronotherapeutics or chronotherapeutic drug delivery, is one technique used to reset the biological clock. It involves progressively phase delaying a person until the circadian oscillator is synchronized with the desired sleep-wake schedule.

(3) Light therapy

The most successful method of shifting one's sleep schedule seems to be exposure to bright light first thing in the morning. This can be achieved by going out in the sunlight, or by sitting in front of a bright light designed for this purpose (typical room lighting is not nearly bright enough). It is important to use a light that has the ultraviolet components filtered out, or eye damage can result.

(4) Pharmacotherapy

Sedative hypnotic drugs are used to maintain normal sleeping time at night. Small doses of central stimulants are used to maintain normal daily activities.

13.3.4   Sleep-walking disorder

13.3.4.1   Overview

Sleep-walking disorder/sleepwalking, also known as somnambulism or noctambulism, is a non-rapid eye movement (NREM) parasomnia characterized by apparently purposive complex motor behavior duringslow-wave sleep (N3) sleep, typically occurs within the first third of the night when slow-wave sleep is most prominent. It is also of importance to evolutionary biologists, as it is not observed in nonhuman primates and is regarded as an acquired behavioral response associated with humanoid differentiation

13.3.4.2   Epidemiology

Sleep-walking disorder affects an estimated 10% of all humans at least once in their lives. It is far more common in kids than in adults. Sleep-walking disorder is most common between the ages of 5 and 12 years and has peak prevalence between ages 4 and 8 years. After adolescence, it usually disappears spontaneously. Occasionally, the disorder persists into adult life.

13.3.4.3   Etiology and pathogenesis

The exact etiology of sleepwalking is not delineated. A number of hypotheses include delay in the maturity of the central nervous system, increased slow wave sleep and sleep deprivation. Sleepwalking may be familial, which show heritable factors may predispose an individual to sleepwalking disorder. Other factors that may bring on sleepwalking disorder include environmental factors, fever, stress and excessive tiredness, etc.

13.3.4.4   Clinical features

Behaviors: typically, there is no physiological forewarning that indicates a sleepwalking episode is about to occur. Sleepwalking episodes may include sitting up in bed, walking around, eating, and in some cases "escaping" outdoors. In their confused state, sleepwalkers may think they are being attacked and may react violently to defend themselves, but rare cases are associated with violent behavior.

Although sleepwalking cases generally consist of simple behaviours, there are occasionally reports of people performing complex or repeated behaviours. Most children do not actually walk, but sit up and make repetitive movements.

Glassy-eyed stare/blank expression: although their eyes are usually open, the expression is dim and glazed over. It may last from 30 seconds to 30 minutes. During a sleepwalking episode, pupils are typically dilated.

Disorientation: the sleepwalker could be confused and perplexed, and might not know why/how they got out of bed; however, the disorientation will go away within minutes. Episodes usually end with patients returning to bed or awakening(briefly) confused and disoriented.

Communication: usually, sleepwalkers do not respond to questions and are very difficult to wake, but sometimes, it is typically gibberish.

Amnesia: sleepwalkers often have little or no memory of the incident, as their consciousness has altered into a state in which it is harder to recall memories. Children sleepwalkerusually do not remember anything that happened during sleepwalking episode.

Sleepwalkers can occasionally harm themselves. Adults with severe problems should be given advice about safety, avoidance of sleep deprivation, and any other circumstances that might make them excessively sleepy(e. g. , drinking alcohol before going to bed).

13.3.4.5 Diagnosis and differential diagnosis

(1)Diagnosis(diagnostic point, ICD-10)

Characterized by one or more of the following episodes: waking up, usually in the first third of the night and walking around; glassy-eyed stare/blank expression; disorientation may last a few minutes; episodes last from a few minutes usually less than 30 minutes; going back to bed or other place for sleeping automatically; amnesia; doing not respond to questions and being very difficult to wake. Having not obviously affect social and vocational function. Exclusion of sleepwalking disorder caused by other physical diseases(e. g. , epilepsy), other mental disorders (e. g. , depression, dissociative (conversion) disorder, schizophrenia) and other sleep disorders(e. g. , sleep terror, nightmares).

(2)Differential diagnoses

Partial-onset seizures: the major consideration in any paroxysmal disorder is to rule out an epileptic basis for the episodes. Frontal lobe epilepsy and temporal lobe seizures can mimic sleepwalking episodes. However, there are certain clinical and EEG features that can help in differentiating sleepwalking from seizures. Usually, sleepwalking episodes occur during first few cycles of N3 sleep as compared with seizures, which often occur during drowsiness of N2 sleep anytime during the night.

13.3.4.6 Treatments

Most cases do not need to be treated.

Nonpharmacologic measures: patients may benefit from education, reassurance, addressing precipitating factors, ensuring a safe environment, and proper sleep hygieneand CBT(see 13. 3. 1. 7 Treatments). As sleepwalkers can occasionally harm themselves, they need to be protected from injury. Doors and windows should be locked. Removal of potentially dangerous objects from the bedroom, clearing the floor obstructions, and allowing the patient to sleep on the ground floor, on a mattress placed directly on floor or in a sleeping bag. Adults with severe problems should be given advice about safety, avoidance of sleep deprivation, and any other circumstances that might make them excessively sleepy (e. g. , drinking alcohol before going to bed).

Pharmacologic measures: refractory cases, recurrent episodes with a risk of injury to self or others are usually an indication for drug treatment. Low-dose benzodiazepine(e. g. , clonazepam) or antidepressant medications may alleviate sleepwalking.

13.3.5　Sleep terror/night terror

13.3.5.1　Overview

Sleep terror, also known as night terror, is episode of screaming, intense fear and flailing while still asleep. Sleep terror disorder is an arousal in the first third of the night during deep non-rapid eye movement (stages 3 and 4) sleep. A sleep terror episode usually lasts from seconds to a few minutes, but episodes may last longer. Sleep terror is sometimes familial. Sleep terror often is paired with sleepwalking and is much less common than nightmares.

13.3.5.2　Epidemiology

The condition begins and usually ends in childhood, but occasionally persists into adult life. Approximately 2% of adults and 20% of young children have sleep terrors. High comorbidity with sleepwalking.

13.3.5.3　Etiology and pathogenesis

Various factors can contribute to sleep terrors, such as sleep deprivation and extreme tiredness, stress, sleep schedule disruptions, travel or sleep interruptions, fever.

13.3.5.4　Clinical features

Case report:

Sarah, female, 12 years old, student, poor sleep quality for 3 months. 3 months ago, Sarah's parents found that Sarah repeatedly screamed and cried during sleep. When her parents woke her up, she sat in the bed, seemed very scared and confused, with short breathe, fast heart beats and heavy sweat. The next day, she couldn't remember what happened last night. She was very healthy in the past.

It is characterized by a sudden arousal with intense fearfulness. Recurrent episodes usually begin with a piercing scream or cry and are accompanied by behavioral manifestations of intense anxiety bordering on panic and marked tachycardia, tachypnea, diaphoresis, and mydriasis. Patients are unresponsive to stimuli, difficulty arousing during an episode, and, if awakened, are confused or disoriented. After a few minutes patients slowly settles and returns to normal calm sleep without awakening. There is little or no dream recall and amnesia for the episodes usually occurs. In rare cases, awakening elicits aggressive behavior.

13.3.5.5　Diagnosis and differential diagnosis

(1) Diagnosis (diagnostic point, ICD-10)

Characterizing by one or more of the following episodes: begin with a frightening scream or shout, sitting up in bed and appear frightened, staring wide-eyed accompanying sweat, breathe heavily, and having a racing pulse, flushed face and dilated pupils; recurrent episodes usually occur in the first third of the night and last form 1-10 minutes; be unresponsive to stimuli; be hard to awaken, and be confused or disoriented if awakened at least a few minutes; have no or little memory of the event the next morning and recollections can be very limited (usually limited to one or two pieces of image); exclusion of sleepwalking disorder caused by other physical diseases (e. g. , epilepsy, brain tumor); exclusion of sleep terror caused by other mental disorders [e. g. , dissociative (conversion) disorder] and other sleep disorders (e. g. , sleepwalking disorder, nightmare).

(2) Differential diagnoses

Nightmare: sleep terror differs from nightmare. The dreamers of a nightmare wake up from the dream and may remember details, but patients who have sleep terror episode remain asleep and usually have no recall of the details of the event and is unresponsive during the episode. However, there are certain clinical and EEG features that can help in differentiating sleep terror from nightmare. Usually, sleep terror occurs during deep non-rapid eye movement(stages 3 and 4) sleep as compared with nightmare, which often occurs in REM sleep.

13.3.5.6　Treatments

A regular bedtime routine and improved sleep hygiene and CBT(see 13.3.1.7 Treatments)have been shown to be helpful. Benzodiazepines and antidepressant medications have been shown to be effective in preventing sleep terror, but the prolonged use should be avoided.

13.3.6　Nightmare disorder/nightmares

13.3.6.1　Overview

Nightmare disorder/nightmares, also known as dream anxiety disorder or dream anxiety attacks, is asleep disorder characterized by frightening or terrifying dreams that result in feelings of extreme fear, horror, distress, or anxiety. The nightmares, which often portray the individual in a situation that jeopardizes their life or personal safety, occur during REM sleep and that often result in full awakening with detailed dream recall. Frequent nightmares are associated with insomnia and poor-quality sleep.

13.3.6.2　Epidemiology

Nightmares are common particularly in children. Peak prevalence is in late adolescence or early adulthood. Approximately 20% of children and 5%-10% of adults may suffer from nightmares. Frequent nightmares are in 1%-2% of adults. The prevalence in women is higher. Nightmares normally start between the ages of 2-5. 10%-50% of children aged 3-6 are estimated to suffer from nightmares. Older people are 20%-50% less likely to have nightmares than young people. Nightmares are seen in at least 50%-70% of posttraumatic stress disorder(PTSD) cases.

13.3.6.3　Etiology and pathogenesis

Traumatic events(e. g. , sexual assault, the death of a loved one) , extreme stress or sleep disturbance may contribute to the onset and maintenance of nightmares. Nightmares may be stimulated by frightening experiences during the day, and frequent nightmares usually occur during a period of anxiety. Mental conditions like post-traumatic stress disorder and other psychiatric disorders have been known to cause nightmares as well. Other causes include fever, psychotropic drugs, and alcohol detoxification. Twin studies suggest that genetic factors may be involved.

13.3.6.4　Clinical features

During the nightmare, the patient may scream and yell out things. Patients are often awakened by these threatening, frightening dreams and can often vividly remember their experience. Most often the dream emotion is anxiety but other emotions like sadness, anger, and disgust can also be the major feature of a nightmare. The most common nightmares are being chased, falling, being paralyzed, the death of close persons, and being late. Upon awakening, patients are un-usually alert and oriented within their surroundings, but may have an increased heart rate and symptoms of anxiety, like sweating. They may have trouble falling back to sleep for fear that they will experience another nightmare. A person experiencing nightmares would hinder the individual from completing everyday jobs efficiently and correctly because of the anxiety and lack of sleep.

13.3.6.5　Diagnosis and differential diagnosis

(1)Diagnosis(diagnostic point, ICD-10)

Recurrent frightening dreams that occur during the second sleep episode; terminate in awakening with vivid detailed recall of the threatening, frightening nightmare; no confusion or disorientation upon awakening; causes clinically significant distress or impairment in functioning; exclusion of nightmares caused by other physical diseases (e. g. , fever) and other mental disorders (PTSD, major depression, anxiety disorders).

(2) Differential diagnoses

Sleep terror: sleep terror occurs earlier night and may initially be unresponsive or disorientated with difficulty waking or bringing to awareness, and has no recollection. However, sleepers of nightmares are often awakened by the dreams which can often be vividly remembered. There are certain clinical and EEG features that can help in differentiating nightmare from sleep terror. Usually, sleep terror occur during deep non-rapid eye movement (stages 3 and 4) sleep as compared with nightmare, which often occur in REM sleep.

PTSD: nightmare is an important clinical feature of PTSD. PTSD is characterized by the development of multiple symptoms after exposure to traumatic events: intrusive symptoms (e. g, nightmares, flashbacks), avoidance, negative alterations in thoughts and mood, and increased arousal. Certain clinical and EEG features can help differentiating nightmare from PTSD. Nightmare often occurs in REM sleep, however, posttraumatic reenactments are replays of a traumatic event which can occur during REM sleep but also during NREM sleep.

13. 3. 6. 6　Course and prognosis

The prognosis is good. The symptoms should resolve as time passes. If the symptoms persist beyond the age of 6, consideration should be given to underlying conditions such as anxiety disorders, affective distress or PTSD.

13. 3. 6. 7　Treatments

(1) Etiological treatment

Daytime stressors should be identified and resolution attempted. Frightening experiences during the day should be reduced and frightening books or TV should be avoided for about 2 hours prior to bedtime. Bedtime should become a safe and comfortable time.

(2) Sleep hygiene and CBT

Stress relief techniques such as meditation, Yoga and exercise may help to eliminate stress and create a more peaceful sleeping atmosphere (see 13. 3. 1. 7 Treatments).

(3) Pharmacotherapy

Reassurance and conservative management is the only treatment required for sporadic nightmares. Antidepressants are often used to treat nightmares in PTSD.

Therapy usually helps to deal with the frightening themes of the nightmares and alleviate the recurrence of the dreams.

13. 4　Sexual dysfunctions

13.4.1　Overview

Sexual dysfunctions, also are known as sexual disorders or sexual malfunctions, are difficulty experienced by an individual during any stage of a normal sexual activity characterized by persistent problems with sexual pleasure or response. Sexual dysfunctions are common and can cause clinically significant distress.

According to the ICD-10, sexual dysfunction disorders(F52) not caused by organic disorder or disease may be classified into lack or loss of sexual desire(F52.0)(including hypoactive sexual desire disorder and sexual aversion disorder/frigidity), sexual aversion and lack of sexual enjoyment(F52.1, anhedonia), failure of genital response(F52.2, including female sexual arousal disorder, male erectile disorder, psychogenic impotence), orgasmic dysfunction[F52.3, inhibited orgasm(male)(female), psychogenic anorgasmy], premature ejaculation(F52.4), nonorganic vaginismus(F52.5), nonorganic dyspareunia(F52.6), excessive sexual drive(F52.7), other sexual dysfunction, not caused by organic disorder or disease(F52.8), unspecified sexual dysfunction, not caused by organic disorder or disease(F52.9).

13.4.2　Epidemiology

Sexual dysfunctions are highly prevalent worldwide although lack of large – scale epidemiologic data. Prevalence estimates of foreign female sexual dysfunctions about 4% –7% and of male sexual dysfunctions about 10%. The occurrence of sexual dysfunctions increases directly with age in both men and women. Although the frequency of symptoms increases with age, personal distress about those symptoms appears to diminish as individuals become older.

13.4.3　Etiology and pathogenesis

Sexual dysfunctions can be lifelong or acquired, generalized or situational, and result from psychological factors, biological and physiological factors, personality, experience, combined factors, and numerous stressors including prohibitive cultural mores, health and partner issues, and relationship conflicts.

13.4.4　The clinical types of sexual dysfunctions

This section discusses non – organic sexual dysfunction, including hypoactive sexual desire disorder (HSDD), male erectile dysfunction(MED), orgasmic dysfunction, premature ejaculation, nonorganic dyspareunia, nonorganic vaginismus.

13.4.4.1　Hypoactive sexual desire disorder

Hypoactive sexual desire disorder, also known as inhibited sexual desire(ISD) or hyposexuality, is considered asexual dysfunction with a lack or absence of sexual fantasies and desire for sexual activity that causes marked distress or interpersonal difficulty. In DSM-5, HSDD has been broken down into two separate conditions: female sexual interest/arousal disorder and male hypoactive sexual desire disorder. HSDD is the most common female sexual dysfunction. Prevalence of HSDD varies from 17% –55% in women and 15% – 58% in men and 5% –15% of women have the problem continuously. Variability is due to different modes of recruitment, age, gender, countries, and culture.

HSDD is characterized by absence of sexual fantasies and desires for sexual activity. The main symptoms for HSDD include the following: absent or reduced interest in sexual activity and sexual thoughts or fantasies; reduced or no initiation of sexual activity; absent or reduced sexual excitement or pleasure during most sexual activity; absent or reduced sexual interest or arousal in response to internal or external cues (such as a partner's attempts to initiate sexual activity); absent or reduced genital or nonessential sensations during sexual activity. Sometimes, HSDD is associated with other mental disorders such as anxiety disorders, depression, personality disorders. In many cases, HSDD may be diagnosed in conjunction with another psychiatric disorder.

According to ICD-10, diagnosis of HSDD requires meeting four specific criteria. Symptoms criteria: deficient(or absent) sexual/erotic thoughts or fantasies and desire for sexual activity. Course criteria: symptoms occurs lasts more than three months. Severity criteria: the symptoms cause clinically significant distress. Exclusion criteria: symptoms not be related to another mental, medical, substance disorder or other relationship circumstances such as severe distress.

There are a variety of products available including biological, physical, psychological treatments which have proven very effective in restoring sex drive. Psychotherapy: CBT, psychoanalysis and individual or couples sex therapy are effective treatment for improving HSDD. Treatment generally focuses more on relationship and communication issues, or education about sexuality. It can be important to let partners understand why low sexual desire is a problem for the relationship because two partners may have different understanding of sex without knowing it. If HSDD is a result of stress, techniques may be recommended to more effectively deal with that. Biological, physical treatment: treatments for the biological and physical causes depend on the individual. For example, changes in medication or diabetes control may be in order. A woman might need to make some lifestyle changes to combat fatigue. Estrogen therapy may be helpful for some women. Testosterone is another hormone that affects the sex drives of both men and women. Testosterone supplementation for some men with low testosterone levels can increase sexual desire. However, testosterone therapy is currently not approved for women by FDA. Two antidepressants [addyi(flibanserin) and bupropion] have been studied to treat acquired, generalized HSDD in pre-menopausal women. The addition of some drugs for underlying conditions — such as levodopa used to treat Parkinson's disease — has been found to help with male sexual desire by increasing production of the neurotransmitter of dopamine.

13.4.4.2   Male erectile disorder

Male erectile dysfunction(MED), also known as impotence, is a type of sexual dysfunction characterized by the inability to achieve or maintain an erection of the penis for satisfactory coitus. MED symptoms might include persistent trouble getting an erection and keeping an erection and reduced sexual desire. It has two subtypes of primary male erectile disorder and secondary male erectile disorder. Primary cases may occur due to a combination of low sexual drive and anxiety about sexual performance. Secondary cases may arise from diminishing sexual drive in the middle-aged or elderly, loss of interest in the sexual partner, anxiety, depression, or organic disease and its treatment. Up to 30 million American men are estimated to frequently suffer from ED, and it strikes up to half of all men between the ages of 40 and 70.

According to ICD-10, diagnosis of MED requires meeting four specific criteria. Symptoms criteria: unable to obtain the erection; unable to maintain the erection until the sexual activity has become satisfying to the couple participating in the partnered activity. Marked decrease in erectile rigidity during sexual activity. Course criteria: symptoms occurs lasts more than three months. Severity criteria: the symptoms cause clinically significant distress in each sexual experience. Exclusion criteria: Symptoms not be related to another mental, medical, substance disorder or other relationship circumstances such as severe distress.

Treatments include biological, physical, and psychological treatments. Psychotherapy is effective for MED. Medication: the first-line specific therapy is now the use of PDE-5 inhibitors — sidenafil(viagra), vardenafil, and tadalafil — which are effective in about 70% of cases. PDE-5 inhibitors have largely supplanted earlier physical treatments for erectile dysfunction(i. e. , intracavernosal injections, vacuum devices, and surgical methods).

13.4.4.3   Orgasmic disorder

Orgasmic disorder, includes female orgasmic disorder and male orgasmic disorder, is difficulty reaching orgasm, even when they're sexually aroused and there's sufficient sexual stimulation. Orgasmic disorder affects approximatelyone in three women. Men orgasmic disorder is much less common than female orgasmic disorder. The main symptoms of orgasmic disorder is the inability to achieve sexual climax. Having unsatisfying orgasms or taking longer than normal to reach climax are also symptoms. Female orgasmic disorder may have difficulty achieving orgasm during either sexual intercourse or masturbation.

According to ICD-10, orgasmic disorder has four specific diagnosis criteria. Criterion A is inability to achieve sexual climax. Criterion B requires that the symptoms must persist for at least six months. Criterion C causes significant distress in almost all(75%-100%) of all sexual encounters. Criterion D is symptoms that could not be related to another mental, medical, substance disorders or other relationship specific circumstances.

Treatment for orgasmic disorder depends on the condition. Psychotherapy is effective. Coital Alignment Technique(CAT) is an adjustment in coital technique designed to improve the ability of male-superior coitus to produce female orgasm. The position combines the intimacy of face-to-face contact with a repositioning of male(the so-called "riding high" variation) so that there is greater contact of the penile shaft with the clitoris and a mutual rocking(rather than thrusting) motion. Medication: in some cases, estrogen hormone therapy(involving taking a pill, wearing a patch, or applying a gel to the genitals)may be used. Testosterone therapy is another option. However, testosterone therapy is currently not approved for female orgasmic disorder by FDA in the United States. Some over-the-counter(OTC) products and nutritional supplements may also help women with orgasmic disorder. Arousal oils, such as Zestra, warm the clitoris and increase stimulation may be beneficial to use during sexual intercourse and masturbation.

13.4.4.4 Premature ejaculation

Premature ejaculation(PE), also known as early ejaculation, rapid ejaculation, rapid climax, premature climax, and(historically) ejaculation praecox, is uncontrolled ejaculation either before or shortly after sexual penetration. There is no uniform cut-off defining "premature", but ICD-10 applies a cut-off of 15 seconds from the beginning of sexual intercourse. The main symptoms are uncontrolled ejaculation either too early or coming too quickly after vaginal or non-vaginal penetration. PE occurs before the person wishes it and may result in unsatisfactory sex for both partners and can increase the anxiety. It is one of the most common forms of male sexual dysfunction. It has probably affected every man at some point in lifetime.

According to ICD-10, diagnosis of PE requires meeting four specific criteria. Symptoms criteria: PE is manifested by ejaculation prior to or shortly after vaginal penetration. In most cases, symptoms criteria will be determined by an individual's interpretation and self-report. Course criteria: symptoms occurs lasts more than three months. Severity criteria: the symptoms must cause clinically significant distress. Exclusion criteria: the sexual disorder is not better explained by another mental, medical, substance-related, or situational condition such as severe relationship distress.

A combination of medication and non-medication treatments is often the most effective method. Psychotherapy is effective for PE. In addition, relaxation techniques or using distraction methods may help somebody delay ejaculation. Medications: drugs that increase serotonin signalling in the brain slow ejaculation and have been used successfully to treat PE. These include selective serotonin reuptake inhibitors(SSRIs), such as paroxetine or dapoxetine, as well as clomipramine. However, SSRIs can cause various types of sexual dysfunction such as anorgasmia, erectile dysfunction, and diminished libido. Stopping the use of alcohol, tobacco, or illegal drugs may improve how well they can control ejaculation.

13.4.4.5 Nonorganic dyspareunia/dyspareunia

Nonorganic dyspareunia is persistent or recurrent genital pain occurring before, during, or after intercourse.

Some patients complain superficial pain at the opening of the vagina or surface of the genitalia when penetration is initiated. Some feel deeper pain in the vault of the vagina or deep within the pelvis upon deeper penetration. Others feel pain in more than one of these places.

Dyspareunia can have many different causes. Pain that is experienced after partial penetration may result from scars, impaired lubrication of the vagina, other painful lesions, or the muscle spasm of vaginismus. Pain on deep penetration strongly suggests pelvic pathology. There is an increase in reported dyspareunia postmenopausally due to hormonally induced physiological changes in the vagina. Dyspareunia can result from tension and anxiety about the sex act. Fear, avoidance, and psychologic distress around attempting intercourse can become large parts of a woman's experience of dyspareunia. Further pain may cause women to avoid coitus. There is some increase in dyspareunia in the immediate postpartum population, but it is usually temporary. Chronic dyspareunia is a common complaint in women with childhood sexual abuse or rape history. Dyspareunia occurs in both women and men. Globally, dyspareunia has been estimated to affect between 8%–21% of women, at some point in their lives. The treatment of dyspareunia depends on what is causing the pain.

13.4.4.6　Nonorganic vaginismus

Nonorganic vaginismus/vaginismus, also called vaginism, is a condition that constriction of the outer third of the vagina due to involuntary pelvic floor muscle tightening or spasm, which interferes with penile insertion and intercourse. Spasms often begin as soon as the penis attempts to enter the vagina. In severe cases constriction occur even when the woman attempts to introduce her own finger.

Li Jing

Chapter 14

Psychosomatic Illnesses

14.1   Introduction

Psychosomatic illnesses refer to a group of somatic diseases, in which psychosocial factors play an important role in the occurrence and evolution. This kind of disease is mainly affected the hypothalamus, and is closely related to the autonomic nervous system and the endocrine function. Psychosomatic medicine studies the relationship among psychological, physiological and social factors with disease processes, from the perspective of biologic−psycho−social medicine. It is a comprehensive medical science, which involves medicine, psychology, social science, and behavioral science. It is an important part of the medical science system.

14.1.1   Definition

Psychosomatic medicine study the relationship between psychological, physiological and social factors in the course of disease. It is a comprehensive medical science, involving medicine, psychology, social science and behavioral science. The concept of psychosomatic medicine consists of a broad and narrow concepts. In a broad concept, it is a study of all human health and disease related to the psychosomatic (including biology, psychology and Sociology). In a narrow concept, it refers to the study of the etiology, clinical manifestation, diagnosis, treatment, rehabilitation and prevention of psychosomatic diseases.

14.1.2   The development of psychosomatic medicine

As early as the Qin and Han Dynasties and ancient Greece, there were related concepts and records of psychosomatic medicine. It was considered that "unity of mind and form", emotions and personality had a great impact on human diseases and health. In 1939, the Journal of Psychosomatic Medicine was published by the American Journal of psychosomatic medicine. In 1943, the American Psychosomatic Medical Association was established. So far, the scientific system of psychosomatic medicine had been formally established. In 1984, there were 1,358 psychiatric hospitals in the United States, of which 869 were all specialized counseling liaison psychiatry services. In 2003, psychosomatic medicine was officially classified as a new branch of the American Society of neuropsychosis. In 2004, it was established as a formal training content by the American Medical Education Committee. The European Association of Consultation–Liaison Psychiatry and Psychosomatics(EACLPP) was formally established in 2000.

In 1960, the Japanese Psychosomatic Society was established. After that, it was renamed the Psychosomatic Society of Japan. The Psychosomatic Medicine Committee of China was established in 1986, and the psychosomatic medicine union of Chinese Medical Association was established in 1993. With the development of medicine, the importance and research of psychosomatic diseases reflect the great transformation of modern biomedicine model to bio–psycho–social medical model. At present, the researches of psychosomatic medicine mainly include basic theory study and clinical application. In basic theory, neuroimmunology has been developed. The mediating mechanism of the occurrence and development of psychosomatic diseases is discussed. It takes an interdisciplinary approach, incoporating sociology, ecology, psychology, physiology, genetics, neuroendocrinology and immunology. In clinical practice, consultation liaison psychiatry and behavioral medicine have been developed.

With the social modernization, the prevalence of psychosomatic diseases is increasing. Clinical psychosomatic diseases account for 25% –35%. Psychosomatic diseases in the medical field account for 32. 2% – 35. 1%, while psychosomatic diseases in the internal medicine follow – up system account for more than 50%.

14. 1. 3　The classification of psychosomatic illnesses

In disease taxonomy, psychosomatic disease is not an independent disease category, and all kinds of diseases are classified into the corresponding diseases of clinical medicine. The classification and scope of psychosomatic medicine are not consistent. The traditional classification which was made by Alexander F. (1934), including hypertension, peptic ulcer, ulcerative colitis, asthma, rheumatoid arthritis, hyperthyroidism and migraine. In recent years, with the development of medicine, more somatic diseases have been attributed to psychosomatic diseases. Modern systemic diseases considered as psychosomatic diseases are as follows.

(1)Cardiovascular system: coronary heart disease, primary hypertension, paroxysmal tachycardia, migraine, Reynold's disease.

(2) Respiratory system: bronchial asthma, hyperventilation syndrome, vascular allergic eyes, hay fever.

(3)Digestive system: peptic ulcers, ulcerative colitis, colonic anaphylaxis, anorexia nervosa and gluttony.

(4)Genitourinary system: menstrual disorders, sexual impotence, depression, nervous polyuria, premenstrual syndrome.

(5)Endocrine system: diabetes, hyperthyroidism, obesity.

(6)Skin: nervous dermatitis, pruritus, alopecia, dermatitis, psoriasis, chronic urticarial.

(7)Musculoskeletal system: rheumatoid arthritis, spasmodic torticollis, and tension headache.

(8)Nervous system: hyperalgesia and autonomic nervous dysfunction.

(9)Others: malignant tumor, pregnancy toxemia.

14. 2　Etiology and pathogenesis

The causes of psychosomatic diseases are complicated. Psychosocial factors and individual psychological qualities are the two important factors that lead to psychosomatic disorders.

14.2.1 Psychophysiological intermediary mechanism

Psychosomatic diseases are closely related to the metabolic endocrine system and the immune system, social psychological factors which play a role in the target organs and make them physiological changes. If the degree of stimulation is too strong or prolonged, the organ is susceptible to physical symptoms or develops into a disease.

14.2.1.1 Autonomic nervous system

The autonomic nervous system is also called immediate response to stress, including the sympathetic and parasympathetic nervous systems. The central nervous system accepts and integrates stress. This impulse is transmitted to the hypothalamus. By stimulating the sympathetic nervous system, the release of a large number of catecholamines in the medulla of the adrenal glands increases the blood flow of heart and brain. The body is alert and sensitive to various stimuli. This leads to higher heart rate, higher blood pressure, faster breathing and slower gastrointestinal peristalsis. It embodies the function of the body to mobilize to deal with the stress factors.

14.2.1.2 Endocrine system

Also known as the long-term response to stress, endocrine glands have a vital function in maintaining the stability of the body environment. It has a complex feedback regulation system and has extensive connections with the autonomic nervous system. In response to stress, such as the secretion of hypothalamic neurohormone, hypothalamic corticotropin releasing factor(CRF), which stimulates the anterior pituitary adrenocorticotropic hormone(ACTH), promote adrenal cortical hormone secretion and enhance the synthesis and metabolism of the body, and the function of the system play an extensive role.

14.2.1.3 Immune system

The immune system helps maintain internal stability and eliminates invasion, but it also causes the risk of allergic reaction and autoimmune diseases. Psychoneuroimmunology is an important research field in psychosomatic medicine. Animal experiments showed that under the stress state, the lymphocytes reduce, synapse reduction, antibody and immunoglobulin production decreased, macrophage activity decreased, T cells mature slowly, expression of immune regulatory genes Bcl-2 and Bax of the rate of change, resulting in immune cell apoptosis. The final result is the reduction of T cell killing effect and the production of lymphokine, the reduction of specific antibody produced by B cells, and the decrease of serum IL-6 and TNF content. The stress can effect immune function by means of: ①hypothalamic regulation; ②the influence of autonomic nerve function on lymphocytes; ③the action of corticosteroids.

14.2.2 Psychological factors

14.2.2.1 Emotion and autonomic nerve function

The symptoms of psychosomatic diseases are mainly manifested in organs or systems controlled by the autonomic nervous system, such as cardiovascular system, digestive system, respiratory system, and endocrine system. Through conditioned reflex or operative reinforcement, the autonomic nervous response is enhanced. The autonomic nervous response further affects the mood, so repeated reinforcement and vicious cycle lead to psychosomatic diseases. Moderate positive emotions are beneficial to promoting physical function and maintaining health. Negative emotions such as anger, resentment and so on are a necessary response for the body to adapt to the environment, but if the intensity is too long, it will have an adverse effect on organ function, eventually leading to disease. For example, long-term distress, fear and disappointment will inhibit gastrointestinal movement and affect digestive function. As time passes, it may lead to diseases like ulcers.

14.2.2.2　Personality

Personality is the most essential psychological characteristic of the individual. Characteristics are the internal basis of psychological conflict induced by psychological conflict. Flanders Dunbar(1935) was the first to associate personality traits with physical diseases. The following are the individual characteristics associated with the common psychosomatic diseases(Table 14-1).

Table 14-1　The relationship between personality traits and psychosomatic diseases

Somatic disease	Related personality characteristics
Coronary artery disease and hypertension	Type A character. It is characterized by a sense of urgency(such as haste in most of the time), competitiveness, and possibly hostility; especially hostility may be related to coronary artery disease
Bronchial asthma	Overdependence
Cancer	Inability to express feelings, bereavement
Migraine and ulcerative colitis	Compulsive personality type
Obesity	Impulsive personality

14.2.2.3　Life events

Psychological mood often changes with social life events. Sely first studied the causal relationship between life events and mental diseases in the United States. Holmes and Rahe(1967) developed a Social Readjustment Rating Scale, including 43 life change events, such as death of a spouse, divorce, unemployment, retirement, and imprisonment. Each group is given a certain score, and a quantitative method is applied to study the social environment and various life events. It is found that the probability and severity of disease are closely related to life events.

14.2.2.4　Individual susceptibility

Under the same psychosocial stimulus, only a few people will suffer from psychosomatic diseases. This indicates that the occurrence of psychosomatic disease is individual difference. The individual's physiological and psychological quality determines the susceptibility, and the physiological quality may be related to the heredity. Psychological quality refers to the individual's value orientation, cognitive level, personality characteristics and social experience. It is closely related to the occurrence of psychosomatic disease.

14.2.2.5　Cognitive evaluation

When there is a stressor, the first response of an individual is to perceive the changes in the situation. Cognitive evaluation of irritable events can change the intensity or nature of stress response. Healthy people are confident that they have the ability to deal with, expect to improve, and the stressors can be a kind of controller, and the stress response is mild.

14.3　Types of psychosomatic disease

14.3.1　Respiratory system psychosomatic disease

14.3.1.1　Bronchial asthma

Asthma is one of the typical psychosomatic diseases in the respiratory system has been recognized. The induction or formation of asthma is related to some negative emotions, such as anxiety, disappointment, distress, anger, fear, and depression.

Through a prospective study of 1,150 adults, the researehers found that poor life satisfaction, stress state, and neuroticism were associated with the onset of asthma. Compared with healthy people, adults with asthma always follow with interpersonal sensitivity, anxiety, fear, depression, hostility, paranoia, or more obsessive−compulsive symptoms, the psychological obstacle will be a predisposing factor for asthma, so it will continue to aggravate.

Studies have shown that 35%−40% of asthmatic patients have been suggested to induce bronchoconstriction and may also be suggested to be relieved, and non−asthmatic people have no such reaction. Patients with unhealthy psychological and psychological disorders have a high mortality rate of asthma attacks. Although some asthma patients didn't receive treatments, their symptoms were significantly relieved, which may be related to the relief of nervousness and the enhancement of safety. The study also found that 40% of asthmatic children aggravated their condition when they cried. Similarly, watching thrillers or being scolded suddenly can also cause asthma attacks.

It is generally believed that negative mood, such as anger, fear, depression and anxiety, can induce or exacerbate asthma. In the process of asthma, negative mood can not only inhibit the hypothalamic neurosecretory cells, but also decrease the secretion of adrenocorticotropic hormone in the hypothalamus. So adrenocortical hormone secretion is also reduced.

The hegative mood can also affect the emotional center and the anterior hypothalamus, thus stimulate the vagus nerve to increase acetylcholine released. Both of these effects can cause asthma attacks. Asthma and bad mood are reciprocal cause and effect, and asthma patients are often in the vicious cycle of the attack−fear−attack.

In addition, the personality of asthmatic patients are characterized by anxiety, excitement, emotional instability, naive, strong dependence and introverted personality. Negative mood and personality defects make the immune function decrease, the sensitivity of the external boundary is enhanced, and asthma is easy to induce and aggravate. When asthma attacks, it can also cause symptoms such as emotional tension and anxiety.

14.3.1.2　Overventilation syndrome

Over ventilation syndrome is the reaction caused by acute anxiety. The pathogenesis is not clear at present. Some over ventilation syndrome can be induced by certain stressor or food, such as emotional stress, work−related stress, coffee and tea. Due to the negative function of the autonomic nervous system, the respiratory dysfunction will become involuntary. This will lead to rapid and light breathing, reduce blood carbon dioxide, and finally cause respiratory alkalosis. The attack will cause rapid heartbeat, palpitations, sweating, dizziness, anxiety, dizziness, limb numbness, and convulsions. The patient has a sense of hypoxia which will make the patient more nervous. Patients recognize these symptoms, but they can't control their overbreathing. Most patients tend to be anxious or hysterical. Attacks can be stopped by giving suggestive psychotherapy or understanding the psychological factors of the disease. Inhaling carbon dioxide can also do the same.

14.3.2 Cardiovascular system psychosomatic disease

14.3.2.1 Primary hypertension

The pathogenesis of hypertension is complex. Although some mechanisms have been revealed, it has not been fully elucidated yet. Primary hypertension is a multifactorial disease. Physical factors such as kidney disease, and nervous system disease, psychological factors such as personality, stress, poor situation, social factors and lifestyle will lead to the onset. In psychological factors, chronic stress is more likely to induce hypertension. Intense anger, insecurity, and severe anxiety can often induce the disease. Many symptoms of hypertension, such as fatigue, dizziness, headache, palpitation, and insomnia, are all seen in anxiety or anger. The character of hypertension patients is overly conscientious, good activity, strong competitive, easy to be excited and annoyed. A large number of studies have found that emotional reactions caused by various stressors can cause repeated blood pressure reactions for people with certain genetic quality, and eventually lead to continuous blood pressure risen. So far, data on hypertension mostly support the combined effect of social situations and personality traits, which can increase the risk of hypertension. However, more researches on clinical, epidemiological and animal experiments are needed. Many drugs (such as adrenal corticosteroids and monoamine oxidase inhibitors) can also cause hypertension, and should be carefully identified in the diagnosis of essential hypertension.

Medication treatment should be carried out when hypertension patients are treated with psychotherapy. When the patient realises his blood pressure rises, it will focus on his own blood pressure, which is one of the causes of anxiety, this moment, antianxiety drugs are often effective. Psychotherapy can help to calm the patient's mood, avoid and eliminate stressful situations.

14.3.2.2 Coronary heart disease

With the progress of medicine, the death spectrum of disease has changed. Cardiovascular and cerebrovascular diseases have become the first major killer. The incidence of coronary heart disease in China has increased by 2-3 times in 10 years, and the incidence of acute myocardial infarction has increased by more than 2 times in 10 years. Psychosocial factors have become a major factor in inducing coronary heart disease, such as interpersonal tension, anxiety and depression, or type A character. According to statistics, in patients with coronary heart disease, the ratio of type A personality is 3 times higher than that of patients with type B personality. In 1979, International Conference of cardiopulmonary and hematology had confirmed that type A character is an independent risk factor of coronary heart disease. Patients with type A personality tend to become excited, angry, and impatient. This will lead to a series of physiological changes, causing a higher blood viscosity and accelerating the formation of thrombus. 1/2-2/3 of myocardial infarction cases have incentives, including emotional, mental stress and manual labor. These negative emotions aggravate coronary artery ischemia and hypoxia state by influencing the mechanism of neuroendocrine.

14.3.3 Digestive system psychosomatic disease: peptic ulcer

The occurrence of gastrointestinal diseases is closely related to the mood. Experiments have proved that the psychosocial factors are related to the occurrence of peptic ulcer, and the duodenum is more obvious than the stomach. A prospective study of the 1950s pointed out the correlation between psychological and physical factors in peptic ulcer. In particular, these studies illustrated the ubiquity of the nonspecific response to stress. Peptic ulcer patients often have their own unique characteristics. These features appear calm, serious, stubborn, and coercion. Peptic ulcer occurs in young and middle-aged people, because in this age group work and rest time is often irregular. Their social and family pressures are relatively high and are often accompanied by negative emotions such as nervousness, anxiety, sadness and resentment. Psychological stimuli can cause brain function disorders, and also stimulate gastric acid and pepsin secretion increased, prompt ulcers. In addition, stress can cause changes in endocrine function, increased secretion of corticosteroids, thereby speed up the formation of ulcers.

14.3.4 Endocrine system and metabolic psychosomatic disease

14.3.4.1 Hyperthyroidism

Epidemiological survey shows that the incidence of hyperthyroidism in China is 3%. Because of the enhanced sympathetic activity, patients often accompanied by neuroticism, hand trembling, and insomnia. About 90% of patients with thyroid enlargement, some also have exophthalmos symptoms.

Recent studies have shown that hyperthyroidism is an endocrine disease induced by mental stimulation on the basis of heredity. Clinical studies have found that about 80% of hyperthyroidism patients have had a sudden or chronic mental stimulus before the onset. Clinical and research shows that Negative emotions liketension, fear, melancholy, and anger can affect the endocrine system function through brain, leading to hyperthyroidism. It was found that the prevalence of hyperthyroidism increased significantly in wartime and natural disaster areas.

Recently, the relationship between related daily life events and the incidence of hyperthyroidism have studied. The results showed that hyperthyroidism patients experienced more stressful events within 12 months before onset.

The pathogenesis of hyperthyroidism by mental stimulation is still unknown.

Recent data show that psychological stress can lead to changes of the immune system function. The change of adrenal cortex hormone and sympathetic nervous system may be the intermediate of the immunosuppressive effect induced by tension. It is also suggested that trauma can cause dysfunction of central nervous system and hypothalamic pituitary adrenal axis, resulting in decreased immune surveillance ability, increased thyroid stimulating immunoglobulin and hyperthyroidism.

The occurrence of hyperthyroidism has a significant correlation with personality characteristics. The personality characteristics of hyperthyroidism studies showed the patients have some common features: excessive responsibility, do not care to sacrifice their own interests, rely on hope and need to be suppressed, excessive fear death, injury, and death in severe fear particularly vulnerable. Recent studies have shown that patients with hyperthyroidism are introverted, unstable, nervous, anxious, depressed, and sensitive to external stimuli. It is believed that personality traits, like autoimmune mechanisms, may be related to the vulnerability of the thyroid tissue in some way.

As a non-specific factor, negative mood can activate genetic or physical susceptibility tendency, and influence thyroid function by affecting the immune system.

Hyperthyroidism has a great influence on patients. Patients often suffer from insomnia, emaciation and temper irritable. This will seriously affect daily life and interpersonal relationships. Female patients may have menstrual disorders and difficult to get pregnant.

Hyperthyroidism also has a great influence on the psychological state of patients. Patients with hyperthyroidism often have the following psychological characteristics. ①Anxiety and irritability. Most patients with hyperthyroidism are multilingual, impulsive, irritable, anxious, prone to insomnia, lack of thought, and memory loss. ②Negative and pessimistic. The course of hyperthyroidism is long and easy to relapse. Some patients lose confidence in the treatment. In this way, there will even be a hyperthyroidism crisis. Therefore, for patients with hyperthyroidism, psychotherapy and self-mood adjustment are important during medication or surgrey. Although hyperthyroidism has a certain genetic tendency, the incidence of female, family history and traumatized people is high, but these are just susceptible factors, and the key lies in their psychological quality and attitude towards life. The patient should be optimistic. Relaxed work and living environment and harmonious family life are helpful for the treatment of hyperthyroidism.

14.3.4.2   Obesity

Modern psychology studies have proved that obesity is a psychosomatic disease. There are many reasons for obesity, but it is generally believed that the main reason is overeating. They often have unhealthy eating habits. They not only eat frequently, but also eat more food, especially those who eat too much carbohydrates and fat. Patients' excessive eating habits are often not due to hunger, but because of impulse to eat. Their unhealthy eating habits are mainly related to psychological factors. Therefore, "eating" symbolizes a kind of self-satisfaction and can relieve anxiety. When people encounter setbacks, worries and anxieties, they will eat a lot to relieve the current pressure. Many obese people feel comfortable when they are overweight, and feel frustrated when restricting their diet to lose weight. A few obese people have the habit of night eating. They are anorexic during the day. Obesity may lead to new internal conflicts and increase new anxieties. These anxieties may need more food to alleviate, which will form a vicious circle.

14.3.5   Reproductive system psychosomatic disease: premenstrual tension syndrome

The patient shows mental and behavioral symptoms before menstruation, and the symptoms disappear after menstruation. The main symptoms are fatigue, irritability, depression, excessive sensitivity, suspicion, unstable mood, breast distending pain, craving, increased appetite and gastrointestinal symptoms before menstruation. The occurrence is related to the imbalance of hormone secretion, and psychosocial factors are also related to the occurrence and development of premenstrual syndrome. The function of the female reproductive system is directly affected by the hypothalamus-pituitary-gonadal axis. Psychosocial factors, mediated by emotional responses, act on the endocrine system of the autonomic nervous system and hypothalamus pituitary gland, and then affect the functional status of female reproductive organs, resulting in the onset.

14.3.6   Nervous system psychosomatic disease: tension headache

Tension headache is also known as muscular contractile headaches. The disease is manifested by the blunt or straining sense of the head. Tension headache is mostly related to stress. Usually, anxiety, depression or mental stress are the psychological factors leading to the continuous contraction of the head and neck muscles. This disease is very common in the clinic. Psychological stress, abnormal mood and severe sleep may lead to abnormal brain blood supply, resulting in cerebral vasospasm and headache.

14.4   Diagnosis and differential diagnosis

The diagnosis needs to combine biomedicine and psychosomatic medicine perspectives.

14.4.1   Biomedical diagnosis

Psychosomatic disease involves various body systems. Psychosomatic diseases such as the circulatory system are still known as coronary heart disease and primary hypertension. Psychosomatic diseases of the digestive system are still known as peptic ulcers and ulcerative colitis.

14.4.1.1 The history

A comprehensive understanding of the history includes major diseases, medical history, personal history, marital and childbearing.

14.4.1.2 Physical examination

The patients may exaggerate the complaints, and their symptoms and signs are inconsistent. This requires detailed physical examination to exclude other diseases.

14.4.1.3 Laboratory examination

The acquisition of auxiliary data, such as disease pathogens, pathological changes and organ functional status, can help clinical diagnosis.

14.4.1.4 Imaging examination

It includes electronic computed tomography(CT), nuclear magnetic resonance tomography(MRI), single photon computed tomography (SPECT), electronic image endoscopy and Doppler color flow phenomenon. These tests can increase the accuracy of biological diagnosis.

14.4.1.5 Autonomic nerve function examination

Since psychosomatic diseases mainly occur in the autonomic innervated organs, the examination of autonomic nervous function is helpful for the diagnosis. The autonomic nerve function examination includes the pressure test of eyeball and carotid artery, skin scratch sign, skin temperature measurement, methacholine test, and drug test.

14.4.2 Psychosomatic medical diagnosis

The diagnosis of psychosomatic disorder is to confirm whether there is a clear psychosomatic relationship between somatic diseases and whether psychosocial factors are important in the process of disease. The diagnostic method of psychosomatic medicine is to use psychosocial, psychosocial, psychophysiology and psychophysiology to confirm the characteristics of psychosomatic diseases.

14.4.2.1 Psychiatric interview

By talking with patients, the physician collects valuable clinical information, and observe their general mental state and speech behavior characteristics.

14.4.2.2 Psychosocial factors

To understand psychosocial factors and severity of patients before onset, the following scales can be applied: social adaptation scale and life events questionnaire. Most patients with psychosomatic diseases have experienced major events affecting life in the past, and this provides a basis for the diagnosis of psychosomatic diseases.

14.4.2.3 Mental examination

The doctor diagnosed whether the patient was in an emotional disorder such as anxiety, depression, hysteria, hypochondriac state, obsessive-compulsive state and so on. Through the spirit of examination, they exclude some serious mental illness, such as schizophrenia, affective disorder, atypical depression and other types of neurosis, and determine the severity of the mood disorders.

14.4.2.4 Psychological test

It is helpful to use the scale to test patients' emotional state, such as anxiety, depression and personality traits. The following are some commonly used scales: Self-rating Anxiety Scale(SAS), self rating Depression Scale(SDS), Hamilton Anxiety Scale(HAMA), Hamilton Depression Scale(HAMD), Eysenck Personality Questionnaire(EPQ) and the Minnesota Multiphasic Personality Inventory(MMPI), symptom checklist 90 (SCL-90)cartel personality test.

14.4.2.5 Personality diagnosis

Personality are relatively stable and persistent, which will potentially affect the external speech and actions of the person, and related to the psychosomatic disease.

14.4.3 Differential diagnosis

14.4.3.1 Identification with neurosis

Neurosis includes anxiety symptoms, obsessive-compulsive disorder, somatoform disorder, neurasthenia and so on. The onset and prognosis of psychosomatic diseases and neuroses are all related to psychological factors and personality characteristics. They need to be differentiated. The key point is that neurosis is not like real psychosomatic diseases.

14.4.3.2 Identification with somatic disease

Psychosomatic diseases and various physical diseases have clear organic pathological changes and pathophysiological processes, which should be identified.

The main point of identification is that psychological factors are the main causes of the psychosomatic disease, or the psychological factors cause the disease to be aggravated, relapsed or deferred. The occurrence of simple physical disease is mainly related to biological or physicochemical factors. Although the symptoms are the same, the cause of the disease is different. For example, renal hypertension is a systemic disease caused by renal insufficiency. Primary hypertension is a psychosomatic disease closely related to psychological factors and without biological causes.

14.4.3.3 Several conditions should be paid attention to in the differential diagnosis of psychosomatic disease

(1) Somatic disease caused by psychological factors.

(2) The cause, deterioration or delayed rehabilitation of somatic disease has a close relationship with psychological factors.

(3) The mental disease is manifested by symptoms similar to the somatic disease.

(4) Mental symptoms of a body disease.

(5) The manic episode caused by lupus erythematosus and the mental disorder in the early stage of hepatic encephalopathy. Patients with chronic bronchitis showed paranoia, and delusional symptoms.

(6) Psychosis and somatic disease occur simultaneously in the same patient.

(7) If schizophrenic patients have hepatitis, there is no direct connection between them. But mental symptoms may affect the treatment and rehabilitation of somatic diseases.

14.5 Treatments

In view of the etiology and pathogenesis of psychosomatic disease, the treatment of psychosomatic disease should be a comprehensive treatment under the model of biologic psychosocial medicine. Under general circumstances, multidisciplinary physicians should be coordinated. The tasks of psychiatrists are providing training, consultation, medication and psychological treatment for special cases.

For the treatment of psychosomatic diseases, the principle of psychosomatic treatment should be followed. First of all, we should take active and effective measures to treat physical symptoms and control the progress of the qualitative pathological process to lay a good foundation for the treatment of psychosomatic diseases. Doctors need to know more about the mental factors, personality traits, behavior patterns, and interpersonal relationships in the family and work place. They should help patients change their previous unhealthy behavior patterns, so as to improve their ability to adapt to social and changeable objective environment, improve interpersonal relationship and eliminate unhealthy emotional reactions.

14.5.1 Medication

In addition to the treatment of various specific diseased organs, most patients with psychosomatic diseases are applicable to anti-anxiety drugs and anti-depressants. At present, the commonly used anti-anxiety drugs are alprazolam and clonazepam. Traditional anti-depressants such as doxepin and amitriptyline are not widely used. They have been replaced by new drugs such as serotonin(5-HT) reuptake inhibitors, buspirone, and Dai Lixin. For refractory cases, small doses of antipsychotics, such as risperidone, olanzapine and quetiapine, can be added on the basis of antidepressants.

14.5.2 Psychotherapy

Psychotherapy is the main treatment for psychosomatic diseases. Doctors should establish good doctor-patient relationship with patients, give patients necessary sympathy and support, and listen patiently to patients' complaints. In this way, you may help them to improve their mood, discover wrong cognition and correct attitude towards disease as well as to improve their family and surrounding environment. The commonly used treatments include psychoanalysis, behavioral therapy, cognitive therapy, Morita therapy, and music therapy. Biofeedback therapy is a relaxation training combined with the instrument to regulate the autonomic nervous system. It has been used to eliminate anxiety and has some obvious effects on psychosomatic diseases.

14.5.3 Traditional Chinese medicine treatment

Doctors in the past time had created many effective prescriptions with a good effect on psychosomatic diseases. For example, Xiaoyao Powder has a good effect on menstrual period or premenstrual tension syndrome.

Acupuncture may be a unique treatment for physical and mental diseases. This method can affect many systems, organs, cells, neurotransmitters, hormones, and receptors. Acupuncture and moxibustion can also affect a number of mental and emotional control centers in the brain, such as the marginal system, and the prefrontal cortex, which can lead to a series of functional adjustment, and can also produce certain comfort effects. This placebo effect is also beneficial to patients.

14.5.4 Others

Other treatments can have certain therapeutic effect including biofeedback therapy, relaxation training, physical therapy, hydrotherapy, qigong and Tai-chi.

14.6　Prevention

Psychosomatic disease is the result of the combination of psychological and biological factors. Therefore, psychosomatic diseases should also be prevented from two aspects at the same time. Psychosocial factors mostly need a long time to cause psychosomatic disease, so the psychological prevention of psychosomatic diseases should start early.

14.6.1　Cultivate a sound character

Personality and psychosomatic diseases are closely related, so the cultivation of personality can be effective in preventing heart disease, for those with obvious weakness of the psychological quality, such as easy to anger, depression, and autistic paranoid tendencies should strengthen the cultivation of the healthy personality early through psychological guidance.

14.6.2　Keep good mood

Maintaining a good mood is conducive to the treatment of psychosomatic diseases. In the encounter of social, work, life, learning and other environmental changes or the impact of life events, appropriate psychotherapy or drug treatment is an important means to prevent the development of the disease.

14.6.3　Lifestyle changes

For those who have obvious bad behavior, such as smoking, drinking, eating too much and lack of exercise, doctors should use psychotherapy to correct their bad behavior. Long-term healthy behavior is the basis of normal body.

14.6.4　Improve the support system and coping ability

There is evidence that people have a low prevalence in a good support environment. For individuals, the ability to solve problems should be developed and a positive response to difficult setbacks should be adopted. For families, there is a need to build a harmonious atmosphere. Social support systems are also important, such as the development of mental health services, psychological counseling and crisis intervention.

14.6.5　Pharmacotherapy

Psychotropic drugs can change the metabolism of the nervous system, and improve emotional and physiological functions. Under the guidance of psychiatrists, the therapy can effectively improve the symptoms.

Niu Qihui, Wang Yali

Chapter 15

Consultation–liaison Psychiatry

15.1 Introduction

15.1.1 Definition of consultation–liaison psychiatry

Consultation–liaison psychiatry(CLP) refers to the psychiatric services specialises in the interface between general medicine and psychiatry. The role of consultation–liaison psychiatrists is not only carrying out psychiatric interviews to patients with psychological or behavioral problems but also providing psychiatric consultations for non–psychiatric medical staffs in the team. Consultation–liaison psychiatrists are also responsible to developing the theoretical foundation of CLP, especially aiming to develop and promote systematic treatments for psychiatric problems of patients with concurrent physical illnesses. Furthermore, consultation–liaison psychiatrists in university teaching hospitals are expected to provide training of basic psychiatric concepts to medical students and residents.

15.1.2 Significance of consultation–liaison psychiatry

The comorbidity of psychotic disorders and medical illness may be one of the most troublesome problems encountered by the primary health care or the general hospital. In fact, about one–third of medical and surgical outpatients in general hospital have physical disease, with one–third are diagnosed with mental disease and the rest have psychosomatic disease.

According to an investigation in China, the prevalence rate of psychotic disorders among inpatients in general hospital setting is approximately 20%, mostly including anxiety disorders, depressive disorders and organic mental disorders.

Due to the limited knowledge of mental illness, the detection of these illnesses has been delayed in both out–patient and in–patient care, which leading to misdiagnosis or missed diagnosis. A report showed that only 15.9% of physicians at general hospitals in shanghai could be correctly recognised mental health difficulties in patients. As a result, some patients with severe somatoform disorders undergo multiple investigations and even surgery before the diagnosis is made. Around 20% of medical and surgical inpatients have anxiety or depression, which are two common reasons for causing a medical condition apparently worsening. Adequate recognition and treatment of the psychiatric disorder should be an integral part of management, since it has been shown to improve outcome.

There is evidence that consultation–liaison psychiatry can improve outcomes and reduce costs of medical care (NHS confederation, 2009). One of the most promising chance to improve productivity in the healthcare is by enhancing the interaction between psychiatrists and physicians. This is a key role of consultation–liaison psychiatry and one that offers a reduction in health care costs. Then, dealing with comorbid psychiatric illness can obtain persistent reductions in admissions to hospital for people with a range of long–term medical conditions, with the associated saving excessive cost of unnecessary investigations and treatment.

15.1.3   Future development

(1) Strengthening consultation–liaison psychiatry service.

(2) Enhancing continued education of psychiatric knowledge in general hospital.

(3) Carrying out researches on consultation–liaison psychiatry.

(4) Promoting the development of the multidisciplinary team, working with other clinical professionals to provide appropiate services for patients with integrated psycho–social–medical method.

15.2   Working scope

15.2.1   Task of consultation–liaison psychiatry

15.2.1.1   Provide consultation–liaison services for non–psychiatric professional clinicians

According to an investigation abroad, about 20% of medical outpatients have mental disorder to varying degrees, of whom with chronic physical illness the prevalence rate of mental disorder is approximately 25%. Some psychological symptoms can be resulted from certain physical illness. For example, patients with malignant tumor may suffer from anger, anxiety, depression and despair etc. ; patients may appear anxious, scared and irritable in different level as a result of surgical treatment, chemotherapy or radiotherapy for the severe medical illness. Faced to difficulty in diagnosing comorbid mental illness, non–psychiatric physicians could apply for psychiatrist's consultation. Thus, psychiatrists could take part into a series of medical procedures, including ward round, curative observation and follow–up.

15.2.1.2   Conduct training of psychiatric knowledge and clinical skill for medical personnel

There is a lack of psychiatric education in medical colleges, and continued medical education in general hospitals. Some doctors even have not paid enough attention to the bio–psycho–social medical model. To achieve transformation of medical model, psychiatrists are available to participate into imparting psychiatric knowledges and clinical skills to relevant medical staff.

(1) Participating in the teaching of psychiatry in medical college, so that medical students can master the etiology, pathophysiological mechanism, clinical manifestations, diagnosis and treatment in mental illness during undergraduate study period.

(2) Developing the mental health knowledge of non–psychiatrists in continued medical education.

(3) Restoring or establishing a clinician's rotation learning systems in the psychiatry department, to learn basic requirement, operation specification and relevant content of psychiatric examination.

(4) Initiating a lecture or forum on basic knowledge of psychiatry for clinicians.

(5) Restoring or establishing a clinical psychiatric case seminar system, to strengthen the connection and communication between clinicians and psychiatrists.

15.2.1.3 Provide mental health related knowledge for patients and families

Many people avoid going psychiatric clinic because of the stigma of mental illness. It is reported that a first-episode psychotic symptom may be misunderstood as a normal phenomenon or a general ideological, emotional problem by 80% of patients or their families, less than 7% of those would make a correct judgement. 35% -56% of patients would not go to psychiatric clinic until one year later after he (she) was ill, which delays timely treatment for the mental disorder. Therefore, it is of great significance to strengthen the publicity and popularization of mental health knowledge.

(1) Give lectures to improve mental health knowledge of patients with mental illness and their families.

(2) Set up boards or website to regularly about signs of recurrence and rehabilitation measures of patients with mental illness, prevention of psychological subhealth, sleep disorders, depression related knowledge.

(3) Carry out regular medical consultations, distribution of psychiatric propaganda materials, face-to-face communication and guidance, to help the families to treat the patient correctly and do a good job in the rehabilitation of patients with mental illness.

15.2.1.4 Scientific research

Scientific research can provide more theoretical basis and practical experience for the development of consultation-liaison psychiatry. The main research contents of the consultation-liaison psychiatry are seen in the following.

(1) The influence of psychosocial factors and psychotic symptoms on the occurrence, development, clinical manifestation, intervention and prognosis of somatic disease.

(2) Psychosocial reaction or abnormal behavior caused by somatic disease.

(3) Effect of psychotherapy or pharmacotherapy on the somatic disease.

(4) Prevalence rate of mental disorder.

(5) Comprehensive evaluation of the medical and teaching work of consultation-liaison psychiatry.

(6) Definition of laws, doctor-patient's rights, responsibilities and obligationsrelated to consultation-liaison psychiatry.

15.2.2 Working type of consultation-liaison psychiatry

15.2.2.1 Patient-centered consultation

The patient-centered consultation is the most common type of consultation. When making a consultation for a patient with mental health problems, such as severe anxiety, depression, a consultation-liaison psychiatrist could do the following.

(1) Making a clear analysis and diagnosis of the patient's problem.

(2) Answering questions proposed by non-psychiatric clinicians, such as whether patients have a mental illness or not; what is the influence of disease on the patient; whether patients need special psychiatric treatment, etc.

(3) Determining the role of consultant who is invited in the procedure of diagnosis and intervention. If there are some works that need to be done by the inviter, he (she) could be clearly informed of how to implement. If the treatment involves consultant, he (she) would follow up the patient on time and closely ob-

serve the development of patients' condition.

(4) The treatment plan should be implemented under the patient's acceptable conditions, with the consent of the inviter or patients' families and the signing of informed consent.

15.2.2.2 Inviter doctor-centered consultation-liaison

Some relationship between doctors and patients is relatively complex. When doctor-patient relationship is broken, patients would not accept the judgement of the nature and severity of the disease from the inviter doctor. Patients with negative emotions are tending to have impulsive behaviours, which might lead to potential threaten to the inviter doctor. Otherwise, other medical professionals do not agree with the management of inviter doctor. As mentioned above, consultation-liaison would adopt inviter doctor-centered model.

15.2.2.3 Medical team-centered consultation-liaison

This type of consultation is usually carried out in the intensive care unit (ICU), not only beneficial to patients, but also to explore and improve collaborative quality of the entire medical team. When a consultation doctor is invited to make recommendations, the doctor should take into account the various interaction between all the members of the medical team, and also between the medical staffs and the patients.

15.2.3 Service pattern of consultation-liaison psychiatry

15.2.3.1 Service pattern based on non-psychiatrist

At present, non-psychiatric physicians are mainly involved in clinical work related to consultation-liaison in the general hospital. The advantage of this model is that non-psychiatrists are trained to provide basic psychiatric service to patients in a short time. But the disadvantage is that non-psychaitrists with limited psychiatric knowledge have difficulty in dealing with more complex psychiatric disease.

15.2.3.2 Service pattern based on the department of psychiatry in general hospital

Some general hospitals have psychiatric department or a professional department providing mental health service. The advantage of it is that mental health providers not only have relatively solid clinical knowledge and skills but also are familiar with the working procedure of the comprehensive hospital.

15.2.3.3 Service pattern based on specialized psychiatric hospital

A comprehensive hospital can invite mental health professionals to take part into recognition and treatment of psychotic symptoms and psychological problems in patients with physical illness. Taking the psychiatric hospital as the main body can be in a variety of ways, such as requesting consultation, visiting together, or holding a seminar.

15.2.3.4 Service pattern based on consultation-liaison center

The consultation-liaison organization is composed of mental health professionals and other related medical professionals (such as neurologist, endocrinologist, psychologist, social workers and health personnel). The advantage of this model is that all kinds of staff can communicate directly and knowledge can be complementary to each other. But running this model requires that relevant personnel have a high degree of specialization and strong coordination ability at the same time.

15.2.4 Service content of consultation-liaison psychiatry in general hospital

15.2.4.1 Psychiatric consultation in various department of the general hospital

In a comprehensive hospital, the mental health problem covers a wide range of patients in all clinical departments. The application of psychiatric consultation may consist of a series of mental health related problems, including the following.

(1) General psychological problems, such as mild anxiety, depression or fear.

(2) Psychological reaction to a variety of procedures of diagnosis and treatment. For example, a woman is fearful before surgical operation.

(3) Psychosomatic disease, like hypertension or gastric ulcer.

(4) Neurosis, such as anxiety disorder, agoraphobia, or obsessive—compulsive disorder.

(5) Physiological disorders related to psychological factors insomnia, anorexia nervosa, or sexual dysfunctions.

(6) Personality disorder and psychosexual disorder paranoid personality disorder or sexual identification disorder.

(7) Organic psychotic disorder, like Alzheimer's disease or vascular dementia.

(8) Psychotic disorder, such as patients with mental illness comorbid somatic disease.

(9) Other mental illness, such as mental retardation, autism, or ADHD.

15.2.4.2 Consultation of other clinical doctors

Long—term usage of antipsychotic can cause damage in cardiovascular, endocrinal, digestive and hematopoietic system. In addition, psychiatric symptoms and some disease (such as neurological disease) are closely related. The diagnosis and treatment of some serious physical disease (such as infectious disease) must be made by the specialist. Therefore, it is necessary to ask the doctor of the clinical department to consult for following conditions.

(1) Disturbance of consciousness, there are some common disorders of consciousness: confusion, delirium, twilight state.

(2) Blood cell abnormalities, leukocytic reduction and granulocytic deficiency caused by clozapine.

(3) Arrhythmia and electrocardiogram abnormality, sinus bradycardia, ST—T abnormality.

(4) Respiratory tract infections, hospital acquired upper respiratory tract infections.

(5) Endocrine disorder, hyperprolactinemia, metabolic syndrome caused byantipsychotics.

(6) Fracture, especially in elderly patients, osteoporosis, bone brittleness.

15.3　Clinical application

Case report:

A 60 - year - old man is brought to the emergency department by ambulance for benzodiazepine overdosage. The man begin to recover after medical personnel's active rescue. He says that he has been feeling low and tired and can not sleep well since his wife died from cerebral apoplexy 3 months ago. He lives alone with few other social contacts, and says that he has not been eating well. He bursts into tears during the interview. The emergency doctor asks whether he has suicide ideation or behaviors, the man says that he desperately misses his wife, he has nothing to live for, his life has been destroyed.

15.3.1　Identification and treatment

15.3.1.1　Delirium, mental disorders secondary to a medical cause

Delirium has often the connotation of a syndrome with multifactorial aetiology, characterized by an acute behavioural decompensation with fluctuating attention in the context of a preexisting vulnerability. Delirium is a clinical condition characterized by a series of clinical features, including circadian rhythm disturbances, impaired attention, visual hallucination, agitation and disorientation. Visual hallucinations are commonly seen in organic mental disorder such as delirium tremens and toxic encephalopathy.

Prompt recognition of delirium is crucial. Delirium may present 3 different clinical types.

(1) Hyperkinetic or overactive, characterized by psychomotor agitation, and, sometimes, illusions and hallucinations.

(2) Hypokinetic or underactive, characterized by psychomotor slowing, drowsiness, reduced response to external stimuli and apathy.

(3) Mixed, characterized by an alternation of the phases of the hyperkinetic and hypokinetic type.

The hyperkinetic variant is easy to diagnose, but it is also the least frequent. The hypokinetic variant is conversely the most common clinical presentation, especially among the elderly, but it is more difficult to diagnose, and is related to a worse prognosis. The symptoms of hypokinetic delirium may in fact be mistakenly attributed to dementia, depression, or sedative drugs, being often considered as a "normal" state in view of age and biological complexity of the patient.

Recently, the consultation—liaison psychiatrist could identify and confirm the presence of delirium not only by specific mental status examination (MMSE), but also confusion assessment method (CAM). Additionally, it is strongly recommended to complete the advanced neurocognitive test for the detection of aphasia, apraxia, and agnosia.

The recognition of a medical etiology is critical as it may have reversible course and need specific treatment. Furthermore, failure to provide treatment may lead to permanent deficits and disability. The consultation—liaison psychiatrist can use a list of delirium risk factors to assess the patients. These include a variety of predisposing factors, such as advanced age, cognitive impairment, depression, sensory impairment, and precipitating factors, such as multiple medications, sleep deprivation, poorly controlled pain, drug toxicity or withdrawal, acute illness and associated abnormal blood values, and the use of physical restraints. The CLP must review all laboratory evaluations and neurodiagnostic test, such as cerebrospinal fluid biochemistry, electroencephalography (EEG) and cranial computer tomography (CT) or magnet resonance imaging (MRI) scan and be prepared for further tests. In general hospital, most cases of delirium are either partially or entirely reversible, most frequent causes include metabolic imbalance, overdose or toxicity of psychoactive drug. This may be supplemented by laboratory biochemical, biotoxicology screening, or serum level of potential psychoactive substance.

Primary treatment of delirium consists of correction of precipitating cause and exacerbating factors. In addition, certain adjustive medication may be useful. Neuroleptics in small doses may be helpful for calming down the agitation of the confused patient. Environmental changes, like providing clocks, familiar objects from home, and frequent orientation from staff or families, would minimize patient's confusion.

Delirium usually has a sudden onset with a fluctuating clinical course thereafter. There is gradual resolution of symptoms with effective treatment of the underlying cause. Symptom resolution may be much slower in the elderly. There is often patchy amnesia for the period of recovery. The mortality is high(-20% of patients will die during that hospital admission, up to 50% at 1 year).

15.3.1.2　Depression

The prevalense of depressive disorders in patients in the general hospital is twice of the general population. In primary care, the prevalence of depressive illness is less than 5%, while in medical outpatients it is between 5%—10% and in medical inpatients it is between 10%—20%. The frequency of depressive illness is raised in those with more severe illnesses, and some conditions (e. g. , cardiac and neurological disorders) show very high rates. Unfortunately, less than 25% of these are diagnosed and only about 50% of those received treatment. When such depression is a reaction to the stress or medical conditions, it may respond to improvement in the patients' clinical condition. However, when symptoms become more severe and impede the patient daily activities or social functioning, psychiatric evaluation should be requested immediately.

There is a tendency to assume that depressed mood in a patient represents an understandable adjustment reaction that does not need treatment. This may bring the patient to needless suffering, because the depression may respond to the use of a depressant medication, in addition to the treatment of some underlying medical problems. Situations for the association of depression and physical illness include:

(1) Physical illness causes the depression.

1) Biological cause: e. g. , hypothyroidism, Cushing disease, Parkinson's disease.

2) Psychological cause: related to loss or change, life events secondary to illness, e. g. , amputation, loss of sexual function. Particularly potent are fatal or potentially fatal, disfiguring, or disabling diseases.

(2) The depression is a side-effect of the treatment for the physical illness.

1) Drug treatments, e. g. , steroids, β-blockers, digoxin, calcium channel blockers, aminophylline, theophylline, NSAIDs, cimetidine, metoclopramide, levodopa, methyldopa, isotretinoin, α-interferon.

2) Disfiguring, painful, or prolonged treatments.

(3) The physical illness is a result of the depression, e. g. , liver failure after paracetamol overdose in context of depressive relapse.

(4) The physical illness and the depression have a common cause, e. g. , stressful life events acting as precipitants to both myocadiac infarction and depression.

(5) The co-occurrence may be coincidental—depressive illness is common and the co-occurrence with other common illnesses can be expected by chance.

The treatment strategy of depression in patients with medical illness involves both psychotherapy and antidepressant medications. Cognitive behavior therapy (CBT) has been strongly recommended to assist many patients and their families in coping with illness. Antidepressant drugs are useful in treating depressed medical patients and can improve mood, appetite, and sleep disorders. Tricyclic agents must be used cautiously in patients with cardiac conduction abnormalities (particularly bundle branch blocks), in patients with delirium or dementia who may become more confused, and in those for whom anticholinergic side effect would be detrimental. Many tricyclic drugs cause orthostatic hypotension and must be used carefully in patients who can not tolerate a decrease in blood pressure. Monoamine oxidase inhibitors should be carefully used in this population, because they have numerous interactions with food substances and other drugs. It has been confirmed to have a wide margin of safety and similar therapeutic effect with typical antidepressants for the new generation antidepressants (e. g. , SSRIs, SNRIs, NaSSa), which are suggested as the first-line antidepressants in medical patients.

15.3.1.3 Anxiety

Anxiety is a common phenomenon in patients and may be viewed as a reflection of their current situation. If anxiety is severe, prolonged, or is interfering with appropriate medical management, it may become a focus of clinical attention. Often patients don't meet all of the diagnostic criteria of anxiety disorder. Thus, it is important to make an individual assessment and make a decision based on symptom severity, social function impairment, and response to the treatment for anxiety.

There are some organic causes of anxiety symptoms.

(1) Neurological (epilepsy, head injury, brain tumour, dementia, encephalitis).

(2) Endocrine (hyperthyroidism, hypothyroidism, Cushing disease, hyperparathyroidism, Addison's disease).

(3) Metabolic (uraemia, electrolyte disturbance, porphyria). SLE (lupus psychosis).

(4) Medications (steroids, levodopa, interferon, anticholinergics, antihypertensives, anticonvulsants, stimulants).

(5) Drug abuse (cocaine, LSD, cannabis, PCP, amphetamines, opioids).

Patients with ischemic heart disease may present episodes of panic and chest pain which are difficult to distinguish clinically from angina; however all investigations for the discrete episode will be normal. The aim of treatment is to help distinguishing symptoms arising as a result of heart disease or panic. The patient who meets the criteria of panic disorder treatment should be instituted with antidepressants. Cognitive therapy may also be useful.

15.3.1.4 Patient management problems

The consultation-liaison psychiatrist may be requested to assist in management of following situations.

(1) Non-compliance with doctor's professional advice that may result in severe medical consequence.

(2) Agitation, disruptive behavior.

(3) Personality, which would interfere with clinical management.

Since many patients' management problems arising out of underlying medical process, recognition and confirmation of these problems are of primary concern. The evaluation of patient's management problems includes consideration of biological, psychological and social factors as they interact in a particular clinical setting. Metabolic disturbance, drug intoxication, and drug withdrawal syndrome are common reason for agitation. The consultation-liaison psychiatrist should provide specific suggestions for immediate control of agitation, including the indications and contradictions for use of restraints, or medications. It is essential to arrange for adequate but unobtrusive help to be available. Physical contact (including physical examination) should not be attempted unless the purpose has been clearly understood by and agreed with the patient. If restraint can not be avoided, it should be accomplished quickly by an adequate number of people using the minimum of force. Staff should not attempt single-handed restraint. Extreme caution is, of course, required if the patient could be in possession of an offensive weapon. Diazepam (5-10 mg) may be useful for patient with panic. Intramuscular lorazepam and intramuscular haloperidol (2-5 mg, repeated) can be used for those who are psychotic and have been exposed to antipsychotics. Haloperidol or olanzapine (oral or intramuscular) is recommended in delirium unless this is secondary to alcohol withdrawal. When the patient becomes calm, medication may be continued in smaller doses, usually three to four times a day and preferably by mouth. Careful observations of the physical state and behavior by nurses are necessary during this treatment. In addition, the consultation-liaison psychiatrist is expected to offer guidelines regarding the legal implications of treating such patients.

The consultation-liaison psychiatrist must assess the extent to which the patient's personality might be contributing to a dysfunctional response to illness. Specific issues, if pertinent, should be discussed along with appropriate management strategies. These patients often engage in struggles with the staff over their own diagnosis and treatment. Appropriate concession to the patients could minimize conflict on critical matters. Uncontrolled schizophrenia and affective disorder, are causes of problems in medical patient management.

In many cases, social dysfunction contributes to patient management problems. Several instances of abrupt departure against medical advice occur through the dysfunction of the interaction of the patient and the treatment team. The consultation-liaison psychiatrist must function as a social system consultant by suggesting ways in which medical treatment protocols can be modified to avoid or overcome management problems.

15.3.1.5 Symptoms with no apparent medical cause

A substantial proportion of patients in primary care will have symptoms for which, after adequate investigation, no cause can be found. Non-specific symptoms without underlying organic pathology are very common and usually transient. Where they become prolonged enough to merit medical attention they may present to any specialty, with presentations such as pain, loss/disturbance of function, and altered sensation. The consultation-liaison psychiatrist has to answer whether there is a conversion disorder, or somatization disorder, or chronic factitious illness, or malingerer.

Patients with somatic symptoms for which no adequate physical cause can be found make up a large and heterogeneous group, including conversion and dissociative disorders, somatization disorder, factitious disorder, malingering. Causative mechanisms of these disorders are currently unclear, but the following may play a part: psychological factors; health beliefs; affective state; underlying personality; autonomic arousal; increased muscle tension; hyperventilation; disturbed sleep; prolonged inactivity; impaired ability to filter afferent stimuli. During the course of psychiatric assessment of these patients, "secondary gain" need to be clarified. Since all illness offer some degree of secondary gain, this mechanism should not be assumed uncritically to "explain" the signs or symptoms. The consultation-liaison psychiatrist should help the patient and the family recognize and prevent secondary gain from impeding recovery.

Conversion and dissociative disorders are characterized by the presence of a psychological conflict, of which the patient is unaware, that produces anxiety, followed by the unconscious "convention" of this anxiety into a somatic sign or symptom that symbolically expressed and resolved the psychological conflict. Hypnosis may be useful both in evaluation and treating this condition.

Somatization disorder is a disorder in which there is repeated presentation with medically unexplained symptoms. Certain patients, usually women, have lifelong patterns of various somatic complaints, so called somatization disorder. Symptoms may occur in any system and are to some extent suggestible. The most frequent symptoms are non-specific and atypical. At all ages, it is associated with significant psychological distress, functional impairment, and risk of iatrogenic harm.

Factitious disorders are those which are intentionally produced or elaborated, with the aim of receiving a medical diagnosis. This simulation may represent a lifestyle indulging in mimicking medical illness. These patients are not the same as malingerers, who pretend to have medical problems to obtain a specific conscious goal(e. g. , obtaining opiate prescription, obtaining legal compensation). Recognition of these two psychological conditions should alert the staff to withhold invasive diagnostic or therapeutic efforts. Treatment can then be focus on psychosocial issues.

Management principles should include: ①assessment; ②diagnosis; ③clear explanation; ④minimization of iatrogenic harm; ⑤empirical use of potentially beneficial treatments; ⑥consideration of involvement in treatment trials. There have been some trials of medication and of cognitive-behavior therapy. Antidepressant medication has been shown to benefit several kinds of medically unexplained symptoms, including fibromyalgia and irritable bowel syndrome. Pain may be helped by tricyclic antidepressants. This benefit occurs especially(but not exclusively) in patients with marked depressive symptoms. Cognitive-behavior therapy is moderately effective in the treatment of non-cardiac chest pain, irritable bowel syndrome, and chronic fatigue syndrome.

15.3.1.6 Patients with suicidal behavior or self-injurious behavior

An increased suicide risk is mostly likely associated with chronic physical illness because of the high risk of depression in this group. For those patients, a recent bereavement, presence of delusions, suicidal ideation, chronic mental illness and a family history of suicide are all associated with a higher risk of suicide.

It is important to remember that risk is not static. It varies between populations, across age ranges, and within individuals over different periods of time. Clinicians and researchers are not terribly proficient at quantifying and predicting risk. The positive predictive value of most methods of assessment (the proportion of individuals identified as high risk by risk assessment measures, who are actually high risk) is low. This means it is very difficult in clinical practice actually to predict which patients will take their lives. Despite this, it is good practice to carry out a risk assessment.

The doctor should consider the following factors.

(1) Always conduct a risk assessment.

(2) Be aware of demographic risk factors.

(3) Be aware of previous psychiatric and behavioral factors, for example previous illness, previous history of deliberate self-harm, alcoholism, a family history of suicide.

(4) Ask about negative mood.

(5) Ask about suicidal thoughts.

(6) Identify the presence of other key symptoms, for example hopelessness and worthlessness.

(7) Ask about suicidal actions.

(8) Be especially vigilant if the patient is a young male, over 50 years of age, or recently discharged from hospital or has a serious mental illness that is relapsing.

(9) Ask about any protective factors, for examples a supportive partner or family member, or supportive accommodation provided by social services.

By the end of assessment the doctor should aim to answer the following questions.

(1) Is there ongoing suicidal ideation? Evidenced by: continuing stated wish to die; ambivalence about survival; sense of hopelessness towards future; clear intent to die at time of act.

(2) Is there evidence of mental illness? Diagnosed in the normal way. Most common diagnoses are depressive illness and alcohol misuse. Be alert to comorbid substance misuse and to the combination of an acute stressor on the background of a chronic condition.

(3) Are there non-mental health issues which can be addressed? Many patients will reveal stressors such as: family or relationship difficulties; life events (particularly relating to previous abuse; school or employment problems; debt; legal problems; problems related to immigration). They can be usefully directed to appropriate local services.

Having assessed the suicidal risk, the obvious first requirement is to prevent patients from harming themselves. These arrangements require adequate staffing and a safe environment. Wards design should minimize the availability of means of self-harm. This includes preventing access to open windows and other places where jumping could lead to serious injury or death, removing ligature points from which hanging could take place (e. g. , by boxing in pipework), preventing access to ward areas in which self-injury would be easier to enact, and removing potentially dangerous personal possessions such as razors and belts. If the risk is high, special nursing arrangements may be needed to ensure that the patient is accompanied.

Although the continued prescribing of antidepressants during the period following an episode of depression reduces the risk of a subsequent episode of depression, a reduction in suicidal behavior has not been demonstrated. However, there is accumulating evidence that lithium prophylaxis reduces suicide rates, and some evidence that clozapine may reduce suicide attempts among people with schizophrenia or schizoaffective disorder.

15.3.2 Other conditions served by consultation–liaison psychiatry

15.3.2.1 Evaluation of patients for suitability for medical or surgical procedures

Every doctor should be aware of the psychological impact of physical disease. Serious physical illness is associated with uncertainty. Clinical practice may exacerbate the patient's anxiety. Other common reactions to physical illness are:

(1) Search for meaning: why has this illness happened to me?

(2) Loss of control: what is going to happen to me?

(3) Failure: I have failed or done something wrong.

(4) Stigma: I am ashamed or embarrassed about my illness.

(5) Fear: am I going to die or have terrible pain?

(6) Secretiveness: I mustn't tell anyone, I must keep it to myself.

(7) Isolation: I am the only person going through this… no one understands.

Relatives and friends of patients with serious physical illness often find it difficult to provide support and help, because they do not know whether or how to talk about the illness. The consultation–liaison psychiatrist is a key figure to provide help.

The consultation–liaison psychiatrist should try to discuss with the patient how he/she feels about the illness. It can be reassuring for patients to realize that their feelings of bitterness or anger are not particularly. The consultation–liaison psychiatrist should encourage the patient to share these experiences with close friends. The role that consultation–liaison psychiatrist could play is to facilitate the patient's natural adjustment to the illness not to make him/her do something that feels strange.

15.3.2.2 Pain

Patients may continue to complain of pain despite analgesic management that is usually effective. This difficult clinical problem may give rise to request for psychiatric consultation. Such consultation requests an awareness that pain is a complex phenomenon involving an interplay of biological and psychosocial factors.

The consultation–liaison psychiatrist should interview these patients with the primary physician, with emphasis on the potential biological basis and the current treatment strategies. The patient is then evaluated for certain psychiatric disorders that is associated with unusual or refractory pain syndromes. Depression should be considered. Since its association with chronic pain may lead to increased preoccupation with the pain and loud complaints, somatoform pain disorder, and factitious disorder.

Psychosocial factors may also play a role in in refractory pain syndrome. Pain have a special meaning for the patients. It may mimic the pain a close relative experienced in a terminal illness. Cultural backgrounds, unresolved mourning, and secondary gain, may play a role in the pain syndrome.

The past few years, pain control techniques besides opioid analgesics have been developed for chronic pain. Nonsteroidal anti–inflammatory drug is effective alternatives to narcotics for many patients. Tricyclic antidepressants, often in low doses, have been effective for chronic pain. Also, new antidepressant (duloxetine) has been approved to treat chronic pain by FDA. Supportive psychotherapy, hypnosis, even placebos have shown effective for some patients with chronic pain.

15.3.2.3 Obesity

The increasing prevalence of obesity is a significant public health concern. Recent data indicates the worldwide prevalence of obesity(body mass index, BMI $\geq$ 30 kg/m^2) has doubled from 1980 to 2008, with 10% of men and 14% of women in 2008. Obesity is a leading risk factor for a number of significant chronic diseases, including increased risk of cardiovascular disease, type 2 diabetes, hypertension, stroke, osteoarthritis and cancer. The prevalence of depression, and associated risk of poor health outcomes, is elevated in an obese population, and further elevated in a treatment-seeking obese population. The highest 12-month prevalence rates of comorbid depression and obesity are found in individuals seeking bariatric surgery, with studies reporting prevalence of 19%-66%.

The high prevalence of depression in an obese population is concerning given the overall impairment to health and risk of chronic diseases associated with either of these disorders independently, and the increased risks associated with them co-existing simultaneously. Consequently, it seems likely that depression may also negatively influence obesity treatment outcomes. A better understanding of the association between comorbid depression and obesity is critical to inform appropriate prevention and intervention strategies.

In a recent systematic review and meta-analysis of longitudinal studies of overweight, obesity and depression, 80% of the studies showed evidence that obesity is prospectively related to depression, while 53% showed evidence that depression is prospectively related to obesity. Obese persons had a 55% increased risk of developing depression over time, whereas depressed persons had a 58% increased risk of being obese. These results highlight the likely bidirectional relationship between obesity and depression.

Markowitz and colleagues identified three risk factors that are consistently found to moderate the risk of depression in obese individuals: severity of obesity, gender and socioeconomic status. They further proposed a model, informed by research evidence, clinical experience and relevant theory, consisting of a series of causal pathways that may explain a bidirectional relationship between obesity and depression. The model suggests that obesity leads to depression via the health and appearance concern pathways, which include constructs such as functional impairment, quality of life, physical activity, experience of stigma, body image, dissatisfaction and dieting behaviours. They further postulate that depression leads to obesity via the direct physiological and indirect psychosocial pathways, which includes constructs such as elevated stress reaction, immunological dysfunction, hypothalamic-pituitary-adrenal axis, negative cognitions, eating dys-regulation and poor adherence to treatment.

Furthermore, some antidepressants and second-generation antipsychotics may induce significant weight gain, such as mirtazapine, olanzapine, clozapine, that should be cautiously take into account by the clinician to reduce potential risk of overweight or obesity for patients with depression or schizophrenia.

15.3.2.4 Persistent postural-perceptual dizziness

Persistent postural-perceptual dizziness(PPPD) is a chronic functional disorder of the nervous system, characterised by non-spinning vertigo and perceived unsteadiness. The symptoms are exacerbated when patients assume upright postures and in situations with complex or moving visual stimuli. The most common provocations are benign circumstances such as standing, walking, looking at traffic or sitting in a busy restaurant, which may be perceived as noxious or threatening. Symptoms of PPPD may be alleviated transiently in moments of distraction and flare fleetingly without apparent provocation.

A UK population-based study of primary care found that 4% of all patients registered with a general practitioner experience persistent symptoms of dizziness, and most of thoseare incapacitated by their symptoms. In UK neurology clinics, 2% of all secondary referrals are diagnosed primarily with vertigo or dizziness, half of which were deemed psychological/functional.

The disorder can have different clinical presentation, such as the primary symptoms of dizziness, unsteadiness and hypersensitivity to self-motion or complex visual stimuli, or the secondary complications of phobic avoidance of provocative situations and functional gait abnormalities. This can lead patients to different medical specialties (otolaryngology, psychiatry, neurology). Historically, the varied presentations resulted in the definitions of various overlapping nosological predecessors of PPPD, such as phobic postural vertigo, space – motion discomfort, visual vertigo, chronic subjective dizziness, psychogenic gait disorder and others. Arguments for differentiation of these disorders remain valid, but PPPD has recently emerged as a unifying and diagnostically unambiguous disorder that has been recognised by the WHO and has been included in the 11th edition of the International Classification of Diseases (ICD-11) and the recently established International Classification of Vestibular Disorders.

PPPD is usually precipitated by episodes of vertigo or unsteadiness of vestibular, neurological or psychiatric origin. These triggers appear to induce involuntary utilisation of high-demand postural control strategies and an over-reliance on visual stimuli for spatial orientation. An initial period of high anxiety and excessive vigilance about the acute physical symptoms appears to perpetuate these reflexive processes, which are then inadequately mollified by interactions among cortical vestibular, visual and threat assessment networks. Maladaptive cognitive-behavioural responses commonly add secondary psychological and functional morbidity, such as fear of falling, anxiety or depressive disorders, and functional gait abnormalities. However, PPPD persists independently of any lesional or structural disease.

For functional dizziness, as in PPPD, vestibular exercises promoting habituation are most apt. These differ from treatments used to promote recovery from structural vestibular disorders. Exercises for PPPD must be started more gently and increased more slowly. Techniques aim at fatiguing abnormal reflexive responses to movement tasks and reducing sensitivity to visual stimuli have shown long term clinical benefit in PPPD. An exercise program that is too aggressive may exacerbate symptoms, causing patients to stop far before they can achieve any benefit. Selective serotonin reuptake inhibitors (SSRIs) and serotonin norepinephrine reuptake inhibitors (SNRIs) showed promising in reducing dizziness and unsteadiness in a majority of patients with chronic dizziness, a previous incarnation of PPPD. Treatment with medications from these two classes of serotonergic antidepressants is supported by multiple prospective, clinical trials, but no randomised controlled trials as yet. Clinical response is usually seen after 8-12 weeks, and, if effective, medication should be continued for at least 1 year. There is limited experience with cognitive-behavioural therapy (CBT) for treating functional dizziness. CBT would be expected to help patients with pronounced fear of falling or fear of dizziness, since it can reduce similar avoidance and safety behaviour in patients with other anxiety disorders.

Undiagnosed or untreated patients can suffer for many years, neurologists need to be familiar with functional dizziness and PPPD, make a firm diagnosis and be aware of the treatment options summarised above. The presence of long duration symptoms does not preclude a good outcome with treatment.

15.3.2.5　Forensic issues

The consultation-liaison psychiatrist is often asked to make a judgment about the competence of patients to refuse or consent to a medical or surgical procedure. This process consists of determining whether the patient has psychiatric disorder that impairs judgment. The standards of competence varies with the risk-to-benefit ratio of the procedure. A patient with moderate organic mental disorder may be competent to consent to a computered tomography scan, but not to major surgery. The determination of competence is a judicial decision, though often based on the psychiatric opinion.

Another forensic issue that shouldn't be ignored is the involuntary admission and treatment of patients with mental disorders. The autonomy of patients with mental disorders has been growing in importance, influenced by an increasing emphasis on individual rights, This viewpoint may undermine the original purpose of involuntary admission and treatment, which is to provide adequate mental-health care to those individuals whose mental disorders interfere with their rational ability to consent or decline treatment.

The United Nations Convention on the Rights of Persons with Disabilities adds a new perspective on non-discrimination and equality. Given this context, legal framework for involuntary admission and treatment, and/or commitment laws pertaining to persons with mental disorder has been reformed in many countries. Involuntary admission and treatment generally have been accepted as a necessary measure to protect patients, others, and society. However, it remains a controversial and complex ethical and legal issue, and sometimes it is difficult to balance the rights of patients with public. Many countries stipulate a number of relevant provisions for involuntary admission and treatment that govern their national or regional mental-health care systems. The principles and procedures of involuntary admission and treatment vary among countries because of different cultures, traditions, economies, and human resources.

The formulation of the criterion for involuntary admission or treatment is a complex and cumbersome process. According to the checklist for Involuntary Admission and Treatment developed by the WHO, the criteria for detention in most countries include similar conditions: the patient must be suffering from a severe mental disorder; and compulsory treatment is necessary in the interest of the patient's health or safety, or the protection of other persons. However, these criteria are not included in all legal frameworks.

The mental-health legislation of China came into effect on May 1, 2013. This wide-ranging mental health law on involuntary admission and compulsory treatment reformulated the key principles of the WHO. The main advantage of the law is to legalize the involuntary placement process, and provide suitable treatment to psychiatric patients. Meanwhile, some disadvantages of the law may be obstacles to practices. First, "current risk" is not clearly defined in the criterion of involuntary admission, which may leave a loophole to the abuse of this clause. Second, the law does not have a specific duration for involuntary admission, thus it seems to be quite diverse to implement throught the country without the national guidline. Finally, the law does not metion whether or not the patient who is a "danger to others" may self-apply for discharge. Like all nations, China still has a long way to go before finding the right balance between protection and control.

Chen Hong

Chapter 16

Child and Adolescent Psychiatry

16.1　Disorders of psychological development

16.1.1　Introduction

The developmental of children's cognition, emotion, behavior, ability and character is called psychological development. All kinds of harmful factors can effect on children's mental development, and all aspects of psychology do not reach the age corresponding level, which is called psychological developmental disorder. In ICD-10 and CCMD-3, Psychological developmental disorders are divided into 3 types: mental retardation characterized by significantly below average intellectual functioning and adaptive behavior; specific developmental disorders with the main clinical manifestations of speech and language, learning skills, motor skills and other developmental delays(specific developmental disorders); pervasive developmental disorders, represented by autism.

16.1.2　Mental retardation

Mental retardation(MR)is a generalized neuro-developmental disorder characterized by retarded intellectual development which begins before 18 years old. The main symptoms are impaired daily skills during child development, including the deficient cognitive function, language skills, motor abilities, and social skills. These clinical features caused by biological, psychological, and social factors, leading to a significantly decreased intelligence level and abnormal adaptive behaviors compared to the same-aged peers. Mental retardation is not only a social-psychological phenomenon, but also a biomedical phenomenon, which is neither induced by education deprivation and audio-visual impairments, nor by primary emotional disorders. Mental retardation is not a disease, but a syndrome. It has no single cause and no consistent disease process, it merely indicates that the individual's intelligence and social adaptability are below a certain level.

The concept of mental retardation was developed by Fitzherbert A. in 1534. He wrote "The patient is a fool from birth, who can't count, doesn't know his parents and age". At the end of the 19th century, people tended to use idiots and fools to refer to people with intellectual disabilities. These words, with contempt and discrimination, were replaced by intellectual disability or mental retardation. In France in 1905, the first intelligence scale was developed, and was applied in the United States as a diagnostic tool of mental retardation three years later, providing a quantitative standard for assessing mental retardation accurately. Since 1921, the American Association for mental retardation has regularly published manuals to discuss the diagnosis and classification of mental retardation, and its diagnostic standard has been decided as below two standard deviations of IQ. In 1959, the fifth edition was published, which explained that mental retardation not only refers to lower intelligence, but also includes the defect of adaptation. The concept is still used today.

In 1930s, the intelligence tests began to be used for diagnosis in China, which was relatively early around the world. It was commonly called deficient brain development, mental mal-development, and intelligence deficits. At present, mental disease classification and diagnostic criteria in China have used the same term of mental retardation with the DSM and the world health organization's international classification of diseases(ICD-10). But recently the DSM-5 has changed the term to be intellectual disability, which initially means disabilities in the intelligence.

16.1.2.1   Epidemiology

Mental retardation affects about 1% -3% of the general population. But the prevalence of mental retardation varies widely in different regions, which may be related to the inconsistency of diagnostic criteria, methods and tools. According to the review of epidemiological studies in United States, the prevalence of mild mental retardation is 0.37% -0.59%, the prevalence of moderate, severe and profound mental retardation is 0.3% -0.4%, and the prevalence of males is higher than females with the ratio of 1.6 : 1. In China, a mental retardation survey of 29 provinces and municipalities in 1987 showed a 1.268% mental disability rate, among which were 1.315% of males and 1.220% of females. From 1985 to 1990, an epidemiology study of mental retardation on 0 to 14 year-old population in 8 provinces in China showed the prevalence was 1.2%, among which the urban prevalence rate was 0.70% and the rural prevalence rate was 1.41%. In 2001, the sample survey of children with disabilities aged 0-6 reported that the prevalence of mental disability in children was 0.931%. According to the fifth survey of population in China in 2000, there were 954,000 children aged between 0 and 6 were intelligence disabled in China. In recent years, the prevalence of mental retardation has been declining, which is mainly related to the preventive measures and the improvement of medical level.

There was a differences in the prevalences of mental retardation between males and females. The males showed higher prevalence than females. The reasons for gender differences include many factors such as the abnormalities of genetic susceptibility in male fetuses, antenatal and neonatal injury. The survey also showed that the disease prevalence is significantly higher in rural areas than in urban areas, which may be related to poor rural medical and health conditions easily causing brain damage, iodine deficiency and other factors. Its prevalence among all age groups showed the highest prevalence in school-age children. The reason might be that the early diagnosis of the infant period for mild mental retardation is relatively difficult, and children's obvious intellectual lag can only be observed after their admission to school when comparing to other peers. Also, some patients with mild mental retardation own better social adaptation, have a certain ability to work, resulting the difficulty to identify in the general population.

16.1.2.2   Etiology and risk factors

From fetus to the age of 18, all factors that affect the development of central nervous system can lead to mental retardation, including biological factors and the social and cultural factors. Most of the disorders are mainly caused by biological factors, and the social and cultural factors follow. About half of the patients with mental retardation have specific biological causes, and most of which are with the moderate to severe mental retardation. Although the majority of patients with mild mental retardation are mainly induced by biological factors, it is difficult to find out the exact causes. The following are several main factors that have been identified.

(1) Genetic factors

It includes autosomal and sex chromosomal abnormalities, such as haplotype, triploid, polyploid, chromosome inversion, deletion, translocation, duplication, ring chromosome and isobaric chromosome. The most prevalent genetic conditions include Down's syndrome, which is caused by the presence of all or part of a third copy of chromosome 21; and Klinefelter's syndrome, which results from two or more X chromosomes in males. Congenital ovarian dysgenesis(Turner) is a female sex chromosome losing an X. In addition, there are superfemale, whose sex chromosome is XXX or XO chimera. It is generally believed that the higher the X aberration of the sex chromosome, the higher the incidence and severity of mental retardates.

In addition, genetic studies have shown that the brittle parts of chromosomes have a relationship with the X-linked intelligence deficits, such as fragile X syndrome. In 1984, Jin Ming et al. reported the results of chromosome examination for 70 children with mental retardation. They found 53.4% of the children carry the chromosome fragile site, in the form of fracture and elliptic shape change, which can be distributed on each chromosome.

(2) Genetic metabolic diseases

The abnormality of DNA molecular structure may decrease the enzyme activity, which is important for the body metabolism, leading to hereditary metabolic diseases. Among them, phenylketonuria, galactosemia, leukodystrophy, nodular sclerosis, neurofibroma and congenital hypothyroidism are more common. In addition, a few mental retardations involve multi-gene inheritance, which are caused by environmental factors based on the accumulation effect of multiple genes.

(3) Congenital craniocerebral deformity

Common diseases are familial cerebellar deformity, congenital hydrocephalus, and araphia.

(4) Adverse factors in perinatal period

1) Maternal characteristics

Older age at conception, malnutrition, smoking, drinking, after strong or long-term stress, having a lasting emotional depression, anxiety.

2) Infection

Infection of various viruses(the most common), bacteria, spirochetes and parasites during pregnancy, such as cytomegalovirus, rubella virus, influenza virus, hepatitis virus, HIV, toxoplasma and treponema pallidum.

3) Medications

Many medications can lead to mental retardation, especially those that affect the central nervous system, endocrine and metabolic systems, as well as anti-tumor and salicylic acid drugs.

4) Poisons

Polluted environment, food and water by harmful substances, such as lead and mercury, organic phosphorus and poisonous gases, which can have adverse effects on the development of the fetus. Women who had serious smoking habits were twice as likely to have a premature birth than non-smoking mothers, and their babies may born with a lower body weight. Excessive drinking during pregnancy can lead to fetal alcohol syndrome, and babies tend to have poor growth, low head and low intelligence.

5) Radiation and electro-magnetic waves

Influence the development of the embryo, which produces malformation and affects the development of the central nervous system.

6) Diseases and complications during pregnancy

Pregnant women suffering from various diseases, like diabetes, severe anemia, kidney disease, thyroid disease, threatened abortion, gestational hypertension, preeclampsia, and multiple pregnancy, which could lead to embryonal hypoxia.

7) Complications during process of labor

Preplacental placenta, early separation of placenta, fetal intrauterine distress, cord around neck, prolonged labor, birth injury, and premature birth.

8) Neonatal diseases

Immature, low birth weight, undiagnosed nuclear jaundice, neonatal hepatitis, neonatal septicemia, fetal craniosynostosis, etc.

(5) Factors in postnatal period

Prior to the development of the brain, various diseases that can affect the development of the brain and socio-cultural factors are related to.

1) Brain damage

Central nervous system infection such as encephalitis and meningitis, intracranial hemorrhage, craniocerebral trauma and cerebral hypoxia (drowning, suffocation, carbon monoxide poisoning, prolonged dyspnea), etc.

2) Infant malnutrition

Since infant brain neurons need rich nutrition, the mental development of infants will be influenced by the lack of breast milk, improper feeding methods, chronic diarrhea and vomiting that can cause severe malnutrition.

3) Environmental factors

Human need a good social environment. Thus, audial or visual impairment and social isolation will decrease the opportunities for children to accept education and interpersonal communication, leading to lack of imitation and retarded mental development.

16.1.2.3   Clinical features and classification

Cases report :

Wang, male, 10 years old, twitching for 4 years with lower intelligence, was sent to the mental health clinic in August 2015.

The patient had a convulsive seizure accompanied with unconscious when he was 6 years old. The duration of the seizure was less than 1 minute and onset every few months. The child develops slowly after his born. When he was over 2 years old, he started to call his parents, and at 5 years old to speak several words. At 2 years old, the patient can stand and at 3 years old can walk. Until 8 years old, he was not bed-wetting. After 9 years old, he was able to dress and take care of himself. He entered the school at 8 years old. The scores of verbal test and math test were 20 - 30. He failed to attend to higher grade twice, so he dropt out of school. He can sweep floor, wash dishes, but can't cook or wash clothes. He is obedient and never go out to play himself. Besides, he did not show other weird behaviors.

The manifestations of mental retardation are mainly developmental delay in intellectual functioning and deficits in social adaptive functioning. According to the severity of the delay in intellectual functioning, deficits in social adaptive function and IQ, the psychiatric classifications describe 4 levels of severity: mild, moderate , severe and profound (Table 16-1) .

Table 16-1   Clinical classification of mental retardation

Classification	IQ	Mental age/years	Adaptation deficits	Benefits from special education
Mild	50~70	9~12	Mild	Obtaining practical skills and practical ability to read and calculate , and to adapt to society under the guidance
Moderate	35~49	6~9	Moderate	Obtaining simple social skills , basic health habits and simple manual skills , but can't progress in reading and calculating
Severe	20~34	3~6	Severe	Obtaining benefits from systematic training
Profound	<20	<3	Profound	Responding to eating training and toilet training

(1) Mild mental retardation

Patients with mild mental retardation , whose IQ are between 50 and 69 , accounted for more than 80% of all mental retardation patients. These patients showed mild social adaption deficits. Generally , their language competence develops well , while their synthetically analytical ability , learning ability , and mathematical ability are impaired. Also , they are hard to achieve the degree of primary school in activities involving the abstract thinking and creativity. Mild patients are generally gentle , quiet and easy to manage. They can participate in social productive labor , but lack initiative and enthusiasm , and tend to show stress respond or psychological disorders when encounter adverse stimuli. They can perform house – work , look after themselves and do unskilled or semi–skilled work. They usually require some support.

(2) Moderate mental retardation

About 10% of the patients are classified as moderate level , whose IQ are between 35 and 49. Their verbal comprehension and application develop slowly and their vocabulary is poor to express the thoughts completely. These patients showed deficit look after themselves ability and motor skills , emotionally lability , impulsive behaviors. Some patients need lifelong monitoring as it is difficult for them to reach to the third–grade level in primary. They develop a certain ability to imitate others. After training , they can learn some simple skills for life and work. Most of them are able to engage in simple , repetitive , and unskilled work. Most patients have emotional interactions with their relatives and those who are in contact with them frequently. Thus , they are able to establish a relatively stable relationship.

(3) Severe mental retardation

3% –4% of the cases are classified as severe level , whose IQ are between 20 and 34. They commonly comorbid with organic diseases and suffer from obvious motor function impairments. Because their low language develop level , they can speak simple sentences. Some patients often repeat the monotonous and aimless movement , such as nodding , rocking body , and running. They are not able to take care of their daily life , nor respond for their behaviors in society. It is possible to improve their ability of looking after themselves under the long and repeated training , and some patients can engage in the safe , simple and repetitive physical labor under the supervision.

(4) Profound mental retardation

1% –2% of the cases are classified as profound level , whose IQ are below 20. Their intelligence levels are very low and most of them have no verbal ability. They are unable to recognize their relatives and suffer from incontinence. These patients usually show obvious biological causes , including severe chromosomal aberrations , inherited metabolic diseases and severe deformities of the central nervous system. Because of a low living capacity, most of them have to depend on others. They can only obtain limited ability to self-care after special training. Most of the patients died of weak survival ability and severe diseases.

16.1.2.4   Comorbidities

Mental disorder in patients with mental retardation is higher than in the general population, with more than 50% as reported. Almost all psychiatric diagnoses are likely to occur in common with mental retardation, such as schizophrenia, mood disorders, epilepsy, and attention deficit/hyperactivity disorder.

(1) Schizophrenia

Mental retardation comorbidity with schizophrenia begins in an average age of 23. The symptoms are similar to the symptoms of schizophrenia without comorbiding mental retardation, which contain withdrawn, rigid, impulsive behavior, inappropriate emotion, apathy, poverty of thought, hallucinations, delusions, logical thinking obstacles. The causes of comorbidity may be genetic factors, suggesting that a defect in some parts of gene may have multiple clinical manifestations.

(2) Mood disorders

The prevalence of mental retardation comorbidity with bipolar disorder is higher than the general population, which is 2% – 12%. But their symptoms are usually atypical. During their manic onset, the patients lack humor, higher speed of thinking, nevertheless, they will show excessive activities, irritability, impulsive and emotional behaviors. Mental retardation comorbidity with depressive disorder is more common, which is characterized by decreased activity, speechless, crying, agitation, insomnia, and weight loss. Due to language barrier in patients with mental retardation, it is more likely to be neglected of their depressive symptoms.

(3) Attention deficit hyperactivity disorder

Hyperactivity is a prominent feature in patients with mental retardation, with a total prevalence of over 20%. The main symptoms are hyperactivity, impulsive behaviors, restless, destructive behaviors, and management difficulty. The central nervous stimulant is effective for children with mild mental retardation, but it is not effective to severe cases.

(4) Autism

It is common in children with mental retardation that comorbided with autism. It has been reported that about 75% of patients with autism have intellectual disabilities, and its clinical symptoms are associated with different levels of intelligence. Patients with mental retardation and autism are characterized by severe social communication disorders and difficulties to acquire language and academic skills. Despite the low level of the intelligence in patients with mental retardation, their communications with others are better, and their emotional reactions to people and surroundings are higher, thus they are easier to accept training, and show better prognosis than patients comorbided with autism.

(5) Epilepsy

Epilepsy is another common disease in patients with mental retardation. Studies have shown that about 20% – 25% of patients with mental retardation show epilepsy symptoms in hospitalization, and at least 15% of epilepsy patients show mental retardation. It is generally believed that the lower the level of intelligence, the greater the degree of epilepsy, the more difficult it is to control seizures, and the more prominent the behaviors and personality disorders will be.

(6) Attack and rigid behaviors

The symptoms of behavioral disorders are common in patients with mental retardation, such as aggressive behaviors, destructive behaviors, stereotyping, and social withdrawal. These patients show shouting, attacking others or self-harming, and some of the patients will move body repeatedly, banging their heads against the wall and sucking fingers.

16.1.2.5　Diagnosis

(1) Diagnostic criteria

1) Significantly lower Intelligence than the average. IQ is two standard deviations below the mean of the population in the individual intelligence test, generally, below 70.

2) Inadequate social adaptability. There are obvious deficiency in the ability to live and perform social duties.

3) The disease started before the age of eighteen.

According to the ICD-10, mental retardation(F70-F79) refers to a disease of retarded or insufficient mental development, and skill impairments in the developmental stage are known as the main characteristics. It is these skills that constitutes the overall level of intelligence, such as cognitive, language, motor and social ability. Developmental delay may occur with or without any other mental or physical conditions.

F70 Mild mental retardations: IQ level 50-69(mental age are 9-12 years old for adults). Although it may be difficult for these patients to learn in school, many adults with mild intellectual disabilities can work and maintain good social relations, even contribute to society.

F71 Moderate mental retardation: IQ level 35-49(mental age are 6-9 years old for adults). It can cause significant developmental delays in childhood, but most patients can develop skills to look after themselves independently after learning, and also the social skills and learning skills. Adult patients need help when living and working in the community.

F72 Severe mental retardation: IQ level 35-49(mental age are 6-9 years old for adults). It can cause significant developmental delays in childhood, but most patients can develop a degree of skills to look after themselves independently after learning, and the social skills and learning skills. Adult patients need help when living and working in the community.

F73 Profound intellectual disabilities: IQ level below 20 (mental age are below 3 years old for adults). These patients are severely limited in their ability to selfcare, self-control, communication and motor ability.

F78 Other mental retardation.

F79 Unspecified mental retardation.

(2) Diagnosing mental retardation

1) Medical history collection

Collecting comprehensive information about prenatal, perinatal and postnatal history, the history of developmental milestones, rising and diseases, as well as the family history, cultural and economic situation, to discover whether there are any adverse factors affecting children's physical and mental development.

2) Physical examination and laboratory examination

Including growth indicators, such as height, weight, head circumference, skin palm fingerprints; endocrine, metabolic examination; EEG; brain X-ray, CT, MRI examination; chromosome analysis. Which are necessary to analyze the etiology of mental retardation.

3) Mental development evaluation

● Intelligence test

It is one of the main evidence for the diagnosis of mental retardation. At present, Gesell Developmental Scale; Wechsler Preschool and Primary Scale of Intelligence(WPPSI); Wechsler Intelligence Scale for Children-Revised(WISC-R); Binet Intelligence Scale, etc. Other scales can be used if necessary, such as the Denver Developmental Screening Test(DDST), Peabody Picture Vocabulary Test, 50 Questions Intelligence

Test, Draw Person test and Raven's Reasoning Test.

Intelligent quotient(IQ) is an indicator of the level of intellectual development. There are two ways of calculating IQ, the ratio IQ and the deviation IQ. Ratio IQ was proposed by L. M. Terman of Stanford University in 1916, when the Stanford–Binet Intelligence scale was revised. Ratio IQ is mental age(MA) divided by the chronological age(CA). Formula: $IQ = MA/CA \times 100$.

Among them, the mental age is the age that is reflected in the intelligence test, and the biological age refers to the actual age. For example, a 7–year–old child who passed the mental test of a 9–year–old group (mental age of 9) had an IQ of 120. The deviation IQ can be calculated by comparing the individual scores in the IQ test with the average scores of normal people of the same age, which was proposed by American psychologist Dr. Wechsler. The IQ scores of each age group are in normal distribution, and the mean and standard deviation of the IQ scores are normal. Deviation $IQ = 100 + 15 \times$ (scores − mean)/standard deviation. The mean value is the average scores of the same age group, and the standard deviation is the average standard deviation of the same age group. For example, there is a 8–year–old child whose Wechsler IQ score is 80. The average score of 8–year–old group is 76, and the standard deviation is 4. Accordingly, the IQ of the child is $100 + 15 \times (80 - 76)/4 = 115$.

In 1983, researchers surveyed a sampling of 2,000 in urban and rural areas in China to revise Wechsler Adult Intelligence Scale. The data showed as follows: $IQ \geqslant 130$ (very superior); IQ 120−129 (excellent); IQ 110−119 (superior); IQ 90−109 (normal); IQ 80−89 (middle and lower); IQ 70−79 (borderline deficiency); IQ <70 (mental retardation).

- Social adaptive behavior assessment

The assessment of social adaptive behaviors is another important basis of diagnosis of mental retardation. The Social Adaptability Scale can be used for 4−12 years old children. If this scale is not suitable, the independent living capacity and extent of social functions of patients can be assessed according to the performance of their peers with the same age and cultural background. The Adaptive Behavior Scale and the Vineland Adaptive Behavior Scale can also be applied.

- Clinical assessment of development

When it is not available to practice the IQ test, clinical assessments of development can be used to gain relatively accurate measures.

16.1.2.6   Differential diagnosis

(1) Temporary developmental delay

Many psychological or physical factors, such as malnutrition, chronic somatic diseases, poor or lack of learning conditions, visual and hearing impairments, may affect children's mental development, leading to mental retardation. If these reasons are removed or corrected, mental development speed can be accelerated in a short term, catching up with the intellectual level of children of the same age, so as to identify with mental retardation.

(2) Characteristic developmental disorder

Specific developmental disorders of language skills, learning skills and motor skills may affect children's intelligence level in the daily life. They often show the learning problem, interpersonal difficulties and deficient social adaptation. According to comprehensive assessments of children development, these children only suffer from a specific developmental disorder instead of general developmental disorders. They show normal levels in other aspects of psychological development, and can complete the study task when the specific impaired skills were not involved. For example, children with a language development disorder can learn in a written way to achieve a comparable level of intellectual achievement. In contrast, for patients with mental retardation, the intelligence and academic performance keep in a stable level.

(3) Schizophrenia

The symptoms of children with schizophrenia affect their normal learning, daily life, interpersonal communication, and other social functions. Patients with schizophrenia have a relatively normal intelligence before disease onset. Schizophrenia also shows a clear process of onset and development, and specific psychotic symptoms, which contribute to the identification with mental retardation

(4) Attention deficit hyperactivity disorder(ADHD)

Due to the lack of concentration and the effects of hyperactivity on learning and social adaptation, the academic performance of ADHD children with normal IQ can be improved through education and drug treatment.

(5) Autism

Most children with autism comorbid with mental retardation. The autism patients present a severe loneliness, lack of emotional reaction to others, interpersonal communication difficulties, rigid behaviors, self-entertaining and special way of attachment. But the patients with mental retardation show better socialization, higher willing to communicate with people, and less language deficits. Importantly, they can perform a role play. It is difficult to identify severe mental retardation from autism.

16.1.2.7 Disease course and prognosis

Patients caused by factors related to birth or perinatal period show the retardation of physical and psychological development after birth, whereas children with a lesser degree of intellectual impairment often be diagnosed after primary school. And for the patients who caused by the post-natal adverse factors for mental development, the pre-disease intelligence level is normal.

Since the pathogenic factors generally cause structural or functional irreversible damage to the brain, it is usually impossible to reduce mental damage or restore normal intelligence. The final level of intelligence and social adaptability of patients was determined by the severity of mental retardation and the acceptance of special education and skill training.

16.1.2.8 Prevention and treatment

(1) Prevention

The prevention is important as mental retardation is difficult to reverse once it occurs.

1) Primary prevention

• Improving the premarital examination, and prenatal care

Regular antenatal examination, prevention of dystocia and urgent production is necessary. In remote poor areas, to prevent injury and infection of the central nervous system in infants is especially crucial. In endemic goiter area, the pregnant women are suggested to add iodine in diets, the newborns are suggested to complete the detection of T_3, T_4, TSH level in cord blood, to prevent the occurrence of endemic(hypothyroidism) cretinism.

• Preventing hereditary diseases

The genetic counseling should be considered when the patients' parents have genetic diseases, children have hereditary diseases or she is elderly mothers. The early detection of neonatal for some congenital metabolic defect disease is important for timely and proper treatment.

2) Secondary prevention

• Regular examination for infants and young children is necessary to recognize the suspicious children, and begin regular visit and early intervention. The examination includes fine motor skills, adaptive behaviors, personal-social behavior and language skills.

• Improve timely education training for children with mental retardation mainly caused by sociocultural or psychosocial factors.

● Applying positive prevention and treatment of all kinds of emotional and behavioral problems in mental retardation patients. To popularize knowledge of mental retardation disease to parents and teachers, making them familiar with the psychological and neurological symptoms of mental retardation children in different period of time and general disposal methods.

3) Tertiary prevention

Reduce disability and improve compensation ability. It mainly includes the counseling and training for daily life and adaptive behaviors to help overcome the difficulties in their behaviors and personality. For the mental retardation patients with physical dysfunction or other deformity, the symptomatic treatments are suggested to restore the best function level and prepare for the future social life and employment.

(2) Treatment

Comprehensive treatments from medicine, education, society and vocational training can be adopted to develop the children's social life ability. And to improve the cooperation of parents, teachers and psychological workers is the premise of the comprehensive treatment.

1) Education training

Education training is carried out by teachers, parents, clinical psychotherapists and occupational therapists. The task of teachers and parents is to enable patients to gain knowledge, daily life skills and social adaptation skills that commensurate with their intellectual level. The psychotherapists use the corresponding psychotherapy for the abnormal emotion and behavior of the patient. And the behavioral therapy is commonly used to correct the abnormal behaviors. When getting education training, patients should be taught properly according to their own intelligence level.

Patients with mild mental retardation generally are capable for primary school (lower grade) education. It is better for them to accept education in ordinary primary school. But if the patient can not adapt to ordinary primary school, they can also go to special education schools. To date, most cities in China have special schools or classes in ordinary primary schools. Teachers and parents should adopt vivid and intuitive methods in the education process, and the same content need to be reinforced repeatedly. The training of daily life ability and social adaptation includes recognizing coins, shopping, making phone calls, going to the hospital, taking public transportation, basic labor skills, avoiding danger and dealing with emergencies, etc. The vocational training can begin during their juvenile period to help them live independently after being an adult.

For the patients with moderate mental retardation, the training should be focused on the self-care ability and social adaption, such as bathing and changing clothes, being polite in communication with others, expressing their requirements and desires properly. Also, the training of language ability is needed.

For the patients with severe mental retardation, the training should be focused on the coordination between the caretaker and patients, as well as simple living ability and self-defence capability. For example, patients should know how to eat, use the toilet, simple language communication to express hunger, avoid injury, etc. It may be helpful to break down each skill into several steps and then gradually reinforce the training repeatedly.

Patients with severe mental retardation are almost unable to gain benefits in education training.

2) Medication

There is a growing trend of applying medication for patients with mental retardation. Drugs are used to control behavior problems such as excessive activity, attention－deficit disorder or other abnormal behaviors. The treatment should be evaluated comprehensively according to the risk of the patient's behavior, the adverse reaction of long-term medication, the neurological examination and previous treatment history of patients.

- Etiology treatment

Suitable for the patients with certain etiological factors. For example, to give diet therapy for galactosemia and phenylketonuria, thyroid hormone replacement therapy for congenital hypothyroidism, the surgery for congenital hydrocephalus and dysrhaphia. Gene therapy has been carried out abroad for some single-gene disorders. However, it is not feasible for wide use for clinic.

- Symptomatic treatment

30% -60% of patients with mental retardation comorbid with psychiatric symptoms, resulting in difficulty of receiving education training. For these cases, the corresponding medication can be used for different psychiatric symptoms.

For patients accompanied by psychomotor excitement, aggressive behavior, self-injury or self-harm, antipsychotic drugs such as haloperidol, risperidone, and aripiprazole can be chosen. The therapeutic dose depending on the patient's age and the severity of psychiatric symptoms.

- Therapy for promoting brain functional development

Including nootropic and drugs improving brain metabolism, such as glutamate, gamma - aminobutyric acid, piracetamide(piracetam), and cerebrolysin. Cerebrolysin has a positive effect on the development of language and motor function, and thus should be used as soon as possible after brain injury or mental retardation.

3) Behavior instruction

For children with mental retardation, individual guidance, independent learning and team training can be applied. Trainers should divide the task into several steps, make proper plans, and help the patients to reach the goal. Behavioral treatment could help the patients to develop normal behavioral pattern, and reduce their attack and self-harming.

4) Parental guidance

Parents should arrange reasonable diets for children, make children cooperate with the treatments, and accept special education, and provide the children a happy family environment and education environment. The method could improve the related knowledge for the parents, which contributes to reduce their anxiety and increase the effect on training.

16.1.3 Autism

Autism is a group of neuro-developmental disorders with the main clinical characteristics that include impairments in two areas of functioning(social communication and social interaction), as well as restricted, repetitive patterns of behavior, interests or activities.

Childhood autism was first discovered by Leo Kanner, a child psychiatrist at Johns Hopkins University in the United States. At the hospital, he observed a five-year-old boy, Donald, showing some strange symptoms. The child seemed living in a world of his own, with an amazing vocabulary but unable to maintain a normal conversation with others. His father said he had a good memory when he was two and a half years old, reciting the verse 23 of the Bible and the names of every American president and vice president, reciting the letters by heart. He rarely talked to people, and often described himself as "you" and "me". Infatuated with rotating sticks, saucepans, and other round objects, he remembered the location of the objects around him clearly, and was irritable even when he changed positions and the habit of life. By 1943, Kanner had met 11 cases similar to Donald, which he first reported the same year. The common characteristics is that: ①extremely isolated and can not develop interpersonal relations with others; ②the development of speech is retarded and the ability of communication with speech is lost; repeat simple game activities and desire to remain the same; lack of imagination of objects and dexterous use of their ability, such as the lack of imaginative games, especially like the rigid placement of objects activities. Kanner named these children "early-onset infant autism." This description is still a main symptom in the diagnosis of autism. Similar cases were subsequently reported in the United States and Europe.

16.1.3.1 Epidemiology

Autism was once considered a relatively rare condition. Recent epidemiological data have radically altered this perception. Based on large surveys in the US, the Centers for Disease Control and Prevention (CDC), estimates the prevalence of ASD as 1 in 68 children, occurring in all racial, ethnic and socio-economic groups, although it is five times more common among boys(1 in 42) that girls(1 in 189). The CDC website also offers data from numerous studies in Asia, Europe and North America showing an average prevalence of ASD of about 1%. A recent survey in South Korea, which screened children in schools, reported a prevalence of 2.6%(3.7% among boys and 1.5% among girls)(Kim et al., 2011). Another study in England estimated the prevalence of ASD at almost 1% in adults(Brugha et al., 2011).

However, epidemiological studies are difficult to compare. They vary in the composition of the population surveyed, recruitment mechanisms, sample size, design, awareness, participation rates, diagnostic criteria, instruments used as well as impairment criteria(Fombonne, 2009). Nevertheless, using the same methodology over ten years, the CDC's Autism and Developmental Disabilities Monitoring Network has found increasing rates of ASD in the US.

16.1.3.2 Etiology

The etiology of Autism is complex, and it is still not clear. The genetic and environmental interactions are related to the following factors.

(1)Genetic factors

Some studies have shown that genetic factors play a crucial role in the pathogenesis of autism, according to estimates of the heritability of autism as high as 90%. The genetic factor(90%) is more important than the environmental factor(10%) in the pathogenesis of the disease. Twin studies have provided strong evidence that the rate of homozygotic twins and heterozygotic twins in autism is 92% and 10%, respectively. The prevalence rate of autistic children was 2%-8%, and there was a phenomenon of family aggregation. The genetic model of this disease is complex, and it is a kind of polygenic genetic disease, which is caused by multiple alleles and environmental factors. So far, it has been found that autism is associated with more than 130 genes and distributed on more than 10 chromosomes. A large number of studies have identified several of candidate genes that may be associated with autism, including *RELN*, *OXTR*, *FOXP* 2, *MET*, *and CNTNAP* 2. In addition, a pair of autistic sibling *NRXN* 1 gene coding exons are found to have heterozygous deletions, and two SNP loci are associated with autistic patients. These genes are involved in synaptic formation and cell adhesion, suggesting that synaptic abnormalities may be one of the important mechanisms of autism. Genome-wide association studies found that $5p15$ *SEMA5A* gene was significantly associated with autism.

Some genetic diseases, such as phenylketonuria and fragile X syndrome, are often accompanied with autism symptoms. Some people think that heredity mainly causes cognitive dysfunction, which is manifested as learning difficulties and serious autism.

(2)Infection and immunization factors

Congenital rubella virus infection and cytomegalovirus infection may be associated with autism, and it is now assumed that these pathogens produce antibodies from the placenta into the fetus. The cross immune reaction with the developing nervous system of the fetus interferes with the normal development of the nervous system, which leads to the occurrence of autism. Therehas also been abnormal immune function in autism, some studies have found that children with autism serum immunoglobulin IgA levels are lower than normal, B cell activation is also reduced. The activation of cytotoxic immunoglobulin – like receptors and HLA receptors increased significantly.

(3) Neurobiochemical aspects

Autism is associated with a variety of neuroendocrine and neurotransmitter disorders. The present study found that about one third of autistic children's blood 5–HT increased. It has also been found that the pineal hypothalamic–pituitary–adrenaline axis is abnormal, which leads to 5–HT, increase of endogenous opioid peptides and decrease of corticotropin secretion. The repetitive behavior was positively correlated with the sensitivity of 5–HT1D receptor, and the increase of 5–HIAA, a 5–HT metabolite, was associated with the severity of the symptoms. The increase of the level of DA metabolite HVA in cerebrospinal fluid is related to the stereotype of the disease.

(4) Neurological aspects

Perinatal brain injury, abnormal electroencephalogram(EEG), soft sign of nervous system and epileptic seizures were found in most of the children with the disease. The underlying biological factors are unknown and may be associated with germ cell mutations, especially in the father's sperm. A number of autistic studies have found that autistic patients have many mutations, four times more likely to occur in their fathers than in their mothers. The study found a dose relationship between some risk factors and the occurrence of autism, such as premature delivery, mother age ≥ 35 years, multiple births. Serious perinatal problems include two main aspects: birth weight and gestation, and anoxia at birth. However, the mechanism of the impact of specific parental age and obstetrical problems on the risk of autism in children is not clear.

(5) Anatomy and Imaging of brain

In recent years, a large number of magnetic resonance studies have been carried out, but due to the heterogeneity of autism in children, the abnormal brain structure and function can not completely explain the symptoms.

Structural magnetic resonance studies have showed that the head circumference and brain volume of autistic children is increased. Follow–up studies found that 70% children had excessive brain growth after birth, but the changes did not last into adolescence and adulthood. Some studies have found that the enlargement of the whole brain is accompanied by the decrease of the cerebellar vermis, the amygdala and the hippocampus. The increase in brain volume was also associated with increased white matter volume in the prefrontal lobe, followed by a decrease in white matter volume during adolescence and adulthood. Diffusion tensor imaging(DTI) revealed extensive abnormalities in white matter fibers. It was found that the anisotropy of frontal lobe and corpus callosum was increased in children aged 2–3 years, but the fraction Anisotropy (FA) value of frontal and occipital junction decreased in children aged 5 years. The FA values of frontal and occipital regions and superior hemispheric arcuate bundles decreased in children aged 10–18 years, while in adolescents, the prefrontal and temporo–parietal areas decreased. Functional magnetic resonance imaging(fMRI) study found that the fronto–parietal, the frontotemporal and the occipito–temporal functional junctions decreased, and found that the prefrontal cortex were damaged. The reduction of local cooperation leads to the disinhibition of neural activity and the enhancement of local cortical connections, while some of the neural regions involved in memory are super developed. In addition, there are the dysfunction of controlling social cognitive function such as the cerebral island, the amygdaloid nucleus, the medial prefrontal cortex, and inferior temporal gyrus.

（6）Theoretical disorders of mind

"Theory of mind" refers to an individual's ability to understand his or her own and others' mental state （including belief, desire, emotion, perception and intention）, to benefit from predictive behavior, and based on the ability to cooperate appropriately. The theory of mind suggests that autistic children lack the ability to understand the mental state of their own and others, leading to obvious social barriers that prevent them from playing hypothetical or role-playing games. Difficult to observe, understand the emotions of others, and the speech to express emotions and feelings.

16.1.3.3　Clinical features

Cases report:

*General information: Li * * , male, birthday: 2009-6-15, 3 years and 2 months old.*

Mother complained: can not speak, do not play with other children.

At present, he can only say Mom and Dad, and a single word, such as eating, walking, he can not distinguish between you and me, sometimes repeat what others have said. When he want something, he will take the adult's hand and go to what he wants. He doesn't play game, he doesn't answer other people's questions, sometimes he answers the wrong questions. He has little eye contact, no contact with his family, no concern when his parents left, and no crying. He was called by his name as if he had not heard it, and there was no reaction. He didn't realize the joys and sorrows of others, and most of the time he liked to play by himself, and it didn't matter whether he had someone to accompany him or not. He doesn't play with other children, he doesn't take the initiative to join the game. He likes round things such as pushing buttons, pushing switches, playing around on his own, and staring at things that go around, such as fans, car wheels, etc. He likes to put toys in rows, and doesn't allow others to move. He asked for a regular route, a picky diet, and a few vegetables of limited variety. He likes to clap his hands. When he is angry, he hits himself on the head or hits others and bites. He is particularly sensitive to the sound of the toilet, the sound of firecrackers, and the logo of his clothes, which must be cut off. He was active, restless, had nothing to do with his family, and liked to watch the weather report. He had not seen a doctor before and had not received any medical treatment. His diet is normal, his defecation and urine are normal, and his sleep is normal.

Autism is mainly manifested in three major symptoms: repetitive, restricted, stereotyped patterns of behavior, activities and interests, language development disorder, impairments in social interaction and social communication. At the same time, there are also corresponding characteristics in intelligence, perception and emotion. Generally, from the age of 1 year and a half, parents gradually found that the children are different from the other children.

（1）Typical symptoms

1）Language development disorder: the level of language development of the patients is significantly lower than that of the children of the same age, which is the main reason for most of the patients to seek medical treatment. Patients usually speak late; speech progress is also slow after speaking. Patients with late onset may have a relatively normal stage of speech development, but after the onset of the disease speech gradually decreased or even completely disappeared. Until the age of two or three, patients still can not say meaningful words and simple sentences, do not use speech to communicate, often with actions or gestures to express their wishes and demands. For children with language, its language form and content are often abnormal. Patients sometimes imitate language or stereotype repeated language, such as "parrot tongue" "advertising language" and echo language. Some patients can not distinguish you, me, he, she and other pronouns. In addition, it is accompanied by the abnormal tone, speed and rhythm of language. Patients may communicate with others in special, fixed forms of speech. Intonation is usually bland and lack of cadence. Lack the active language, can't express one's wish or narrate a thing in the language which has already mastered, can not propose the topic voluntarily, or can only rely on the rigid speech to carry on the communication, repeatedly tells the same thing. Most of the patients showed language backwardness or language retrogression after normal language development.

2) Impairments in social communication: patients can not establish normal interpersonal communication skills with others. Babies show no eye contact with others, poor expression, lack of expectations for parents and others to embrace and caress, when being caressed will not show a happy expression. Apathy, "defiant", no intention to communicate, no appropriate body language, such as nodding head. They can not distinguish the relationship with others, can not establish a normal attachment with their parents, and can not establish a normal partnership with their peers. Treating strangers and acquaintances in the same way. Lack of interest in interacting and playing with children of the same age does not draw attention to what they mean through their eyes and voices, does not share happiness with others, and does not seek comfort. They will not comfort or care about others' physical discomfort or unhappiness, can not play imaginative and role-playing games, and it is difficult to learn and follow the general social rules. They don't fit together in group activities.

3) Repetitive, restricted, stereotyped patterns of behavior, activities and interests: patients are not interested in the activities, games, toys of normal children, but rather like to play some non-toy items. Such as wheels, bottle caps or electric fans. Enjoy watching TV commercials, weather reports, certain music or sounds. Patients are often obstinately demanding that routine activities be maintained, that habits be fixed, and that changes in the environment be feared or rejected. Like to listen to a sound or music repeatedly, always look at, touch the same thing, regular sleep time, go to school in the same way. If these fixed activities are changed or stopped, the patient will show a very unpleasant and anxious mood, and even act of resistance. The patient may have repeated routine actions, such as rolling over and over, shaking the whole body, turning in circles, playing with switches, running back and forth, arranging toys and building blocks.

(2) Intelligence deficit

50% – 75% of autistic patients are accompanied by different degrees of Intelligence deficit. The patients' intelligence development is unbalanced in different aspects, and the operational intelligence quotient is higher than verbal intelligence quotient, and the mechanical memory and spatial vision ability related problems show better performance. On the other hand, the achievement of the subject which depends on the ability to grasp the meaning is relatively poor. For example, some autistic patients have a fairly good memory for calendars and train timetables. The gap between their best and worst abilities is very large, but the best abilities of most patients are still lower than the corresponding level of children of the same age. According to the intelligence development level of autistic patients, it can be divided into high intelligence type with normal intelligence level or near normal intelligence level and low intelligence type with obvious intelligence damage.

(3) Perception impairment

Most autistic children have sensory abnormality. For example, some patients are slow to feel pain, and some are slow to respond to very strong sound stimuli, but sensitive to certain sounds, and often can't wait to plug their ears when they hear them.

Some patients with visual abnormalities, as shown by the fear of certain visual images, or like to use a special way to look at certain items; like squint, inverted vision. Many patients like to watch luminous objects or rotating objects, and often lick certain objects with their tongues. Patients generally move freely, running back and forth tirelessly, which is often the main concern of parents and doctors, and is often misdiagnosed as ADHD. Tantrums, attacks, self-injuries and destructive behaviors are common in autistic children and may be associated with incorrect parenting patterns.

(4) Other psychiatric and neurological symptoms

Patients often amuse themselves, their emotional response and the surrounding environment do not coordinate. Some patients are emotionally unstable and irritable. There is also the possibility of self-injury, and attacks. Most patients had attention deficit and hyperactivity syndrome, and about 20% of the patients had tic symptoms. Patients can have symptoms of terror, even panic attacks and hallucinations.

The patients with better language ability, higher intelligence quotient and older age often have compulsive symptoms, self-injury, impulsive and aggressive behavior. Some patients also often have eating problems or sleep disorders such as partial food, food rejection and dissimilar food.

About one third of the patients with EEG abnormalities, 12% to 20% of patients with seizures, mainly the type of major seizures, low intelligent patients with a higher incidence.

16.1.3.4   Diagnosis

If the patient has symptoms before 3 years old, such as qualitative impairments in social interaction and socialcommunication, speech retardation, Repetitive, restricted, stereotyped patterns of behavior, activities and interests and other clinical manifestations. Autism can be differential with schizophrenia, mental retardation and other general developmental disorders in children.

A small number of patients with atypical clinical manifestations, such as only some of the core symptoms of autism, or autism after three years of age, can be diagnosed as atypical autism. However, this type of patient should be followed up until a definitive diagnosis is made.

Some clinical evaluation scales can be used to assist in diagnosis, to understand the severity of symptoms, and to evaluate the therapeutic effect. Commonly used rating scales include Autism Behavior Checklist and Clancy Autism Behavior Scale.

(1) Autism rating scales

1) Autism behavior scale(ABS) is a parent rating scale with a total score of more than 53 for suspected autism and 67 for diagnosed.

2) Clancy Autism Behavior Scale(CABS), which is assessed by doctors, can be diagnosed as autistic if the score is more than 30.

3) The Children Autism rating scale(CARS) is a parent rating scale with a total score of more than 14 for suspected autism.

4) Autism Diagnostic Interviews(ADI-R). At present, the diagnostic scale is widely used in foreign countries, and some hospitals in our country have also carried out the examination. ADI is a semi-fixed diagnostic interview tool compiled by Rutter M in 1980s. It is widely used in clinical practice after revision. It is a powerful indicator for diagnosis of autism in foreign countries. Interview by trained psychiatrist, the principal guardian of the child was asked to describe the specific behavioral details of the child for each item. The Chinese version is revised by Dr. Yanqing Guo and Dr. Xiaoling Yang. ADI-R is a diagnostic interview tool with good diagnostic validity and high reliability. But the interview time is long, often takes about 2 hours.

5) Autism Diagnostic Observation Scale(ADOS). It is a diagnostic tool used with ADI-R. There are some specific operational situations, professional observers need to operate according to the specific situation of certain props, while observing and recording and evaluating the response of children. ADI-R collects all the information necessary for autism from a medical history perspective, while ADOS gives professionals the most direct basis from a psychiatric examination.

(2) Assessment of intellectual development

The Stanford Binet Intelligence scale (SBIS) and the Wechsler Intelligence scale for Children (WISC) can be used to evaluate children's intelligence and cognitive function.

Denver developmental screening test (DDST). For early detection of mental development problems in children aged 2 months to 6 years. It is possible to evaluate the social, fine motor, large motor and speech development of children aged 2 months to 6 years old, and to assist in diagnosis.

Peabody Picture Vocabulary Test (PPVT). It has been widely used to study the intelligence of children with normal mental retardation emotional disorders or physiological disorders. It also plays a role in the auxiliary diagnosis of children with autism.

(3) Auxiliary examination

According to the clinical manifestations, there are corresponding auxiliary examinations, including EEG, imaging, genetics, metabolic screening and so on to determine the diagnosis and exclusion of other diseases.

(4) Autism diagnostic criteria

Autism diagnostic criteria according to ICD-10:2),3),4) with a total of at least 6 items.

1) Developmental abnormalities or damage occur before three years of age, at least in one of the following areas: ①understanding or expressing language in social communication situations; ②selective social attachment or interactive interaction; ③functional or symbolic games.

2) At least two aspects of the following performance of mutual social interaction anomalies: ①do not properly use body language such as gaze, facial expression, body posture and gestures to adjust social interaction; ②failing to develop peer relationships related to things, activities, emotions, which are shared with peers; ③lack of social interaction, and improper reaction to others' emotion, or do not depend on social situation to adjust behavior, or fail to integrate social, emotional and communication behavior properly; ④lack of sharing emotion.

3) Qualitative barriers to communication (at least 1 out of 4): ①language development is sluggish or does not have spoken language, and there is no attempt to use non-spoken language to assist communication; ②not to initiate or maintain a continuous exchange of information; ③the use of language in a fixed, repeated or specific manner; ④lack of all kinds of spontaneous masquerade games or social imitation games.

4) Restrictive, repetitive, fixed and rigid behaviours, interests and activities (at least 1 out of 4): ①to persevere in the interest of repeated strictures; ②obsessive attachment to nonfunctional conventions or rituals; ③rigid or repetitive movements; ④attachment to parts or non-functional components of articles.

16.1.3.5 Differential diagnosis

(1) Mental retardation

The main clinical manifestations of autism are social communication disorder and language development disorder. Most of the patients are accompanied by mental retardation. The intelligence deficit of autism lies in the unbalanced development of different aspects of intelligence, the scores of each component of intelligence test are different, and mental retardation is a comprehensive intelligence deficit. The scores of the intelligence tests were generally low.

(2) Schizophrenia

Autistic patients can be associated with some psychiatric symptoms, easily confused with schizophrenia. Autism is a disease from infancy, with social communication, language backwardness as the main clinical manifestations, drug treatment is ineffective. The onset of schizophrenia is mostly in school age, mainly manifested in hallucinations, thinking rupture and delusion, and other core symptoms of schizophrenia, with normal language and intellectual development. Antipsychotic drugs can effectively improve clinical symptoms.

(3) Asperger syndrome

The etiology is not clear, belongs to one of the extensive developmental disorders, there are also social communication disorders, limited, repetitive, stereotyped interest and activity. According to the diagnostic criteria of DSM-Ⅳ, patients with Asperger syndrome (AS) generally have no language delay. They have normal or close to normal oral expression ability, can use body language and other means to communicate. There was no significant delay in cognitive development, age-appropriate self-care life skills and adaptive behavior. Their deficiencies in social interaction and stereotypical patterns of interest and behavior are similar to autism. But it is difficult to distinguish from high-functioning autism. Some experts think the two diseases are basically the same. However, there are still some patients with Asperger syndrome, whose characteristics are obvious and can be distinguished from autism and high function autism.

The prevalence rate of Asperger syndrome is 15/100,000-5/10,000, males are more than females, the ratio of male to female is (3-4) : 1. The disease starts late, progresses slowly and lasts life long. Patients do not have eye contact, facial expression, and body posture. There are no cognitive development, self-care ability and adaptive behavior defects.

(4) Heller syndrome

Also known as childhood disintegrating disorder, it is one of the generalized developmental disorders from 2 to 3 years of age, characterized by rapid retrogression of various abilities, including speech function, interpersonal skills, motor skills and self-help. The clinical manifestations include social communication disorder, poor ability of language expression and understanding, limited, repetitive, stereotyped interest and activity style, general loss of interest in the surrounding things and so on. But Heller syndrome has 3-4 years of normal development stage before onset, after the onset, a variety of functions appear obvious and rapid retrogression, based on which, it can be distinguished from autism.

(5) Rett syndrome

Rett syndrome is an X-linked neuro-developmental condition that affects girls almost exclusively. It is a kind of generalized developmental disorder with similar clinical manifestations to autism. The main point of distinguishing from autism is that the nervous system symptoms and signs of Rett syndrome are more prominent, such as ataxia, dystonia, scoliosis or kyphosis, and development delay. Half of the patients developed severe motor impairment after reaching adolescence due to spinal cord atrophy.

Generally, the development of maternal pregnancy and perinatal period is normal, the head circumference of birth is normal, and the psychomotor development is normal at 5 months after birth. The patient developed the disease from 5 to 30 months. The acquired language and hand motor skills were gradually lost. The hands were placed in front of the chest as "rubbing hands" "washing clothes", and the face presented "social smile". Gradually decline in intelligence, language understanding and expression of decline or loss of ability, walking instability. Often accompanied by seizures.

16.1.3.6   Course and prognosis

Chronic onset, in which some patients before the age of 3 years have psychological retardation, have never reached the developmental level of normal children of the same age. A few patients had normal psychological development before onset, and the phenomenon of developmental regression appeared after onset. The symptoms of some patients improved gradually with the increase of age, but it is difficult to reduce the symptoms such as poor language expression, lack of communication with others, self-injury behavior and rigid movements.

The prognosis of autism depends on the severity of the condition, the intelligence level of the child, the availability of communicative language before the age of 5, the timing and extent of educational and therapeutic interventions. The higher the intelligence level of children, the younger the age of intervention, the higher the intensity of training and the lighter the degree, the better the therapeutic effect. So we advocate training as soon as possible, seize the best opportunity to improve the ability of children as much as possible. The majority of untreated autistic children have a poor prognosis, with more than half developing a lifelong intellectual disability. At home and abroad, many children have basically returned to normal through education and training, and more and more autistic children are getting better and entering ordinary schools. However, there may still be certain barriers to varying degrees throughout life.

16.1.3.7　Treatments

Since the etiology of autism in children is not yet clear, there is no specific treatment. Autism is an incurable disease. To improve the core symptoms, promote the development of intelligence, cultivate the ability of self-care and independent living, and reduce the degree of disability, we should adopt comprehensive intervention measures such as education intervention, behavior correction, drug therapy and so on.

(1) Educational training

The aim of education is to teach them useful social skills, such as the ability to take care of themselves in daily life, the ways and techniques of dealing with people and the use of public facilities, and basic survival skills. Educational training is an individualized training, which needs to make a detailed treatment plan according to the specific symptoms and degree of each patient. The younger the child starts training, the better, and easier to fix the acquired skills. In the process of education, we must pay attention to the role of parents and persevere.

(2) Behavioral and psychological correction

To promote the socialization and language development of autistic children, the emphasis of language training is to promote the children's spontaneous language, expand the scope of communication and ability.

1) Applied behavior analysis therapy (ABA therapy): according to the principle of behaviorism, ABA therapy adopts the techniques of positive reinforcement, negative reinforcement, differentiated reinforcement and punishment to correct all kinds of abnormal behaviors of autistic children and promote the development of the ability of children in different aspects. In the training, each child's training project (task) is divided into the simplest elements, and then presented to the child, let them complete gradually. The main steps include the trainer's command, the child's response, and the trainer's response and pause.

①Evaluate the behavior and ability of the children and analyze the target behavior. ②Decomposing the task and strengthening the training step by step, and only carrying out the training of a certain decomposing task within a certain period of time. ③ Promote the children to complete the decomposing task by reward. Reinforcement is mainly food, toys and verbal, body posture praise, reinforcement with the progress of children gradually receding. ④Using the technique of hint and concealment. According to the ability of children, give them different degrees of tips or help, and with the children to learn the content of proficiency gradually reduce tips and help. ⑤Break between two training sessions. Through the above steps to train children's attention skills, imitation skills, receptive language skills, expressive language skills and social skills.

2) Language training: one of the main disorders of autistic children is language communication disorder. Autistic children without speech ability are trained to use simple gestures, pictures and words. For

autistic children with difficult pronunciation training to do tongue exercise, oral massage, and so on, to promote the development of language skills.

(3) Medication

Medication can not change the course of autism, and lack of specificity. But drugs can eliminate the psychotic symptoms, emotional instability, attention deficit and hyperactivity, impulse and compulsion, which is conducive to protect the safety of the patient or others, smooth implementation of education and training and psychotherapy.

The commonly used drugs are as follows.

1) Antipsychotic drugs such as risperidone, are approved by the Food and Drug Administration of the United States in 2006 for the treatment of persons aged 5-16 with autism. Drugs can reduce patients' irritability, self-injury and aggressive behavior. The initial dose was 0.25-0.50 mg, twice per day. Then adjust the dose according to the condition. The effective dosage is between 0.5-2.5 mg.

2) All antidepressants were not approved to treat autism spectrum disorder. For anxiety, depression, obsessive-compulsive symptoms of patients over 12 years old, as appropriate to the symptomatic treatment, can choose antidepressants such as fluoxetine, and sertraline.

3) Drugs for attention deficit hyperactivity disorder(ADHD): including methylphenidate and tomoxetine, suitable for patients over 6 years of age with ADHD. Patients with autism have poor tolerance to drugs, should use lower doses, and closely observe the side effects of drugs.

16.2   Behavioral and emotional disorders

16.2.1   Introduction

Behavioral and emotional disorders in children and adolescents begin with childhood and adolescence, the symptoms may gradually alleviated or disappear with age, but if they do not receive treatment and intervention in time, these symptoms may persist into adults. It can affect the social adaptability of adult, and it is frequently related to severe co-morbidities such as substance abuse, personality disorders, crime and other issues.

The main behavioral and emotional disorders in childhood and adolescence are including: attention deficit and hyperactivity disorder, conduct disorder, tic disorders, emotional disorder especially in childhood, social dysfunction in children, non-organic enuresis and faeces, feeding disorders and transvestites, stereotypical dyskinesia and stuttering.

16.2.2   Attention deficit hyperactivity disorder

Attention deficit hyperactivity disorder is a common neurodevelopmental disorder in childhood. The main performance is that attention is easily dispersed, difficulty in concentration, excessive activity regardless of the situation, emotional impulse and accompanied by cognitive impairment and learning difficulties. Their attention level is often lower than that of children of the same age, and their intelligence level is the same or close to that of their peers. It is a chronic disease and has a significant functional impact on children, such as learning difficulties, poor performance, poor motor coordination, low self-esteem and poor relationships with family and peers. Without timely treatment, some children will have symptoms for life. ADHD also had a high risk of other mental disorders, 30%-50% of the patients with destructive behavioral disorders, 15% – 75% with mood disorders, 8% – 30% with anxiety disorders, 6% – 92% with learning difficulties and 7% with tic disorders.

16.2.2.1 Conceptual evolution

As early as 1845, Hoffmann described the excessive activity of children as a pathological condition. In 1937, Bradley pointed out that this is a special form of behavior disorder in children, and the use of amphetamine treatment has achieved some results. In 1947, Strauss et al took brain injury as an important cause and named it "brain injury syndrome". In 1949, Clements said the brain damage was mild, also known as "mild brain damage syndrome". In 1966, Gessel claimed ADHD was not mild brain damage, but "mild brain dysfunction. " The World Health Organization named it "hyperactivity syndrome" in the 9th edition of the International Classification of Diseases and "hyperactivity disorder" in the tenth edition. The third edition of the American Psychiatric Association's Diagnosis and Statistical Manual of Mental Disorders has difficulty concentrating attention based on the most common and prominent symptoms of ADHD. Renamed as "attention deficit disorder with hyperactivity or attention deficit disorder without hyperactivity", the 4th edition is called attention deficit/hyperactivity disorder, divided into inattention, hyperactive/impulse and combined type. The fifth edition coincides with the forth edition. Whether it is hyperactivity disorder or attention deficit disorder, the terms are not related to the cause of disease, but a description of symptom.

16.2.2.2 Epidemiology

The prevalence rate is generally 3% –5% , and the ratio of male to female is (4–9) ∶ 1. Cross–cultural studies have found that ADHD occurs in almost all countries and cultural backgrounds. There are differences in prevalence among different countries and socio–economic and cultural classes, with less than 1% reported prevalence in the UK, 5% –20% in the Netherlands and 5% –10% in the United States in the 1970s and 1980s. The prevalence rate of ADHD in school age children reported in Japan is 1. 3% and 13. 4%. The prevalence rate of ADHD in 7 large studies was 4. 3% or 5. 8%. In addition, the study found that many ADHD children were families with separated or divorced parents, low financial status of their fathers and inconsistent parenting methods.

The symptoms of attention deficit/hyperactivity disorder appeared basically in preschool, but were most prominent at the age of nine. ADHD is often associated with learning difficulties and behavioral problems. In general, more than 65% children have one or more co–infections. The comorbidity often leads to severe damage to social function, reduced clinical efficacy and poor prognosis. In order to make the academic level of children with attention deficit and hyperactivity disorder reach their intellectual level, about 20% patients need special education and 15% of them need special behavior correction services.

16.2.2.3 Etiology and pathogenesis

The etiology and pathogenesis are still unclear. It is considered to be a syndrome caused by a variety of biological, psychological and social factors.

(1) Biological factors

1) Genetic factors

● Control study found that most parents of ADHD patients had hyperactive history in childhood, the prevalence of siblings in ADHD children was 3 times higher than that in control group, and affective psychosis was also more common. In addition, fathers of ADHD children are more likely to develop antisocial personality traits or alcohol dependence, and mothers are more likely to suffer from hysteria. If ADHD children are associated with behavioral disorders, their adult relatives have higher rates of personality disorders, alcohol addiction, and hysteria.

- Study of foster children, Cantwell(1975) and Morrison and Stewart(1973) found that the birth parents of ADHD children were more likely to be diagnosed with ADHD. The biological parents of ADHD children had more antisocial personality, alcohol dependence and hysteria than those of adoptive parents or control children. Biological parents are more likely to have a history of childhood hyperactivity and behavioral disorders and mental disorders. Van den Oord et al. (1994) also proved that genetic factors play an important role in the study of their consanguineous and unrelated relatives.

- The prevalence of hyperactivity disorder in monozygotic twins is 5 times higher than dizygotic twins, and the consistency of hyperactivity and attention disorder in monozygotic twins is much higher than dizygotic twins. O'Connor (1980) and Martin (1984) reported that the consistency of hyperactivity disorder in monozygotic twins was 100, while that in dizygotic twins was much lower. In recent years, Gemini studies have also reported that the main variable for attention disorder, hyperactivity and impulsive symptoms is associated with genetic factors(an average of about 80%) (Faraone 1996, Gjone 1996). Some scholars also reported that the identical rate of ADHD in monozygotic twin children was about 80%, while that of dizygotic twins was only 29%.

- Study on heritability: Stevenson analyzed 91 pairs of female twins and 105 pairs of identical twins by multivariate regression. The heritability of hyperactivity and attention deficit was 0.75 and 0.76 respectively. Explain again the effect of heredity on the disease. Levy F studied 1,938 twin families. According to DSM-IV standard, the consistency rate of proband, the heritability of monozygotic twins and siblings were calculated, and the result was 0.75-0.91.

- Several research groups in molecular genetics have used several large families to study the molecular genetics of children with ADHD and their family members. Biederman et al carried out quantitative genetic analysis of large families in Boston, suggesting that a single gene might explain the disease. Other scholars believe it is polygenic. The earliest molecular genetic studies on ADHD suggest that ADHD is associated with dopamine receptor gene polymorphism. The initial focus was on the D_2 receptor gene, which some researchers believe is also associated with alcohol dependence, tic and so on. Other scholars have referred to such problems as reward deficiency syndrome. Lahoste(1996) reported that the proportion of D_4 receptor 7 repeat alleles in ADHD children was higher than that in control group. Bailey et al. 1997, Swanson(1998) repeated this result. Sunohahara et al. (1997) and Faraone (1999) obtained similar results in adult ADHD. Comings D. E et al. (1996) reported that ADHD was a polygenic inheritance, which was related to $D\beta H$, DTI gene and D_2 receptor gene. There may also be some inconsistent results, which may be related to the different phenotypes of selected ADHD. Barkley RA(1998) et al predict that molecular genetic research on ADHD in children may be a fruitful field at the same time or after the completion of the human genome.

2) Metabolic factors

Studies on catecholamine metabolism, animal experiments and human studies suggest that children with ADHD are mainly abnormal in catecholamine pathway. The determination of adrenaline and dopamine concentrations in urine, serum and cerebrospinal fluid supports the hypothesis that the replacement rates of dopamine and adrenaline decrease. Animal experiments showed that after injecting newborn rats with 6-hydroxydopa and selectively destroying the dopamine pathway, these rats had obvious hyperactivity and difficulty in walking. When given psychotropic substances, they improve the ability to complete learning tasks, reduce the level of activity, with the aging of rats, activity can be reduced, but learning defects still exist. A similar phenomenon can be observed in children with ADHD.

3）Neurobiochemical factor

Neurobiochemical studies showed that there was no significant difference in dopa β－hydroxylase, monoamine oxidase and catecholamine oxygen－methyltransferase between children with ADHD and healthy children. The results of the metabolites of norepinephrine and dopamine are inconsistent. There is a consistent view on the decrease of 3－methoxy－4－hydroxybenzene glycol（MHPGs）in children with ADHD.

4）Neuroanatomical factor

Some neuroanatomists examined hyperactivity children and their siblings, found that the blood flow in the basal ganglia and the midbrain increased in hyperactive children after application of Ritalin, but the blood flow in anterior cortex decreased especially in the motor area of the cerebral cortex. Brain imaging techniques have also demonstrated cortical atrophy in young people with a history of ADHD, although previous CT studies have not found any difference between hyperactive children and normal children. But new imaging techniques, such as PET, have consistently found changes in brain function, especially in the prefrontal region. These findings are important because the functions of the frontal and cortical motor areas are important for maintaining attention, controlling impulses, and regulating aggression and motor activity.

Seidman（1999）reviewed the MRI findings of 13 studies（202 boys and 14 girls）and found that the common abnormalities were in the corpus callosum and the caudate nucleus. The main abnormalities of corpus callosum were anterior（parietal sheath）, posterior（parietal）or decreased volume of both. The volume of the caudate nucleus was reduced to unilateral or bilateral, and only one study reported an increase in volume. The volume of the globus pallidus and the right anterior were also reduced. One study found that the whole volume was reduced by（4.7%）and especially on the right side by（5.2%）. These findings are consistent with early theoretical models.

（2）Environmental factors

The role of family and social factors in the development of ADHD is not clear. Studies have shown that maternal smoking, drinking or other medications during pregnancy are harmful to the development of the embryonic brain. Nicotine may damage developing nerve cells. Many fetuses with alcohol syndrome have the same hyperactivity, attention deficit and impulsive performance as children with ADHD after birth. Drugs affect the normal development of brain receptors, which in part help transmit input signals from the skin, eyes and ears and assist in controlling responses to the environment. Toxins in the environment can also disrupt brain development or signal processing in the brain, causing ADHD.

（3）Pathological mechanism

PET studies have found that the density of dopamine receptor is related to the development of children, and the specific change of dopamine receptor density is not mature until adolescence. The prefrontal cortex is thought to be the dopa pathway in prefrontal lobe in hyperactive children. Neuropsychological studies suggest that prefrontal lobe function is immature in hyperactive children and that prefrontal cortex is related to impulsive and aggressive behavior of children. Local cerebral blood flow study found that the frontal lobe and caudate nucleus were mainly involved. Studies have shown that medication increases blood flow in basal ganglia and midbrain, while decreases blood flow in motor area. Other studies focus on the thalamus, the reticular activation system and the anterior midbrain tract. There were also some differences in neuroendocrine between hyperactive children and normal controls. The study found that growth hormone responses to amphetamine or Ritalin were different in hyperactive children. It is further demonstrated that hyperactivity and normal children have biological differences. The study of skin electrical and evoked potential found that the arousal level of hyperactivity disorder children was insufficient, which was related to antisocial behavior and behavior disorder.

Psychological research also found that children with ADHD had higher social thresholds. Both of positive and negative reinforcement, hyperactive children are not easy to accept, general rewards and punishments are not easy to restrain and correct this kind of children's behavior problems. Studies have shown that taking Ritalin or other neuroactive drugs, hyperactivity children's social threshold were reduced, positive or negative reinforcement levels were adjusted, which laid the foundation for behavior correction. These psychological, physical and pharmacological studies provide a theoretical framework for explaining why children with hyperactivity can not learn from life events. Therefore, this kind of children are difficult to follow social norms, prone to academic difficulties and interpersonal tension and social adaptation obstacles.

(4) Neuropsychological and neurobiological hypotheses

Viginia Douglas(1972) emphasizes attention shift and impulse control, leading to the concept of attention deficit disorder. Jeffrey Matter(1980) suggested that the symptoms of hyperactivity in children were related to the anterior lobe dysfunction. Paul Wender (1971) proposed the hypothesis of reduced catecholamine activity in caudate nucleus and pleasant center. Setterand Cantwell(1974) proposed the hypothesis of cortical arousal insufficiency. All these ideas still influence the research direction of imaging and functional imaging. At present, some studies mainly focus on cognition and brain.

In 1997, Barkley suggested that the main flaw in ADHD was executive functions, including working memory, inhibition, and planning damage. Executive function depends on the reticular structure regulated by the forebrain cortex. Voller(1991) and Heilman(1991) suggest that the right side defect(attention deficit has hemispheric dominance) involves the prefrontal cortex and basal ganglion. Molecular genetic studies have shown that the polymorphism of ADHD and dopamine gene may also be a complex disease involved in the interaction between genes and environment.

16.2.2.4   Clinical features

Case report:

Wang, male, 8 years old. He was very active since childhood. He didn't listen carefully in class, and his parents had difficulty in bringing him up. In July 2016, his parents brought him to the mental health specialist children's clinic for treatment. The history was reported by from his mother. The child showed hyperactivity since young. He was able to walk around 1 year old, liked to climb everywhere, not afraid of danger, often fell. When he got any toys, he took them apart and broke them. He was never afraid of strangers. When he visited his relatives and friends, he opened others' drawers and cabinets and rummaged around. At the age of 6, he went to school and never paid attention to his class and homework. He always made small moves, teased his classmates, played mischief, and often clashed with his classmates. Speaking in class is undisciplined and often interrupted the order of the class. He didn't concentrate during doing homework, will be attracted to other things, need parental supervision. His things were messy, often lost stationery, umbrellas and other supplies, or school to forget what to bring. Parents once wanted to help him develop some hobbies, but no matter what he was learning, he was impatient and could not persevere. Grumpy, what needs to be met immediately, or entangled endlessly. His academic achievement is average, in the past year there is a downward trend, no lying, theft and other bad behavior. Since childhood sleep is less, seems to be overworked. Partial eclipse. Defecation and urine are normal.

The symptoms of ADHD are varied and often have different clinical manifestations depending on age, environment and attitude towards the people around them.

(1) Attention deficit

Attention deficit is the main symptom of the disease, it is difficult for the patient to concentrate during classes, doing homework or other activities. The patient is easily distracted by external stimuli, or often constantly shift from one activity to another. Patients do not pay attention to the details of the activities, often lead to careless errors. In conversation with adults absent-minded, as if not listening. Often avoid or be unwilling to engage in tasks that require sustained focus for a longer period of time, and are not able to complete these or other assigned tasks on time. Patients often lose their toys, stationaries or other personal belongings and forget their daily activities.

(2) Excessive activity

The patient often appears very restless, has many small movements, twists in the seat, leaves the seat without authorization in the classroom or other request quiet occasion, runs around or climbs. Lack of thinking, disregard for the consequences, and acting on a whim before action is often accompanied by a fight or dispute with a partner, which can result in adverse consequences. On any occasion, patients are particularly talkative, or interrupting other people's conversations. He can't wait to answer the teacher's questions, he'll rush to disturb the company's game, and he won't be able to wait in line patiently.

(3) Emotional instability and impulsive willfulness

ADHD children often over-react to unpleasant stimuli because of a lack of restraint, causing them to hurt or destroy things on impulse. Their needs must be satisfied at once, otherwise they will cry and lose temper. Their mood is unstable, they shout or coax for no reason, and they have no patience to do anything. Impulsive willfulness is a prominent and frequent symptom of ADHD. Therefore, some scholars regard it as a main symptom.

(4) Learning difficulties

The intelligence level of most ADHD children is normal, some of them are in critical state, which may be related to the lack of concentration during the test. Some ADHD patients have perceptual difficulties, for example, when copying pictures, they often can not distinguish the relationship between theme and background, can not analyze the combination of graphics, nor can they integrate each part of the figure into a whole. Some ADHD children read "6" as "9", or "b" as "d", even unable to distinguish between left and right. The change of the former belongs to comprehensive analysis difficulty, while the change of the latter belongs to the obstacle of spatial location. In addition, they also have dysfunctions in reading, spelling, writing, or language expression. Children with ADHD answer questions without careful thinking and are not fully aware of it. At the same time, attention deficit and hyperactivity will affect the efficiency of class attendance, the speed and quality of homework, resulting in poor academic performance, lower than their intellectual level.

(5) Neuro-developmental abnormalities

The patients had poor development of fine movement, coordinated movement and spatial position perception. Such as turning over, pointing to the movement, laces and buttons are not flexible, left and right also difficult to distinguish. A few patients have some problems, such as delayed language development, poor language expression, low intelligence and so on.

(6) Conduct disorders

30% -58% of ADHD patients suffered from conduct disorders. Conduct disorders are characterized by aggressive behavior, such as verbal abuse, assault, wounding, vandalism, mistreatment of others and animals, sexual assault, robbery, or acts that do not conform to ethical and social norms. Such as lying, truancy, vagrancy, arson, theft, cheating and molestation.

Generally speaking, the fluctuation of clinical symptoms of ADHD is sometimes related to different situations and activities of children. It is most difficult for them to maintain their attention when doing homework, doing activities that require a lot of repetition or great effort, and doing things that are not novel.

Symptoms of inattention and hyperactivity in attractive, new or unfamiliar environments can be alleviated. The maintenance of attention is significantly better in a continuous and direct reinforcement process than in a delayed reinforcement procedure. When the guidance is necessary to repeat, ADHD children complete the task, their attention maintenance is not a problem. There is little difference between ADHD children and healthy children in the absence of particularly strict norms and strict disciplinary requirements. The fluctuation of the symptoms with the situation shows that the severity of symptoms in children with ADHD is affected by the environment and has a high interaction with them.

(7) Clinical features in adulthood

DSM-5 clearly points out that children and adults share a set of diagnostic criteria for ADHD. Compared with ADHD in children, the clinical features of adult ADHD are as follows.

1) Over-activity

Restless can not adhere to quiet activities such as reading, often in a state of activity, inactive feel irritable.

2) Attention deficit

The patients' attention is easily distracted, by other stimuli, and it is difficult for them to concentrate even if they deliberately try to exclude external stimuli. They often lose their minds or forget their previous plans.

3) Disorganization

Lack of planning and organization often unable to complete work. There is no organization and no clear direction in various activities, problem solving, and scheduling.

4) Emotional instability

Perceived by others as a tendency to change emotions like teenagers, such as from emotional normality to depression or happiness or even excitement. They describe themselves as often overwhelmed, upset, and dissatisfied. Patients may also show an emotional outbreak, suddenly lose their temper, they also feel afraid of this, easily irritated or often in a state of irritation. When there are or no external stimuli, these mood changes suddenly without corresponding physiological changes.

5) Emotional overreaction

The intensity and duration of the response to stimuli is beyond normal, characterized by excessive depression, uncertainty, anxiety and even anger, and often feel a sense of crisis when facing and dealing with problems. Difficult to cope with, easy to argue with others.

6) Impulsiveness

They seek for temporary happiness, regardless of the consequences, and make rash and quick decisions. The lighter interrupts the conversation, drives dangerously, and purchases impulsively; the heavy is similar to mania or antisocial personality disorders such as animal abuse and stealing from the mall. Poor ability to work, and reckless establishment of relationships, such as multiple marriages, separations or divorces.

16.2.2.5 Diagnosis

ADHD is diagnosed by an assessment of child's behavioral and mental development. It often takes into account feedback from parents and teachers with most diagnoses begun after a teacher raises concerns.

ADHD diagnoses 18 symptom entries as follows.

(1) Six (or more) of the following attention-deficit symptoms, which have occurred frequently, have lasted for at least six months to the extent of maladaptation and are not commensurate with their stage of development.

Inattention: ①failure to focus on details, or careless errors in school homework or other activities; ②it is difficult to continue to focus on work or game activities; ③when talking to him(her), it seems that they are not listening; ④it is difficult to comply with instructions or unable to do homework, family work or work (not as a result of opposing sexual behavior or inability to understand the content of instructions); ⑤difficulties in organizing planning and activities; ⑥avoid or be unwilling to do tasks that require constant brainstorming(e. g. , school or homework); ⑦loss of essential items for work or activity(such as toys, workbooks, pencils, books or stationery); ⑧be easily distracted by external stimuli; ⑨forget everything in daily life.

(2)Six(or more) of the following hyperactivity and impulsive symptoms occur frequently and have lasted for at least six months to the extent of maladjustment and are not commensurate with their stage of development.

1)Hyperactivity

①Fidgeting constantly or awkwardly on the seat; ②they will leave their seats at will in the classroom or on other occasions where they must continue to sit; ③run around or climb high and low in inappropriate situations(in adolescents or adults, only subjective feelings can not calm down); ④it is difficult to play quietly or participate in leisure activities; ⑤always moving, as if driven by the motor as unstoppable.

2)Impulsivity

①Many words; ②answer the question before it is finished; ③in games or group activities, it is difficult to wait for rotation; ④interrupt or interfere with others(e. g. , by interrupting or interrupting a person's game).

DSM−5 diagnostic criteria: if the child begins to develop obvious attention deficit and/or hyperactivity, impulsive symptoms before the age of 12, and in more than two occasions, such as school, family and other settings, these clinical manifestations. It can be diagnosed as attention deficit hyperactivity disorder (ADHD) if it lasts for more than 6 months and has adverse effects on social function(such as academic achievement, interpersonal relationship). The DSM diagnosis divided 18 symptomatic criteria into two dimensions and three subtypes. In 9 attention deficit symptoms, if 6 or more, the diagnosis of attention deficit is the main type; in 9 hyperactive impulses, the diagnosis of hyperactivity/impulse was mainly based on 6 or more hyperactive impulses. If both conditions are met, the diagnosis is combined. The number of diagnostic items for adult ADHD was 5.

ICD−10 diagnostic criteria: it is emphasized that attention deficit and hyperactivity/impulse symptoms exist simultaneously. There are six or more attention deficit symptoms, three or more hyperactivity symptoms and one or more impulsive symptoms. It has lasted for at least 6 months and has reached a level of maladaptation that is not commensurate with its stage of development for at least 6 months.

16.2.2.6　Differential diagnosis

(1)Mental retardation

Patients may be accompanied by attention deficit and hyperactivity. But the mental structure of the patients with attention deficit and hyperactivity disorder is unbalanced and some of the intelligence factors are low. Through treatment, attention to improvement, academic performance can be improved to the level of intelligence. But the mental retardation children's intelligence score is generally below 70, the performance is the overall intelligence decline and the social adaptation ability is generally low. Their academic achievement is consistent with their intelligence level, and they also have language and motor retardation, and their judgment ability, understanding ability and social adaptation ability are all on the low side.

（2）Conduct disorders

Children with obvious violations of their age in accordance with the social norms or moral norms, harm the personal or public interest, there is a strong aggressive behavior. 30% –58% of ADHD patients suffered from conduct disorders.

（3）Emotional disorders

Some children with emotional disorders also have symptoms of psychomotor arousal and attention deficit, which are difficult to distinguish from ADHD children. Children with mood disorders overlap with ADHD children because they all have chronic unhappiness, depression and negative reactions from parents, classmates, teachers and playmates. They were also restless about positive reinforcement such as praise and love, and mothers' rewards did not change the reinforcement thresholds of these children. The first and main symptom of the patients with emotional disorders is emotional problems. The course of disease is in the form of attack and the duration is short. Attention deficit and hyperactivity disorder showed long–term persistent attention deficit and excessive activity.

（4）Tic disorders

The main manifestation is involuntary rapid, transient and irregular twitch of the head and face, limbs or trunk muscles, such as eyebrow, shoulder shrug, neck tilting, waving, pedaling and twisting, etc. At the same time may be accompanied by involuntary vocal twitching, prone to be mistaken for hyperactivity or naughty. It is easy to find the characteristics of tic symptoms through careful mental examination, and distinguish them from attention deficit and hyperactivity disorder. However, about 20% patients with tic disorder are associated with attention deficit and hyperactivity disorder.

（5）Schizophrenia

The early stage of schizophrenia, patients may not observe school discipline, too much activity, attention loss in class, decline in academic performance, and so on. However, schizophrenia will gradually appear the characteristic symptoms of schizophrenia, such as hallucinations, delusions, emotional indifference, isolation, strange behavior, and so on, but ADHD will not appear these symptoms.

（6）Autism

Autistic patients are mostly accompanied by hyperactivity, impulse and attention disorder, but autistic patients also show interpersonal communication and communication difficulties, speech disorders, interest and activity limitations and other symptoms.

（7）Chronic social and environmental problems

The broken family environment makes it difficult for children to concentrate on serious study and life. Children living in such environments have many symptoms of ADHD, whether they are caused by poor parental role models or because parental education is inconsistent and recriminating each other. For these children, adverse signs of social and family circumstances may help to distinguish them from the general ADHD. Chaotic families may have one or more children with severe hyperactivity. ADHD symptoms may co-exist with a broken family atmosphere or may be secondary to adult families with alcohol dependence, anti-social personality, and separation and conversion disorders. Once children are placed in a stable, consistent and complete family and social environment, their symptoms disappear completely. In this case, ADHD diagnosis can not be made easily.

16.2.2.7   Course and prognosis

Nearly half of the patients had been ill before the age of 4, but many of them went to the hospital after primary school because of attention deficit resulting in learning difficulties, or because they showed serious behavioral problems. ADHD is not limited to childhood diseases, many symptoms can continue into adolescence, and even adulthood. Some studies have reported that about 20% school age children diagnosed clinically as ADHD gradually disappear after puberty, and up to 70% –80% of them will continue to have this disorder in adults. 65% of them will continue into adulthood. 20% –30% of the patients not only had clinical symptoms, but also had antisocial behavior, substance dependence, alcohol dependence and other problems. The probability of substance use disorder in ADHD patients was 30% –43%, about 2 times of that in the general population(8% –15%). ADHD patients had earlier smoking and alcohol consumption, higher rates of puberty smoking than normal, and a significantly higher risk of drug addiction. The ratio of non–alcoholic substance dependence of ADHD was 12% significantly higher than that of normal control 3%. 32% –53% of adult patients with ADHD had ever had alcohol addiction and abuse, and 8% –32% of them were associated with another drug addiction or abuse at the same time. Follow–up studies also found that ADHD was more likely to develop into alcohol, drug and nicotine dependent patients in early adulthood with a ratio of 2.0(1.3–3.0). The factors that lead to poor prognosis include combined disorder, dyslexia, emotional disorder, poor family and social psychological factors, low intelligence and so on.

16. 2. 2. 8　Treatments

The methods of treatment include counseling and medications. Counseling includes cognitive behavior therapy, family education, physical training, and social skills training. The curative effect of combined therapy is better than that of single treatment.

(1)Counseling

1)Cognitive behavioral therapy

ADHD children have many problems in daily life besides the main symptoms, such as the difficulty of developing and maintaining relationships with other children and the poor basic life skills of ADHD children. Therefore, cognitive behavioral therapy is used to meet the needs of children's emotional and social development. Behavior therapy uses the principle of conditioned reflex, when the correct behavior occurs in training, reward; when incorrect behavior occurs, give punishment, combined with the principle of reward and punishment, such as token, activity reward and temporary isolation. Cognitive behavior therapy is effective in controlling hyperactivity, impulsive control and aggressive behavior. Through language self–control, self–guidance, role rehearsals, self–reward and self–praise, the skill improves social interaction and improves and corrects children's behavioral problems. This kind of training is carried out by the combination of family, outpatient and school, the curative effect can be outstanding and steady. Short–term treatment is better than long–term treatment.

2)Family education

In most families with problematic children, parents always blame children for problematic behavior, and there is a lack of effective or pertinent communication between parents and children. Parents need special help to understand the etiology, symptoms and behavioral habits of ADHD. Parents should take good measures to limit certain behaviors of their children, give priority to understanding and encouragement, and ensure adequate sleep and proper nutrition. School and family should have consistent discipline. Instruct children to do some housework and take some responsibility. In short, parents need to master consistent, positive, effective behavior correction.

3)Physical training

Children with hyperactivity can benefit from progressive body training programs. Because they have difficulty in communicating in the collective activities of the team, it is easy to make the sports activities become their negative experience. The physical training program is individual exercise, which can guide them to control impulses and aggression, make them listen to guidance, enhance self – esteem and self–

confidence. Body training includes weightlifting, fitness, track and field sports, swimming, tennis and other items, so that the appearance and feeling of the body in good condition to improve physical activity. A good teacher—student relationship can promote physical training, promote better self—control, self—discipline and self—esteem of hyperactive children. In recent years, the training method of sensory integration in the treatment of hyperactivity disorder in children is based on the nerve needs of children, leading to the appropriate response to sensory stimulation training, can reduce hyperactivity, impulse and other behaviors.

4) Social skills training

Children with ADHD also have some interpersonal problems. Through behavior training, such as demonstration, role playing, to improve children's social and communication skills, so that children learn more effective ways of expression, improve social skills and develop good habits.

(2) Medication

Many medications have been shown to be effective and safe for childrenwith ADHD. Medications can be divided into stimulants and non—stimulants.

1) Stimulant medications are the pharmaceutical treatment of choice, the representative drug is methylphenidate. The mechanism of methylphenidate is to increase the release of dopamine and norepinephrine from presynaptic node and inhibit its reabsorption. Methylphenidate is available in immediate release and extended release preparations (Methylphenidate OROS ®). Immediate release methylphenidate reaches plasma peak levels in 1–3 hours after ingestion. The effects last approximately 4 hours; thus it is necessary to take medicine 2 or 3 times a day. Methylphenidate significantly reduces hyperactivity and impulsive symptoms, improves attention, the effective rate is 70% or 80% . The immediate release methylphenidate, also known as Ritalin, was used at the initial dose of 5 mg/d, the Maximum daily dose is 60 mg. The commonly used dose was 0. 3 – 0. 6 mg/kg per day, starting with small dose. Methylphenidate OROS ® releases about one quarter of the amount immediately and the rest during the next 9 hours. The effect can last 12 hours. This kind of preparation only require a once—a—day dosage schedule.

Side effects of methylphenidate include loss of appetite and weight loss, nausea, abdominal pain, difficulty in falling asleep, emotional instability, and irritability. The long – term treatment had no significant effect on the growth and development of children under the condition of ensuring adequate nutritional intake and regularly measuring their height and weight. The use of high—dose stimulants may produce symptoms such as euphoria and excitement, and the patient's tolerance to drugs will also increase, with the risk of substance dependence and substance abuse. The occurrence of such problems can be reduced by strict drug management, proper dose, intermittent medication and so on.

Stimulant therapy for attention deficit and hyperactivity disorder may induce or aggravate tic symptoms, but the symptoms can disappear after withdrawal. If twitch symptom is light, or appear only when patient is emotional tense, can continue to use. If twitch symptom is serious need to change to use other medicine. When tic symptoms are very serious or associated with Tourette syndrome, the combination of stimulant and antipsychotic drugs should be used.

At present, there are few studies on the long—term efficacy of central stimulant. The Swanson divided all children into 3 categories. The first group (34%) showed a gradual improvement in symptoms, and by 36 months the effect of drug therapy was becoming more and more evident. The second group (52%) : at the beginning, the symptoms improved significantly, and the curative effect remained stable over time. The third group (14%) : the first treatment was effective, and later came back to the pre—treatment symptom level. The main influencing factors are the advantages of social demography and behavior. The second kind of children is more stable than the first and third groups of children at the beginning of the study, their parents' marriage is more stable, their intelligence quotient is higher, and the score of behavior problems is lower. They had relatively good social functions and were initially more assigned to drug or combination therapy groups.

2) Non-stimulant medications: tomoxetine is a selective norepinephrine reuptake inhibitor, which acts by blocking the presynaptic membrane norepinephrine transporter. Non-stimulants can control attention deficit hyperactivity and impulsive symptoms, improve cognitive function such as response inhibition, and improve attention and executive function. Imaging evidence suggests that topoxetine improves inhibition and control by enhancing the activity of the right inferior frontal gyrus, and blood drug concentrations are related to the activation of the right inferior frontal gyrus. Topoxetine is safe and effective, as effective as methylphenidate. It covers the improvement of night symptoms and can be used in simple or refractory ADHD. It is better for ADHD patients with tic disorder, substance abuse, destructive behavior or emotional disorders. The side effects of tomoxetine are similar to those of stimulants

3) Clonidine and guanfacine are alpha-2 agonists with demonstrated efficacy in the treatment of ADHD. They are the second line therapy for ADHD. These medications can also be used for patients with comorbid tic disorders or Tourette's syndrome, in which its efficacy seems to be higher.

4) Tricyclic antidepressants such as imipramine, have also been shown to reduce ADHD symptoms. Nevertheless tricyclic antidepressants are associated with significant side effects, are less effective than stimulant medications and should be used only after failure to respond to two or three stimulants and atomoxetine. Tricyclic antidepressants can interfere with cardiac conduction and can cause sudden death; itis important that patients are monitored with electrocardiogram beforeand during treatment.

16.2.3　Conduct disorder

Conduct disorder is a mental disorder onset in childhood or adolescencethat presents itself through a repetitive and persistent pattern of behavior in which the basic rights of others or major age-appropriate norms are violated. It's a behavior disorder frequently seen in childhood or adolescence. Some symptoms are non-criminal actions, andothers are criminal. These actions are often called antisocial behaviors at home and abroad, including continual lying, pilferage, hooky, fleeing from home, fighting and premarital licentiousness, or criminal behaviors like rape, arson, robbing and murder. These antisocial behaviors may be shown early during 5-6 years old, but more often in adolescence. Some of these behaviors are obviously antisocially in 12, with most of them happening during 15-16, while it's rarely to find them over 16. The diagnosis can be made based on the anti-social behaviors last at least half a year.

16.2.3.1　Epidemiology

According to the Chinese researches, the prevalence rate is between 1.45% and 7.35%, which is higher among men than that among women with a ratio from 3 : 1 to 12 : 1 and reaches peak in 13 years old. Researches in England showed that the prevalence rate was 4% among children aged 10-11. In the US, the rate is 6%-16% among male under 18 while that among female is 2%-9%, and the rate among people in city is higher than that among people in village.

16.2.3.2　Etiology

The cause of conduct disorder is complicated that biological, psychological, social and developmental factors have different effects on its occurrence, advancement and duration. This is because antisocial behaviors are complex, relating to one's physical conditions and psychosocial qualities of biology, as well as his attitude toward growth environment, in particular his family and the society. It'snecessary to understand the cause and severity in different levels, in which there is biological reasons, social and family atmosphere and physical conditions. The cause of conduct disorder contains many aspects of culture, civilization, education and others. Therefore, it's not because the act of a simple factor but interplays betweenmany negative stimulators that a person has conduct disorder.

(1) Biological factors

In recent years, many researchers found that biological factors had, in part, influences on conduct disorder. Systematic investigations and studies on conduct disorder among children and adolescents and juvenile crime from Institution of Mental Health, Peking University proved that children and adolescents with conduct disorder, when compared with those in control arm, had much more deficits in craniocerebral trauma, perinatal diseases or injuries, and central nervous system infections not only in life histories but during perinatal and infant periods. Many researchers have found that parents whose children have conduct disorder, having mental illness, retarded mental development and dementia in three generations than those from control group. According to the studies, conduct disorder is related to No. 2 and No. 19 chromosomes. Polymorphic expression of some genes related with conduct disorder are related to inattention, hyperactivity and offensive. It is reported that the interaction between DR2 and DR4 genes is related to conduct disorder. In addition, researches of adults, teens and children who have antisocial and offensive behaviors shows that their monoamine neurotransmitters may have disorders. For instance, there is disorder of 5-HT level on teens with conduct disorder. Many perspective studies show that pregnancy smoking will enhance the risk of giving birth to a baby who behaves as conduct disorder during childhood and adolescence.

(2) Social environment and family

Many scholars have been emphasizing that most teenagers with conduct disorder come from families at a low stage of economy. Family is the most important factor about conduct disorder because family is a key environment where children and teenagers are affected. As longitudinal studies show, some 30% teenagers get conduct disorder out of some nonsocial factors like family and school. Bad family environment has high correlation with conduct disorder, especially adolescent crimes. One cause is physical abuse in childhood, which affects cognition, emotion and modulation of neuro hormones. Lacking of love and warm relationship with parents is related with adolescent crimes. Therefore, some preventions and therapies need cooperation of family and school, as well as community. Family factors contain:

1) Unharmonious family

There are severe conflicts or quarrels for long. Family members live in negative atmosphere for long. Major members separate temporally or permanently, even divorce.

2) Poor relationship between parents and children

In 1969, Bolwly presented great importance of relationship between parents and children during childhood, which has huge influence on health mental development and form of normal social relations. Mccord did a study for 30 years on children from broken families aging between 5-15. He found that 61.8% of those boys doing crime at adolescence were lack of love from mother, while only 21.6% of them doing crime who had love from mom. This result told that it's not because of broken family itself but whether there is a tight relation between mom and child that leads to the problem.

3) Little or useless management from parents

Parents don't limit their children to their behaviors and ignore them. According to a research about the reason to adolescent crimes in China in 1987, teenagers absolutely left by family, school and society had very high rate (more than 95%) of crime. Those teens, who loss educations from family and school, and have no occupations, are more likely to commit a crime.

4) Improper management from parents

It's a key point to form conduct disorder and adolescent crimes that parents are too strict with their children, brutal to or give corporal punishment. Scholars also find that there is a significant if parents play "good cop, bad cop", or they have different opinions.

5) Bad social interactions

Many teens aren't eager to commit a crime at first. However, they make bad friends during social interactions. Affected by those bad friends, they start to act illegally. Therefore, bad social interaction is a mediator of conduct disorder. This fact tells us not only the naivety of adolescent crime, but that bad interaction is an important reason for it. In addition, through bad social interactions, teenagers affect themselves and form criminal groups.

16.2.3.3　Clinical features

Case report:

Wang, a 12-year-old boy, lies, steals, fights and runs away from home for several days. In the second grade of primary school, he lived with his father ever since his parents divorced, he had little contact with his mother and other relatives. In addition to daily work, his father often plays cards with his workmates, and seldom cares about him. He began to cheat for snacks under the pretext of paying school fees, and then stole money or valuable products from his classmates. He didn't want to study, did not finish his homework, often skipped classes, fought with his classmates, and occasionally abused animals. Dismissive of the advice of the teacher's neighbors. He shrugged off the advice of his teacher and neighbors.

(1) Antisocial behavior

Antisocial behavior refers to the behavior that violate moralities or social standards, including telling lies, stealing, extorting or robbing others, rape or having obscene actions, bullying, setting fire, escaping from school or home, staying overnight outside against parents, joining in gangs and committing crimes.

(2) Aggression

Offending to others and their possessions, such as fighting, teasing others by hitting and torturing, abusing the weak, disabled and animals, destroying others' or public possessions. They vent their harm and contradiction in these offensive ways when in a deep mood. In male, there are many physical offenses while oral offenses in female.

(3) Oppositional defiant disorder

The patients show obvious actions of disobedience, defiance and provocation toward adults, especially their parents. These actions are more likely to be seen on children under 10 years old. Performances are telling lies to avoid punishment, to lose temper easily, grudge against others, trying to revenge on others, ignoring commands, blaming others out of own faults, quarreling with others, defiance to parents and teachers, interfering others, violating school rules and refuse criticism.

(4) Comorbidity

Patients of conduct disorder often have ADHD, depression, anxiety, instable emotion and are easily irritated. They can also have development disorders, such as low ability in expression and understanding, having difficulties in reading, bad coordination and low IQ. Those patients are usually self-centered, like to blame and control others. They attract attentions on purpose and argue for their mistakes. They are selfish and cold-blooded.

Symptoms vary in different ages, sex and development levels. Lies, steals and offenses are happened at early stage, followed by severe illegal behaviors, containing house invasion, rape and robbing. Males are more likely to have conduct disorder since childhood. Symptoms differ in different sex. There are more confrontations in male than in female. Behaviors of conduct disorder in male are offense, steal, damage to public properties and at school, while that in female are lie, escaping from school and home, substance abuse and prostitution.

16.2.3.4   Diagnosis

According to ICD-10(1992), the diagnosis is based as follows.

(1) Excessive levels of fighting or bullying.

(2) Cruelty to other people or animals.

(3) Severe destructiveness to property.

(4) Fire-setting.

(5) Stealing.

(6) Repeated lying.

(7) Truancy from school and running away from home.

(8) Unusually frequent and severe temper tantrums.

(9) Rebellious provocation.

(10) Long-lasting severe disobedience.

If any one of these behaviors, last at least six months and exclude other mental illnesses, is sufficient for the diagnosis.

16.2.3.5   Differential diagnosis

(1) Attention deficit hyperactivity disorder

These patients may out of attention deficit hyperactivity disorder (ADHD), fight with others or act against rules at school, as well as have resistant and offensive words or acts after frustration. However, patients with ADHD have obvious deficits in attention. These deficits can be adjusted by central stimulants or other treatments, which differs from conduct disorder. If a person with ADHD has comorbidity of conduct disorder, diagnosis of them should be made together.

(2) Mental retardation

These patients are easily instigated by others because they lack intelligence and judge and control of their behaviors. Therefore, they are expected to do something against the law, offensive or resistant. But there is firm evidence to prove a person having lower IQ and adaptation to the society.

(3) Schizophrenia

Patients may show illegal, offensive or antagonistic behaviors. However, it's only parts of all clinical performances. Those patients also have core symptoms like hallucinations, delusions and other mental disorders. After antipsychotic medication, those symptoms that include behavior disorders are reduced or disappeared.

(4) Disorder of affection

Children who suffer from anxiety or depression may have offensive or agonistic behaviors. But they are in elevated or depressed mood obviously while abnormal behavior is just one of the clinical performance. Symptoms disappear after medication.

16.2.3.6   Progress and prognosis

Some patients develop problems in behavior gradually after their parents' divorce, transfer to another school and making bad friends with conduct problems. At the beginning, these problems rarely and discontinuously happen in a light degree. If not stopped or intervened in time, behavior problems are gradually strengthened and fixed, forming persistent or repeated behavior disorders. Childhood onset (symptoms start before the age of 10) has more confrontational behavior, longer course of disease and worse prognosis than the adolescent onset. Partnerships can have an important impact on children's behavioral development. Gender is also an important factor leading to the persistence of symptoms. The prevalence of antisocial behavior in women is significantly lower than that in men, and the incidence of early onset and adult crime in men is significantly higher than that in women. Children with speech or executive dysfunction are vulnerable to isolation, resulting in increased destructive behavior or academic weariness, which leads to the duration of the course of behavioral disorders.

Only a few patients have good prognosis, while most of them have poor prognosis. The poor prognoses are: the behavior problem is difficult to eliminate, the relationship between parents and children or the relationship between teachers and students is bad, the study is difficult or dropped out of school, which can't be accepted by the normal children and adolescents, to form gangs with hooligans in society to carry out illegal and criminal activities. Some patients' behavior problems continue into adulthood, resulting in adult employment, marriage, interpersonal relations and other difficulties, about half of them in adulthood with criminal behavior or antisocial personality disorders.

16.2.3.7 Therapy

It's hard to treat conduct disorder without an independent and effective way. It's important to find out and interfere in early stage and to concentrate on biological, psychological and social factors. At present, education and psychological therapy are mostly used, while medication has lower efficacy. Interferences are as follows.

(1) Psychological education to parents. Adjusting behavior disorders in conduct disorder, in particular antisocial behaviors. Training parents' skills of behavior therapy to improve children's positive behaviors. Training of family association and solving problem.

(2) Building communications between home and school to deal with bad behaviors and score at school.

(3) Training of children social skills.

(4) Consultant for parents about marriage and psychological disorders.

1) Family therapy

It's useful only with parents actively participating in. Contents of family therapy are as follows. ①Coordinating the relationship between family members, in particular between parents and children. ②Redressing parents' attitudes toward children's bad behaviors in neglect or hard punishment. ③Training parents to talk with their children in proper ways, educating them by strengthening good acts and slight punishment. ④Reducing family conflicts.

2) Behavior therapy

It's a key point to change social cognition deficits, such as communication skills, ways to solve problems, control of impulse and emotional management, on patients. According to their age and clinical performance, positive strength, extinction or game therapy can be used. The goal is to extinct their bad acts gradually and form a normal pattern of behavior so as to improve adaptation to society. In recent years, a new therapy called "training of problem solving skills", which is based on the theory that children with conduct disorder have deficits on cognition, such as communication skills, ways to solve problems, control of impulse and emotional management have been widely used. There are four steps to conduct the therapy.

Step 1: help children understand what the problem is, by recurring it in mind.

Step 2: make plans to get the result.

Step 3: carry out the plan.

Step 4：evaluate the result.

This method has more efficacy than other psychological therapy in reducing antisocial behaviors and increasing prosocial behaviors.

3）Community therapy

Family therapy isn't fit for those patients with severe disorder of family functions. Therefore，community interference，can be conducted to help those children. In addition，some interference can be made at school，such as training of social and learning skills to improve academic performance，improve their self-esteem and correct the behavior. Repelled by mates is associated with offensive actions and bad performance in learning with behavior problems. Management and treatment can be concerned about improving mate relationships，such as train of life skills，encouraging them to talk with each other，improving their communication abilities.

4）Medication

There's no particular medication but to use different drugs toward symptoms accordingly. Patients showing severe impulsivity and offensive behavior should be treated withchlorpromazine，haloperidol or carbamazepine in low doses. Patients with ADHD can be treated with central stimulants like methylphenidate or phenylisohydantoin. Patients with depression or anxiety can be treated with antidepressant or antianxiety.

16.2.4　Tic disorder

Tic disorder is a group of complex chronic neuropsychiatric disorders that mainly occur in childhood. It has some form of involuntary，rapid，repetitive non-rhythmic movement or（and）sudden vocal tic without purpose. Tic has an insupportable experience，but it can usually be self-contained for a period of time，aggravated by stress，and disappears during sleep. As a result of exercise and/or vocal tic，patients will lack self-esteem and have a negative impact on family life，social image and job performance. And patients are often have compulsive，impulsive and hyperactive behavioral and emotional disorders. The prevalence of tic disorder is 6% -12%. According to the age of onset，course of disease，clinical manifestations and accompanied vocal tic，it can be divided into three clinical types：transient tic disorder，chronic motor or phonation tic disorder and Tourette syndrome.

16.2.4.1　Epidemiology

Most tic disorders occurs in school age. Motor tic often occurs before 7 years old，and the onset of vocal tic is usually after 11 years old. The prevalence rate of school-age children with tic disorder is 12% -16%，transient tic disorder is 4% -6% and chronic tic disorder is 1% -2%. The lifetime prevalence of Tourette syndrome is 0.3% -0.8%. The prevalence of twitch disorder is 2.42‰ in the population aged 8-12 years in China. The prevalence of males is higher than females with the ratio of 2 : 1 to 4 : 1.

16.2.4.2　Etiology and risk factors

The etiology of tic disorder is unclear. The main causes of Tourette syndrome，chronic motor disorder and vocal or phonic tics are biological factors and genetic factors. Transient tic disorder may be the biological and/or psychological factors as the main cause. If biological factors are dominant，it is easy to develop chronic tic disorder or Tourette syndrome. If psychological factors are the main factors，it may be temporary stress or emotional reaction，and the symptoms will disappear naturally in a short period of time.

（1）Genetic factors

Genetic factors have been confirmed to be associated with the etiology of Tourette syndrome，but the genetic pattern is unclear. Family studies have found that 10% -60% of the patients have positive family history. Twin studies have confirmed that the rate of syndromes of monozygotic twins（75% -90%）is significantly higher than that of dizygotic twins(20%). The study found that the incidence of tic disorder in foster relatives was significantly lower than that in blood relatives. Relatives of patients with Tourette syndrome were more prone to chronic tic disorder, obsessive−compulsive disorder, attention deficit and hyperactivity disorder.

(2)Physical factors

The onset of the disease, is caused by local physical disease irritation and produce tic. For example, conjunctivitis or trichiasis stimulation causes the blink; upper respiratory tract infection results in nasal aspiration and facial twitch. However, when the local disease causes are removed, tic symptoms continue to exist.

(3)Psychological factors

The life events can cause tension and anxiety and induce tic symptoms. These stimuli may also lead to exacerbation of tic symptoms.

(4)Neurobiochemical factors

Tourette syndrome is related to the excessive release of dopamine or the hypersensitivity of postsynaptic dopamine D_2 receptor, hyper function of central noradrenergic system, endogenous opioid peptide, and 5−HT. The clinical use of neuroprotective drugs and other drugs acting on the dopamine system can successfully control the twitch of Tourette syndrome. In contrast, dopaminergic agonists such as levodopa, levo−benzenebutylamine, and Ritalin tend to exacerbate tic symptoms. It has been suggested that the etiology of Tourette syndrome may be related to the defect of dopamine system, however. It is not clear what role the different subcortical and subcortical Bardoan receptor subtypes play.

(5)Neuroimmune factors

In recent years, it has been suggested that 20%−35% of Tics is associated with autoimmune damage after infection. There has been a lot of research on the relationship between groupa hemolytic streptococcal infection and group a hemolytic streptococcus infection. Some patients with Tourette syndrome may have aggravated tic symptoms when eating seafood, food pigment and food additives, but the specific mechanism still needs to be further studied.

(6)Other

Some patients had perinatal complications, such as labor injury, asphyxia, premature delivery, low birth weight, and a few had a history of head injury. Inmonozygotic twins, babies with lower body weight are more likely to develop twitch disorders. Maternal adverse events during pregnancy can increase the risk of children suffering from tic disorders such as stress events and adverse environment pregnancy early serious nausea vomiting symptoms. The level of androgen before birth has a significant and lasting effect on the development of nervous system function. Androgen and sex−related factors may contribute to the gene expression of Tourette's syndrome through its effects on the nervous system.

Although the etiology of tic disorder is related to many factors, such as heredity, infection, biochemistry, immunity, and social psychology, the specific etiology and the special manifestation and severity of the specific disease still need to be further explored.

16.2.4.3　Clinical features

Case report:

The boy is a 9−year−old, third−grade student. He involuntarily cleared his throat and shrugged his shoulders for a year and a half. The patient had an uncontrollable voice of clearing his throat for no reason a year and a half ago and relieved spontaneously after 3 months. And 2 months ago, he began to shrug, nod, crooked mouth and shout. He was very distressed and blamed for being out of control in class. There is a sig-

nificant increase in the frequency of occurrence before the examination or participating in the competition, or when parents pay special attention to it, to the point that it happens every 4 minutes. The patient was born prematurely, premature rupture of membranes at delivery, neonatal score of 9, and normal growth and development in childhood. There was no family history of neuropsychiatric diseases and no other positive findings in physical examination.

(1) Basic symptoms

Tic symptoms are mainly characterized by movement tic or vocal tic, including simple or complex tic. These tic behaviors can occur in one or more parts of the body. The simple forms of tic include blink, nose shrug, crooked mouth, shrug, shoulder rotation or slanting shoulder, and complex forms include jumping, running and slapping yourself. Simple forms of vocal tic include clearing the throat, roaring, snorting, and canine barking, while complex forms include repetitive language, imitation language, foul language and so on.

The characteristics of occurrence are involuntary, sudden, rapid, repetitive and non-rhythmic, which can be suppressed in a short period of time, but can not be controlled for a long time. Attacks are more frequent under psychological stimulation, emotional stress, physical illness or other stress conditions, and symptoms are relieved or disappeared during sleep.

(2) Clinical types

1) Transient tic disorder, also known as tic disorder, is the most common type. The main performance is simple movement tic. Often occurs first in the head and face, such as blinking, nose, mouth, side look, shaking his head, oblique neck and shrug. A few are characterized by simple vocal tic, such as clear voice, cough, snorting, barking or "ah" "oh" and other monotonous sounds. Some cases can also be seen in multiple parts of the complex movement tic, such as jumping, running and slapping themselves, and so on. In some cases, tic is fixed to one part of the body, while in others, the twitch part often changes from one to the other. For example, the onset of the disease is only blinking, lasting for a month or two, and then relieves. Other cases may present multiple motor tic symptoms, such as frowning, and upper limb tic. Children tend to ignore their tic symptoms or try to hide them. Some children who have strong and repeated symptoms of blinking, sniffing and clearing their throat often go to the department of ophthalmology, otolaryngology and other departments to see a doctor, and treat them according to myopia, trachoma, conjunctivitis, and pharyngitis. This type of tic disorder is most common in children aged 4-7 years of early school age, and is more common in boys. Tic symptoms occur repeatedly in one day for at least 2 weeks, but generally not more than a year, with no serious consequences. At present, there is no good clinical method to predict whether twitch will reduce, heal or worsen.

2) Chronic motor or vocal tic disorder: most patients showed simple or complex motor tic. A few patients show simple or complex vocal tic, generally there is no movement tic and vocal tic at the same time. In addition to the head, face, neck and shoulder muscles, tic also often occurs in the upper and lower limbs or trunk muscle group. Symptoms usually persist. In some cases, motor tic and phonation tic alternately appeared in the course of the disease. For example, the initial performance is a simple frown and kick, lasting half a year to ease, followed by a clear voice tic. Tic may occur daily or intermittently. The most common tic is movement, especially the face, head and neck, and limbs. The course of chronic tic disorder is continuous, often more than one year. Symptoms of chronic motor or phonation tic disorders are relatively constant, lasting for several years or even for life. Some studies have found that some tic symptoms can be alleviated in late adolescence. Adults may show only chronic motor or vocal tic residual symptoms.

3) Tourette's syndrome: is also known as vocal and multiple motor combined tic disorders. It is a chron-

ic neuropsychiatric disorder which impairs children's physical and mental development and cognitive function to varying degrees. Further impact on social adaptation, or even delayed disability.

Tourette syndrome is the most representative type of tic disorder. It has the most complex and severe clinical manifestations and is the most difficult to diagnose and treat. Initial symptoms usually occur before puberty, 5-8 years old. It is characterized by progressive movement and vocal tic. The first symptom is simple movement tic, most of which are intermittent facial muscle tic, a few of the initial symptoms are simple phonation tic. With the progress of the course of the disease, the number of tic body parts increased, gradually involving the shoulder, neck, limbs or torso, the form of expression also developed from simple twitch to complex twitch. A single movement tic or vocal tic can develop into both, the frequency also gradually increased. The intensity of tic varies so much that a small twitch can only be felt by the patient himself, while a severe twitch can be detected by others and even hurt themselves and their surroundings. In a few cases, violent motor tic(such as self-beating, scratching, etc.) may lead to lip injuries, disfigurement, and blind pestle and eyes. About 30% of patients had coprolalia or obscene behavior, mostly around puberty. Tic occurred every day in most patients with intermittent tic in a few patients, but the symptoms were relieved for less than 2 months in the same year. The duration of the disease is prolonged, which has a great impact on the social function of the patients.

(3) Other symptoms and co-morbidity

Some patients also show by repetition of language and action, imitation of language and imitation of action. Tic disorders are often associated with multiple diseases. The effects of these co-infections are often greater than the symptoms themselves and should therefore be taken into account in assessing the condition and in developing treatment protocols. Among the children with tic disorder, 20% -60% had obsessive-compulsive personality and symptoms accompanied by Tourette syndrome, including obsessive-compulsive attitudes and obsessive-compulsive movements. The symptoms were repeated check and check, ritual action, sniffing and licking, repeated scrubbing, repeated aimless action, etc. About 50% children were associated with attention deficit and hyperactivity disorder. There was no correlation between hyperactivity disorder and tic severity, but children with attention deficit hyperactivity disorder were more likely to develop psychological problems and destructive behaviors. Tic disorders can also be associated with emotional instability or irritability, destructive and aggressive behavior, and sleep disorders. The use of central stimulant may induce tic symptoms or aggravate the original tic symptoms. The incidence of self-injury was 33% - 44% . There are many forms of self-injury, such as head-bumping, finger biting, scratching the skin and so on. In severe cases, it even causes permanent self-harm.

(4) Laboratory examinations

50% -60% of the children had abnormal electroencephalogram(EEG) , most of them were in the middle of frontal lobe. 10% patients with Tourette syndrome show brain structure abnormalities in CT scan, such as brain atrophy, and PET studies showed increased glucose utilization in bilateral basal ganglia, frontal cortex, and temporal lobe.

16.2.4.4 Diagnosis

Childhood began to appear motor tic and vocal tic, excluding other reasons caused by, can be diagnosed as tic disorder. After that, the clinical types of tic disorders were determined by course of disease, clinical manifestation and whether accompanied by vocal tic.

The following is ICD-10 diagnostic criteria.

(1) Transient tic disorder

1) Occurs in childhood and early adolescence, most commonly in children aged 4-5 years.

2）Recurrent, involuntary, repetitive, rapid, aimless, single or multiple motion tic, or vocal tic. Common manifestations are blinking, grimacing, and head tic.

3）Tic symptoms can be controlled in a short period of time(minutes to hours) and disappear after falling asleep.

4）Tic symptoms occur several times a day, almost daily, for at least 2 weeks, but not more than one year.

5）Exclude muscle spasms caused by extrapyramidal nervous system diseases and other causes.

（2）Chronic motor or vocal tic disorder

1）Repetitive, involuntary, rapid, aimless tic, no more than 3 groups of muscles at 1 time.

2）During the course of the disease, there has been movement tic or vocal tic, but the two do not exist at the same time; in weeks or months, the intensity of the tic does not change.

3）Tic symptoms can be controlled in several minutes to several hours; the period of illness lasts at least 1 year.

4）Before the age of 21.

5）Exclude chronic extrapyramidal neuropathy, myoclonus, hemifacial spasm and psychosis.

（3）Vocal and multiple motor combined tic disorders

1）The disease onsets before the age of 21, mostly between the ages of 21 and 15.

2）Recurrent, involuntary, rapid and aimless tic that affects many groups of muscles.

3）Multiple tic and vocal tic occur simultaneously.

4）Tic symptoms can be controlled for several minutes or hours.

5）The intensity of symptoms varies within weeks or months.

6）Tic occurs several times a day, almost daily. The course of disease was more than 1 year, and the remission of symptoms in the same year was not more than 2 months.

7）Elimination of chorea, hepatolenticular degeneration, seizure of myoclonic seizures, drug-induced involuntary movement and other extrapyramidal diseases.

16.2.4.5　Differential diagnosis

（1）Nervous system diseases

Chorea minor, hepatolenticular degeneration, epileptic myoclonus and other neurological diseases have motor disorders. However, these diseases not only have limb or torso motor abnormalities, but also have nervous system symptoms, signs, laboratory tests positive findings, and generally no vocal twitching. The corresponding treatment can effectively improve the symptoms.

（2）Obsessive-compulsive disorder

The patient's compulsive movements are similar to those of tic disorders. But obsessive compulsive symptoms are conscious movements, patients know subjectively that their actions are meaningless, unnecessary, have the desire to overcome. The existence of self-compulsion and anti-compulsion makes patients feel anxious and painful. Some compulsive actions are secondary to compulsive thoughts, while tic disorders lack these characteristics.

（3）Hysteria

Children with hysteria can show twitchy or spasmodic behavior, but hysteria patients have definite strong psychological factors as the etiology, and the changes of symptoms are related to psychological factors. Remove psychological factors, and the corresponding psychotherapy symptoms can be completely alleviated. Tic disorders are aggravated in stressful situations, but tic symptoms also exist without psychological factors.

(4) Acute dystonia

This is a side-effect of antipsychotic drug. Manifested as the sudden increase in the tension of the local muscles, lasting for a period of time after a temporary remission, mostly occur in the neck and face, and also the limbs. Tic disorders are rapid, repetitive, rigid muscle twitches that can be self-controlled and stop for a short time. They can be identified according to their characteristics. However, when patients with tic disorders have side-effects of haloperidol therapy, they need to be carefully examined and differentiated. There is a need to prevent the misconception of acute dystonia caused by drugs as an exacerbation of tic symptoms, which can lead to more serious side effects.

16. 2. 4. 6　Course and prognosis

The prognosis of transient tic disorder is good, and the symptoms gradually alleviat or disappear in a short time. Symptoms of chronic movement or vocal tic persist, but have little effect on life, learning and social adaptation. The prognosis of Tourette's syndrome is poor and it takes a long time to take medicine to control the symptoms. Once treatment is stopped, the symptoms recur. Co-morbidity attention deficit and hyperactivity disorder, behavioral disorder and depression has a great impact on the patients' daily life, academic performance and social adaptability. The majority of Tourette's syndrome patients gradually improved in the late adolescence, a few continued into adulthood, or even lifelong.

16. 2. 4. 7　Treatments

Before treatment, the patients' psychological, social, educational and occupational suitability must be evaluated thoroughly, and the treatment should be selected according to the clinical type and severity. Collection the detailed information and the data of symptom can play an important role for treatment. The Yale tic severity scale is a reliable quantitative instrument for evaluating tic symptoms. Chronic twitch and Tourette syndrome are chronic diseases, so it is very important for patients and families to receive long-term and effective treatment from clinicians.

The treatment of tic disorder should be based on timely comprehensive treatment, including drug therapy, psychotherapy, diet adjustment and environmental therapy. Patients with transient tic disorder or mild symptoms are only treated with psychotherapy. Chronic motor or vocal tic disorder Tourette syndrome, or tic symptoms seriously affected daily life, mainly drug treatment, combined with psychological treatment. If due to psychological factors, we should actively remove psychological factors.

(1) Drug therapy

1) Treatment for tic symptoms

Haloperidol: the curative effect of this medicine is remarkable, the effective rate is 60% -90%. The first dose is 0. 5-1. 0 mg, once or twice a day, and if the effect is not good for 3-7 days, the dosage should be increased. The dose range is 1-10 mg/d. Drugs mainly have sedation and extrapyramidal side effects. If adverse reactions occur, they should be dealt with in a timely manner.

Tiapridea: the effective rate is about 76% -87%. The side-effects of extrapyramidal system are rare. It is suitable for patients over 7 years old. The commonly-used dose was 50-100 mg, 2 times or 3 times per day. The common side-effects include drowsiness, fatigue, dizziness, gastrointestinal discomfort, excitement, and insomnia.

Benzimidazoline: it is also known as clonidine, a central α_2 receptor agonist, and an antihypertensive drug. It can excite the presynaptic α_2 receptor and act on the central dopamine neurons and the norepinephrine system, thus relieving the twitch symptoms. The effecency is 20% or 70%. The oral dose is 0. 05 mg/d, divided into 2 - 3 times. Posterior ear patch 2 mg/sheet, half or 1sheet a time, once every 6 days. This medicine can also treat attention deficit hyperactivity disorder, so it is especially suitable for children with attention deficit hyperactivity disorder. Side effects include lethargy, hypotension, dizziness, dry mouth. People with heart disease may have arrhythmias or aggravated arrhythmias. Blood pressure and electrocardiogram should be monitored regularly during use.

Currently, clonidine transdermal patch is mainly used to replace the traditional oral dosage form. There are three sizes: 1 mg/sheet, 1.5 mg/sheet, 2 mg/sheet. According to the body weight, they were given 1 mg/sheet for 20−40 kg weight, 1.5 mg/sheet for 41−60 kg, and 2 mg/sheet for > 60 kg. The patch can be used once for 7 days to release the drug to the body at a constant speed, so it is convenient to use. And there is no peak and valley of blood drug concentration phenomenon, can give full play to drug efficacy, reduce adverse reactions.

Risperidone: risperidone has been reported to be effective in patients over 15 years of age. The initial dose is 0.25−0.50 g/d, twice a day. If the symptoms are not significantly alleviated after 1−2 weeks, the dose can be increased slowly. 0.25−0.50 mg is added every 3−7 days. The dosage range is 0.5−6.0 mg/d. The main side effects are sedation and extrapyramidal reaction.

Guanfacine: is also known as chlorobenzene, it is a new type of central α_2 receptor agonist, which belongs to the same class as clonidine. The drug has good efficacy and tolerance for hyperactivity, attention deficit and tic symptoms, and is more suitable for the treatment of Tourette syndrome with attention deficit hyperactivity disorder. Because the drug action is concentrated in the brain prefrontal lobe, it has the improvement to the attention, the working memory, and the sedation, the hypotensive effect is less than clonidine. The initial dose of guanofaxine is 0.5 mg, which is added once every 3−4 days. The total amount of guanofaxine is 0.5−3.0 mg, and is given orally 2−3 times a day. The common side-effects are mild sedation, fatigue and headache.

Atypical antipsychotics: new atypical antipsychotics have fewer side-effects and are more acceptable than classic antipsychotics. At present, new antipsychotics can effectively control tic symptoms include risperidone, quinthiapine, olanzapine, aripiprazole, and ziprasidone. The risk of delayed dyskinesia is significantly lower than that of classic antipsychotics, but some drugs still have side effects such as acute dystonia, sedentary inability, and restlessness. In recent years, aripiprazole has been used for the treatment of Tourette's syndrome. Chinese studies showed that aripiprazole is effective in children with Tourette syndrome. The total effective rate is 87% and the cure rate is 47% at the end of 8 weeks. The adverse reactions are relatively mild, showing transient gastrointestinal discomfort, and palpitations, without obvious sedative effect. The initial measurement of aripiprazole is 2.5 mg/d. Within 2 weeks, the dosage is increased according to the state of illness and tolerance. The dose is constant at the end of the 4th week, and the maximum dose is less than 20 mg/d. The method of administration is one time in the morning and evening or only one time in the morning or evening.

2) Treatment of comorbidity

Obsessive-compulsive disorder: clomipramine, sertraline, and fluvoxamine. The general situation is to be used in combination with drugs that treat tic symptoms.

Attention deficit hyperactivity disorder (ADHD): tumoxetine clonidine and guanofaxine is the first choice. If the curative effect is not remarkable, can choose antidepressant drug.

Self-injury behavior: fluoxetine can reduce the behavior of self-injury, but the mechanism is not clear.

(2) Psychotherapy

Psychotherapy is the main method to prevent the recurrence of disease and reduce complications, including family therapy, cognitive therapy and behavioral therapy. The purpose of family therapy and cognitive therapy is to adjust the family system so that patients and families can understand the nature of the disease and the causes of the fluctuation of symptoms. And eliminate the negative factors that may have effect on symptoms in interpersonal environment, reduce the anxiety and depression secondary to tic symptoms, and improve the social function of patients. Cognitive behavior therapy is beneficial to obsessive–compulsive disorder associated with tic disorder. Behavior correction is beneficial to impulses and hyperactivity disorder associated with tic disorder. There are many different behavioral treatments. For example, massed negative practice, habit reversal training, self–monitoring, relaxing exercises, and biofeedback. However, further evaluation and verification of the effectiveness are still needed.

(3)Diet therapy and environmental therapy

In addition to medication and psychotherapy, it is also necessary to properly arrange daily rest time to avoid overstrain and fatigue. Appropriate participation in certain sports and recreational activities to maintain a relaxed and happy mood. Food additives may be associated with excessive activity and learning difficulties in children. Caffeinated drinks can exacerbate tic symptoms. In this end, these children should avoid the use of food additives, pigments, caffeine and salicylic acid.

16.2.5　Emotional disorder in childhood

Children and teenagers' emotional disorders starts in childhood, with the main clinical manifestations of anxiety, fear, obsession, depression and shyness. It affects the normal social function or be accompanied by some physiological reactions. Childhood emotional disorder relates to social psychological factors, children development and life situation, characterized by abnormal emotions, such as anxiety, fear, force, or shy. These emotions in patients are more severe and last longer than normal children, affecting their daily life and study. In China, the prevalence rate of emotional disorder is 17.7%, specially, females are more than males, and urban prevalence is higher than in rural areas.

16.2.5.1　Etiology and risk factors

The occurrence of emotional disorders in children is related to a variety of factors, which are the result of the interaction between biological factors, children's temperament, individual characteristics and environmental factors. Genetic susceptibility, timidity, sensitivity of children, parents'excessive protection or too strict management, inappropriate education, and the body diseases are factors that cause children's emotional problems. When children encounter some psychological stress factors, such as fighting, being blamed, learning overload, fatigue, first time to kindergarten, new term beginning, and transfer, they tend to suffer from emotional disorders.

16.2.5.2　Clinical features

(1)Separation anxiety disorder

Cases report:

A child, male, 3 years old, is lively and lovely, has been raised by the mother herself. The mother started to send him to kindergarten 3 months ago. From the first day in the kindergarten, the child cried, holding his mother's clothes, refusing to eat and take a nap, even refusing to drink water. He cries all day long and looking for mother, the teacher can't stop the crying. In the afternoon, he often stands in front of the gate of the kindergarten and waits for his mother, doesn't play with other children. When he gets back home, he follows his mother, fearing that his mother would leave him. The child often screams "mom" during sleep.

The main reason for the formation of separation anxiety disorder(SAD) is the chronic unadapted anxiety caused by the disengagement of familiar environment or attachment. The excessive anxiety will occur when children are separated from the relatives they are attached to, especially their mothers, also the grandparents, fathers, and other caregivers. Before the age of 6, it appears that children will worrythat they may get hurtor the parents will never return, if they are separated from their attachment objects. Children are anxious when their attachment objects are not around, feeling terrible situations will happen, such as being lost, kidnapped, killed, orhospitalized, even never see a loved once again.

There are 3 stages of separation anxiety disorder: first, children show resistance, crying, rejection, and being extremely painful; then children show the emotional reactions such as helplessness, sadness and disappointment; in the end, they appears to be normal, showing apathy and indifference, but the child may have physical symptoms such as rejection of school or abdominal pain. The consistent symptoms that occur in all children are significant social impairments and unstable clinical manifestations. Every time a separation occurs, there is a headache, nausea, vomiting and other somatic symptoms, or the children will refuse to go to school. The symptoms can also be characterized by overly emotional reactions during or after separation, such as restlessness, crying, anger, pain, indifference or social withdrawal. Theyare not willing to go to bed at night without the company of attachment objects, or have separate nightmares repeatedly that even wake them up many times.

(2)Phobic anxiety disorder

Cases report:

Meng, female, 13 years old, is an Grade 8 student. She started being anxious about the examinations. Each time just before the examination, she would appear dizziness and irritability. Although she had studied hard to prepare for the examination each time, and every exam score was good, she still feel anxiety and fear before the exam, and began to worry there will be various problems during the exam. Therefore, she grasped all the time to review. But her performance is not very prominent. A few days before the exam, she will show a lot of symptoms such as diarrhea, panic, irritability and loss appetite. Recently, the school informed that there will be an exam in the whole district. Meng is very afraid, worry that something will affects the exam.

Phobic anxiety disorder in childhood is a child's excessive fear of the general objective things or situations in daily life. The prevalence rate is 2% –5%. Generally the prevalence rate of females is more than males. The disorder commonly occur in preschool children, who show too much fear of certain things and situations. There are 2 types: first, fear of physical injury, such as death and bleeding; second, fear of natural events, such as fear of darkness or animals. All patients' symptoms can be relived in early adolescence, and the prevalence rate is only 2% at age 11.

When exposed to the specific objects of fear, the patient will show a series of reactions in cognition, emotion, behavior, movement and physiology. Sometimes patients appear catastrophic response, feeling threatened and extreme fear, and show autonomic nerve dysfunction, including higher or lower heart beats, pale face, sweating, and urine incontinence. In this case, their first reaction is to try to escape quickly from what they fear. Children usually are not able to aware that their fear is excessive and unreasonable, and they will be anxious, crying, astonished, or tightly hold others, sometimes even show the facial expressions of fear or the body trembling. Parents think the children are too concerned about the objects or situations they fear.

(3)Social phobia

Cases report:

Wu, female, 14 years old. She considers herself to be a weirdo, being too shy. For more than two years, she have never talked more with people. She dares not look straight into their eyes when talking with others. Every time she talks, she will blush and stare down at the toes. Her heart beats speed up, and her body gets goose bumps, as if the whole body was shaking. She doesn't want to get in touch with her classmates. Be-

cause she thinks others hate her and regard her as a weirdo. She mostly afraid to contact the boys. As long as there is a boy, she will be nervous even in the dormitory. She is also afraid of teachers. In the class, she would feel relaxed only when the teacher turn his back to the students. As long as the teacher faces the class, she dares not to look at the blackboard. Because of tension, she can not understand the learning contents. It's worse that she starts to be unnatural when speaking in front of her friends and neighbors. Because of these problems, she seldom goes to social places, reducing the contacts with people. She have tried to overcome this problem, by reading a lot of psychological books, guiding herself according to social skills, convincing herself, and controlling herself. However, they did not work. She complained that the problem had seriously affected her development, including declining academic performance, failed communication with others, and classmates' alienation.

Children show fear, anxiety, and avoidance of a new environment or stranger. In a new environment, or with a stranger(including peers), some children will be constantly nervous, shy and embarrassed, and pay too much attention for their behaviors. Also, some childrenwould feel pain and discomfort when they enter a new environment. In these situations, they will cry and refuse to talk. The patientsare afraid to speak or performon the stage, and to go to a place where there are crowded people. In these cases, they show social avoidance behaviors, but have a good social relationship with their family or acquaintance. The core symptom of social phobia is the excessive anxiety that occurs in one or more social situations, and all children will have the same symptoms.

1) Avoiding social situations that they are afraid of, and showing intense anxiety and depression when they can't avoid them.

2) Physical anxiety response has no corresponding organic pathological basis.

3) The anxiety response not only occurs in the process of getting along with adults, but also in the process of getting along with their peers.

(4) Selective mutism

Cases report:

A 4-year-old girl was attacked by a neighbor's dog. The child was sent to an emergency department by the owner of the dog.

On the second day of hospitalization, the child was in a depressive state and had mild withdraw from the contact with people. Her psychical and mental conditions have been evaluated. During the consultation of doctors, the child was visibly irritable and refused to engage in any conversation. She used nonverbal communication, including gestures and shaking head, which were not present before the dog attack. On the sixth day of the hospitalization, the child first spoke to her mother and asked, "Where were you when the dog attacked me?"

Fifteen days after the injury, the child was discharged from the hospital. After 2 months, her mental conditions were monitored. During that time, the child refused to talk to the doctor and other children in the neighborhood, but only used gestures to communicate. Nevertheless, she can conduct normal conversation at home. Her memory of being attacked by a dog remains clear. 6 weeks later, when talking about dogs, the child repeatedly showed traumatic memories. During this period, the little girl showed persist avoidance of the event-related ideas and conversations. More strikingly, her parents reported that the child was still avoiding contact with the dog's owner and avoiding the location where the dog attacked. Besides, her feelings of alienation for neighbors remain. She was overly alert when she was alone, showing intense anger and anxiety, and being difficult to concentrate.

In 1994, the American psychological association concluded that the prevalence of selective mutism in children was less than 1%. Kamulainen and Bergman's epidemiological investigation about selective mutismfound that the prevalence is between 0. 2% –20% , and the majority of children's symptoms last for more than a year. Some research has shown that girls with selective mutism were more than boys, in a ratio of 2 ∶ 1. At present, psychological factors are considered to be the main cause of this disorder.

Selective mutism(SM) is a kind of anxiety disorder in early childhood and adolescence. The disorder usually begins in 3–5 years old. The main characteristic is that the children remain silent on certain occasions while keep normal language functions in other situations. The disorder most likely to occur during school, kindergarten or moving, immigration, and during other life changes. Also, insome cases the symptoms develop gradually. The severityof the symptoms need to be assessed from the generalization of mutism, the degree of mutism(whether to use pen, eyes and gesture to communicate), and accompanying emotional behavior problems. The complaint of this disorder is mainly "the child don't talk in specific occasions". Because of the silence and behaviors of avoiding the specific occasion in the children with selective mutism, others would describe these children as aloof or don't listen to teachers' instruction, but generally they will not be complained as these characteristics.

Its manifestations mainly include:

1) Can't speak in situations where verbal communication is required, while in other situations it is normal.

2) Last over a month.

3) No language disorders, no problems caused by speaking a foreign language(or different dialects).

4) The causes are related to admission or change of school, relocation or social interaction that affect the children's life.

5) No developmental or mental disorders such as autism, schizophrenia, mental retardation.

(5) Depression

Cases report:

Wang ,female ,12 years old ,has been brought up by her grandmother. In the Grade 3 of primary school, her brother was born. Thus her mom and dad were busier and less contacted. Meanwhile ,fights in the family increased. One morning ,her grandma and mother quarrelled with each other for trifle things. The next morning ,the grandma committed suicide by ingesting pesticide. Wang didn't cry during the entire funeral and neighbors in the village considered Wang as a cold child. Since then Wang talked less than before. She was often late for school ,didn't pay attention to the class. She used to play with classmates ,but now she was always alone and refused to join her classmates. She was in depressive mood and the teacher's education did not work. When the teacher taught the text of Hans Christian Andersen's "little match girl" ,she said she was like a little match girl whom no one loved ,and wanted to live a happy life in heaven with her grandmother.

The core symptoms of depression in children and adolescence are similar to adults, but they also have their own characteristics due to developmental factors. The prevalence of depression among children and adolescence is increased with age. The prevalence of depression is about 0. 3% in the pre–school age ,2% in childhood and 1. 5% –9% in adolescence, while the cumulative incidence of depression is up to 20% at the end of adolescence. In clinic, the causes of depressive symptoms in some adolescents are unknown.

Childhood depression lasts for an average of 7 months, and 40% of the initial onset of depression can be remitted without treatment. The patients who did not recovery are likely to have chronic depressive disorder, while the patients in remission still have higher recurrence rates and risk of mood disorders. Previous evidence suggests that if a parent has depressive disorder, especially onset before the age of 30, the risk of recurrent depression in a child is significantly increased. Compared with mood disorders in adults, childhood mood disorders are more likely to be chronic and develop into bipolar disorder.

There are three typical clinical symptom clusters in childhood depression.

1) Emotional disorders: characterized by low mood, no happy feeling, remorse, sad, no interest in playing, low self-esteem, crying, irritability, self-harm and suicidal thoughts/behaviors. Some children have symptoms that are not typical, and their parents may ignore them. Somatic injuries caused by self-injury and suicide tend to be misdiagnosed as accidents in other hospital departments. Children who are depressed may often cry, response slowly to external stimuli, move slowly, and suffer from loss of appetite and poor sleep. School-age children can use words to describe their mood, such as "bad mood" and "I can't do anything when I grow up".

2) Behavioral disorder: in the state of depression, children can show externalized behavioral problems, such as hyperactivity, inattention, and lower grades; being undisciplined, impulsive, rebellious, disruptive and other disciplinary actions such as playing truant, fighting, and having bad relationships with peers. Or the child may appear to be internalized behavioral problems such as loneliness, withdrawal or not playing with children.

3) Somatic symptoms: the younger the patient is, the more psychic symptoms there will be. The common symptoms include sleep disturbance, decreased/increased appetite, headache, dizziness, stomachache, fatigue, chest tightness, and shortness of breath.

16.2.5.3 Diagnosis

Patients show the clinical symptoms as described above, which persist for more than a month, and reach to the serious degree that cause disturbance in patients'living, learning, and social activities. After ruled out the broad developmental disorders, schizophrenia, affective disorders, seizure disorder, generalized anxiety disorder, the child can bediagnosed as mood disorders.

16.2.5.4 Differential diagnosis

(1) Depressive disorder

Patients with depressive disorder is unwilling to interact with people and unwilling to speak. Children have obvious depressive experience, silence situation is not specially appointed to some object or scene.

(2) Autism

Patients with autism can be clinically manifested as speech and social communication deficits. However, autistic refusal to speak has no feature of scene and object selection. There are obstacles in their ability of speech comprehension and expression. Sometimes there are spontaneous speech when refusing to speak. Narrow interest and rigid behavior are existed at the same time.

(3) Schizophrenia

Patients with schizophrenia can show isolation and withdrawal, according to its clinical symptoms, such as hallucinations and delusions, it is not difficult to identify.

16.2.5.5 Course and prognosis

In addition to social phobia, the emotional problems in children and adolescents can be remitted to normal after months and years if they get appropriate treatments. Some patients' symptoms developto chronic process, persisting into adolescence, and a tiny minority of cases persisting into adulthood. If the patients co-morbid with oppositional defiant disorder, attention deficit hyperactivity disorder or poor family conditions, their prognosis will be poor. The average duration of social phobia is about 20 years, and is generally not self-alleviating. About 25% of patients relieved with age. In the cognitive-behavioral group therapy forthe patients with social phobia, the effect can be predicted. The higher the degree of depression, the morethe avoidant personality characteristics and the shorter the treatment period, the poorer treatment effects will be. Although the change of negative self-evaluation frequency is related to the social phobia symptoms, it can not predict the treatment effect.

16.2.5.6   Treatments

The main treatment is psychotherapy, and medication is not usually required. In some cases, small doses of anti-anxiety or anti-depressants can be used.

(1) Psychological treatment

The methods of psychotherapy include supportive psychotherapy, family therapy, cognitive behavioral therapy and game therapy.

Supportive psychotherapy is characterized by helping children to make good use of their potential " resource" and ability, reducing the setback, changing their views and feelings of frustration, guiding them appropriate methods, providing emotional support, to help children go through the crisis andto deal with the difficulties and frustration effectively. The therapist should build a good therapeutic relationship, listen to the patient's complain of their inner experience, express sympathy to patient's pain appropriately, guide patients to make full use of their potential to adapt to the environment, arouse the positivity of patients, and enhance the confidence of overcoming the emotional disorder. At the same time, the therapist should assist patients to re-evaluate and understand the stress they encounter, and encourage patients to use available resources and supports to alleviate their response to frustration.

The purpose of family therapy is to change the way of interaction between family members, to change the relationship pattern related to the problem of children, and to let parents give children more emotional communication and supports. Family therapy begins with understanding the structure and function of the family, and negotiate appropriate space and privacy boundaries for the family members. The treatment must also assess the likelihood of a parent's mood disorder, and if so, parents are advised to receive medication and marital therapy.

Cognitive behavioral therapy is the preferred treatment for children and adolescents with mild depression symptoms. The therapist should be aware that children should be the center of the treatment. The treatments require that children and therapists work together to solve current problems, rather than only therapist's efforts. By letting children keep a diary and assigning homework, therapists teach the children to monitor and record their thoughts and behaviors. Cognitive behavior therapy is also a very effective psychological therapy for children with anxiety disorder. For children with anxiety disorders, the main points of the therapy are desensitization, gradually prolonged exposure, self-management, and cognitive strategies. Therefore, the cognitive therapy can help children recognize the anxiety, distinguish the physical anxiety response, and develop strategies for coping with anxiety symptoms. Methods of behavioral therapy are exposure, role-playing, relaxation training and reinforcement.

Due to the immature language expression, the undeveloped cognitive level, and the limited comprehension ability of young children, they are not suitable for cognitive therapy and the better effect can be achieved by using game therapy instead. In the game therapy, the therapist let the children freely choose the game to fully express their emotion. Through the method of game therapy, the therapist can observe the child's behavior and understand the inner thoughts of the child, which is the bridge between the therapist and the child. And by playing games, children can relax, express their emotions naturally and relieve their depression and anxiety.

(2) Medication

Drug therapy is only a secondary treatment for anxiety and phobias in a few of patients. Selective serotonin reuptake inhibitors fluoxetine, sertraline and fluvoxamine are choice drugs for treatment of children's separation anxiety disorder. For treating phobias, fluoxetine, fluvoxamine treatment have significant effects, and other drugs also have certain effects such as paroxetine, Dorset, etc.

To date, the US and Chinese drug administration agencies have not approved any drugs to treat the selective musim of children. Combined drug therapy may be considered for some refractory cases. Selective serotonin reuptake inhibitors, such as fluoxetine and fluvoxamine, can significantly relieve symptoms. And dosage should start at a low dose.

SSRIs are choice drugs for treatment of childhood depression. Commonly used are sertrin, citalopram, fluvoxamine, paroxetine, venlafaxine, hydrochloric acid anfepion, minazole and nefazolone.

Sun Li

Chapter 17

Personality and Personality Disorders

17. 1　Introduction

17.1.1　Personality

The term personality comes from the ancient Greek "persona". Persona, originally refers to the actor's mask in Latin. Personality is defined as the set of stable, predictable, habitual behaviors, cognitions and emotional patterns that evolve from social and environmental factors.

Many approaches have been taken on to study personality, including biological, cognitive, learning and trait based theories, as well as psychodynamic, and humanistic approaches. Personality psychology is also divided among the first theorists, with a few influential theories being posited by Sigmund Freud, Alfred Adler, Abraham Maslow, Hans Eysenck, Carl Rogers, and Gordon Allport.

The origins of personality included genetic influences, childhood experience, parental behavior patterns, early family and school education, social environment.

Personality can be determined through a variety of tests. However, dimensions of personality and scales of personality tests vary and often are poorly defined. Examples of such tests are: Minnesota Multiphasic Personality Inventory(MMPI), Big Five Inventory(BFI), Neurotic Personality Questionnaire KON - 2006, Eysenck's Personality Questionnaire(EPQ), or Rorschach inkblot test.

Gaining an understanding of a patient's personality is important in psychiatry. Different personalities predispose to some psychiatric disorders, and they may account for unusual features of a psychiatric disorders. They may also explain how a patient approaches treatment, and dictate different strategies for establishing and maintaining a healthy therapeutic relationship.

17.1.2　Personality disorders

Personality disorders(PD) are severe disturbances in the characterological condition and behavioural tendencies of the individual usually associated with significant distress or disability.

The two major systems of classification are the ICD-10 and the DSM-5. Both have deliberately merged their diagnoses to some extent, but some differences remain. For example, ICD-10 does not include narcissistic personality disorder and schizotypal personality disorder. ICD-10 uses the term "anankastic" is used, whereas "obsessive-compulsive" is used in DSM-5. In ICD-10 the term "dissocial" is used, whereas in DSM-5 the term "antisocial" is used. In ICD-10, the term "anxious" is used, whereas "avoidant" is used in DSM-5.

The ICD-10 classification listes under the code F60 as follows. Specific personality disorders (F60): paranoid personality disorder (F60.0); schizoid personality disorder (F60.1); dissocial personality disorder (F60.2); emotionally unstable personality disorder (F60.3, impulsive type and borderline type); histrionic personality disorder (F60.4); anankastic personality disorder (F60.5); anxious (avoidant) personality disorder (F60.6); dependent personality disorder (F60.7); other specific personality disorders including (F60.8); personality disorder, unspecified (F60.9).

17.1.3　Diagnosis of personality disorders

The ICD-10 provides 6 criteria for general personality disorder. ①Markedly disharmonious attitudes and behavior, involving usually several areas of functioning, e. g. , affectivity, arousal, impulse control, ways of perceiving and thinking, and style of relating to others. ②The abnormal behavior pattern is enduring, of long standing, and not limited to episode of mental illness. ③The abnormal behavior pattern is pervasive and clearly maladaptive to a broad range of personal and social situations. ④The above manifestations always appear during childhood or adolescent and continue into adulthood. ⑤The disorder leads to considerable personal distress but this may only become apparent late in its course. ⑥The disorder is usually, but not invariably, associated with significant problems in occupational and social performance. These general criteria should be met by all personality disorders before a more specific diagnosis can be made.

For different cultures, it may be necessary to develop specific sets of criteria with regard to social norms, rules and obligations.

The ICD-11 classification of Personality Disorders focuses on core personality dysfunction, while allowing the practitioner to classify 3 levels of severity (mild, moderate, and severe) and the opinion of specifying one or more prominent trait domain qualifiers.

17.2　Classification of personality disorders in ICD-10

17.2.1　Paranoid personality disorder

17.2.1.1　Overview

Paranoid personality disorder (PPD) is a personality disorder characterized by paranoid delusions and a pervasive, long-standing suspiciousness and generalized mistrust of others.

17.2.1.2　Epidemiology

Paranoid personality disorder occurs in 2.0% -4.0% of the general population, and between 0.7% and 2.4% of the adult US population. Paranoid personality disorder usually appears in early adulthood and presents in a variety of contexts. It is more common in men. Paranoid personality disorder typically decreases in intensity with age and with many people experiencing few of the most extreme symptoms by the time they are in their 40s or 50s. Higher incidence is in family members of schizophrenics.

17.2.1.3　Etiology and pathogenesis

A combination of biological, psychosocial and environmental factors may lead to paranoid personality disorder. Studies suggest that genetic factors contribute to paranoid traits and a possible genetic link between paranoid personality disorder and schizophrenia exist. Paranoid personality disorder is modestly heritable and shares a portion of its genetic and environmental risk factors with other personality disorders. In addition, psychological factors(such as coping skills, personality and temperament) and social factors(such as family, friends, environment) are important to paranoid personality disorder. Psychologist view paranoid personality disorder as a result of an underlying belief that other people are unfriendly in combination with a lack in self-awareness.

17.2.1.4 Clinical features

Case report:

The patient, was a 45-year old male who grew up in a difficult family with two siblings. He often suspected his wife had an affair, forbade his wife to have private affair. So his marital affection broke. He said, "although she denied it again and again, and other relatives said no, I just worried that she would betray me. If she dared to betray me, I would not let her feel better." He had no friends, no harmonious relationship with colleagues. He always thought he has been treated unfairly and suspected that people around him would betray and hurt him.

Patients with paranoid personality disorder are hypersensitive, unwarranted, offensive, hostile, easily insulted, and habitually relate to the world by vigilant scanning of the environment for clues or suggestions that may validate their fears or biases. Other symptoms include pervasive distrust of others(including friends, family, partner or spouse, the characterized as being pathologically jealous; believing(without reasoning) that others are malevolent and cheating; being hypersensitive to criticism; becoming detached or isolated; having trouble working with others.

Paranoid personality disorder may appear as a prodrome to schizophrenia; these individuals are at risk for agoraphobia, obsessive-compulsive disorder, depression, and substance abuse.

However, these individuals with paranoid personality disorder often don't believe that their behavior is abnormal and irrational.

17.2.1.5 Diagnosis and differential diagnosis

(1) Diagnosis

It is a requirement of ICD-10 that a diagnosis of any specific personality disorder also satisfies a set of general personality disorder criteria.

Paranoid personality disorder is characterized by at least 3 of the following symptoms: ①excessive sensitiveness to setbacks and rebuffs; ②tendency to bear grudges persistently; ③suspiciousness and a pervasive tendency to distort experience by misconstruing the neutral or friendly actions of others as hostile or contemptuous; ④a combative and tenacious sense of personal rights out of keeping with the actual situation; ⑤recurrent suspicions regarding spouse or sexual partner, without justification; ⑥excessive self-aggrandizing, persistent self-referential attitude; ⑦preoccupation with unsubstantiated "conspiratorial" explanations of events. Course criteria: this disorder usually begins in early adulthood and presents in a variety of contexts. Severity criteria: symptoms must cause significant difficulties in relationships, occupational and social performance. Exclusion criteria: exclusion of symptoms caused by other physical diseases(e. g. , gross brain damage); or psychiatric disorders(e. g. , schizophrenia, borderline personality disorder).

(2) Differential diagnoses

Paranoid schizophrenia: both are paranoia, suspicious, hypersensitive, hostile. However, unlike patients with paranoid schizophrenia, patients with paranoid personality disorder do not have any fixed delusions and hallucination.

17.2.1.6　Course and prognosis

The disorder usually has a chronic course, causing lifelong marital and job-related problems. Some patients who accept treatment can hold a job and maintain healthy relationships. However, they must continue treatment throughout the lifetime, because there is no cure for paranoid personality disorder. Symptoms of paranoid personality disorder will continue, but can be managed with care and support.

17.2.1.7　Treatment

Treatment for paranoid personality disorder can be challenging, because patients with paranoid personality disorder don't see their symptoms as unwarranted and have intense suspicion and mistrust of others. If an individual is willing to accept treatment, psychotherapy, antidepressants, antipsychotics and anti-anxiety medications are helpful.

Psychotherapy: as with most personality disorders, psychotherapy is the treatment of choice. It should not be surprising that there has been little outcome research to suggest which types of treatment are most effective with this disorder. It is likely that a therapy which emphasizes a simple supportive client-centered approach will be most effective. Other psychotherapies, such as family or group therapy, are not recommended. Long-term prognosis for this disorder is not good.

Medications: medications are usually contraindicated for this disorder, since they can arouse unnecessary suspicion that will usually result in noncompliance and treatment dropout. Antidepressants such as SSRIs or anti-anxiety medication such as alprazolam is appropriate to prescribe for severe depression or anxiety that interferes with normal daily functioning. Antipsychotics may be appropriate if a patient has severe impulsion, attack, agitation or delusion which may result in self-harm or harm to others, or social dysfunction.

17.2.2　Schizoid personality disorder

17.2.2.1　Overview

The term "schizoid" was suggested by Kretschmer(1936). Schizoid personality disorder(SPD) is a personality disorder characterized by a lack of interest in social relationships, a tendency towards a solitary or sheltered lifestyle, seclusive coldness, detachment, apathy, and prone to engage in excessive fantasy.

Schizoid personality disorder is not the same as schizophrenia or schizoaffective disorder, but there is some evidence of links and shared genetic risk between schizoid personality disorder, schizophrenia, schizotypal, and paranoid personality disorder. Thus, schizoid personality disorder is considered to be a "schizophrenia-like personality disorder".

17.2.2.2　Epidemiology

The prevalence rates of schizoid personality disorder in the general population are approximately 3% – 5%. This disorder is slightly more common in males than in females. There is an increased prevalence of schizoid personality disorder in relatives of people with schizotypal personality disorder and schizophrenia.

17.2.2.3　Etiology and pathogenesis

The direct heritability estimates of schizoid personality disorder range from 50% –59%. Twin studies with schizoid personality disorder traits such as low sociability and warmth suggest these are inherited. Genetically, this disorder is linked with schizophrenia. Evidence for dysregulation of dopaminergic pathways in these patients exists. In general, prenatal caloric malnutrition, premature birth and a low birth weight are risk factors, which may contribute to the development of schizoid personality disorder. Those who have experienced traumatic brain injury may be also at risk of schizoid personality disorder. Some psychologists had emphasized that excessively perfectionist, unloving or neglectful parenting could play a role.

17.2.2.4　Clinical features

Case report:

The patient, male, 21 years old. He had an introverted personality since childhood. He rarely communicated with others, had no friends, and was indifferent to everyone, including his parents. He seemed to be interested in nothing, but often did something weird in his own, making others confused and uncomfortable.

Persons with schizoid personality disorder are often aloof, indifferent, detached and cold, which causes trouble in establishing relationships or expressing their feelings. Some patients appear extremely callous. They are seclusive, solitary and separative from others. Patients are introspective prone to fantasy, and interested in intellectual matters, but show little sense of enjoyment or pleasure in the activities that most people enjoy.

Schizoid personality disorder can be first apparent in childhood and adolescence with poor peer relationships, solitariness, and underachievement in school. This may mark these children as different and make them subject to teasing.

17.2.2.5　Diagnosis and differential diagnosis

（1）Diagnosis

It is a requirement of ICD-10 that a diagnosis of any specific personality disorder also satisfies a set of general personality disorder criteria.

Specific diagnosis criteria of schizoid personality disorder. Must be present symptoms criteria:

At least four of the following criteria: ①emotional detachment, coldness or reduced affect; ②limited capacity to express feelings; ③consistent preference for seclusiveness and apathy; ④little interest in personal relationship; ⑤indifference; ⑥little interest in sexual relationships; ⑦taking little sense of enjoyment or pleasure in the activities; ⑧indifference to social norms and conventions; ⑨excessive preoccupation with introspection and fantasy. Course criteria: this usually begins in early adulthood and presents in a variety of contexts. Severity criteria: symptoms must be present to the extent that they cause significant difficulties in relationships, occupational and social performance. Exclusion criteria: exclusion of symptoms caused by other physical diseases(e. g. , gross brain damage); exclusion of symptoms caused by other psychiatric disorders(e. g. , schizophrenia, schizotypal personality disorder).

（2）Differential diagnoses

Schizophrenia: patients with schizoid personality disorder do not have any disturbance of thought such as fixed delusions or hallucinations.

Schizotypal personality disorder: patients with schizoid personality disorder do not have the same eccentric behavior or magical thinking seen in patients with schizotypal personality disorder. Schizotypal patients are similar to schizophrenic patients in terms of odd perception, thought, and behavior.

17.2.2.6　Course and prognosis

Schizoid personality disorder is usually chronic and long-lasting mental conditions, and is not expected to improve with time without treatment; some of schizoid personality disorder may develop into major depression. However, many remains unknown because it is rarely encountered in clinical settings.

17.2.2.7　Treatments

People with schizoid personality disorder rarely seek treatment. There are little data on the effectiveness of various treatments on it because it is seldom seen in clinical settings. However, if an individual is willing to accept treatment, psychotherapy and medication may be helpful.

17.2.3 Dissocial personality disorder

17.2.3.1 Overview

Dissocial personality disorder (DPD), which is also called antisocial personality disorder (DSM-5, APD), is a personality disorder characterized by failure to adhere to social norms, deceit, manipulation of others, and violation of the rights of others. An impoverished moral sense or conscience is often apparent, as well as a history of crime, legal problems, or impulsive and aggressive behavior. Dissocial personality disorder is different from delinquency, asociality or antisocial behavior.

17.2.3.2 Epidemiology

Dissocial personality disorder occurs 3% in men and 1% in women in general population. The prevalence of the disorder is even higher in selected populations such as prisoners, patients in alcohol or other drug abuse than in the general population. There is a higher incidence in poor urban areas but no racial difference. Dissocial personality disorder begin in childhood or early adolescence and continuing into adulthood. Patients with dissocial personality disorder usually have a history of conduct disorder symptoms prior to age 15.

17.2.3.3 Etiology and pathogenesis

Dissocial personality disorder is seen to be caused by a combination and interaction of biological or genetic and environmental influences. Genetically, it is the intrinsic temperamental tendencies as determined by their genetically influenced physiology. Environmentally, it is the social and cultural experiences of a person in childhood and adolescence encompassing their family dynamics, peer influences, and social values.

Genetic factors: research into genetic associations in dissocial personality disorder is suggestive that dissocial personality disorder has some or even a strong genetic basis. Twin studies have reported significant genetic influences on antisocial behavior and conduct disorder. In the specific genes that may be involved, the gene that encodes for monoamine oxidase A (MAO-A) and for the serotonin transporter (SCL6A4) are interested in their correlation with dissocial personality disorder. Various other gene candidates for dissocial personality disorder have been identified by a genome-wide association study published in 2016. Several of these gene candidates are shared with attention-deficit hyperactivity disorder, with which dissocial personality disorder is comorbid.

Biological factors: Testosterone is a hormone that plays an important role in aggressiveness in the brain. Studies show criminals who have committed violent crimes tend to have higher levels of testosterone than the average persons do. One of the neurotransmitters that have been discussed is serotonin (5-HT). Low levels of behavioral inhibition may be mediated by serotonergic dysregulation in the septohippocampal system. Brain structure deregulation, specifically within the prefrontal cortex and amygdala, plays an important role. This may underlie the low arousal, poor fear conditioning, and decision-making deficits described in antisocial personality disorder.

Environmental factors: Some studies suggest that the home and social environment have contributed to the development of antisocial behavior. The parents of these children display antisocial behavior, which can lead children to an emotional bond that may contribute to dissocial personality disorder.

Confusing discipline regimens, child abuse, and inadequate supervision have been associated with development of dissocial personality disorder. The socio-cultural perspective of clinical psychology views disorders as influenced by cultural aspects. There is also a continuous debate as to the extent to which the legal system should be involved in the identification and admittance of patients with preliminary symptoms of dissocial personality disorder.

17.2.3.4　Clinical features

Case report:

The patient, male, 20 years old, unmarried, unemployed. He was the only child in the family and his parents doted on him very much. Since young, he began to squander money, did not listen to the discipline, and liked to play tricks on classmates, such as put dead rat and cockroaches in girls' schoolbag. In junior high school, he smoked, drank, and stolen money, often absent from school. He dropped out of high school due to repeated extortion and school bullying. He broke up with his girlfriend. He was so angry that he stabbed the girl's mother and was detained now.

The main clinical features of dissocial personality disorder are impulsive aggression, violate the law, no guilt, and social maladjustment.

Patients with dissocial personality disorder behave violently, impulsively aggressively, hostilely, irascibly and recklessly, failing to consider or disregarding the consequences of their actions. They may repeatedly disregard and jeopardize their own safety and others and place themselves and others in danger, and can lash out violently. Their behaviors are mostly driven by accidental motivation, emotional impulse, or instinctive desire, without planning or premeditation. Some of patients may lie, deceive, manipulate of others, fail to adhere to social norms, violate of the rights of others, and even violate the law. Individuals are prone to alcohol or substance abuse and addiction. Many patients with have extensive histories of conduct problems such as attacks, theft, lie, deception, smoking, drinking and drug abuse. Antisocial behavior and criminal infractions are before adulthood or before 18 years old. About 25%–40% of youths with conduct disorder will be diagnosed with dissocial personality disorder in adulthood.

Individuals with dissocial personality disorder are contrary to usual moral and ethical standards and cause a person to experience continuous conflict with society. They show no social responsibility or morality, and are indifferent to others. They are lack of empathy and remorse for others, and have a callous attitude to those they have harmed. Patients ignore the rights of others, can not keep loyalty to sociality or to others, is unable to experience guilt or to learn from past behaviors, is impervious to punishment, and tends to rationalize his or her behavior or to blame it on others.

Social maladjustment is an important characteristic of psychopathic patients. Dissocial personality disorder often depart from social norms. People with this disorder typically can't fulfill responsibilities related to family, work or school. Their attachments and emotional bonds are weak, and interpersonal relationships often revolve around the manipulation, exploitation, and abuse of others. They may have difficulties in sustaining and maintaining them while they generally have no problems in establishing relationships. Family relationships are often strained due to their behavior and the frequent problems that these individuals may get into.

17.2.3.5　Diagnosis and differential diagnosis

(1) Diagnosis

It is a requirement of ICD−10 that a diagnosis of any specific personality disorder should also satisfie a set of general personality disorder criteria.

Specific diagnosis criteria of dissocial personality disorder: it is characterized by at least 3 of the following. ①Callousness: unconcern for the feelings or problems of others. ②Irresponsibility: gross and persistent attitude of irresponsibility and disregard for social norms, rules, and obligations. ③The impairments in personality functioning: incapacity to maintain enduring relationships, although having no difficulty in establishing them. ④Impulsivity: behaving violently, impulsively aggressively, hostilely, irascibly and recklessly without a plan or consideration of outcomes. ⑤No guilt: lack of guilt or remorse to profit from experience, particularly punishment. ⑥Marked readiness to blame others or to offer plausible rationalizations for the behavior that has brought the person into conflict with society. Those diagnosed with dissocial personality disorder must be at least 18 years old. Exclusion of antisocial behavior caused by bipolar disorder or schizophrenia.

(2) Differential diagnoses

Drug abuse: it is necessary to ascertain which came first. Patients who began abusing drugs before antisocial behavior started may have behavior attributable to the effects of their addiction.

17.2.3.6　Course and prognosis

Dissocial personality disorder usually has a chronic course, but some improvement of symptoms may occur as the patient ages. Many patients have multiple somatic complaints, and coexistence of substance use disorders and/or major depression is common. There is addition of morbidity from substance use, trauma, or suicide.

17.2.3.7　Treatments

Dissocial personality disorder is considered to be among the most difficult personality disorders to treat. Psychotherapy is generally ineffective. Studies have shown that outpatient therapy is not likely to be successful. Pharmacotherapy may be used to treat symptoms of anxiety or depression, but use caution due to high addictive potential of these patients.

17.2.4　Emotionally unstable personality disorder

Emotionally unstable personality disorder includes impulsive type (impulsive personality disorder) and borderline type (borderline personality disorder).

17.2.4.1　Borderline personality disorder

(1) Overview

Borderline personality disorder (BPD) is characterized as an instability of interpersonal relationships, self-image, and emotions. Borderline personality disorder belongs to both ICD-10 (F60.3) and DSM-5 (a subtype of cluster B personality disorder), but the diagnostic criteria of ICD-10 differ slightly from that of the DSM-5 system used.

(2) Epidemiology

The prevalence of borderline personality disorder is about 1%-2% in the general population, which occur three times more often in women than in men. It begins in early adulthood and is present in a variety of situations. Among the diagnostic personality disorders, borderline personality disorder is about 30%-60%.

Borderline personality disorder is estimated to contribute to 20%-25% of psychiatric inpatients and 10% of psychiatric outpatients. The overall prevalence of borderline personality disorder in the US prison population is thought to be 17%. Substance abuse among people with borderline personality disorder is estimated at 38%.

(3) Etiology and pathogenesis

The causes of borderline personality disorder are complex and may involve genetics, neurobiological, environmental, and social factors.

Genetic factors: the heritability of borderline personality disorder has been estimated at 40%. Studies of twins and families suggest that borderline personality disorders seem to be more strongly influenced by genetic effects than other mental disorders such as eating disorders, depression, bipolar disorder. Moreover, twin, sibling, and other family studies indicate partial heritability for impulsive aggression. Trull et al. found that gene on chromosome 9 was linked to borderline personality disorder features.

Biological factors: biological factors may play a role. ①Brain abnormalities: a number of studies in borderline personality disorder have found patients had brain abnormalities. For example, neuroimaging studies have reported findings of reductions in the brain regions involved in the regulation of stress responses and emotion, affecting the hippocampus, the orbitofrontal cortex, and the amygdala, amongst other areas. The hippocampus, and amygdale tends to be smaller, the prefrontal cortex tends to be less active, and the hypothalamic–pituitary–adrenal axis(HPA axis) is released in response to stress in people with borderline personality disorder. ②Neurobiological factors: borderline personality disorder of women may be predicted by changes in estrogen levels throughout the menstrual cycles. In addition, serotonin that helps to regulate mood, may be dysfunctionrelated to borderline personality disorder.

Psychological and factors: ①childhood trauma. Studies show that patients with borderline disorder usually have childhood trauma, including physical abuse, sexual abuse, and domestic violence, neglect, etc. Patients with borderline disorder are more likely to report having been verbally, emotionally, physically, or sexually abused by caregivers of either gender. ②Psychological factors(e. g. , temperament, personality shaped by their environment and coping skills that deal with stress) and social factors (e. g. , how people interact in their early development with family, friends, and other children). may contribute to borderline personality disorder.

Environmental factors: an unstable family environment predicts the development of the disorder, while a stable family environment predicts a lower risk.

(4)Clinical features

Case report:

The patient, female, 17 years old. She had been emotionally unstable since junior high school. She often felt depressed, and sometimes lost her temper. She had no stable friends, rarely played with classmates, and often complained that her parents were indifferent to her and were unwilling to buy things for her. She often quarreled with her parents for this, and sometimes her parents also scolded her. She was used to hiding in the corner and cutting her arms with a knife until blood flew out. And she said that it wasn't hurt at all, but was very relief and only pain would make her feel alive. She was always telling about her unhappy childhood, had no hope for the future, and was immersed in her sad experience. Her relationship with her boyfriend was also unstable. Shortly after a fierce quarrel with her parents, she jumped off the building and got a fracture.

The symptoms of borderline personality disorder include: impulsivity, emotional instability, significant separation anxiety, unstable relationships, and self–identity disturbance.

Emotions: the main characteristic of borderline personality disorder is unstable, strong and fluctuating emotion, which generally manifests as unusually intense emotional responses to environmental triggers, with a slower return to a baseline emotional state. Borderline patients feel occasional intense joy, sometimes exceptionally enthusiastic, idealistic, joyful, and loving. However, they are especially prone to dysphoria, depression, anxiety, and distress. Sometimes they may feel overwhelmed by negative emotions such as severe depression, guilty/shame, worry, anger, and are also especially sensitive to feelings of rejection, criticism, isolation, and failure.

Behavior: impulsive behavior or aggression is common. Self–harming or suicidal behavior is common in patients with borderline personality disorder. Self–harm rates is 50% –80% and the lifetime risk of suicide is 3% –10% among patients with borderline personality disorder. The most common method of self–harm is cutting. Bruising, burning, head banging or biting are common. Alcohol and drug abuse are also common, as the patient attempt to self-adjust their distressing emotions.

Separation anxiety: many patients with borderline personality disorder have separation anxiety issues. Patients with borderline personality disorder are described as "walking into life with the umbilical cord and looking for places to connect". They are intense abandonment fears and inappropriate anger, even when faced with a realistic time-limited separation or when there are unavoidable changes in plans. They try to do everything possibly to avoid separation situations such as begging or even suicide. The fear of loneliness and lack of self-soothing ability often require the use of stimulative behaviors and substances such as promiscuity, drinking, and drug to relieve the emptiness and loneliness. These abandonment fears are related to an intolerance of being alone and a need to have other people with them.

Interpersonal relationships: the typical pattern is unstable intense interpersonal relationships, such as idealizing someone and then suddenly believing the person doesn't care enough or is cruel. Borderline patients strive for affection and intimacy in insecure, ambivalent or, avoidant patterns in relationships, as a result, they are regularly disappointed and conflicted, and may exhaust their partners with the intensity of emotional demands.

Self-identity disturbance: patients with borderline personality disorder tend to have trouble seeing a clear picture of their identity. In particular, they tend to have difficulty knowing what they value, believe, prefer, enjoy and self-esteem. For example, they are lack of thought and answer about such questions, "who am I? what am I? where am I going", etc., which let them feel empty and lost.

(5) Diagnosis and differential diagnosis

1) Diagnosis

It is a requirement of ICD-10 that a diagnosis of any specific personality disorder also satisfies a set of general personality disorder criteria.

Specific diagnosis criteria of borderline personality disorder: The impulsive type criteria must be met with at least two of the following in addition. The impulsive type criteria: at least three of the following must be present, one of which must be: ①liability to outbursts of violence or anger, with inability to control the resulting behavioural explosions; ②marked tendency to quarrelsome behaviour and to conflicts with others, especially when impulsive acts are thwarted or criticized; ③marked tendency to act unexpectedly and without consideration of the consequences; ④unstable and capricious mood; ⑤difficulty in maintaining any course of action that offers no immediate reward. At least two of the following in addition: ①liability to become involved in intense and unstable relationships, often leading to emotional crises; ②disturbances in and uncertainty about self-image, aims, and internal preferences(including sexual); ③chronic feelings of emptiness; ④excessive efforts to avoid abandonment; ⑤recurrent threats or acts of self-harm.

Most patients with borderline personality disorder are able to work if they find appropriate jobs and their condition is not too severe. Patients may be found to have a disability in the workplace, if the condition is severe that the behaviors of sabotaging relationships, engaging in risky behaviors, or intense anger prevent the person from functioning in their professional role. Exclusion of symptoms caused by other physical diseases(e. g., gross brain damage); exclusion of symptoms caused by other psychiatric disorders(e. g., schizophrenia, dissocial personality disorder).

2) Differential diagnoses

Schizophrenia: unlike patients with schizophrenia, patients with borderline personality disorder do not have frank psychosis(may have transient psychosis, however, if they decompensate under stress or substance abuse).

Bipolar disorder: borderline personality disorder is often confused with bipolar disorder because both have similar symptoms such as mood instability, irritability impulsion, and aggressive behaviour. However, they are significantly distinct disorders. Bipolar disorder is a subtype of anxiety disorder while borderline personality disorder is a subtype of personality disorder. Mood swings experienced in borderline personality disorder are rapid, brief, moment – to – moment reactions to perceived environmental or psychological triggers. Bipolar disorder is characterized by alternation of mania and depression.

(6) Course and prognosis

Course and prognosis is variable, but many patients develop stability in middle age.

With treatment, most patients borderline personality disorder can relief from distressing symptoms. In addition, patients also achieve high level of psychosocial functioning overall though vocational achievements are generally more limited compared with those with other personality disorders. For example, patients with remitted symptoms are more likely to have good relationships with at least partner or parent, good sustained work and school history. Substance abuse, eating disorders, and major depression are commonly coexisted with borderline personality disorder. The risk of suicide is higher and suicide rate is approximately 10%, which is 50 times more than the general population.

(7) Treatments

Psychotherapy is the primary treatment for borderline personality disorder. Patient's personality can play an important role during the therapeutic process. CBT is also a type of psychotherapy used for treatment of borderline personality disorder. Recent research has shown that patients with borderline personality disorder undergoing dialectical behavior therapy (DBT) and psychodynamic approaches exhibit better clinical outcomes.

Medications are useful for treating comorbid disorders, such as anxiety and depression, aggression, attack, etc. Antipsychotics such as haloperidol, flupenthixol, aripiprazole and olanzapine may reduce anger, suicidal behavior, psychotic paranoid symptoms. The mood stabilizers such as valproate semisodium, lamotrigine, topiramate may ameliorate depression, interpersonal problems, anger, impulsivity anxiety and psychiatric pathology. Antidepressants such as amitriptyline may reduce depression.

Short-term hospitalization has not been found to be more effective than community care for improving outcomes or long-term prevention of suicidal behavior in those with borderline personality disorder.

17.2.4.2　Impulsive personality disorder

(1) Overview

This section discusses impulsive personality disorder. The code of ICD – 10 for impulsive personality disorder is F60.3. Impulsive personality disorder is not separately included in DSM-5, although several features match the criteria for borderline personality disorder.

(2) Etiology and pathogenesis

The cause of dependent personality disorder is unknown. However, it is believed to involve a combination of genetic, biological, psychosocial and developmental factors.

Physiological causes: a large number of experiments show that the attack behavior has physiological basis. Some studies suggest that the delayed development of the cerebellum and the neural obstruction that transmit pleasure may make it difficult to feel pleasure and safety, which may lead to aggression.

Psychologicalcauses: aggression is related to role identification, inferiority, low self-esteem, etc.

Family causes: generally, aggression is related to family education. Coddled and scolded children tend to be aggressive? In addition, children imitate the parent's attack behavior.

（3）Clinical features

Case report:

A 24-year-old male went to jail twice for theft, provocation and trouble. He is very impulsive and irritable. In the first month after imprisonment, he quarreled and fought with others twice for no reason. His mood is unstable. His violent tendency is obvious, and self-control is poor. In the past, he competed for a seat in an internet safe and beat, hit a stranger for no reason. When asked why, he said "I don't know. Whoever is not good to me, I will repay twice. Although sometimes I regret about my actions, I just can't control my temper."

Patients with impulsive personality disorder are irritable, difficult to control their emotions, and are liable to outbursts of unrestrained anger which they subsequently regret for. The sudden outbreak of impulsive and aggressive behaviors are also very common. Sometimes, they may use physical violence, causing serious harm. Unlike people with dissocial personality disorder, they do not generally have difficulties in relationships.

（4）Diagnosis and differential diagnosis

1）Diagnosis

It is a requirement of ICD-10 that a diagnosis of any specific personality disorder should also satisfy a set of general personality disorder criteria.

Specific diagnosis criteria of impulsive personality disorder: impulsive type criteria: at least 3 of the following must be present, 1 of which must be: ①liability to outbursts of violence or anger, with inability to control the resulting behavioural explosions; ②marked tendency to quarrelsome behaviour and to conflicts with others, especially when impulsive acts are thwarted or criticized; ③marked tendency to act unexpectedly and without consideration of the consequences; ④unstable and capricious mood; ⑤difficulty in maintaining any course of action that offers no immediate reward.

2）Differential diagnoses

Manic episode: impulsive personality disorder and manic episode have similar symptoms, such as irritability, impulsion, and aggressive behaviour. However, they are significantly distinct disorders. Manic episode is a subtype of mood disorder, while impulsive personality disorder is a subtype of personality disorder. Irritability, impulsion, and aggressive behaviour in borderline personality disorder are rapid, brief, moment-to-moment reactions to perceived environmental or psychological triggers. Manic episode is characterized by heightened mood, flight of ideas and hyperactivity.

（5）Treatments

Treatments for dependent personality disorder include psychotherapy and medication.

Psychotherapy is the primary treatment for impulsive personality disorder and may be beneficial.

Medications are useful for treating aggression and attack. Antipsychotics such as haloperidol, flupenthixol, aripiprazole and olanzapine may reduce impulsive and aggressive behaviour. Antidepressants such as amitriptyline may reduce depression.

17.2.5　Histrionic personality disorder

17.2.5.1　Overview

The definition histrionic personality disorder(HPD) has gone through many changes. It was first named as hysteria, and then hysterical character and hysterical personality disorder, which is listed as in the DSM-5. The code of ICD-10 code for histrionic personality disorder is F60.4. Histrionic personality disorder is included in both ICD-10 and DSM-5, but the criteria are somewhat different.

Histrionic personality disorder is characterized by a pattern of excessive emotional expression and attention seeking, including inappropriate seductiveness and an excessive need for approval. Patients with histrionic disorder are lively, dramatic, vivacious, enthusiastic, and flirtatious.

17.2.5.2　Epidemiology

Histrionic personality disorder occurs between 1.0%–3.0% in general population and 10%–15% in inpatient and outpatient of mental health institutions. The prevalence of histrionic personality disorder in women is four times than men. It usually begins in early adulthood and presents in a variety of contexts.

17.2.5.3　Etiology and pathogenesis

The exact causes of histrionic personality disorder is unknown, but many researchers believe that both learned and inherited factors play a role in its development. Traits such as extravagance, vanity, and seductiveness of hysteria may be inherited, while other traits may be due to a combination of genetics and environment, including childhood experiences. Psychoanalytic explanations relate this disorder either to failure to resolve oedipal conflicts or to oral conflicts. Freud believed that lustfulness was a projection of the patient's lack of ability to love unconditionally and develop cognitively to maturity, and that such patients were overall emotionally shallow. He believed the reason for being unable to love could have resulted from a traumatic experience, such as the death of a close relative, or divorce of one's parents.

17.2.5.4　Clinical features

Patients with histrionic personality disorder exhibit attention–seeking behavior and excessive emotionality. They are dramatic and extroverted, but unable to form long–lasting, meaningful relationships. They are often sexually inappropriate and provocative.

Self–dramatization is a striking feature, and may include overreaction, emotional instability, excitability, self–centeredness, and over–dependence on others. They are more likely to look for being the center of attention and ask others focus on them above all things and become uneasy and unappreciated when they are not the focus, which leads to social and romantic relationship problems(e. g. , divorce or separation) due to jealousy and lack of trust. Exaggerated responses are common among patients with histrionic personality disorder, which suggests that a person can be more likely to be theatrical and upset with different types of things or theatrical behavior, even suicide attempts. Their rapidly shifting emotional states may appear superficial or exaggerated to others. They seek intimacy and can be inappropriately seductive. Patients with histrionic personality disorder are more seductive. They are often inappropriately behave in a seductive manner even if they should not be doing so. A big part of this seductiveness can involve a person is overly concerned with appearance. This concern with appearance may end up being extreme and rough for someone to handle and can cause a person to develop an unrealistic self–impression. Patients have shortlived enthusiasms and easily influenced by others, especially by figures of authority.

17.2.5.5　Diagnosis and differential diagnosis

(1) Diagnosis

It is a requirement of ICD–10 that a diagnosis of any specific personality disorder also satisfies a set of general personality disorder criteria.

Specific diagnosis criteria of histrionic personality disorder by ICD–10:①histrionic personality disorder characterized by: continuous seeking for appreciation, excitement and attention; self–indulgence; theatricality; self–dramatization; shallow and labile affectivity; exaggerated expression of emotions; suggestibility; easily hurt feelings; egocentricity; lack of consideration for others. ②This usually begins in early adulthood and presents in a variety of contexts. ③Patients with histrionic personality disorder are usually high–functioning, both socially and professionally. ④Exclusion of symptoms caused by other physical diseases(e. g. , gross brain damage); exclusion of symptoms caused by other psychiatric disorders [e. g. , mood disorders (manic episodes) , dissociative disorders, borderline personality disorder].

(2) Differential diagnoses

Borderline personality disorder: patients with borderline personality disorder are more likely to suffer from depression and brief psychotic episodes and attempt suicide. Patients with histrionic personality disorder are generally more functional than patients with borderline personality disorder.

17.2.5.6　Course and prognosis

The disorder is usually chronic, with some improvement of symptoms with aging.

17.2.5.7　Treatments

Psychotherapy such as supportive therapy, problem−solving therapy, interpersonal therapy, group therapy, cognitive therapy is the treatment of choice. Medication does little to affect the personality disorder, but may be helpful with symptoms such as anxiety and depression.

17.2.6　Anankastic personality disorder

17.2.6.1　Overview

ICD−10 uses the term anankastic personality disorder(APD) , whereas DSM−5 uses the term obsessive−compulsive personality disorder (OCPD). Kahn (1928) used this term to avoid the implication that anankastic personality disorder is linked to obsessive−compulsive disorder. The diagnostic criteria of ICD−10 differ slightly from that of the DSM−5 system used. Anankastic personality disorder is characterized as orderliness, perfectionism, control over other or environment, excessive attention to details, at the expense of flexibility, efficiency, and openness to experience.

17.2.6.2　Epidemiology

Anankastic personality disorder occurs ranging from 2.1% to 7.9% in the general population. Study found a prevalence rate of 7.9% in the US. Men are twice more likely to be diagnosed with anankastic personality disorder than women. It may occur in 8% −9% of psychiatric outpatients. The pattern begins at early adulthood and presents in variety of contexts.

17.2.6.3　Etiology and pathogenesis

The exact cause of anankastic personality disorder is unknown. However, it is believed to involve a combination of biological, psychosocial and environmental factors. Genetic theory suggests that the DRD_3 gene may be related to anankastic personality disorder and depression, particularly in male patients. But genetic concomitants may lie dormant until triggered by negative life events of those who are predisposed to anankastic personality disorder. These negative life events include childhood trauma such as physical, sexual abuse, or psychological trauma and adulthood experience. Based on the environmental theory, anankastic personality disorder is a learned behavior.

17.2.6.4　Clinical features

Case report:

The patient, female, 30 years old, secretary. She is a perfectionist, checking over and over again at work, afraid of making mistakes, and not assured of what others have done. All the documents given to her, she would check verbatim for typos, line spacing, font size, etc. Besides, she was strictly observe discipline, did not understand flexibility, and asked others to follow her own ideas.

The symptoms of anankastic personality disorder include: ①paying attention to minor details. These individuals become so preoccupied with unimportant details, that they are often unable to complete simple tasks in a timely fashion. ②Perfectionism. Patients with anankastic personality disorder have a pervasive and unreasonable pattern of perfectionism, which eventually interfere with completing the normal work or task at hand and makes their lives and work as a burden. ③Excessive doubt and scrupulousness. Patients with anankastic personality disorder feel extremely doubt and caution so that they are indecision and examine repeatedly. ④Excessive morality. Patients with anankastic personality disorder are often excessively moral, conscientious and undue preoccupation with productivity to the exclusion of pleasure and interpersonal relationships. They can appear humourless and ill at ease when others are enjoying themselves. ⑤Rigidity and stubbornness. They are so excessive pedantic and unduly adherence to social conventions, customs, rules or regulations that they have a pervasive pattern of inflexibility, may lack imagination, and fail to take advantage of opportunities. On the other hand, they appear stiff and unreasonable insistence that others exactly submit to them, or unreasonable refuse others to do their things. They are often successful professionally but have poor interpersonal skills and are lack adaptability to new situations. They usually avoid change and prefer a familiar routine. They may be stubborn and controlling and generally thrifty, sometimes to the point of being miserly. They may hoard objects and money. ⑥Anankastic personality disorder is considerable similarities and overlap with eating disorders, Asperger's syndrome, and obsessive – compulsive disorder (OCD).

17.2.6.5   Diagnosis and differential diagnosis

(1) Diagnosis

It is a requirement of ICD-10 that a diagnosis of any specific personality disorder also satisfies a set of general personality disorder criteria.

Specific diagnosis criteria of anankastic personality disorder. Symptoms criteria: it is characterized by at least 4 of the following: ①preoccupation with details, and rules; ②perfectionism that interferes with normal task completion; ③excessive conscientiousness, cautiousness, and exclusion of pleasure and interpersonal relationships; ④rigidity, and stubbornness; ⑤excessive adherence to social conventions; ⑥unreasonable insistence and unreasonable reluctance to allow others to do things; ⑦feelings of excessive doubt and caution; ⑧intrusion of insistent and unwelcome thoughts or impulses. Course criteria: this usually begins in early adulthood and presents in a variety of contexts. Severity criteria: symptoms of anankastic personality disorder may cause varying level of distress for varying length of time(transient, acute, or chronic), and may interfere with the patient's occupational, social, and romantic life. Exclusion criteria: exclusion of symptoms caused by other physical diseases; exclusion of symptoms caused by other psychiatric disorders(e. g. , eating disorders, Asperger's syndrome, obsessive–compulsive disorder and other personality disorders).

(2) Differential diagnoses

Narcissistic personality disorder: both disorders involve assertiveness and achievement, but the patients with narcissistic personality disorder are motivated by status, whereas anankastic personality disorder patients are motivated by the work itself.

Obsessive–compulsive disorder(OCD): anankastic personality disorder is often confused with obsessive–compulsive disorder. Some anankastic personality disorder individuals do have obsessive–compulsive disorder; however, they are significantly distinct disorders. Obsessive–compulsive disorder is a subtype of anxiety disorder while anankastic personality disorder is a subtype of personality disorder. Patients with anankastic personality disorder need to check things repeatedly, or have certain thoughts repeatedly without recurrent obsessions or compulsions. Patients do not generally feel the need to repeatedly perform ritualistic actions and usually find pleasure in perfecting a task. On the contrary, patients with obsessive–compulsive disorder need to check things repeatedly, or have certain thoughts repeatedly with recurrent obsessions or compulsions. Patients do generally feel the need to repeatedly perform ritualistic actions and usually more distressed after their actions. Obsessive–compulsive disorder patients can be aware of their problems and wish that their thoughts and behaviors would go away. There is a greater anxious associated with obsessive–compulsive disorder.

17.2.6.6　Course and prognosis

The course and prognosis are unpredictable. Some patients can have comorbid obsessive–compulsive disorder(most do not) and eating disorders.

17.2.6.7　Treatments

Treatments for anankastic personality disorder include psychotherapy and medication. If patients do not agree with the diagnoses of anankastic personality disorder, treatment will be complicated or impossible.

Cognitive behavioral therapy, behavior therapy or self–help may be helpful to anankastic personality disorder. Cognitive analytic therapy is an effective form of behavior therapy.

Medications are not usually suggested alone for anankastic personality disorder. Antidepressants such as SSRIs is appropriate to be useful for depression or anxiety.

17.2.7　Anxious(avoidant) personality disorder

17.2.7.1　Overview

ICD–10 uses the term "anxious" while DSM–5 uses the term "avoidant". The code of ICD–10 for anxious personality disorder(APD) is F60.6. DSM–5 called avoidant personality disorder(AVPD) is a subtype of cluster C personality disorder. Although anxious(avoidant) personality disorder is included in both ICD–10 and DSM–5, the criteria are somewhat different. Anxious(avoidant) personality disorder is a personality disorder characterized by a pattern of persistent tension, social inhibition and avoidance.

17.2.7.2　Epidemiology

Anxious personality disorder occurs in about 2.4% of general population with equal frequency in females and males. It is a prevalence rate of 2.36% in the American general population. It occurs in 14.7% of psychiatric outpatients. The pattern begins in early adulthood and is present in variety of contexts.

17.2.7.3　Etiology and pathogenesis

The exact cause of anxious personality disorder is unknown. However, it is believed to involve a combination of genetic, biological, psychosocial and environmental factors. Specifically, inherited characteristics such as behavioral inhibition, fear, shyness, and withdrawal may give an individual a genetic predisposition towards anxious personality disorder in childhood and adolescence. In addition, childhood emotional neglect and peer group rejection are both associated with an increased of anxious personality disorder development. Some researchers believe that a combination of high sensitivity coupled with adverse childhood experiences may rise the risk of anxious personality disorder.

17.2.7.4　Clinical features

Case report:

The patient, female, 24 years old, freelancer. She was unwilling to deal with people, afraid of being criticized, denied or excluded. She lacked personal attractiveness or inferiority, behaved restrainedly with strangers, avoided going to public, and couldn't work normally after graduation from college so that chose to be a freelancer.

Patients with anxious personality disorder display a pattern of severe social anxiety and social inhibition. They feel pervasive and persistent tension and apprehension with preoccupied with the possibility of rejection, or criticism, disapproval, and worry that they will be embarrassed or ridiculed. Their fear of rejection is so overwhelming that it affects all aspects of their lives. They feel insecure, low self-esteem, socially inferior, unappealing, and socially inept. They are hypersensitive to negative evaluation that begins in early adulthood and presents in a variety of contexts. So, they are cautious about new experiences, avoid social activity, risk, and contacting with others. They have few close friends and isolate from relationships, but they are not emotionally cold. They are extremely shy and easily got injured despite a strong desire for companionship, and they avoid interpersonal contact or keep a certain distance from the people around them despite a strong desire for intimacy. Anxious personality disorder is similar and overlapping with anxiety disorders, and obsessive-compulsive disorder, depression, post-traumatic stress disorder, etc.

Patients withanxious personality disorder are prone to self-harm. Particularly, patients with anxious personality disorder comorbidity of post-traumatic stress disorder have the highest risk of self-harming behavior. Substance abuse (e. g. , heroin, alcohol, benzodiazepines) are also common in individuals with avoidant personality disorder.

17.2.7.5　Diagnosis and differential diagnosis

(1) Diagnosis

It is a requirement of ICD-10 that a diagnosis of any specific personality disorder also satisfies a set of general personality disorder criteria.

Specific diagnosis criteria of anxious personality disorder. Symptoms criteria: it is characterized by at least four of the following: ①persistent and pervasive feelings of tension and apprehension; ②preoccupation with being criticized or rejected; ③belief that one is socially inept; ④restrictions in lifestyle because of need to have physical security; ⑤unwillingness to become involved with people unless certain of being liked; ⑥avoidance of social activities and associated features are hypersensitivity to rejection and criticism. Course criteria: these symptoms usually begin in early adulthood, present in a variety of contexts, and occur in most situations. Severity criteria: symptoms are so overwhelming that it affects all aspects of their lives. Exclusion criteria: exclusion of symptoms caused by other physical diseases; exclusion of symptoms caused by other psychiatric disorders(e. g. , anxiety disorder, post-traumatic stress disorder, obsessive-compulsive disorder, dependent personality disorder, borderline personality disorder).

(2) Differential diagnoses

Social anxiety disorder: anxious personality disorder is often confused with social anxiety disorder. Both involve anxiety, fear and avoidance of social situations, however, they are significantly different. Social anxiety disorder is a subtype of anxiety disorder while anxious personality disorder is a subtype of personality disorder. Social anxiety disorder is characterized by a significant amount of fear in one or more particular setting(e. g. , speaking in public) with physical symptoms including excessive blushing, trembling, excess sweating and rapid speech. Avoidant personality disorder is an overall fear of rejection and a sense of inadequacy.

However, a patient can be diagnosed disorders concurrently if both criterias are met.

17.2.7.6　Course and prognosis

Anxious personality disorder is usually chronic and long-lasting mental condition although may remit with age. Some patients can have comorbidity of anxiety and depressive disorders. Comorbidity and Substance abuse may significantly affect prognosis.

17.2.7.7 Treatments

Treatments for anxious personality disorder include psychotherapy and medication. If patients do not agree with the diagnoses of anxious personality disorder, treatment will be complicated or impossible.

Psychotherapy, including assertiveness and social skills training is most effective. Group therapy, cognitive therapy, and exposure treatment may also be beneficial.

Appropriate medications such as antidepressants (e.g. ,SSRIs) may be prescribed for co-existing condition, such as anxiety disorder and major depression.

17.2.8 Dependent personality disorder

17.2.8.1 Overview

Dependent personality disorder(DPD) is the code of F60.7 in ICD-10, and it is categorized as a cluster C personality disorder in DSM-5. Although dependent personality disorder is included in both ICD-10 and DSM-5, the criteria are somewhat different. Dependent personality disorder is a personality disorder that is characterized by a pervasive psychological dependence on other people. This personality disorder is a long-term condition in which people depend on others to meet their emotional and physical needs, with only a minority achieving normal levels of independence.

17.2.8.2 Epidemiology

Dependent personality disorder occurs in approximately less than 1% of the general population. The disorder is diagnosed more often in females than males.

Evidence should that dependent personality disorder is inherited. Individuals with a history of physical diseases and anxiety disorders are more susceptible to acquiring this disorder. It usually becomes apparent in young adulthood or later as important adult relationships form.

17.2.8.3 Etiology and pathogenesis

The cause of dependent personality disorder is unknown. However, it is believed to involve a combination of genetic, biological, psychosocial and developmental factors, which is called biopsychosocial model of causation. A twin study (2004) suggests a heritability of 0.81 for developing dependent personality disorder. Another study(2012) estimated that between 55% and 72% of the risk of the condition is inherited from one's parents. In addition, psychological factors(e.g. ,coping skills, personality and temperament) and social factors(such as family, friends, and environment) are important to dependent personality disorder.

17.2.8.4 Clinical features

Case report:

The patient ,female ,35 years old ,tailor ,married for 10 years. She was always worried about being abandoned by her husband and obeyed everything that her husband arranged. In the past three years ,the husband had an affair. Half a year ago ,the husband took his lover to live with the patient and their daughter. The husband and his lover slept in one bedroom and the patient took his daughter to another. The patient had to take care of people ,she cooked and washed clothes for them. Two days ago ,the husband and the lover left and decided not to come back. The patient was in a trance ,unable to work ,unable to sleep at night.

Patients with dependent personality disorder have poor self-confidence, fears of being abandoned. They have excessive needs to be taken care of due to excessively dependent. They avoid responsibility and allow others to take responsibility for basic or important decisions in their lives or may need excessive help to make decisions. They are so difficult in making decision that they require parents or spouses to make all of the decisions for them. Such as what to do or where to go. They are often protected by support from a more energetic and determined parents or partner. When a close relationship ends, they frantically seek another relationship to replace the previous one or need medical help. They have great difficulties in getting angry with those they depend on. They are unduly compliant, but are unwilling to make direct demands on other people. They are lack of vigour and self-reliance, and feel uncomfortable or helpless when alone.

17.2.8.5　Diagnosis and differential diagnosis

（1）Diagnosis

It is a requirement of ICD-10 that a diagnosis of any specific personality disorder also satisfies a set of general personality disorder criteria.

Specific diagnosis criteria of dependent personality disorder. Symptoms criteria: it is characterized by at least 4 of the following: ①preoccupation with poor self-confidence, fears of being abandoned; ②subordination of one's own needs to those of others; ③incapacity to make everyday decisions; ④allowing others to take responsibility for basic or important decisions for them; ⑤unwillingness to make even reasonable demands; ⑥feeling uncomfortable or helpless when alone. Associated features may include perceiving oneself as incompetent, helpless, and lack of stamina. Severity criteria: symptoms must be present to the extent that they cause significant difficulties with employment. Exclusion of symptoms caused by other physical diseases; exclusion of symptoms caused by other psychiatric disorders(e. g. , mood disorders, anxiety disorders, borderline personality disorder, anxious personality disorder).

（2）Differential diagnoses

Borderline personality disorders: patients with DPD usually have a long-lasting relationship with one person on whom they are dependent. Patients with borderline personality disorders are often dependent on other people, but they are unable to maintain a long-lasting relationship.

17.2.8.6　Course and prognosis

Dependent personality disorder is usually chronic conditions. Some patients are prone to express anxiety and depression, particularly after loss of person on whom they are dependent.

17.2.8.7　Treatment

Treatment for dependent personality disorder include spsychotherapy and medication. Psychotherapy including psychodynamic therapy, CBT, interpersonal therapy, group therapy, family therapy and couples therapy may be beneficial. Appropriate medications such as antidepressants(e. g. , SSRIs) may be prescribed for co-existing condition, such as anxiety disorder and major depression.

Li Jing

Chapter 18

Psychosexual Disorders

18.1 Introduction

Psychosexual disorder is also called sexual deviation, which refer to a sexual problem that is a psychological, rather than physiological in origin. The definition of psychosexual disorder depends on the particular society and culture in which the behavior exists. A behavior may be considered deviant by one society, but accepted by another. In addition, the time when the behavior exists also affects the range of psychosexual disorder. Once homosexuality is considered to be a disorder while now it's just a special sexual orientation. Societies define those sexual practices that do not result in healthy, no harming, sexual contact as undesirable and in need of change. Those individuals who engage in sexual behaviors outside this definition are subject to criminal action. Those behaviors that cause harm to others, such as sexual contact with children or physical punishment, are universally defined as abnormal or sexual deviant. However, the sexual behaviors, which are not harmful to others, are not clearly defined.

18.2 Overview

The systematic investigation of sexual preference disorders began in the 1870s. Richard von Krafft–Ebing, a German psychiatrist credited with formally introducing the study of sexology as a psychiatric phenomenon in his notable work, psychopathia sexualis(psychopathy of sex). The textbook was the first of its kind recognizing the variation within human sexuality, such as: nymphomania, fetishism, and homosexuality. It laid the groundwork for the development of research and treatment in this area that has taken place over the past century. Psychologists started to research the sexual variations and coined the term paraphilia to refer to the sexual variations. Krafft–Ebing is considered the founder of medical sexology, he is the predecessor of Sigmund Freud and Havelock Ellis. Havelock Ellis(1859—1939), an English physician and writer who studied human sexuality, wrote extensively about sexual disorders. Sigmund Freud had contributed to the idea of psychosexual disorders and furthered research of the topic through his ideas of psychosexual development and his psychoanalytic sex drive theory.

In this chapter we discuss the main features of the 3 categories of disorders affecting sex and gender that are recognized in ICD-10 and DSM-Ⅳ, namely, gender identity disorder, abnormalities of sexual preference(paraphilia) and sexual dysfunction.

Gender identity refers to one's sense of being male or female. When this sense of identity is at variance with an individual's anatomical sex, that person is said to have a gender identity disorder. Sexual preference disorders are uncommon, but they take many forms and have forensic implications. Sexual dysfunction denotes impaired or unsatisfying sexual enjoyment or performance. They are subdivided, according to the stage of the sexual response, into disorders of sexual desire, disorders of sexual arousal, and disorders of orgasm. There are also categories for the painful conditions vaginismus and dyspareunia.

Psychosexual disorder has some differences and relationships with personality disorder. Patients with psychosexual disorder are usually character introverted, but mostly have good social life. Except for the abnormal sexual behaviors, they don't have other unusual behaviors or antisocial behaviors.

Patients with psychosexual disorder violating the social rules are not all moral corruption or sexual hyperthyroidism. Actually, most patients have low libido, even can't have normal sexual behavior. This sometimes may cause disharmony, even broken in family relations. The patients have fully recognizable ability and normal ethics. They fell guilty after the abnormal behavior, but can't control themselves. The patients usually have the following character traits, inward, shy, quiet, tender, withdrawn or femininity. There are some male patients will have prejudice against women and revenge after self-esteem impaired.

Psychosexual disorder is not equals to sexual crime. Sexual crime includes more illegal behaviors more than those caused by psychosexual disorder, like insulting, raping, prostitution and so on. There are no other abnormal mental activities besides the sexual behaviors. If the patients put distorted sexual impulses into action and cause illegal behaviors, they have full responsibility or limit responsibility.

In different culture, the public recognition of sexual behavior and sexuality differs greatly. Masturbation used to be one of the sexual abnormalities generally, but now is considered to be normal sexual behavior. It happens throughout life. The incidence of men is 96% while women is 94% (Yule M. , 2017). Although masturbation itself is harmless, but the unfriendly attitudes of the around people make the ones who have masturbation feel guilty. It will affect the sexual behavior. Masturbation is considered to be a kind of disease if it inhibits the normal sexual behavior, happens publicly, or causes obsessive-compulsive thoughts.

Since 1973, American Psychiatric Association no longer considers homosexuality as a pathologic disorder, but a variant of human sexuality. The same as heterosexuality, homosexuality is also a result of complex biological and environmental factors. The factors affect the person to form some preference in selecting companion.

18.3   Epidemiology

18.3.1   Sexual preference disorder/paraphilia

Paraphilic sexual interests are common in general population. In a provincial survey, nearly half of the sample expressed interest in at least one paraphilic category, and approximately one-third had experience with such a practice at least once. Voyeurism, fetishism, frotteurism, and masochism interested both male and female(Joyal C. , 2017). A high interest in BDSM-related activities in the general population was found because 46. 8% of the total sample had ever performed at least one BDSM-related activity while

12.5% of the total population indicated performing at least one BDSM−related activity on a regular basis (Holvoet L. ,2017).

The majority of paraphilia studies are conducted on people who have been convicted of sex crimes. In a Turkey research on cases who were sent to Istanbul Forensic Medicine Institute(FMI) by the judicial organs,the male subjects are 97.4% ,39.7% of them are 19−29 years old,10% of them are over age 60, 59% of the subjects are single,36.5% of them are unemployed,71.7% of the incidents have no physical disorder. The paraphilia type of the incidentsare pedophilia(60.3%), exhibitionism(8.1%), pedophilia and exhibitionism(7.5%) and fetishism(5.9%). It was determined that there were more than one paraphilia type in 40 incidents(13%). Paraphilic incidents do not seek for help or are exposed to psychiatric assessment only when they face a criminal inquiry. It suggests that there are more paraphilic incidents in the society than what we encounter.

Since the number of male convicted sex offenders far exceeds the number of female convicted sex offenders,research on paraphilic behavior in women is consequently lacking. However,there have been some studies on females with paraphilia. Sexual masochism has been found to be the most commonly observed paraphilia in women,with approximately 1 in 20 cases of sexual masochism being female. Many acknowledge the scarcity of research on female paraphilia. Some researchers argue that an underrepresentation exists concerning pedophilia in females. Due to the low number of women in studies on pedophilia,most studies are based on "exclusively male samples". Peak incidence is between 15−25 years old. Tend to have other and the frequency decreases with age. The majority of epidemiologic data derive from clinical populations. The frequency of paraphilic behaviors is difficult to obtain because individuals are reluctant to report their sexual fantasies and behaviors.

In paraphilic populations,the frequency reported is deviated from the reality. Some paraphili as are more likely to come to the attention of others because they involve another person(such as pedophilia or exhibitionism). Those paraphili as whose behavior is criminal tend to be over represented in clinical populations. They lead to mandatory reporting and court−ordered treatment frequently. However,those who do not involve other people are less likely to be discovered,such as fetishism. The estimated prevalence of fetishism is 1%−18% in men,and the disorder is very rare in women. There are no exact data on natural history or treatment outcome. The prevalence of transvestitism is estimated to be around 1%. Onset usually occurs at around of puberty(5−14 years).

18.3.2　Gender identity disorder

Estimated rates of transgender identity range from different countries. The prevalences of MTF and FTM transsexuality are about 3.97 and 8.20 per 100,000 people in Japan,respectively,making the MTF−to−FTM ratio about 1 : 2(Baba T_x ,2011). In Serbia,the sex ratio is close to 1 : 1(Vujovic S_x ,2009). The estimated prevalence of transgender identity in the Netherlands in 2015 was 1 : 3,800 for men(transwomen) and 1 : 5,200 for women(transmen)(Wiepjes C_x ,2018). In New Zealand high−school students, 1.2% reported being transgender(Clark TC,2014). The frequency of transsexual applications lay between 2.1 and 2.4 per 100,000 German adult population,while the sex ratio was 2.3 : 1 in favor of male−to−female transsexuals(Weitze C_x ,1996). It is estimated that about 0.005%−0.014% of people assigned male at birth and 0.002%−0.003% of people assigned female at birth would be diagnosed with gender dysphonia,based on 2013 diagnostic criteria,though this is considered a modest underestimate. Studies indicate people who transition in adulthood are up to three times more likely to be male assigned at birth,but that among people transitioning in childhood the sex ratio is close to 1 : 1.

Most clinical centers report a sex radio of 3 to 5 male patients for each female patient. Many adults with gender identity disorder may have qualified for gender identity disorder in childhood. However, some longitudinal study of several dozen boys with gender identity disorder found some three-fourths to emerge as homosexual or bisexual young men and only one to emerge as probably transsexual.

18.3.3 Sexual orientation disorder

4%–5% people prefer homosexuality all lifelong. Since 1973, American Psychiatric Association no longer considers homosexuality as a disease.

18.4 Etiology and pathogenesis

Many theories have been proposed to explain abnormalities ofpsychosexual disorders, none of which are supported by good evidence.

18.4.1 Biological factors

The development of atypical sexuality, homosexuality, or gender identity disorders, has taken on an increasing biological basis in research.

18.4.1.1 Heritable factors

Twin studies support that the homosexuality has heritable basis. Familial heterosexuality cases discover there is relationship between the behavior and heritable factors. Paraphilias is linked with abnormal brain activity or structure, or with genetic predisposition. Neuroanatomical and neuroimaging studies of sex offenders indicate that congenital or acquired brain damage is overrepresented. A study shows father and child co-existing gender identity disorder or gender identity disorder and transvestism could not be explained simply by evoking role modeling because the children did not know of the father's atypical gender behavior before they themselves manifested atypical gender behavior.

Researches showed a significant skewing in the sex ratio in families of homosexual men, such that there were fewer maternal uncles than aunts. Male–to–female transsexual has a significant excess of maternal aunts to uncles. No differences from expected parity are found for female–to–male transsexuals or on any paternal side. An explanation for these findings invokes genomicimprinting(Green R_x,2000).

18.4.1.2 Embryology

The sexual action tends to be male type with the existence of androgens in the embryonic period. It tends to be homosexuality with the lack of androgens before birth. Hirschfield thought the imbalance of gonadal endocrine is the cause of homosexuality.

Handedness is manifest during the first trimester of pregnancy, and there is evidence that it is related to prenatal sex steroid levels. Some studies showed male and female transsexuals were more non–right handed than male and female controls.

Substantial research has found homosexual males to be later in the birth order, with more older brothers but not with more older sisters. The hypothesis explaining these findings is a progressive maternal immunization to the male fetus through the H–Y antigen in successive pregnancies, modifying the later–born male's psychosexual development. Girls with gender identity disorder are significantly more likely to be early born than controls and were born early compared to sisters but not to brothers. Thus, these findings are the inverse of the studies of the boys(Zucker K_x,1998).

18.4.1.3　Monoamine hypothesis

A monoamine hypothesis for the pathophysiology of paraphilic disorders was first reported in 1997 by Kafka. It's based on four converging lines of empirical evidence. First, the monoamine neurotransmitters, dopamine, norepinephrine, and serotonin serve a modulatory role in human and mammalian sexual motivation, appetite, and consummatory behavior. Second, the sexual effects of pharmacological agents that affect monoamine neurotransmitter can have both significant facilitative and inhibitory effects on sexual behavior. Third, paraphilic disorders appear to have axis I comorbid associations with nonsexual psychopathologies that are associated with monoaminergic dysregulation. Last, pharmacological agents that enhance central serotonergic function in particular have been reported to ameliorate paraphilic sexual arousal and behavior.

18.4.1.4　Somatic factors and diseases

Those with congenital virilizing adrenal hyperplasia overproduce adrenal androgen in utero, and, as girls, they are rougher and tumble in play, less interested in dolls, and more likely to be considered tomboys than girls who do not have the disorder. Atypical levels of sex hormones before birth and the attendant effects of specific sex-typed behaviors may modify the child's early social experiences.

Rodent studies have shown that prenatal exposure to the anticonvulsive Phenobarbital(Bellatal) and phenytoin(Dilantin) alters sex-steroid hormones levels, resulting in unmasculinized sexual differentiation. 3 of 243 prenatally exposed anticonvulsant subjects were transsexuals and had undergone sex-reassignment-surgery(Dessens A. B. ,1999).

Reports describe polycystic ovaries as more common in female-to-male transsexuals than in the typical female population. Prevalence of hyperandrogenism, including the polycystic ovary syndrome, in female-to-male transsexuals is high. It has been related to metabolic syndrome. Prevalence of hyperandrogenism was 49.4%(73.7% were cases of the polycystic ovary syndrome), prevalence of the polycystic ovary syndrome in the overall sample was 36.4%, and prevalence of metabolic syndrome was 38.4% and 51.7%(according to ATP-III and IDF criteria respectively)(A. Becerra-Fernández,2014). Insulin-resistant is also common in female-to-male transsexuals,30.1% Among the untreated group(Baba T_x,2011).

The occurrence and development of psychosexual disorder are related to the human gonadal activity stage. It starts in the adolescent stage. The activity ofpsychosexual disorder becomes steady with the age growing to menopause. Psychosexual disorder that begins in middle age or later may be secondary to some organic disorders, or to their treatment. For example, dopamine agonists that are used to treat Parkinson's disease are associated with a range of abnormal sexual behaviors.

18.4.1.5　Central nervous system involvement

The size of a small area of the bed nucleus of the striaterminalis(BNST) was the same in male-to-female transsexuals as in nontranssexual females. Evidence against the size difference being a result of long-term estrogens treatment was that men with prostate cancer treated with estrogens had a normal male BNST. Additionally, there was one female-to-male transsexual in whom the size was typical of men. A further study discerned whether the first reported difference was based on a neuronal count difference or was a reflection of a difference in vasoactive intestinal polypeptide(VIP) innovation from the amygdale, which was used as a marker. The number of somatostatin-expressing neurons of male-to-female transsexuals was similar to that of women. For the female-to-male transsexuals, the number was in the typical male range(Kruijver F_x,2000).

18.4.2 Psychological factors

18.4.2.1 Psychodynamic theory

The theory indicates that psychosexual disorder is the result of heterosexual development failure in the normal developmental process and usually happens in men. It comes from the threaten of being separated and castrated in the early childhood when the children have Oedipus complex. With the function of psychological defense mechanism, psychosexuality degenerate to the naive development stage of early childhood. The development of heterosexuality is thwarted. It is hard to achieve the procreation function of sex that is the mature development type. Sexual impulses stay at the immature state.

Additional psychodynamic models propose factors that increase the child's insecurity or anxiety about the self. Factors that make a child likely to develop gender identity disorder may reside in dynamic factors within the parents that permit them to tolerate the child's cross–gender behavior and, perhaps, within the child, for example, activity levels and sensitivity, which make cross–gender activities more salient.

18.4.2.2 Psychological development stage theory or psychoanalytical theory

Freud divided the human libido development into five stages namely, oral stage, anal stage, phallic stage, latent stage and genital stage. It is considered that psychosexuality will stay at some stage if the development can't proceed smoothly. There is another situation that one degenerate from a superior stage to a lower stage after some frustration. These result in the psychological abnormalities and cause kinds of neurosis and psychosis. Freud recognized that abnormal sexual activities were the reappearance and continuing of their childhood appearances.

Psychoanalysts generally theorize that these conditions represent a regression to or a fixation at an earlier level of psychosexual development, resulting in a repetitive pattern of sexual behavior that is not mature in its application and expression. Another psychoanalytic theory holds that these conditions are all expressions of hostility in which sexual fantasies or unusual sexual acts become a means of obtaining revenge for a childhood trauma. The persistent, repetitive nature of the paraphilia is caused by an inability to erase the underlying trauma completely. Indeed, a history of childhood sexual abuse is sometimes seen in individuals with paraphilias.

In small samples, male–identified women have been reported to have mothers who are removed in affect from their children, frequently by depression, and fathers who do not support their daughter's femininity. In some cases, the girl was seen as being a substitute husband to treat the mother.

18.4.2.3 Jung's collective unconsciousness theory

Collective unconsciousness seems to be a collection of psychological archetypes which is the key concept in Jung's analytical psychology theory. The archetypes represent the genetic images formed from the surviving of early stage ancestors or animal ancestors. Jung assumes that there is some innate or potential images in human heart.

18.4.2.4 Behaviorism

Behaviorism uses social learning theory to explain the essence and pathogenesis of sexual abnormalities. They think the abnormal sexual activities are learned imperceptibly like other normal activities. Some sexual preference disorders are formed from the conditioned reflex theory. Nonsexual objects can become sexually arousing if they are frequently and repeatedly associated with a pleasurable sexual activity. Sexual preference is shaped by events and reinforcements during development. The development is not usually a matter of conditioning alone; there must be some predisposing factor, such as difficulty forming person-to-person sexual relationships or poor self-esteem. The incorrect sex educations from parents or adverse social effects are also meaningful. Some parents guide children to develop to the opposite sex out of their own preference and expectations, like dressing up boys into girls or dressing up girls into boys. Children tend to develop into the opposite sexual psychology if they grow up with the opposite sex around.

18.4.2.5 Personality factors

There are some personality factors, such as inward, inflexible, inferiority, implied, weak communication skills and so on. People with inward, unstable, neurosis, psychotic shy, sensitive, suspicious, timid, depressed or anxious personality tend to degenerate to childhood when they are faced up with dilemma or sexual frustration. They use forgotten childhood sexual way to ease psychological problems in adult and catharsis their sexuality. It presents as psychosexual disorder activities.

18.4.2.6 Integration theory

The theory advocates explaining psychological disorder with integration of different theories. It thinks that the cognition and belief to sex are important in the occurrence and development, so are the attitude and behavior to sex. The theory emphasizes that the social culture, family environment and individual socialization factors all need to take into consideration when integrated different kind of theories.

18.4.3　Social and environmental factors

18.4.3.1 Parents' attitudes to sexual activities

If parents forbid and reject all sexual activities including touching, children will feel guilty and shame which inhibit the children's ability to enjoy sex in the future life and affect the healthy development of adults' relationship.

Usually, children receive more positive responses when acting as the same sex and prefer to same-sex playmates. Fraternal separation occurred earlier in families with gender identity disorder boys than in families with control boys. Additionally, fathers of gender identity boys recall spending less time with their sons than do fathers of control boys. The boys with gender identity disorder are perceived by their parents as having been "beautiful" during infancy.

18.4.3.2 Social culture

Different culture may hold different view to sexual behaviors. In some societies, homosexuality is unacceptable while in some others it is acceptable. Homosexuality may be more common in the later societies.

In some cultures, love and sex are separated. People establish emotional connection within their own social class or circle. They have sex activities with the co-called inferior people like prostitute but have no emotional connections or affinity. When people have psychosexual disorder, they feel guilty in the sexual activity with spouse. Only in the sexual relationship or sexual activity without any gentle or care, can they feel sexual satisfy.

18.5　Clinical features

18.5.1　Sexual preference disorders/paraphilia

Paraphilia is the experience of intense sexual arousal to atypical objects, situations, fantasies, behaviors, or individuals. Such attraction may be labeled as sexual fetishism. No consensus has been found for any precise border between unusual sexual interests and paraphilic ones. Abnormalities of sexual preference can be divided into two groups—abnormalities of the object of the person's sexual interest, and abnormalities in the preference of the sexual act. Abnormalities of the sexual object include pedophilia and fetishism. Abnormalities of preference of preference of the sexual act include exhibitionism, voyeurism, and autoerotic asphyxia.

18.5.1.1　Fetishism

Case report:

Liu, male, 25 years old, married. The relationship with his wife is good. He has a private suitcase, not allowing others to see. His wife opened his suitcase someday when he was on a business trip. There were used brassiere and female underpants inside, even with semen stain on them. Liu admitted he stole the brassiere and female underpants afterwards. The female underwear evokes Liu's sexual arousal and urges him to steal them. Only by stealing female underwear can he achieve sexual excitement. Liu prefers to achieve sexual excitement by masturbation with playing female underwear rather than by sexual intercourse with his wife.

In sexual fetishism, the preferred or only means of achieving sexual excitement are inanimate objects or parts of the human body that do not have direct sexual associations. The objects are usually from heterosexual personal items. It happens usually in the adolescence. The objects that evoke sexual arousal are many and varied, but for each individual there is usuallyonly a small number of such objects. The objects, like brassiere and underpants, are collected to achieve sexual excitement. Some others are obsessed with parts of the human body, like fingers, toes, hair, and nails. Contact with the object or body parts causes sexual excitement, which may be followed by solitary masturbation or by sexual intercourse that incorporates the fetish. The disorder merges into normal sexual behavior, but is considered to be abnormal when the behavior takes precedence over the usual patterns of sexual intercourse. Fancy for the sexual appliances which are used to stimulate genital is not fetishism. Only in the situation that fascination is the most important or only way achieving sexual excitement, fetishism is diagnosed.

18.5.1.2　Transvestic fetishism/fetishistic transvestism

Case report:

Male, 32 years old, unmarried. He has been dressed up with his elder sister's clothes since childhood until high school. He usually wears female clothes, like red sweater, red coat, brassiere, or red high-heeled shoes. He thinks it's beautiful to wear female clothes and feels pleasant. Though he is laughed by others, he won't change it. He knows himself is male and doesn't have the intent to change gender.

Transvestic fetishism generally experience sexual arousal when cross-dressing. Transvestic fetishism ranges from the occasional wearing of a few articles of clothing of the opposite sex to complete cross-dressing. Transvestic fetishism is rare among women, and the description below applies to men. Transvestic fetishists generally experience sexual arousal when cross-dressing, and the behavior often terminates with masturbation. In the beginning, clothes may be worn only in private places. Gradually the clothes are worn in public, either underneath male outer garments or in some cases without such precautions against discovery. Cross-dressing is performed to achieve sexual excitement. If the act is forbidden, one will become obviously upset. Transvestic fetishists are in no doubt that their gender conforms to their external sexual characteristics. Most are heterosexual and many have sexual partners. Once they achieve sexual excitement, cross-dressed clothes are taken off. Sexual arousal may diminish with aging, so that the person dresses mainly in order to feel feminine.

18.5.1.3 Exhibitionism

Case report:

Male, 42 years old, scientist, married. He usually pretends to urinate beside the public toilets, fences or remote alley and exposures his genital to females passing by. He asks them to watch and masturbate during exposure. The ages of females ranges from 12 to 60 years old, mainly adolescent and middle-aged. Most ladies are scared and run away. Some ignore him. He was put into jail for two years but still had impulse to exposure when he saw females. He was regret and asked the doctor to cut off his genital.

Exhibitionism is the act of exposing in a public or semi-public context those parts of one's body that are not normally exposed—for example, the breasts, genitals or buttocks, but without any attempts at further sexual activity with the other person. The act of exposure is usually preceded by a feeling of mounting tension. Most exhibitionists choose places from which escape is easy or remote corners, and suddenly reveal their penis to the other person, from whom the exhibitionist seeks to evoke a strong emotional reaction. This reaction is interpreted by the exhibitionist as sexual interest, although it may in fact be shock, fear, or laughter. This distorted interpretation is accompanied by a state of intense excitement. The more intense the situation is, the more excited the exhibitionists are and the more satisfied they feel. The exhibitionists usually don't have the desire of sexual intercourse. Some men masturbate during exposure; others do so afterwards. Organic diseases should be taken into consideration if the action happened in the middle-aged for the first time.

18.5.1.4 Voyeurism

Case report:

Male, 21 years old, unmarried. He often observes the sexual activity of his neighbors and masturbates during observing secretly. He does it repeatedly but doesn't desire to engage in sexual activity with the woman he observes.

Voyeurism refers to observing the sexual activity or intimacy acts of others repeatedly as a preferred means of sexual arousal. The voyeur also spies on women who are undressing or without clothes, but does not attempt to engage in sexual activity with them. Although the voyeur usually takes great care to hide from the women whom he is watching, he often takes considerable risks of discovery. Voyeurism is usually accompanied or followed by masturbation. Watching porn videos or albums to achieve sexual excitement is not considered to be voyeurism.

18.5.1.5 Frotteurism

Case report:

Male, 37 years old, married. He was accused for rubbing penis against strange female's body on bus or in the crowd for several times. He felt regret but couldn't stop doing this. His family accompanied him to see the doctor for help.

Frotteurism is a paraphilic interest in rubbing, usually one's pelvic area or erect penis, against a non-consenting person for sexual pleasure. It may involve touching any part of the body, including the genital area. It generally happens in a crowded place. There is no further desire to have sexual intercourse or expose genitals. A person who practices frotteuristic acts is known as a frotteur.

18.5.1.6 Sexual sadism disorder

Case report:

Male, 46 years old, married. He could only get sexual arousal by biting and clamping his wife before sexual intercourse. He was accused by his wife because he forced her to kneel down and bark like a dog.

Sexual sadism refers to the achievement of sexual arousal habitually, and in preference to heterosexual intercourse, by inflicting pain on another person, by bondage, or by humiliation. The acts may be symbolic, causing little actual harm, like punching and kicking, whipping, biting, pinching, clamping, scalding, electric shock and so on. There are other ways, like posturing sex partners into some miserable ways or ask them to kneel down and bark like a dog. Extreme examples are the rare "lust murders", in which the killer inflicts mutilations on the genitalia of his victim. In these rare cases, ejaculation may occur during the sadistic act, or later during intercourse with the dead body (necrophilia). People with sexual sadism disorder are at an elevated likelihood of having paraphilic sexual interests.

18.5.1.7　Sexual masochism disorder

Case report:

Male, 32 years old, married. He was jailed due to rape and got married 5 years ago. Every time before sexual intercourse, he takes off his wife's clothes and whips her to achieve sexual excitement. He asks his wife to scratch his buttock and bite his lips.

Sexual masochism disorder is the condition of experiencing recurring and intense sexual arousal in response to enduring moderate or extreme pain, suffering, or humiliation. In normal sexual activities, there is also sexual gratification from the experience of pain. Only when the experience of suffering or humiliation becomes the exclusive or necessary way, it can be defined as disorder. The suffering may take the form of being beaten, trodden upon, or bound, or the enactment of various symbolic forms of humiliation. Masochism, unlike most other sexual deviations, occurs in both women and men.

18.5.1.8　Pedophilia

Case report:

Male, 62 years old, married. He often asked the 6-year-old girl in the neighborhood to have dinner at his home. Several times later he began to fondle the little girl and forbade her to tell her parents. He was jailed due to fondle a strange 5-year-old girl in a secret park corner.

In contrast to the generally benign effects of fetishism on others, pedophilia has serious forensic and clinical implications. Pedophilia is repeated sexual activity (or fantasizing about such activity) with prepubertal children as a preferred or exclusive method of deriving sexual excitement. Pedophiles usually choose a child aged between 6 years and puberty, but some prefer young children. The child may be of the opposite sex (heterosexual pedophilia) or the same sex (homosexual pedophilia). Pedophiles use the way of exhibitionism, raping, or fondling. It is almost exclusively a disorder of men, although female cases are recognized. Some pedophiles approach children within their extended family, or in their professional care, while others befriend unrelated children. With younger children, fondling or masturbation is more likely to occur than full coitus, but sometimes young children are injured by forcible attempts at penetration. There are rare and tragic cases of pedophilia associated with sexual sadism. Special attention should be paid that some male Alzheimer patients will perform as pedophilia in early stage.

18.5.1.9　Necrophilia

Necrophilia is a sexual attraction or sexual act involving corpses. In most countries, although sex with a corpse is not explicitly, a person who has sex with a corpse may be convicted under the law.

18.5.1.10　Zoophilia

Case report:

Male, 21 years old, unmarried. He came to the doctor with his dog. He was hurt when he had sexual intercourse with his dog. He told the doctor this was not the first time he had sexual activity with dog. He could get sexual arousal easier with dogs than his girlfriend. He felt regret and wanted to change this.

Zoophilia involves having sexual intercourse with animals as a preferred or exclusive practice for achieving sexual excitement even though they have the chance to have sexual intercourse with other adults. They usually choose domestic animals or birds.

In some remote area or places lack of sexual partners, some people choose animal for sexual intercourse to relieve sexual desire. They are not truly zoophilia. Once they leave the environment, they will have normal sexual activities and abandon the way with animals. Although sex with animals is not outlawed in some countries, in most countries, bestiality is illegal under animal abuse laws or laws dealing with buggery or crimes against nature.

18.5.1.11 Obscene phone call

Case report:

Male, 45 years old, unmarried. He called a lot every day. If the person who picked up the call was a female, he would pretend to be a researcher to invest the details of her sexual intercourse. He got sexual arousal by this way and masturbated during the call.

An obscene phone call, as the term is commonly used, is an unsolicited telephone call where a person derives sexual pleasure by using sexual or foul language to an unknown person. Making obscene calls for sexual pleasure is know as telephone scatologia and is considered a form of exhibitionism. It is generally considered to be a form of sexual harassment. Obscene phone callers are often male, feel inadequate, have feelings of isolation, have trouble forming relationships and consider making obscene phone calls to be the only way that they can sexually express themselves. Some pretend as birth control officials or researchers to invest the details of others' sexual act, and masturbate during the call.

18.5.2 Gender identity disorder

Gender identity disorder refers to strong and persistent preference for living as a person of the opposite sex and disgust to personal anatomic gender. They have a strong desire to change their gender.

Inner gender identity is subjective feeling of personal gender characteristic, which means one clearly senses "I'm a man" or "I'm a woman". Gender identity is the personal feeling of the distinction between man and woman. Gender role is objective. It's the public express to one's gender, male, female, or bisexuals. For exactly a person, gender role is the degree of one's expression of being a man or a woman to the public. Mostly gender identity and gender role are the same. For gender identity disorder patients, they experience greatly uncoordinated of their anatomic gender and gender identity.

18.5.2.1 Gender identity disorder of children

Case report:

A 17-year-old anatomical girl referred to a gender identity clinic reported feeling different from other girls since childhood, though unable to identify the reason then. She enjoyed playing with both gender, but generally preferred the companionship of boys. She preferred wearing unisex or boyish clothes, and resisted wearing a skirt or dress. Everyone referred to her as a tomboy. Pubertal changes were unwelcome. She tried to hide her breast by wearing loose fitting tops and stooping forward. Menses were embarrassing and poignantly reminded her of her femaleness, which was becoming increasingly alienating. As sexual attractions evolved, they were exclusively directed to female partners. She began socializing in lesbian circles but did not feel comfortable there and did not consider herself lesbian but a man. For sexual partners, she wanted heterosexual women and wanted to be regarded as a man.

It usually happens in the early childhood, usually 2 years old, and fully developed in the adolescence. Children perform effeminate behavior in boys and masculine behavior in girls. They focus on the clothes and activities of the opposite sex. They insist themselves to be the opposite sex, and have negative emotions to their own gender. For example, a girl insists she will grow a penis and becomes a boy, so she stands to urinate. On the contrary, a boy tries to squat down to urinate and want to remove his penis and scrotum. This disorder is rare, while the situation in which gender role is not the same as normal style is more common. These two should be distinguished. If a girl performs like a boy or a boy has some effeminate behaviors, the diagnosis is not sure enough. The diagnosis of gender identity disorder of children is made only in the situation male or female identity is totally confused. It is not gender identity disorder of children if it happens in the adolescence.

18.5.2.2 Dual-role transvestism

Case report:

Female, 16 years old, unmarried. She was raised up with her brothers. The friends of her were mostly boys. She knew she was a girl but often wore boyish clothes to be similar with the boys around. In this way she felt less isolated.

Dual-role transvestism involves people who wear clothes of the opposite sex to gain temporary membership of the opposite sex, but are neither transvesticfetishists (seeking sexual excitement) nor transsexuals (wishing for a change of gender and sexual role). The key point of differential diagnose is that cross-dressing doesn't evoke sexual excitement in dual-role transvestism. This disorder includes gender identity disorder, but not includes transsexualism or transvstitism.

18.5.2.3 Transsexualism

Case report:

Male, 23 years old, unmarried. He was raised up as a girl and dressed female clothes. He played with girls since childhood. He felt uneasy when got older and realized he was a boy. He convinced he should born to be a girl. His study was affected because he felt uneasy with some limitations. He was depressed asked the doctor for help in altering his appearance. He didn't have any other psychotic symptoms and difficulties in communication with female classmates.

Transsexual people have an overpowering wish to live as a member of the opposite gender to their anatomical sex, and seek to alter their bodily appearance and genitalia. There are two characteristics. One is sustained existing and intense self gender identity disorder. Transsexual people have a strong conviction, which usually starts before puberty, of belonging to the gender opposite to that to which they were assigned. The other is strong disgusting and unacceptable to their anatomical sex. They strongly demand to change their anatomical sex. Male-to-female transsexuals are more common than female-to-male transsexuals. Many transsexual people will self-harm or mutilation if they can not have surgery. Some male-to-female transsexuals even castrate themselves. These threats should be taken seriously because they indicate extreme distress, and are sometimes carried out. Sometimes it will have serious consequences.

Male-to-female transsexuals usually originate in the childhood. They are addicted in girls' game and fancy to be a girl. They avoid some seemingly rough games and comparatively competitive activities. They feel miserable about the physical changes in the adolescence and seek opportunities to have transsexual surgery. Many male-to-female transsexualstry to play female role in public, like dress up female clothes, so that they can live and work like women. Some are not satisfied just dress up. They even take estrogen to get more stable adjustment. A few male-to-female transsexuals want to have transsexual surgery at any prize. The decision to have surgery will bring serious social problems to the transsexuals and ethical issues to the doctors. Follow-up studies show transsexual surgery may have positive function to help the transsexuals live happier, but only for those who have already been diagnosed transsexuals definitely and tested in ordinary life as the opposite sex for 1–2 years. Before the surgery, the transsexuals have to change their postures and voices to get the public approbation. Some researches indicate participating gender supportive teams are helpful to transsexuals. There is a special situation that some male homosexuals, schizophrenia patients or serious personality disorder patients will also ask for transsexual surgery, but the surgery can not satisfy them in any aspect physically, socially or psychologically.

Female-to-male transsexualsare increasing nowadays. They may ask for surgeries of mastectomy, hysterectomy and ovariectomy, or they will ask for taking androgens to change voices and make muscle and fat distribution masculine permanently. They will also ask to implant artificial penis through plastic surgeries. As well as male-to-female transsexuals, female-to-male transsexuals who want to have transsexual surgery also need to meet the technical and ethical standards and live as man for more than 1 year. Artificial penis surgery is not satisfying as artificial vagina surgery. There will be many complications in the process of extending urethra into artificial penis.

18.5.3 Sexual orientation disorder

Sexual orientation disorder originates deferent kinds of disorders in the sexual development and sexual orientation. The sexual activity itself may stay normal. But some people also have psychological disorder in the sexual development and sexual orientation, like one doesn't want to be like this or hesitated and anxious, depressed and painful. He or she seeks for treatment to change the situation.

According to the diagnosis criteria of ICD – 10, sexual orientation disorder is not a disorder any more. Only when it is accompanied with psychological disorders, it is considered to be a disorder. The most common form is homosexuality.

18.6 Diagnosis and differential diagnosis

The exact cause of the disease is not clear yet. The diagnosis is made according to the detailed history, life experience and clinical manifestations. Before making the diagnosis, organic diseases should be excluded and examinations like sex hormones and chromosomal aberration are necessary.

18.6.1 Risk factors

(1) Frustrated heterosexuality.
(2) Disturbed by major life events.
(3) Influence from obscene pornography. The original damage is to strongly evoke the watchers' sexual desire and make them consistently masturbation. The secondary damage is distorting one's understanding of sexual problems and increasing the offensive to women.
(4) Special sexual preference or interests in the childhood or adolescence.
(5) Sexual experiences in the childhood.

18.6.2 Diagnosis key points

(1) Unlike normal people, the sexual arousing behaviors are obviously abnormal in the sexual partners selecting and sexual activities. The behaviors are stable and hard to correct. They are not occasional.
(2) The consequences of the behaviors damages personally and social, but the behaviors could not be

controlled.

(3) The patients have insight to distinguish the behaviors. They know the behaviors are not meeting the social standard. Under the pressure of law and public opinion, they would try to avoid the behaviors.

(4) Except for the abnormal activities due to psychological disorders, the patients' social function is good and has no obvious personality disorders.

(5) There is no mental retardation.

18.6.3　Diagnostic criteria(ICD-10)

18.6.3.1　Sexual preference disorder

(1) Fetishism(F65.0)

The ICD-10 defines fetishism as a reliance on non-living objects for sexual arousal and satisfaction. It is only considered a disorder when fetishistic activities are the foremost source of sexual satisfaction, and become so compelling or unacceptable as to cause distress or interfere with normal sexual intercourse. The ICD's research guidelines require that the preference persists for at least 6 months, and is markedly distressing or acted on.

(2) Transvestic fetishism/fetishistic transvestism(F65.1)

The wearing of clothes of the opposite sex principally to obtain sexual excitement and to create the appearance of a person of the opposite sex. Fetishistic transvestism is distinguished from transsexual transvestism by its clear association with sexual arousal and the strong desire to remove the clothing once orgasm occurs and sexual arousal declines. It can occur as an earlier phase in the development of transsexualism.

Transvestic fetishism is a psychiatric diagnosis applied to those who are thought to have an excessive sexual or erotic interest in cross-dressing; this interest is often expressed in autoerotic behavior. It differs from cross-dressing for entertainment or other purposes that do not involve sexual arousal, and is categorized as a paraphilia in the Diagnostic and Statistical Manual of the American Psychiatric Association. There are two key criteria before a psychiatric diagnosis of "transvestic fetishism" is made.

1) Individuals must be sexually aroused by the act of cross-dressing.

2) Individuals must experience significant distress or impairment-socially or occupationally-because of their behavior.

(3) Exhibitionism(F65.2)

A recurrent or persistent tendency to expose the genital to strangers(usually of the opposite sex) or to people in public places, without inviting or intending closer contact. There is usually, but not invariably, sexual excitement at the time of the exposure and the act is commonly followed by masturbation. When exhibitionistic sexual interest is acted on with a non-consenting person or interferes with a person's quality of life or normal functioning, it can be diagnosed as exhibitionistic disorder in DSM-5.

(4) Voyeurism(F65.3)

A recurrent or persistent tendency to look at people engaging in sexual or intimate behavior such as undressing. This is carried out without the observed people being aware, and usually leads to sexual excitement and masturbation.

The DSM-Ⅳ defines voyeurism as the act of looking at "unsuspecting individuals, usually strangers, who are naked, in the process of disrobing, or engaging in sexual activity". The diagnosis would not be given to people who experience typical sexual arousal simply by seeing nudity or sexual activity. In order to be diagnosed with voyeuristic disorder the symptoms must persist for over 6 months and the person in question must be over the age of 18.

(5) Pedophilia(F65.4)

The International Classification of Diseases(ICD-10) defines it as a sexual preference for children of prepubertal or early pubertal age. Pedophilia is termed pedophilic disorder in DSM-5, and the manual defines it as a paraphilia involving intense and recurrent sexual urges towards and fantasies about prepubescent children that have either been acted upon or which cause the person with the attraction distress or interpersonal difficulty. In order to be diagnosed with voyeuristic disorder the symptoms must persist for over 6 months and the person in question must be over the age of 18.

(6) Sadomasochism(sadism/masochism)(F65.5)

A preference for sexual activity which involves the infliction of pain or humiliation, or bondage. If the subject prefers to be the recipient of such stimulation this is called masochism; if the provider, sadism. Often an individual obtains sexual excitement from both sadistic and masochistic activities.

Sexual sadism disorder is the term employed by the current version of DSM-5. It refers to the "recurrent and intense sexual arousal from the physical or psychological suffering of another person, as manifested by fantasies, urges, or behaviors". It is classified as one of the paraphilias, called an algolagnic disorder, which is one of the "anomalous activity preferences". The formal diagnosis of Sexual Sadism Disorder would apply if the individual has acted on these urges with a nonconsenting person or if the urges cause significant distress to the individual, or impairment in social, occupational, or other important areas of functioning.

(7) Multiple sexual preferencedisorders(F65.6)

Sometimes more than one sexual preference disorders occur in one person and there is none of first rank. The most common combination is fetishism, transvestism and sadomasochism.

(8) Other sexual preference disorders(F65.8)

The diagnostic criteria for frotteuristic disorder are: over a period of at least 6 months, recurrent and intense sexual arousal from touching or rubbing against a nonconsenting person, as manifested by fantasies, urges, or behaviors; the individual has acted on these sexual urges with a nonconsenting person, or the sexual urges or fantasies cause clinically significant distress or impairment in social, occupational, or other important areas of functioning.

18.6.3.2　Gender identity disorder

(1) Gender identity disorder of children(F64.2)

A disorder, usually first manifest during early childhood(and always well before puberty), characterized by a persistent and intense distress about assigned sex, together with a desire to be(or insistence that one is) of the other sex. There is a persistent preoccupation with the dress and activities of the opposite sex and repudiation of the individual's own sex. The diagnosis requires a profound disturbance of the normal gender identity; mere tomboyishness in girls or girlish behaviour in boys is not sufficient. Gender identity disorders in individuals who have reached or are entering puberty should not be classified here but in F66.

Exclude: egodystonic sexual orientation(F66.1), sexual maturation disorder(F66.0).

(2) Dual-role transvestism(F64.1)

The wearing of clothes of the opposite sex for part of the individual's existence in order to enjoy the temporary experience of membership of the opposite sex, but without any desire for a more permanent sex change or associated surgical reassignment, and without sexual excitement accompanying the cross-dressing.

Gender identity disorder of adolescence or adulthood, nontranssexual type.

Exclude: fetishistic transvestism(F65.1).

（3）Transsexualism（F64.0）

A desire to live and be accepted as a member of the opposite sex, usually accompanied by a sense of discomfort with, or inappropriateness of, one's anatomic sex, and a wish to have surgery and hormonal treatment to make one's body as congruent as possible with one's preferred sex.

18.6.4   Differential diagnose

18.6.4.1   Other diseases

Patients with brain organic diseases, schizophrenia, or mental retardation also have abnormal sexual activities. But the abnormal sexual activities are part of the manifestations of the diseases, but not original.

18.6.4.2   Situational sexual abnormalities

Situational sexual abnormalities mean the abnormal sexual activities only happen in some situations, like ocean voyage, imprisoned, or separated from sexual partner. When the situation changes, the abnormal sexual activities disappear.

18.6.4.3   Atypical behaviors

Children with a gender identity disorder must be distinguished from other gender-atypical children, such as tomboyism girls or sissy boys.

18.6.4.4   Sexual crime

From the motivation of behaviors, sexual crime is acquired after birth and because of moral corruption. Sexual assault of sexual preference disorder is the result of innate factors and environmental effect.

Spying, rubbing or fondling is temptation behaviors in the sexual crime. If the victim is afraid to resist, the criminal will continue to sexual assault. The patients with sexual preference disorder use spying, rubbing or fondling to achieve sexual excitement instead of sexual intercourse. Because they have already gain sexual satisfaction, there will be no further sexual assault.

There are usually plans before sexual crime. The criminals hide and eliminate evidences after sexual assault and pretend to be innocent or deny their criminal behaviors after being caught. The patients with sexual preference disorder implement sexual assault because of impulse and uncontrollable compelling. They are usuallylack of plans and easily to be caught. They won't deny for the behaviors and hope to be controlled by law. The practices show prorate punishments contribute to control sexual assault.

18.6.5   Associated features

Psychosexual disorder may be associated with other diagnosis. Although a few gender identity disordered patients have a history of major psychosis, including schizophrenia or major affective disorder, most do not. A variety of personality disorders may be found in patients with gender identity disorder, particularly borderline personality.

18.7   Course and prognosis

Paraphilic behaviors emerge in adolescence and early adulthood. In general paraphilic behaviors are chronic. Although it has shown that individuals may cross over from one paraphilia to another, the overall course of paraphilic behavior is chronic. Because of the early onset and repudiated biological priming of the paraphilias, they are often difficult to treat.

For children, peer ostracism can make school attendance difficult. They may drop out, depression may develop, and drug use may begin. For adults, male-to-female transsexual husband may require the fantasy that he is the woman and the partner is a man, or that they are both women. The clinical picture commonly results in marital.

From a systematic review, the majority of male-to-female transsexuals seemed satisfied with the pitch-raising surgery. However, none of the studies used a control group and randomization process (Van Damme S. ,2016). In studies, 90. 2% were satisfied of male-to-female patients (Hess J. ,2014) and 88% of female-to-male patients (Falcone M. ,2018) were satisfied with the reassignment and without regret. Regret was associated with failure by the patient to carry out the real life experience and a poor surgical result. One outcome study that included a random assignment as surgically treated and a waiting-list control group supports postoperative improvement in social integration, sexual adjustment, and psychological symptomatology with surgical intervention.

A study on postoperative functioning of young adult transsexuals who had undergone sex-reassignment surgery conclude that starting sex-reassignment procedures before adulthood resulted in positive postoperative functioning. Improvements in psychological functioning were positively correlated with postsurgical subjective well-being (de Vries A. ,2014). A systematic review showed improvement in psychological functioning compared with baseline after initiating hormone therapy in transgender adults, especially in male to female participants (White Hughto J. M. ,2016). Less gender dysphoniais reported in follow-up. Postoperatively, they functioned socially and psychologically well. Long-term follow-up shows, 98% of all Danish transsexuals who officially underwent sex-reassignment surgery, one in three had somatic morbidity and approximately 1 in 10 died (Simonsen R. ,2016). Furthermore, total mortality was 51% higher than in the general population in the MtF group, mainly from increased mortality rates due to suicide, acquired immunodeficiency syndrome, cardiovascular disease, drug abuse, and unknown cause. In female-to-male transsexuals, total mortality and cause-specific mortality were not significantly different from those of the general population (Asscheman H. ,2011).

18.8　Treatments

Treatments for psychosexual disorder are difficult. Once the disorder forms, it's difficulty to completely correct. The patients and their family are all miserable. Symptomatic and supportive treatment is helpful. In addition, the abnormal behaviors might ease after menopause.

18.8.1　Counselling

Counselling should deal with the full range of options available. It emphasizes the need to set realistic goals and to consider the full consequences of anycontemplated changes, both for the person concerned and for their family, including and children.

18.8.2　Psychotherapy

Psychotherapy is the first choice for psychosexual disorder. Review the psychological development process and understand the factors that cause the abnormal sexual activities. Patients may realize how and when they become abnormal and try to correct. The efficacy depends on how urgent the patients want to change and whether they are miserable because of the psychosexual abnormalities. The common psychother-apies are psychoanalytic therapy and cognitive–behavioral therapy.

18.8.3   Pharmacotherapy

Psychosexual disorder is a kind of psychological disorder. The efficacy of using pharmacotherapy alone is limited and questioned. Review the history and present status of pharmacotherapy using in psychological disorder. The reasons taken into consideration are as follows. ①Decrease the sexual desire and abnormal sexual impulses, and to enhance the controllable ability. ②Change the mandatory and over–valued abnormal sexuality. ③Ease the depression and anxiety of the patients, so that the psychotherapy can be carried out successfully. The commonly–used medicines include antiandrogen, estrogen, antianxiety drugs, antidepressant, and antipsychotics.

18.8.4   Psychosexual disorders

18.8.4.1   Sexual preference disorder

Empirical evidence for treatment of individuals with paraphilias is derived from studies of sex offenders. Measurement of outcome is flawed, with recidivism rates underestimating actual recurrence of the pathological behavior. The majority of treatment efficacy studies are conducted on incarcerated or civilly committed offenders. They only represent a unique population with treatment outcomes that may not generalize to the nonincarcerated or community residing sex offender. Many studies do not differentiate between types of offenders. The ethical and public safety implications of a well–designed study with a matched, randomly assigned control group impede its design.

(1) Biological treatment

The scientific basis of biological treatment in disorder of sexual preference is the reduction of sexual behaviors by decreasing testosterone levels. Testosterone is produced by the testes that is responsible for the development of secondary sex characteristics in men. Testosterone helps maintain sex drive, the production of sperm cells, male hair patterns, muscle mass, and bone mass. Testosterone strongly influences both male and female sexual drive and the resultant sexual behavior.

(2) Surgical treatment

Surgical treatment for sex offenders consist of 2 types: neurosurgery and castration. The neurosurgical procedure involves stereotaxic removal of parts of the hypothalamus to disrupt production of male hormones and decrease sexual arousal and impulsive behaviors. This procedure had significant adverse effects and was considered largely ineffective. Surgical castration is the removal of the testes. The effect of surgical castration is to globally reduce available androgen by the removal of the testes.

Controversy exists as to whether surgical castration should be offered as a treatment, as chemical castration achieves the results and spares the procedure.

(3) Pharmacologic treatment

Anti–androgens: anti–androgen treatment refers to treatment with drugs used to block production or interfere with the action of male sex hormones. Cyproterone acetate(CPA; Androcur) and medroxyprogesterone(MPA; Depo–Provera) are the 2 most commonly used anti–androgen medications. Both CPA and MPA are synthetic progesterones that reduce the serum level of testosterone and diminish sexual preoccupation and urges, making self–control easier. A meta–analysis of anti–androgen studies by Grossman and colleagues report a spectrum of differences between patients treated with anti–androgens and those not treated, with recidivism rates as low as 1% for treated patients and as high as 68% for untreated patients(Grossman

L. , 1999). The side-effects of antiandrogen include, weight gain, hyperglycemia, hot and cold flashed, liver dysfunction, hypertension, muscle cramps, phlebitis, gastrointestinal complaints, and feminization. Long-term sequelae of antiandrogen treatment are unknown for the studies are mostly less than 8 years.

Hormonal agents: leuprolide (Eligard) and triptorelin (Trelstar) are hormonal agents referred to as long-acting GnRH agonists. These agents inhibit the secretion of luteinizing hormone with a resulting decrease in plasma testosterone levels and libido. They produce a chemical castration. A meta-analysis of pharmacotherapy of disorder of sexual preference was reported on a sample of 118 treated patients that patients previously treated with other agents like CPA, MPA, or SSRIs reported better effects when taking luteinizing hormone-releasing hormone (LHRH) agonists. The side effects associated with GnRH agonists include decreased bone mineral density or osteopenia, weight gain, hyperglycemia, diabetes, hypertension, and insomnia. The most common side effects are erectile/ejaculatory problems and gynecomastia. GnRH agonists include leuprolide and triptorelin may be more effective, better-tolerated alternatives to antiandrogen treatment.

For the female-male patients, treatment is composed of testosterone, most commonly esters of testosterone. For the male-female patients, treatment consists of estrogens. These estrogens are frequently associated to an anti-androgen (cyproterone acetate) in the pre-reassignment phase. Avoiding the hepatic way, transdermal form is recommended. The most frequent secondary effects of hormonal treatments is venous thromboembolism. It is essential and necessary to conduct endocrinological follow-up.

SSRIs: although the pharmacologic mechanism is poorly understood, SSRIs have been shown to be effective in reducing paraphilic symptoms. Greenberg and colleagues demonstrated that sertraline (Zoloft), fluvoxamine (Luvox), and fluoxetine (Prozac) are equally effective in reducing paraphilic symptoms. But there are insufficient data to conclude that SSRIs are equally efficacious as antiandrogens or hormonal agents.

(4) Psychological treatment

Cognitive approaches described the concept of cognitive distortions (minimizations, excuses, justifications) as one factor that may maintain offender behavior. Relapse prevention and the sexual assault cycle are theoretical models purporting to describe the cognitions and behaviors of sex offenders before, during, and after their abusive acts. The majority of sex offender treatment programs offer a combination of cognitive behavioral and relapse prevention therapies. Recidivism rates from cognitive and behavioral treatment programs range from 3% to 31% depending on the study. A meta-analysis found that cognitive behavioral treatment and antiandrogen treatment were comparable in their treatment effects and significantly more effective than behavioral treatmentalone (Codispoti V. L. , 2008).

(5) Models of treatment

Treatment programs are based on recent research that reveals that imaginal desensitization, masturbatory reconditioning, victim empathy, anger management, cognitive distortions, social skills training, remorse, responsibility training, and relapse prevention are integral components of a treatment program. The acceptable treatments were individual psychotherapy, social skills training, and group therapy.

18.8.4.2 Gender identity disorder

(1) Children

One strategy of therapy looks at the child's level of cognitive development. A child who does not like the activities usually associated with his or her sex concludes that being the other sex is the only solution. Alternate way should be introduced. Boys need to know that they can participate in sedentary play with other boys and girls. Girls need to know that they can play with sports.

A boy with a gender identity disorder has a strained relationship with his father. The boy gravitates towards his mother's activities for his father's absence.

At present, there is no convincing evidence that psychiatric or psychological intervention for children with gender identity disorder affects the direction of subsequent sexual orientation. Transsexualism, however, may be affected.

(2) Adolescents

Adolescents whose gender identity disorder has persisted beyond puberty present unique treatment problems, like how to manage the rapid emergence of unwanted secondary sex characteristics.

Young persons whose previous gender identity disorder has remitted may experience new conflicts that may be a source of anxiety in the adolescent.

Hormone therapy for gender identity disorder are usually conducted in 2 phases. First, hormones with reversible effects, that is, antiandrogens for male-to-female transsexuals and progestins for female-to-male transsexuals, were administered; second, estrogens to feminize the male-to-female transsexuals and androgens to masculineze the female-to-male transsexuals were administered. The sixth(2001) and the seventh (2011) versions of the standards of care for the health of transsexual, transgender, and gender nonconforming people of World Professional Association for Transgender Health(WPATH) recommend that transsexual adolescents[Tanner stage 2, (mainly 12 – 13 years of age)] are treated by the endocrinologists to suppress puberty with gonadotropin-releasing hormone(GnRH) agonists until age 16 years old, after which cross-sex hormones may be given.

(3) Adult

Adult patients are usually severe and intractable. They often present with straight forward requests for hormonal and surgical sex reassignment that is often the best solution. There is controversy with respect to the timing of introducing endocrine treatment of transsexuals. Once the social transition has been effected, hormone treatment can be introduced. The intervention should be supervised by an endocrinologist. The real life experience is typically 1–2 years of full-time cross-gender living.

Persons born male are typically treated with daily doses of oral estrogen. These hormones produce breast enlargement. Other major effects of estrogen treatment are testicular atrophy, decreased libido, and diminished erectile capacity. There also may be a decrease in the density of body hair and, perhaps, an arrest of male pattern baldness. Side effects can be elevated levels of prolactin, fasting blood sugar, and hepatic enzymes. Smoking is a contraindication of endocrine treatment, as it increases the risk of deep vein thrombosis and pulmonary embolism.

Biological women are treated with monthly or two weekly injections of testosterone. The clitoris enlarges to three or four times its pretreatment length and is often accompanied by increasing libido. Hair growth changes to the male pattern, and a full complement of facial hair may grow. Male pattern baldness may develop, and acne may be a complication.

Sex reassignment surgery for a person born anatomically male consists principally of removal of the penis, scrotum, and testes; construction of labia; and vaginoplasty. Postoperative complications include urethral strictures, rectovaginal fistulas, vaginal stenosis, and inadequate vaginal depth. There are also other operations, such as augmentation mammaplasty, thyroid cartilage shaving, cricothyroid approximation procedure, facial contour surgery. A study shows, in penile inversion vaginoplasty for transgender women, the most frequently observed intraoperative complication was rectal injury. Major complications comprised three rectoneovaginal fistulas(Buncamper M. E. ,2016).

Female-to-male patients typically first undergo bilateral mastectomy, and then the construction of a neophallus. Concurrently with phalloplasty, patients may undergo hysterectomy and ovarienctomy. Phalloplasty by Gottlieb and Levine's free radial forearm flap technique is used in female- to - male transsexuals. The rate of total flap failure was 3%. Urinary fistulae and strictures are common reasons. The number of postoperative complications, such as bleeding, thrombosis of the flap requiring revision, or delayed wound healing was considering the high rate of nicotine abuse reasonable(Wirthmann A. ,2018).

Kuang Li

Chapter 19

Suicide and Crisis Intervention

19.1　Introduction

Suicide is among the ten leading causes of death in most countries for which information is available, and the rate is increasing. Over the last three decades, several countries have reported a considerable increase in the number of young men who kill themselves. Although in recent years there have been some signs that this trend may be reversing. The subject is important to all doctors who may at times encounter people who are at risk for suicide, and who may also at times be involved in helping family members or others after a suicide. The importance of the subject is reflected in national and international initiatives for suicide prevention.

For every suicide, it is estimated that more than 30 non-fetal episodes of self-harm occur. Depression, substance misuse, and other mental health problems are more common in people who deliberately harm themselves, and the rate of suicide in the following an episode of deliberate self-harm (DSH) is 60 - 100 times that of the general population. The rate of suicide is also raised in the period following discharge from impatient psychiatric care. for these reasons, psychiatrists need to be particularly well informed about the nature of DSH and suicidal behavior, and about strategies aimed at their prevention.

19.1.1　Definitions

19.1.1.1　Suicide

Most contemporary definitions of suicide rely on two elements: a precise outcome(death) and a prerequisite(the intention or wish to die), as it can be seen in the operational definition proposed by the World Health Organization: for the act of killing oneself to class as suicide, it must be deliberately initiated and performed by the person concerned in the full knowledge, or expectation, of its fatal outcome.

19.1.1.2　Attempted suicide

An act with nonfatal outcome, in which an individual deliberately initiates a non-habitual behavior that, without intervention from others, will cause self-harm, or deliberately ingests a substance in excess of the prescribed or generally recognized therapeutic dosage, and which is aimed at realizing changes which the subject desired via the actual or expected physical consequences.

The definition is descriptive and does not take the person's intention into consideration, neither is the distinction between serious and non-serious suicidal attempts is applied. Given the fundamental importance of outcomes from a public health perspective, this terminology was adopted in 1992 by the International Classification of Diseases, 10th edition (ICD-10), in the category "Intentional self-harm", which includes "purposefully self-inflicted poisoning or injury; and suicide (attempted)".

19.1.1.3 Suicidal ideation

Suicidal ideation is thoughts of serving as the agent of one's own death. Suicidal ideation may vary in seriousness depending on the specificity of suicide plans and the degree of suicidal intent.

19.1.1.4 Suicidal intent

Suicidal intent is subjective expectation and desire for a self-destructive act to end in death.

19.1.1.5 Deliberate self-harm

Deliberate self-harm is willful self-inflicting of painful, destructive, or injurious acts without intent to die.

19.1.2 Epidemiology

Approximately 0.5%–1.4% of people die from suicide, a mortality rate of 11.6 per 100,000 persons per year. Suicide resulted 842,000 deaths in 2013 up from 712,000 deaths in 1990. Rates of suicide have increased by 60% from the 1960s to 2012, withthese increases seen primarily in the developing countries. Globally, as of 2008—2009, suicide is the tenth leading cause of death. For every suicide that results in death are between 10 and 40 attempted suicides.

Suicide rates differ significantly between countries and over time. As a percentage of deaths in 2008 it was: 0.5% in Africa, 1.9% in South–East Asia, 1.2% in America and 1.4% in Europe. Rates per 100,000 were: China 12.7, the United States 11.4, the United Kingdom 7.6, Australia 8.6, Canada 11.1, South Korea 28.9 and India 23.2. It was ranked as the 10thleading cause of death in the United States in 2009 at about 36,000 cases a year, with about 650,000 people seen in emergency departments yearly due to attempting suicide. The country's rate among men in their 50s rose by nearly half between 1999 to 2010. Lithuania, Japan and Hungary have the highest rates. Around 75% of suicides occur in the developing countries. The countries with the greatest absolute numbers of suicides are China and India, accounting for over half the total suicide death. In China, suicide is the 5th leading cause of death.

The leading method of suicide varies among countries. The leading methods in different regions include hanging, pesticide poisoning, and firearms. These differences are believed to be in part due to availability of the different methods. Hanging is the most common method in most of the countries, accounting for 53% of the male suicides and 39% of the female suicides.

Worldwide, 30% of suicides are estimated to occur from pesticide poisoning, most of which occur in the developing countries. The use of this method varies markedly from 4% in Europe to more than 50% in the Pacific region. It is also common in Latin American due to easy access of the farming populations. In many countries, drug overdoses account for approximately 60% of suicides among women and 30% among men. Many are unplanned and occur during an acute period of ambivalence. The death rate varies by method: firearms 80%–90%, drowning 65%–80%, hanging 60%–85%, car exhaust 40%–60%, jumping 35%–60%, charcoal burning 40%–50%, pesticides 6%–75%, and medication overdose 1.5%–4%. The most common attempted methods of suicide differ from the most common successful methods; up to 85% of attempts are via drug overdose in the developed world. In China, the consumption of pesticides is the most common method.

19.1.3 Features of suicide

19.1.3.1 Gender differences

Globally as of 2012, death by suicide occurs about 1.8 times more often in males than females. In Western countries, males die three to four times more often by means of suicide than do females. This difference is even more in those over the age of 65, with tenfold more in males than females dying by suicide. Suicide attempts and self-harm are between two and four times more frequent among females. Researchers have attributed the difference between attempted and completed suicides among the sexes to male using more lethal means to end their lives. However, separating intentional suicide attempts from non-suicidal self-harm is not currently done in the United States when gathering statistics at the national level. In most countries of the world, the sex ratio(male to female) of completed suicides is around 3 : 1, and at the same time, women attempt suicide approximately three times more often than men. However, studies in China present a different picture. Studies in local samples show that the male : female ratio of suicide is about 1 : 1, while most other studies show that women committed suicide more often than males.

Due in part to social stigmatization and the resulting depression, people whose gender identity does not align with their assigned sex are at a high risk of suicide. A number of reviews have found an increased risk of suicide among transgender, lesbian, gay, and bisexual people. The rate among transgender people of attempted suicide is between 30% and 50%.

19.1.3.2 Age difference

For all demographic groups, suicide is rare before puberty, though mass media reports that suicide among young people has increased in recent years. Generally, rates increase in nearly direct proportion to age, with the highest suicide rates in the elderly and a peak in the 19−34 age group. Studies in Western countries reveal that the suicide rate of adolescents and young has increased since 1950. Studies in China show that the age distribution of suicide follows the general picture of Western countries, but that the peak suicide rate in the 15−34 age group is much higher. According to a widely cited study suicide is the leading cause of death in individuals between 15−34 years of age, accounting for 18.9% of all deaths(Phillips et al. 2002). The average suicide rate of this age group was 26.0/100,000 from 1995 to 1999, while at the same stage the average suicide rate of the group aged 60−84 was 68.0/100,000.

19.1.3.3 Difference between rural and urban residents

In China, almost all epidemiological studies reveal that the suicide rate of rural residents is 3−5 times higher than that of their urban counterparts. Generally, the suicide rate is over 25/100,000 in Chinese rural areas, much higher than the world average. A methodological question of this comparison is that suicide statistics only covered regular residents in cities. Currently, we don't know how the urban suicide rate will change if suicide of mobile workers from rural areas are counted.

19.1.4 Explanations of the unique features of suicide in China

To summarize, the main feature of suicide in China is that rural females have a higher suicide rate than expected according to statistics from many areas across the world. Although there has been no systematic investigation of this unique pattern of suicide, several theories have been put forward to explain the phenomena. First, the availability of pesticides and other poison substances may convert a significant proportion of rural female suicide attempters into completed suicides. In Western countries, suicide attempts in females are more numerous than in males, and the usual method is poisoning by different types of medications. In China, the equivalent means for poisoning are pesticides, which are a lot more toxic and more often lead to suicide. Limiting access to poisons, thus has been suggested to be a priority in suicide prevention in China by many domestic and international researchers.

Second, the health care system in Chinese rural areas is often not qualified when a suicide attempter needs emergency rescue. Clinics in villages are accessible to most suicide attempters, but there is barely any equipment or technology to rescue individuals with pesticide ingestion. Health care providers in village clinics generally receive less than 2 years of medical training. About half of the health stations and all county general hospitals can provide qualified emergency service to suicide attempters, but in many cases, suicide attempters have died before they are sent to such institutions for help, as there is no convenient transportation available and the distance to qualified institutions is often too far.

Third, mental health service is not available in most Chinese rural areas. Less than 50% of counties (the population size of most counties vary from 300,000 to 1,500,000) have a mental hospital providing basic service to patients with psychotic disorders. Most rural health care providers only receive three years or less of medical education and have very limited knowledge and skills in mental health. As a result, it is estimated that only 5% of patients with depression and 30% of the patients with schizophrenia receive systematic treatment. There has been no crisis intervention and suicide prevention in Chinese rural areas until today.

Finally, socio-economic and cultural variables such as stigmatization, pressure on delivering male babies, poverty due to low educational level and low socio-economic status may contribute to distress and to the high suicide rate of rural women.

19.2 Risk factors

Factors that affect the risk of suicide include mental disorders, drug misuse, psychological states, cultural, family and social situations, and genetics. Mental disorders and substance frequently co-exist. Other risk factors include having previously attempted suicide, the ready availability of a means to take one's life, a family history of suicide, or the presence of traumatic brain injury. Socio-economic problems such as unemployment, poverty, homelessness, and discrimination may trigger suicidal thoughts. 15%-40% of people leave a suicide note. Genetics appears to account for between 38% and 55% of suicidal behaviors.

19.2.1 Biological factors

19.2.1.1 Biological markers

Developing sensitive prediction models for suicide and suicide attempt is crucial for prevention but is difficult due to the multiplicity of contributory risk factors and the low base rate of suicidal behavior. Anomalies are several biological systems have been associated with suicidal behavior in mood disorders and prospective biological studies, while not yet conclusive, suggest some potential for prediction based on biological measures. Meta-analysis of prospective studies of completed suicide shows that cerebrospinal fluid (CSF) 5-hydroxyindoleacetic acid (5-HIAA) levels and dexamethasone non-suppression yielded odds ratios for prediction of suicide of 4.48 and 4.65 respectively. Given the multi-determined nature of suicidal behavior no one biological index will be adequate to predict suicidal behavior, however including multiple biological markers in a model, for example CSF 5-HIAA and dexamethasone response, in order to assess both trait and state related risks may increase predictive power. Including more than one tests result in some trade-off of sensitivity(requiring a positive result on any single test)versus specificity(requiring a positive result on more than one test). Therefore, also integrating other biological tests reviewed elsewhere, into multivariate predictive models alongside clinical and genetic risk factors to develop still more sensitive and specific predictive models, is a major challenge for this field of research.

19.2.1.2   Neuroimaging of suicidal behavior

Consistent evidence implicates serotonin system dysfunction in the neurobiology of suicidal behavior. Neuroimaging studies link brain structure and function in vivo and contribute to our understanding of neural pathways. Areas of the prefrontal cortex and limbic structures are targeted in neuroimaging studies of suicidal behavior, which have focused on structural, hemodynamic, metabolic, and neuroreceptor changes in the brains of suicide attempters. Neuroimaging studies have revealed that signal hyperintensities, perfusion and metabolic abnormalities, processing of affect and serotonin receptor and transporter changes, may each play a role. Knowledge regarding the neurobiology of suicidal behavior must rely on study designs utilizing robust methodologies, including improve patient and control group selection, improved neuroimaging techniques, and adequate statistical analysis to enhance the validity, consistency, and conclusiveness of the data. Ongoing development of new radioligands and imaging methodologies promise to enhance our ability to delineate the neurobiology of suicidal acts.

19.2.1.3   The genetics of suicide

More systemic approaches are needed when interpreting "local" alterations, since e. g. , the prefrontal cortex-hippocampus-central amygdala-HPA tend to function as one operational unit, by the effects of many functional interactions wherein each part contributes in its unique manner. Furthermore, more/novel(biological) endophenotypes, which better reflect these interactions, may be informative(novel, "common denominators"), such as long-term potentiation in hippocampus/BDNF levels and other subreceptor intracellular processes. Novel psychobiological pathways identified may shed light on the interacting processes related to stress response, as identified by e. g. , genome-wide approaches. The temporal aspects of stress exposure, i. e. , duration and time point in development, are also of crucial importance in the shaping of the suicidal brain; therefore, this aspect of environmental exposure must be continuously included. In all this, the influence of the individual's genetic set-up must be determined at all stages of discovery, since it is of major importance for the function of all neurobiological process. To summarize, it seems that suicidal vulnerability appears through changes in the brain's neurobiology, which occur in its development, being influenced by environmental exposures and the genetic set-up of the individual, and that such changes may produce life-lasting psychobiological alterations of brain structure and function, e. g. , epigenetic mechanisms. To this end, progress in the field is continuing to evolve rapidly and knowledge emanate with greater detail from the original discoveries described here, enabling the development of better tools for prevention, diagnosis and treatment of suicidality in the future.

19.2.1.4   Mental disorders

Mental disorders are often present at the time of suicide with estimates ranging from 27% to more than 90%. In Asia, rates of mental disorders appear to be lower than in Western countries. Of those who have been admitted to a psychiatric unit, their lifetime risk of completed suicide is about 8.6%. Half of all people who die by suicide may have major depressive disorder; having this or one of the other mood disorders such as bipolar disorder increases the risk of suicide 20-fold. Other conditions implicated include schizophrenia(14%), personality disorders(8%), bipolar disorder, obsessive-compulsive disorder, and posttraumatic stress disorder. Others estimate that about half of people who complete suicide could be diagnosed with a personality disorder with borderline personality disorder being the most common. About 5% people with schizophrenia die of suicide. Eating disorders are another high risk condition.

19.2.1.5 Medical conditions

There is an association between suicidality and physical health problems such as chronic pain, traumatic brain injury, cancer, kidney failure(requiring hemodialysis), HIV, and systemic lupus erythematous. The diagnosis of cancer approximately doubles the subsequent risk of suicide. The prevalence of increased suicidality persisted after adjusting for depressive illness and alcohol abuse. Sleep disturbances such as insomnia and sleep apnea are risk factors for depression and suicide. In some instances the sleep disturbances may be a risk factor independent of depression. A number of other medical conditions may present with symptoms similar to mood disorders, including hypothyroidism, Alzheimer's disease, brain tumors, systemic lupus erythematous, and adverse effects from a number of medications (such as beta blockers and steroids).

19.2.2 Psychological factors

It is reported that psychiatric disorders are present in at least 90% of suicides. Depression is the most frequently cited illness linked with suicide, followed by schizophrenia, alcohol abuse disorder, other substance abuse disorders and personality disorder. Recent life stresses such as a loss of a family member or friend, loss of a job, or social isolation(such as living alone) increase the risk. Those who have never married are also at greater risk. Being religious may reduce one's risk of suicide. This has been attributed to the negative stance many religions take against suicide and to the greater connectedness religion may give. Some may take their own lives to escape bullying or prejudice. A history of childhood sexual abuse and time spent in foster care are also risk factors.

In China, retrospective studies utilizing the official death registry report that less than one-third of all suicides have a diagnosis of mental disorders. These studies underestimate the prevalence of mental disorders among those who commit suicide because disorders remain under-diagnosed and under-reported in the death registry. Recently, more rigorous psychological autopsy studies show that about two-thirds of all suicides have a diagnosis of mental disorder. This figure is still much lower than those reported in Western countries.

19.2.3 Social factors

Comparisons of the rates of suicide between and within different countries have been conducted over a period of many years. Many studies have demonstrated that areas with high unemployment, poverty, divorce, and social fragmentation have higher rates of suicide. Such studies can not be used as a means of examining the characteristics of individuals who kill themselves, but they do provide important information about factors within society that may affect the rate of suicide. Another social factor that appears to affect rates of suicide is media coverage of suicide. Suicide and attempted suicide rates were shown to increase after television programs and films depicting suicide. High-profile suicides sometimes affect the means and timing of a suicide. The precise nature of the media content may also be influential in increasing or decreasing the risk of imitative behavior.

19.2.4 Substance use

Substance abuse is the second most common risk factor for suicide after major depression and bipolar disorder. Both chronic substance misuse as well as acute intoxication are associated. When combined with personal grief, such as bereavement, the risk is further increased. Substance misuse is also associated with mental health disorders.

Most people are under the influence of sedative−hypnotic drugs(such as alcohol or benzodiazepines) when they die by suicide with alcoholism present in between 15% and 61% of cases. Use of prescribed benzodiazepines is associated with an increased rate of attempted and completed suicide. The prosuicidal effects of benzodiazepines are suspected to be due to a psychiatric disturbance caused by side effects or withdrawal symptoms. Countries that have higher rates of alcohol use and a greater density of bars generally also have higher rates of suicide. 2.2%−3.4% of those who have been treated for alcoholism die by suicide at some point in their life. Alcoholics who attempt suicide are usually male, older, and have tried to take their own lives in the past. In adolescents who misuse alcohol, neurological and psychological dysfunctions may contribute to the increased risk of suicide.

The misuse of cocaine and methamphetamine has a high correlation with suicide. In those who use cocaine the risk is greatest during the withdrawal phase. Those who used inhalants are also at significant risk with around 20% attempting suicide at some point and more than 65% considering it. Smoking cigarettes is associated with risk of suicide. There is little evidence as to why this association exists; however it has been hypothesized that those who are predisposed to smoking are also predisposed to suicide, that smoking causes health problems that subsequently make people want to end their life, and that smoking affects brain chemistry causing a propensity for suicide.

19.3 Assessment of patients with suicidal behaviors

19.3.1 Overview

The assessment of the suicidal patient is an ongoing process that comprises many interconnected elements. In addition, there are a number of points during patients' evaluation and treatment at which a suicide assessment may be indicated.

The ability of the psychiatrist to connect with the patient, establish rapport, and demonstrate empathy is an important ingredient of the assessment process. For suicidal patients who are followed on an ongoing basis, the doctor−patient relationship will provide the base from which risk and protective factors continue to be identified and from which therapeutic interventions, such as psychotherapies and pharmacotherapies, are offered.

At the core of the suicide assessment, the psychiatric evaluation will provide information about the patient's history, current circumstances, and mental state and will include direct questioning about suicidal thinking and behaviors. This evaluation, in turn, will enable the psychiatrist to identify specific factors and features that may increase or decrease the potential risk for suicide or other suicidal behaviors. These factors and features may include developmental, biomedical, psychopathologic, psychodynamic, and psychosocial aspects of the patient's current presentation and history, all of which may serve as modifiable targets for both acute and ongoing interventions. Such information will also be important in addressing the patient's immediate safety, determining the most appropriate setting for treatment, and developing a multiaxial differential diagnosis that will further guide the planning of treatment.

Although the approach to the suicidal patient is common to all individuals regardless of diagnosis or clinical presentation, the breadth and depth of the psychiatric evaluation will vary with the setting of the assessment; the ability or willingness of the patient to provide information; and the availability of information from previous contacts with the patient or from other sources, including other mental health professionals, medical records, and family members. In some circumstances, the urgency of the situation or the presence of substance intoxication may necessitate making a decision to facilitate patient safety (e. g. , instituting hospitalization or one-to-one observation) before all relevant information has been obtained. Furthermore, when working with a team of other professionals, the psychiatrist may not obtain all information him-or herself but will need to provide leadership for assessment process so that necessary information is obtained and integrated into a final assessment. Since the patient may minimize the severity or even the existence of his or her difficulties, other individuals may be valuable resources for the psychiatrist in providing information about the patient's current mental state, activities, and psychosocial crises. Such individuals may include the patient's family members and friends but may also include other physicians, other medical or mental health professionals, teachers or other school personnel, and other settings where the patient resides.

19.3.2　Conduct a thorough psychiatric evaluation

The psychiatric evaluation is the core element of the suicide risk assessment. This section provides an overview of the key aspects of the psychiatric evaluation as they relate to the assessment of patients with suicidal behaviors. Although the factors that are associated with an increased or decreased risk of suicide differ from the factors associated with an increased or decreased risk of suicide attempts, it is important to identify factors modulating the risk of any suicidal behaviors. Table 19-1 presents important domains of a suicide assessment.

Table 19-1　Characteristics evaluated in the psychiatric assessment of patients with suicidal behavior

(1) Current presentation of suicidality

1) Suicidal or self-harming thoughts, plans, behaviors, and intent

2) Specific methods considered for suicide, including their lethality and the patient's expectation about lethality, as well as whether firearms are accessible

3) Evidence of hopelessness, impulsiveness, anhedonia, panic attacks, or anxiety

4) Reasons for living and plans for the future

5) Alcohol or other substance use associated with the current presentation

6) Thoughts, plans, or intentions of violence toward others

(2) Psychiatric illnesses

1) Current signs and symptoms of psychiatric disorders with particular attention to mood disorders (primarily major depressive disorder or mixed episodes), schizophrenia, substance use disorders, anxiety disorders, and personality disorders (primarily borderline and antisocial personality disorders)

2) Previous psychiatric diagnoses and treatments, including illness onset and course and psychiatric hospitalizations, as well as treatment for substance use disorders

(3) History

1) Previous suicide attempts, aborted suicide attempts, or other self-harming behaviors

Continue to Table 19-1

2)Previous or current medical diagnoses and treatments, including surgeries or hospitalizations

3)Family history of suicide or suicide attempts or a family history of mental illness, including substance abuse

(4)Psychosocial situation

1)Acute psychosocial crises and chronic psychosocial stressors, which may include actual or perceived interpersonal losses, financial difficulties or changes in socioeconomic status, family discord, domestic violence, and past or current sexual or physical abuse or neglect

2)Employment status, living situation(including whether or not there are infants or children in the home), and presence or absence of external supports

3)Family constellation and quality of family relationships

4)Cultural or religious beliefs about death or suicide

(5)Individual strengths and vulnerabilities

1)Coping skills

2)Personality traits

3)Past responses to stress

4)Capacity for reality testing

5)Ability to tolerate psychological pain and satisfy psychological needs

19.3.3   Specifically inquire about suicidal thoughts, plans, and behaviors

In general, the more an individual has thought about suicide, has made specific plans for suicide, and intends to act on those plans, the greater will be his or her risk. Thus, as part of the suicide assessment it is essential to inquire specifically about the patient's suicidal thoughts, plans, behaviors, and intent. Although such questions will often flow naturally from discussion of the patient's current situation, this will not invariably be true. The exact wording of questions and the extent of questioning will also differ with the clinical situation. Examples of issues that the psychiatrist may address in this portion of the suicide assessment are given in Table 19-2.

Table 19-2   Questions that may be helpful in inquiring about specific
aspects of suicidal thoughts, plans, and behaviors

(1)Begin with questions that address the patient's feelings about living

1)Have you ever felt that life was not worth living?

2)Did you ever wish you could go to sleep and just not wake up?

(2)Follow up with specific questions that ask about thoughts of death, self-harm, or suicide

1)Is death something you've thought about recently?

2)Have things ever reached the point that you've thought of harming yourself?

(3)For individuals who have thoughts of self-harm or suicide

1)When did you first notice such thoughts?

2)What led up to the thoughts(e. g. , interpersonal and psychosocial precipitants, including real or imagined losses; specific symptoms such as mood changes, anhedonia, hopelessness, anxiety, agitation, psychosis)?

3)How often have those thoughts occurred(including frequency, obsessional quality, controllability)?

4)How close have you come to acting on those thoughts?

Continue to Table 19-2

5) How likely do you think it is that you will act on them in the future?

6) Have you ever started to harm(or kill) yourself but stopped before doing something(e. g. ,holding knife or gun to your body but stopping before acting,going to edge of bridge but not jumping)?

7) What do you envision happening if you actually killed yourself(e. g. ,escape,reunion with significant other,rebirth,reactions of others)?

8) Have you made a specific plan to harm or kill yourself? (If so,what does the plan include?)

9) Do you have guns or other weapons available to you?

10) Have you made any particular preparations(e. g. ,purchasing specific items,writing a note or a will,making financial arrangements,taking steps to avoid discovery,rehearsing the plan)?

11) Have you spoken to anyone about your plans?

12) How does the future look to you?

13) What things would lead you to feel more(or less) hopeful about the future(e. g. ,treatment,reconciliation of relationship,resolution of stressors)?

14) What things would make it more(or less) likely that you would try to kill yourself?

15) What things in your life would lead you to want to escape from life or be dead?

16) What things in your life make you want to go on living?

17) If you began to have thoughts of harming or killing yourself again,what would you do?

(4) For individuals who have attempted suicide or engaged in self-damaging action(s) ,parallel questions to those in the previous section can address the prior attempt(s). Additional questions can be asked in general terms or can refer to the specific method used and may include:

1) Can you describe what happened(e. g. ,circumstances,precipitants,view of future,use of alcohol or other substances, method,intent,seriousness of injury)?

2) What thoughts were you having beforehand that led up to the attempt?

3) What did you think would happen(e. g. ,going to sleep versus injury verses dying,getting a reaction out of a particular person)?

4) Were other people present at the time?

5) Did you seek help afterward yourself,or did someone get help for you?

6) Had you planned to be discovered,or were you found accidentally?

7) How did you feel afterward(e. g. ,relief versus regret at being alive)?

8) Did you receive treatment afterward(e. g. ,medical versus psychiatric,emergency department versus inpatient versus outpatient)?

9) Has your view of things changed,or is anything different for you since the attempt?

10) Are there other times in the past when you've tried to harm(or kill) yourself?

(5) For individuals with repeated suicidal thoughts or attempts

1) About how often have you tried to harm(or kill) yourself?

2) When was the most recent time?

3) Can you describe your thoughts at the time that you were thinking most seriously about suicide?

4) When was your most serious attempt at harming or killing yourself?

5) What led up to it, and what happened afterward?

(6) For individuals with psychosis, ask specifically about hallucinations and delusions

1) Can you describe the voices (e. g. , single versus multiple, male versus female, internal versus external, recognizable versus nonrecognizable)?

2) What do the voices say (e. g. , positive remarks versus negative remarks versus threats)? (If the remarks are commands, determine if they are for harmless versus harmful acts; ask for examples)?

3) How do you cope with (or respond to) the voices?

4) Have you ever done what the voices ask you to do? (What led you to obey the voices? If you tried to resist them, what made it difficult?)

5) Have there been times when the voices told you to hurt or kill yourself? (How often? What happened?)

6) Are you worried about having a serious illness or that your body is rotting?

7) Are you concerned about your financial situation even when others tell your there's nothing to worry about?

8) Are there things that you've been feeling guilty about or blaming yourself for?

(7) Consider assessing the patient's potential to harm others in addition to him-or herself

1) Are there others who you think may be responsible for what you're experiencing (e. g. , persecutory ideas, passivity experiences)? Are you having any thoughts of harming them?

2) Are there other people you would want to die with you?

3) Are there others who you think would be unable to go on without you?

19. 3. 3. 1 Elicit the presence or absence of suicidal ideation

Inquiring about suicidal ideation is an essential component of the suicide assessment. Although some fear that raising the topic of suicide will "plant" the issue in the patient's mind, this is not the case. In fact, broaching the issue of suicidal ideation may be a relief for the suicidal patient by opening an avenue for discussion and giving him or her an opportunity to feel understood.

In asking about suicidal ideas, it is often helpful to begin with questions that address the patient's feelings about living, such as, "how does life seem to you at this point?" "have you ever felt that life was not worth living?" or "did you ever wish you could go to sleep and just not wake up?" If the patient's response reflects dissatisfaction with life or a desire to escape it, this response can lead naturally into more specific questions about whether the patient has had thoughts of death or suicide. When such thoughts are elicited, it is important to focus on the nature, frequency, extent, and timing of them and to understand the interpersonal, situational, and symptomatic context in which they are occurring.

Even if the patient initially denies thoughts of death or suicide, the psychiatrist should consider asking additional questions. Examples might include asking about plans for the future or about recent acts or thoughts of self-harm. Regardless of the approach to the interview, not all individuals will report having suicidal ideas even when such thoughts are present. Thus, depending on the clinical circumstances, it may be important for the psychiatrist to speak with family members or friends to determine whether they have observed behavior or have been privy to thoughts that suggest suicidal ideation. In addition, patients who are initially interviewed when they are intoxicated with alcohol or other substances should be reassessed for suicidality once the intoxication has resolved.

19.3.3.2 Elicit the presence or absence of a suicide plan

If suicidal ideation is present, the psychiatrist will next probe for more detailed information about specific plans for suicide and any steps that have been taken toward enacting those plans. Although some suicidal acts can occur impulsively with little or no planning, more detailed plans are generally associated with a greater suicide risk. Violent and irreversible methods, such as firearms, jumping, and motor vehicle accidents, require particular attention. However, the patient's belief about the lethality of the method may be as important as the actual lethality of the method itself.

If the patient does not report a plan, the psychiatrist can ask whether there are certain conditions under which the patient would consider suicide(e. g. , divorce, going to jail, housing loss) or whether it is likely that such a plan will be formed or acted on in the near future. If the patient reports that he or she is unlikely to act on the suicidal thoughts, the psychiatrist should determine what factors are contributing to that expectation, as such questioning can identify protective factors.

19.3.3.3 Assess the degree of suicidality, including suicidal intent and lethality of plan

Regardless of whether the patient has developed a suicide plan, the patient's level of suicidal intent should be explored. Suicidal intent reflects the intensity of a patient's wish to die and can be assessed by determining the patient's motivation for suicide as well as the seriousness and extent of his or her aim to die, including any associated behaviors or planning for suicide. If the patient has developed a suicide plan, it is important to assess its lethality. The lethality of the plan can be ascertained through questions about the method, the patient's knowledge and skill concerning its use, and the absence of intervening persons or protective circumstances. In general, the greater and clearer the intent, the higher the risk for suicide will be. Thus, even a patient with a low-lethality suicide plan or attempt may be at high risk in the future if intentions are strong and the patient believes that the chosen method will be fatal. At the same time, a patient with low suicidal intent may still die from suicide by erroneously believing that a particular method is not lethal.

19.3.3.4 Understand the relevance and limitations of suicide assessment scales

Although a number of suicide assessment scales have been developed for use in research, their clinical utility is limited. Self-report rating scales may sometimes assistin opening communication with the patient about particular feelings or experiences. In addition, the content of suicide rating scales, such as the Scale for Suicide Ideationand the Suicide Intent Scale, may be helpful to psychiatrists in developing a thorough line of questioning about suicide and suicidal behaviors. However, existing suicide assessment scales suffer from high false positive and false negative rates and have very low positive predictive values. As a result, such rating scales can not substitute for thoughtful and clinically appropriate evaluation and are not recommended for clinical estimations of suicide risk.

19.3.4 Establish a multiaxial diagnosis

In conceptualizing suicide risk, it is important for the psychiatrist to develop a multiaxial differential diagnosis over the course of the psychiatric evaluation. Studies have shown that more than 90% of individuals who die by suicide satisfy the criteria for one or more psychiatric disorders. Thus, the psychiatrist should determine whether a patient has a primary axis Ⅰ or axis Ⅱ diagnosis. Suicide and other suicidal behaviors are also more likely to occur in individuals with more than one psychiatric diagnosis. As a result, it is important to note other current or past axis Ⅰ or axis Ⅱ diagnoses, including those that may currently be in remission.

Identification of physical illness(axis Ⅲ) is essential since such diagnoses may also be associated with an increased risk of suicide as well as with an increased risk of other suicidal behaviors. For some individuals, this increase in risk may result from increased rates of comorbid psychiatric illness or from the direct physiological effects of physical illness or its treatment. Physical illnesses may also be a source of social and/or psychological stress, which in turn may augment risk.

Also crucial in determining suicide risk is the recognition of psychosocial stressors(axis Ⅳ), which may be either acute or chronic. Certain stressors, such as sudden unemployment, interpersonal loss, social isolation, and dysfunctional relationships, can increase the likelihood of suicide attempts as well as increase the risk of suicide. At the same time, it is important to note that life events have different meanings for different individuals. Thus, in determining whether a particular stressor may confer risk for suicidal behavior, it is necessary to consider the perceived importance and meaning of the life event for the individual patient.

As the final component of the multiaxial diagnosis, the patient's baseline and current levels of functioning are important to assess(axis Ⅴ). Also, the clinician should assess the relative change in the patient's level of functioning and the patient's view of and feelings about his or her functioning. Although suicidal ideation and/or suicide attempts are reflected in the Global Assessment of Functioning(GAF) scoring recommendations, it should be noted that there is no agreed-on correlation between a GAF score and level of suicide risk.

19.3.5　Estimate suicide risk

The goal of the suicide risk assessment is to identify factors that may increase or decrease a patient's level of suicide risk, to estimate an overall level of suicide risk, and to develop a treatment plan that addresses patient safety and modifiable contributors to suicide risk. The assessment is comprehensive in scope, integrating knowledge of the patient's specific risk factors; clinical history, including psychopathological development; and interaction with the clinician. The estimation of suicide risk, at the culmination of the suicide assessment, is the quintessential clinical judgment, since no study has identified one specific risk factor or set of risk factors as specifically predictive of suicide or other suicidal behavior.

While risk factors are typically additive(i. e. , the patient's level of risk increases with the number of risk factors), they may also interact in a synergistic fashion. For example, the combined risk associated with comorbid depression and physical illness may be greater than the sum of the risk associated with each in isolation. At the same time, certain risk factors, such as a recent suicide attempt(especially one of high lethality), access to poison, and the presence of a suicide note, should be considered serious in and of themselves, regardless of whether other risk factors are present.

The effect on suicide risk of some risk factors, such as particular life events or psychological strengths and vulnerabilities, will vary on an individual basis. Risk factors must also be assessed in context, as certain risk factors are more applicable to particular diagnostic groups, while others carry more general risk. Finally, it should be kept in mind that, because of the low rate of suicide in the population, only a small fraction of individuals with a particular risk factor will die from suicide.

Risk factors for suicide attempts, which overlap with but are not identical to risk factors for suicide, will also be identified in the assessment process. These factors should also be addressed in the treatment planning process, since suicide attempts themselves are associated with morbidity in addition to the added risk that they confer for suicide.

Case report:

Mr. S. was an 85-year-old male whose wife died about a month later after placement in a community nursing home. Mr. and Mrs. S. had no children. Mr. S. was also the last one alive out of five siblings. The only support system Mr. S. had was a nephew by marriage and his nephew's wife who had recently moved about 2 hours away. With his wife's death and the relocation of Mr. S. 's nephew, he had lost his support system.

Mr. S. had multiple diagnoses including depression, substance abuse (alcohol), arthritis, and a history of bladder cancer with intermittent hematuria, hypertension, and hylerlipidemia. He had four vessel coronary artery bypass grafting in 1989. In 2003, he had placement of four cardiacstents, and in 2004, insertion of implantable cardiac defibrillator. He also suffered from hearing loss, mild dementia, and herpes zoster that left him with residual, chronic pain. Other than a mildly elevated lipid panel, his lab results were essentially within normal limits. A recent echocardiogram showed his ejection fraction was decreased to 30% (a normal ejection fraction is between 55% to 65%).

The nurse conducted a short form Geriatric Depression Scale on admission in which Mr. S. scored 12/15 representing depression. Mr. S. had been diagnosed and treated for depression 2 years ago when his wife's health had worsened.

19.4 Suicide prevention

Suicide prevention strategies focus on reducing the risk factors and intervening strategically to reduce the level of risk. Risk and protective factors, unique to the individual can be assessed by a qualified mental health professional. Some of the specific strategies used to address are: crisis intervention; structured counseling and psychotherapy; hospitalization for those with low adherence to collaboration for help and those who require monitoring and secondary symptom treatment; supportive therapy like substance treatment, psychotropic medication, family psychoeducation and access to emergency phone call care with emergency rooms, suicide prevention hotlines, etc. ; restricting access to lethality of suicide means through policies and laws; creating and using crisis cards, an uncluttered card formatted readably that describes list of activities one should follow in crisis still the positive behavior responses settles in the personality; person–centered life skills training. For example problem solving; registering with support groups like alcoholics anonymous, suicide bereavement support group, religious group with flow rituals; therapeutic recreational therapy that improves mood; motivating self–care activities like physical exercise's and meditative relaxation. Psychotherapies that have shown most successful or evidence based are dialectical behavior therapy (DBT), it has shown to be helpful in reducing suicide attempts and reducing hospitalizations for suicidal ideation and cognitive therapy (CBT), it has shown to improve problem–solving and coping abilities. In young adults who have recently thought about suicide, cognitive behavioral therapy appears to improve outcomes. Economic development through its ability to reduce poverty may be able to decrease suicide rates. Efforts to increase social connection, especially in elderly males, may be effective. The World Suicide Prevention Day is observed annually on September 10 with the support of the International Association for Suicide Prevention and the WHO.

19.4.1 Interventions

Many methods of intervention have been developed to intercede before suicide is attempted. The general methods include: direct talks, screening for risks, lethal means reduction and social intervention.

19.4.1.1 Direct talks

The WHO has noted a very effective way to assess suicidal thoughts is to talk with a person directly, to ask about depression, and assesssuicide plans as to how and when it might be attempted. Contrary to popular misconceptions, talking with people about suicide does not plant the idea in their heads. However, such discussions and questions should be asked with care, concern and compassion. The tactic is to reduce sadness and provide assurance that other people care. The WHO advises to not say everything will be all right nor make the problem seem trivial, nor give false assurances about serious issues. The discussions should be gradual and specifically executed when the person is comfortable about discussion his or her feelings. ICARE(identify the thought, connect with it, assess evidences for it, restructure the thought in positive light, express or provide room for expressing feelings from the restructured thought) is a model of approach used here.

19.4.1.2　Screening

Screening to detect those at risk of suicide may be one of the most effective means of preventing suicide in children and adolescent. There are various screening tools in the form of self-report questionnaires to help identify those at risk such as the Beck Hopelessness Scale or the Geriatric Depression scale for older people. There is however a high rate of false-positive identification and those deemed to be at risk should ideally have a follow-up clinical interview. The predictive quality of these screening questionnaires has not been conclusively validated so it is not possible to determine if those identified at risk of suicide will actually commit suicide. Asking about or screening for suicide does not create or increase the risk.

19.4.1.3　Suicide prevention by lethal means reduction

Means reduction, reducing the odds that a suicide attempter will use highly lethal means, is an important component of suicide prevention. This practice is also called "means restriction". Researchers and health policy planners have theorized and demonstrated that restricting lethal means can help reduce suicide rates, as delaying action until depression passes. In general, strong evidence supports the effectiveness of means restriction in preventing suicides. There is also strong evidence that restricted access at so-called suicide hotspots, such as bridges and cliffs, reduces suicides, whereas other interventions such as placing signs or increasing surveillance at these sites appears less effective.

19.4.1.4　E-health intervention for suicide prevention

Many people at risk of suicide do not seek help before an attempt, and do not remain connected to health services following an attempt. E-health interventions are now being considered as a means to identify at-risk individuals, offer self-help through web interventions or to deliver proactive interventions in response to individuals' posts on social media. E-health interventions for suicide prevention can be classed into three categories. First, the Internet can be used to help individuals self-screen: to identify whether they might be at risk for suicide or a mental health problem. Through screening and feedback, it may be possible to increase service use, by directing at-risk individuals who would not otherwise seek help to access appropriate evidence-based online programs or to access traditional mental health services. Second, web applications, both guided and unguided, have been developed to provide psychological interventions to assist in reducing suicidal behavior and lowering suicidal ideation. Guided interventions involve a therapist or a researcher assisting the user through the program either through email or over the telephone, whereas unguided are self-help, automated programs which can be initiated and used directly by the public. The third type of intervention is one where a person is considered to be at risk of suicide because of the nature of their social media use. Here, status updates, comments or posts indicative of suicide ideation are used to classify those at risk. Such content can be identified in real-time by other users or by computerized language processing and progress in this area has accelerated.

19.4.1.5　Social intervention

American National Strategy for Suicide Prevention promotes and sponsors various specific suicide prevention endeavors.

(1) Developing groups led by professionally trained individuals for broad-based support for suicide prevention.

(2) Promoting community-based suicide prevention programs.

(3) Screening and reducing at-risk behavior through psychological resilience programs that promotes optimism and connectedness.

(4) Education about suicide, including risk factors, warning signs, stigma related issues and the availability of help through social campaigns.

(5) Increasing the proficiency of health and welfare services a responding to people in need. e. g. , sponsored training for helping professionals, Increased access to community linkages, employing crisis counseling organizations.

(6) Reducing domestic violence and substance abuse through legal and empowerment means are long-term strategies.

(7) Reducing access to convenient means of suicide and methods of self-harm. e. g. , toxic substances, poisons, handguns.

(8) Reducing the quantity of dosages supplied in packages of non-prescription medicines, e. g. , aspirin.

(9) School-based competency promoting and skill enhancing programs.

(10) Interventions and usage of ethical surveillance systems targeted at high-risk groups.

(11) Improving reporting and portrayals of negative behavior, suicidal behavior, mental illness and substance abuse in the entertainment and news media.

(12) Research on protective factors and development of effective clinical and professional practices.

19.4.1.6　Postvention

Postvention is for people affected by an individual's suicide, this intervention facilitates grieving, guides to reduce guilt, anxiety, and depression and to decrease the effects of trauma. Postvention is also provided to intervene to minimize the risk of imitative or copycat suicides, but there is a lack of evidence based standard protocol. But the general goal of the mental health practitioner is to decrease the likelihood of others identifying with the suicidal behavior of the deceased as a coping strategy in dealing with adversity.

19.4.2　Special groups

19.4.2.1　Older people

In most countries the highest rate of suicide is among people aged over 75 years. The most frequent methods are hanging among men, and drug overdose among women. In addition to active self-harm, some older adults die from deliberate self-neglect(e. g. , by refusing food or necessary treatment). As in younger age groups, depression is a strong predictor of suicide in the elderly. Other risk factors are social isolation and impaired physical health, although the latter may act in part through causing depression. Personality is also important, especially anxious and obsessional traits.

19.4.2.2　Adolescents

Suicide rates among adolescents have increased in recent years. A psychological autopsy study showed that about 70% of adolescents who killed themselves had had psychiatric disorders, mainly depressive and personality disorders, which were sometimes comorbid. Many of them had misused alcohol or drugs. The suicide was often the culmination of long – term difficulties with relationships and other psychosocial problems. Approximately two–thirds of these individuals had made a previous suicide attempt.

Optimal treatment of children and adolescents with suicidal behavior requires a continuum of services including emergency intervention, outpatient, home–based, day and inpatient treatment. In practice, however, this is often not possible due to lack of resources.

The first step in managing suicidality is to make sure that the child or adolescent at risk is safe and receives support. The management strategy depends on the level and changeability of risk and assessment confidence.

At the emergency department, young persons who have made a suicide attempt should be assessed by an experienced mental health professional, including interview with parents or relatives and a thorough risk assessment. Before discharge, it is essential to have prepared a plan to deal with crisis, making sure that supporting contact(e. g. , telephone) is available 24 hours a day.

In addition, a no–suicide contract may be helpful(formulated as a commitment by the patient and not as an insurance for the mental health professional since there is no empirical evidence that no–suicide contracts are actually effective). A no–suicide contract usually includes:①confirmation that the patient is not to endanger his life during short period(e. g. , the next day, until the next session with the therapist) ;②a commitment by the patient to adhere to the therapy;③a commitment by the patient to comply with the contingency plan.

The management of suicidality in youth requires clear communication with the young person and family. This also holds for contact with the school, which should always be attempted after obtaining permission from the young person and family.

19. 5　Crisis intervention

Crisis intervention is an immediate and short–term psychological care aimed at assisting individuals in a crisis situation to restore equilibrium to theirbiopsychosocial functioning and to minimize the potential for long–term psychological trauma. Crisis can be defined as one's perception or experiencing of an event or situation as an intolerable difficulty that exceeds the person's current resources and coping mechanisms.

The priority of crisis intervention and counseling is to increase stabilization. Crisis interventions occur at the spur of the moment and in a variety of settings, as trauma can arise instantaneously. Crises are temporary, usually with short span, no longer than a month, although the effects may become long–lasting. Crisis intervention is the emergency and temporary care given an individual who, because of unusual stress in his or her life that renders them unable to function as they normally would, in order to interrupt the downward spiral of maladaptive behavior and return the individual to their usual level of pre–crisis functioning.

19. 5. 1　Crisis

Crises can occur on a personal or societal level. Personal Trauma is defined as an individual's experience of a situation or event in which he/she perceives to have exhausted his/her coping skill, self–esteem, social support, and power. These can be situations where a person is making suicidal threats, experiencing threat, witnessing homicide or suicide, or experiencing personal loss. While a person is experiencing a crisis on the individual level it is important for counselors to primarily assess safety. Counselors are encouraged to ask questions pertaining to social supports and networks, as well as give referrals for long term care.

Societal or mass trauma can occur in a number of settings and typically affects a large group or society. A counselor's primary concern when called to these types of crisis is to assess people's awareness of resources. Individuals experiencing trauma in large scales need to be aware of shelters that offer food and water; places that meet their basic necessities for survival.

19.5.2　Signs of crisis

Counselors are encouraged to be aware of the typical responses of those who have experienced a crisis or currently struggling with the trauma. On the cognitive level they may blame themselves or others for the trauma. Often the person appears disoriented, becomes hypersensitive or confused, has poor concentration, uncertainty, and poor troubleshooting. Physical responses to trauma include: increased heart rate, tremors, dizziness, weakness, chills, headaches, vomiting, shock, fainting, sweating, and fatigue. Some emotional responses the person may experiences consist of apathy, depression, irritability, anxiety, panic, helplessness, hopelessness, anger, fear, guilt, and denial. When assessing behavior some typical responses to crisis are difficulty eating and/or sleeping, conflicts with others, withdrawal from social situations, and lack of interest in social activities.

19.5.3　Universal principles of crisis intervention

While dealing with crisis, both personal and social, there are five basic principles outlined for intervention. Victims are initially at high risk for maladaptive coping or immobilization. Intervening as quickly as possible is imperative. Resource mobilization should be immediately enacted in order to provide victims with the tools they need to return to some sort of order and normalcy, in addition to enable eventual independent functioning. The next step is to facilitate understanding of the event by processing the situation or trauma. This is done in order to help the victim gain a better understanding of what has occurred and allowing him or her to express feeling about the experience. Additionally, the counselor should assist the victim (s) in problem solving within the context of their situation and feelings. This is necessary for developing self−efficacy and self−reliance. Helping the victim get back to being able to function independently by actively facilitating problem solving, assisting in developing appropriate strategies for addressing those concerns, and in helping putting those strategies into action. This is done in hopes of assisting the victim to become self−reliant.

19.5.4　General approach

A general approach of crisis intervention integrates numerous assessment tools and triage procedures. Roberts 7 stage crisis intervention model, SAFER−R model and Lerner and Shelton's 10 step acute stress and trauma management protocol creates one comprehensive model for responding to crisis that can be utilized in most all crisis situations.

19.5.4.1　Roberts 7 stage crisis intervention model(the ACT model)

The Assessment Crisis Intervention Trauma Treatment(ACT) model of crisis intervention developed by Roberts outlines a three−stage framework. It is important to note that this should be followed as a guide not to be followed rigidly. The first step is the assessment stage; this is done by determining the needs of victims, other involved persons, survivors, their families, and grieving family members of possible victim(s) and making appropriate referrals when needed.

3 types of assessment need to be conducted.

（1）The first is triage assessment, which is an immediate assessment to determine lethality and determine appropriate referral to one of the following: emergency inpatient hospitalization, outpatient treatment facility or private therapist, or if no referral is needed.

（2）A crisis assessment also needs to be completed which consists of gathering information regarding the individual's crisis state, environment, and interpersonal relationships in order to work towards resolving the current crisis. This step helps facilitate development of an effective and appropriate treatment plan.

（3）The last area of assessment includes a biosocial and cultural assessment. This would be completed by using systematic assessment tools to ascertain the client's current level of stress, situation, present problem, and severe crisis episode.

The goal of the crisis intervention stage of Robert's ACT model is to resolve the client's presenting problems, stress, psychological trauma, and emotional conflicts. This is to be done with a minimum number of contacts, as crisis intervention is intended to be time limited and goal directed.

（1）Intake and assessing the person who is in crisis/suffering from the after effects of crisis

Stage one of the seven step approach focuses on assessing lethality. The clinician is to plan and conduct a thorough biopsychosocial and lethality/imminent danger assessment; this should be done promptly at the time of arrival. Once lethality is determined one should establish rapport with the victim(s) whom the clinician will be working with.

（2）Exploring the crisis situation of the person

The next phase is to identify major problem(s), including what in their life has led to the crisis at hand. During this stage it is important that the client is given the control and power to discuss their stories in his or her own words.

（3）Understanding the coping style employed by the person

While he or she is describing the situation, the intervention specialist should develop a conceptualization of the client's "model coping style", which will most likely need adjusting as more information unfolds. This is referred to as stage three.

（4）Confronting feelings, exploring emotions and challenging the maladaptive coping style

As a transition is made to stage four, feelings will become prevalent at this time, so dealing with those feelings will be an important aspect of the intervention. While managing the feelings, the counselor must allow the client(s) to express his or her story, and explore feelings and emotions through active listening and validation. Eventually, the counselor will have to work carefully to respond to the client using challenging responses in order to help him or her work past maladaptive beliefs and thoughts, and to think about other options.

（5）Exploring solutions and educating the client in best practices of coping

At step five, the victim and counselor should begin to collaboratively generate and explore alternatives for coping. Although this situation will be unlike any other experience before, the counselor should assist the individual in looking at what has worked in the past for other situations; this is typically the most difficult to achieve in crisis counseling.

（6）Developing a concrete treatment plan/structure of activities and reassuring the clients newly gained healthy perspective

Once a list has been generated, a shift can be made to step six: development of a treatment plan that serves to empower the client. The goal at this stage it to make the treatment plan as concrete as possible which could be followed by the client and implemented as an attempt to make meaning out of the crisis event. Having meaning of the situation is also an important part of this stage because it allows for gaining mastery.

(7)Follow-up

Step seven is for the intervention specialist to arrange for follow-up contact with the client to evaluate his or her post crisis condition in order to make certain resolution towards progressing. The follow-up plan may include "booster" sessions to explore treatment gains and potential problems.

19.5.4.2 SAFER-R model

The SAFER-R Model is a much-usedmodel of intervention with Roberts 7 Stage Crisis Intervention Model. The model approaches crisis intervention as an instrument to help the client to achieve his or her baseline level of functioning from the stage of crisis. This intervention model for responding to individuals in crisis consists of 5+1 stages.

They are: ①stabilize, ②acknowledged, ③facilitate understanding, ④encourage adaptive coping, ⑤restore functioning or, ⑥refer.

19.5.4.3 Lerner and Shelton's 10 step acute stress and trauma management protocol

A comprehensive view of how to treat the trauma consists of ten stages outlined by learner and Shelton (2001). These 10 steps relate similar to the crisis intervention steps.

(1)The first step is to assess for danger/safety for self and others, this means for the victim, counselor, and others who may have been affected by the trauma.

(2)Then consider the physical and perceptual mechanisms of injury.

(3)Once injury is assessed the victim's level of responsiveness should be evaluated.

(4)If any medical needs are there, it should be addressed.

(5)The individual who witnessed or is experiencing a crisis, should be observed to identify his or her signs of traumatic stress.

(6)After the assessment of the situation is completed the counselor should introduce his or her self, state their title and role, and connect with the individual by building rapport.

(7)A good rapport building allows for a more fluid approach in grounding the individual, this can be done by allowing the client/person to tell their story.

(8)The interventionist provides support through active and empathetic listening.

(9)Normalize, validate, and educate the individual's emotions, stress and adaptive coping styles.

(10)Finally, the intervention specialist is to bring the person to the present, describe future events, and provide referrals as needed.

After the crisis situation has been assessed and crisis interventions have been applied, the aim is at eliminating stress symptoms, thus treating the traumatic experience.

Kuang Li

Chapter 20

Somatotherapy for Mental Disorders

20.1　Introduction

Somatotherapy includes pharmacological therapy and physical therapy. Pharmacological therapy is the method that use psychiatric drugs change the thinking, abnormal behavior and mood of the patients. Psychotropic drugs are divided into traditional psychotropic drugs or the first generation of psychotropic drugs, and new psychotropic drugs or the second generation of psychotropic drugs. Many new drugs developed since late 1980s, with less adverse reactions, and is well-tolerated, known as the second generation of new psychotropic drugs or psychotropic drugs. Physical therapy refers to various psychiatric treatments except the psychotropic medication and psychological treatment, some of these methods were used before drug treatment, which proved to be effective and are still used now. Such as improved electroconvulsive therapy, it plays an important role in the clinical treatment of mental disorders, which has remarkable curative effect and good security. This chapter mainly introduces several physical treatment techniques, such as electric convulsive therapy, repetitive transcranial magnetic stimulation treatment, and some other physical therapies.

20.2　Psychotropic drugs treatment

20.2.1　Overview

Psychotropic drugs refers to drugs acting on the central nervous system, and psychotropic drug therapy is the treatment by application of psychotropic drugs to change the abnormal behavior, mood or thinking. At the beginning of the 1950s, the first synthetic chlorpromazine for the treatment of mental disorders emerged and ushered in a new era of modern psychotropic drugs. Over the past decades, a variety of drugs with different structure were developed, which greatly improve the treatment and prognosis of mental illness.

According to the clinical characteristics, psychotropic drugs are included:

(1) Antipsychotic drugs

It's a kind of drugs acting on the central nervous system, regulating neurotransmitter function, used for the treatment of schizophrenia and other psychotic symptoms.

(2) Antidepressant drugs

It's a kind of drugs through increased central neurotransmitters, which used for the treatment of various depression.

(3) Mood stabilizer or antimanic drugs

It's a kind of drugs used for treatment of mania and bipolar disorder.

(4) Anxiolytic drugs

It includes drugs which used for the treatment of the anxiety.

In addition, there are also psychostimulants for children suffer from attention deficit hyperactivity disorder (ADHD) and nootropic drugs to improve the circulation of the brain, and the metabolism of nerve cells.

The following principles should be followed in the clinical application of psychotropic drugs .

(1) The choice of psychotropic drugs for each patient should consider the gender, age, physical condition, first episode or recurrence, medical conditions, the use of other drugs and other factors of the patients.

(2) According to the main symptoms to select medicine, every psychiatric symptoms have diverse clinical manifestations, they are differences in different periods of disease symptoms or different patients. We choose appropriate drugs according to the symptoms in patients with the disease and the characteristics of the symptoms.

(3) The initial dose of antipsychotic drugs is small, according to the tolerance of patients with gradual dose titration. In order to obtain early curative effect, we can appropriate accelerate the speed of titration for the little side-effect and well tolerated patients. For antidepressants and anxiolyticdrugs, most of the initial dose is a therapeutic dose and don't require titration. When the drug dose reach the treatment range, it should be closely observed to determine an effective low dose as a therapeutic dose for the patients. When the full course of enough dose treatment is not effective, the treatment plan should be considered adjusting.

(4) Psychotropic drug have immediate release, sustained-release formulations, and long-acting injection. The choice of appropriate dosage form should be according to the patient's age, severity of disease, whether actively cooperate with the treatment and some special requirements, so as to improve patient compliance.

(5) Comprehensive evaluation of the efficacy and safety of the treatment, the choice of drugs should befollowed the above mentioned principles. Once the application of psychotropic drugs, not only to observe the remission of patients'symptoms, but also should closely observe and detect adverse reactions, so as not to appear serious adverse reactions, which will affect the tolerance and compliance of patient.

20.2.2　Antipsychotic drugs

20.2.2.1　Classification

Antipsychotic drugs include two categories: the first generation antipsychotics and second generation antipsychotic drugs, which are used to treat schizophrenia and other related mental disorders (Table 20-1).

(1) First generation antipsychotics (classical antipsychotic drugs or traditional antipsychotic drugs): the first generation antipsychotic drugs mainly act on D_2 receptor of central nervous system, which include

four categories.

1) Phenothiazines, include chlorpromazine, thioridazine, perphenazine, fluphenazine, trifluoperazine.

2) Thioxanthenes, include fluorine thioxanthenes, chlorprothixene.

3) Butyrophenones, include haloperidol, penfluridol.

4) Benzamides, such as sulpiride.

According to the clinical characteristics, the first generation antipsychotic drugs can be divided into two categories: low potency drugs and high potency drugs. The former with chlorpromazine as a representative, which has strong sedative effect, anticholinergic effect, toxicity to cardiovascular and liver, extrapyramidal side effect is fewer, and high dose for treatment. The latter with haloperidol as a representative, which is prominent for anti-hallucinations and delusions, weak sedative effect, weak toxicity to cardiovascular and liver, low dose for treatment, extrapyramidal side-effect is reavier.

The first generation antipsychotic drugs have some limitations. The negative symptoms improved were not obvious for some patients; 30% patients with positive symptoms improvement are not ideal. The incidence rates of extrapyramidal side effects are high, which cause a poor compliance. The first generation antipsychotic drugs can't effectively improve cognitive function, and the drug anti cholinergic effects may cause deterioration of memory. The patient's long-term social function were not improved, and affect the quality of work and life.

(2) Second generation antipsychotics have higher 5-serotonin type 2 (5-HT2) receptor blocking effect, namely dopamine(DA) receptor and 5-HT2R antagonist. They have higher selective effect on the mesolimbic system than the nigrostriatal system. Representative drugs like clozapine, olanzapine, quetiapine, ziprasidone, risperidone and its derivatives paliperidone, and so on. The second generation antipsychotic drugs are effective in positive symptoms, negative symptoms, cognitive function and emotional symptoms. They have small extrapyramidal side-effects, which increase patient compliance.

According to pharmacological effects, second generation antipsychotics are divided into 4 categories.

1) 5-HT and DA receptor antagonists(serotonin-dopamine, antagonists, SDAS), such as paliperidone, risperidone, ziprasidone and sertindole.

2) The multi receptor agonist(multi-acting receptor targeted agents, MARTAs), such as clozapine, quetiapine, olanzapine.

3) Selective D_2/D_3 antagonists, such as amisulpride.

4) D_2, 5-HT1A receptor partial agonists and 5-HT2A receptor antagonists, such as aripiprazole.

The side effects of second generation antipsychotics are mainly manifested in the following aspects.

1) EPS(the extrapyramidal reaction), the EPS incidence rate of second generation antipsychotics is relatively low, often occurs in high doses, such as risperidone, ziprasidone, amisulpride, aripiprazole.

2) The high blood prolactin cause menstrual disorders or lactation, such as risperidone and amisulpride.

3) Prolong the QTc interval of ECG, mainly in ziprasidone. In clinical, QTc extended >500 ms, or than the basic value increased >60 ms, can increase the risk of TDP(torsade de pointes), and cause the possible occurrence of sudden cardiac death.

4) Weight gain, clozapine and olanzapine are the most obvious. Ziprasidone and aripiprazole are less likely to cause weight gain. Weight gain is due to increased appetite and reduced activity, which are prone to diabetes, hyperlipidemia and hypertension. Life style intervention should be taken to patients.

Table 20-1　Classification and dosage range of common antipsychotic drugs

Classification of drug	Dosage range/(mg/d)	Half-life/hours
(1) First generation antipsychotics		
1) Phenothiazines		
Chlorpromazine	300-600	24
Thioridazine	300-600	24
Perphenazine	16-64	10
Trifluoperazine	15-50	24
Fluphenazine	5-20	33
Fluphenazinedecanoate	12.5-50 mg/2 weeks	
2) Thioxanthenes		
Chlorprothixene	300-600	30
3) Butyrophenones		
Haloperidol	5-20	21
Haloperidol decanoate	50-200 mg/4 weeks	
Penfluridol	20-120 mg/week	
4) Benzamides		
Sulpiride	600-1,200	8
5) Dibenzoxazepine		
Loxapine	30-100	4
(2) Second generation antipsychotics		
1) Benzisoxazole		
Risperidone	2-8	24
Paliperidone	3-12	
Paliperidonepalmitate	39-234 mg/4 weeks	
2) Benzisothiazole		
Ziprasidone	80-160	7
3) Dibenzodiazepines		
Clozapine	150-600	12
Olanzapine	10-20	33
4) Dibenzothiazepine		
Quetiapine	300-750	6
5) Benzamides		
Amisulpride	400-1,200	12
6) Quinolinone		
Aripiprazole	10-30	75

20.2.2.2 Mechanism of action

Antipsychotic drugs mainly act by blocking dopamine receptors and 5-serotonin receptors in the brain and have an antipsychotic effect, and they also produced various side effects. The blocking characteristics of antipsychotic drugs are described as follows.

(1)The blocking-effect of dopamine receptor is mainly blocking the D_2 receptor. There are 4 projection pathways in the dopaminergic system of the brain. The mesolimbic and subcortical pathways are associated with antipsychotic effects; the nigrostriatal pathway is associated with extrapyramidal side-effects; the tuberoinfundibular pathway from the hypothalamus to the pituitary is associated with the side-effects of elevated prolactin levels.

(2)The blocking-effect of 5-serotonin receptor is mainly blocking the 5-HT2A receptor. 5-HT blockers have potential antipsychotic effects. The high $5-HT2A/D_2$ receptor blocking ratio leads to lower extrapyramidal symptoms and improved negative symptoms.

(3)The blocking-effect of adrenergic receptors is mainly blocking the $\alpha-1$ receptor. It can produce sedation, orthostatic hypotension, tachycardia, sexual dysfunction, delayed ejaculation and other side-effects.

(4)The blocking-effect of cholinergic receptors is mainly M1 receptors, which can produce a variety of anticholinergic side effects, such as dry mouth, constipation, dysuria, blurred vision, and memory disorders. Histamine receptors blocked are mainly the H_1 receptors, which can produce side-effects of sedative and weight gain.

(5)Aripiprazole is different from the first generation and the second generation of antipsychotic drugs, which is a stabilizer of 5-HT-DA system. Aripiprazole has a weak excitatory effect on the postsynaptic dopamine D_2 receptor. When the activity of DA is too high, the activity of DA can be lowered and the positive symptoms of schizophrenia are treated by aripiprazole. The drug has partial activation on the DA receptor of presynaptic membrane, and it can treat the negative symptoms of schizophrenia.

Aripiprazole has a blocking effect on the postsynaptic membrane 5-HA2A receptor, which has a balance effect on the function of 5-HT and DA system, reducing the production of EPS and improving the efficacy of schizophrenia. The drug also has a partial effect on the 5-HT1A of postsynaptic membrane. In addition, aripiprazole has a certain affinity for D_3, D_4, muscarinic M receptor, α-adrenergic and histamine H_1 receptors.

Antipsychotic drugs have a broad range of pharmacological effects. In addition to the above receptor blocking related effects, they also have the effect of strengthening other central inhibitors, such as antiemetic, reduce body temperature, induce epilepsy, and the impact on the heart and blood system.

20.2.2.3 Clinical application

The therapeutic effect of antipsychotic drugs include:①antipsychotic effect, include anti hallucination, delusional effect(treatment positive symptoms) and activation(treatment negative symptoms);②non-specific sedation;③prevention of disease recurrence.

(1)General principles of antipsychotic drugs' clinical application

1)Indications

Antipsychotic drugs are mainly used to control a variety of psychotic symptoms, such as hallucinations, delusions, psychomotor excitement. Therefore, antipsychotic drugs are mainly used to treat various types of schizophrenia, prevent relapse of schizophrenia, and control manic episodes. And they also can be used for other organic or no-organic mental disorders with psychotic symptoms.

2) Contraindication

Severe cardiovascular diseases, liver diseases, kidney diseases, and severe systemic infections are prohibited. Hypothyroidism, adrenal insufficiency, myasthenia gravis, angle closure glaucoma, and previous history of drug allergy are also prohibited. The patients with low white blood cells, the elders, pregnant women and lactating women should be cautious.

3) Early diagnosis and treatment

Once diagnosed with schizophrenia, antipsychotic medication should be started immediately. Delayed treatment often misses the best treatment opportunity, leading to poor prognosis.

4) Single drug use and drug combination

For first-episode schizophrenia, the first choice is monotherapy. The effect of enough dose and course treatment is poor. Consider change another different mechanism of antipsychotic drugs or drug combination. For refractory schizophrenia, the combination therapy is recommended, and 2 drugs are selected should with different mechanisms, the dosage of the two drugs should be reduced.

5) Course of treatment

The treatment of schizophrenia advocates the whole course of treatment, which include acute stage treatment, consolidation stage treatment and maintenance period treatment.

(2) Usage and dosage

1) The choice of drugs

The choice of drugs mainly according to the side-effects and symptoms. There is no significant difference in the therapeutic effect of antipsychotic drugs in the treatment of enough dosage and course. Patients with excitement should be used antipsychotic drugs with strong sedative effect, or injection, such as haloperidol and chlorpromazine. Due to the minor side-effects and good tolerability, the second generation of antipsychotic drugs has partially replaced the first generation of antipsychotic drugs in clinical practice.

2) Stages of drug therapy

The treatment of schizophrenia should follow the principle of the whole course of treatment, which includes acute stage, consolidation stage and maintenance stage.

● Acute phase treatment

The acute phase of schizophrenia includes the first onset, recurrence, and the aggravation of the disease patients demonstrate. The symptoms of agitation, hallucination, mental disorder, behavior disorder and hostility attack, and the treatment should be regarded as acute phase treatment. The goal of acute phase treatment is to relieve psychotic symptoms as soon as possible, including positive symptoms, negative symptoms, emotional symptoms, behavioral symptoms and cognitive symptoms. Try to achieve clinical recovery.

Specific measures in the treatment of acute stage: ①for schizophrenic patients, should be early diagnosis and early treatment, which is directly related to the prognosis and rehabilitation treatment; strictly implement the whole course treatment, choose appropriate antipsychotic drugs; health education for the patients and their families, get the cooperation of family members, provide good family support for patients, and ensure the patients complete the course of treatment. ②For patients with recurrent schizophrenia, the past treatment should be inquired in detail, and the past drugs with the best curative effect should be selected. The dosage of drugs and the duration of maintenance therapy should be appropriately improved, and change another medicine or combination of drugs can be considered to ensure the best curative effect. Patients and their families are still informed of the treatment cycle and prognosis of the disease, informing the importance of maintenance therapy, which can improve patient compliance and get good support of the family members.

Pay attention to the following aspects in the treatment of acute stage: complete physical condition assessment of patients before treatment, selection of indications, contraindications excluded, routine physical examination, examination of the nervous system, blood routine, blood biochemical (including liver and kidney function) and electrocardiogram; the first medication should be started in small dose titration, and avoid serious adverse reactions; as far as possible a single medication, avoid the frequent replacement of drugs. If patients with severe symptoms, difficult to manage, to cause harm to the society, and the guardian should be advised to let patients in hospital treatment. The treatment period is about 6-8 weeks in the acute phase.

● Consolidation therapy

After the acute phase treatment, patients entered a relatively stable period, and the mental symptoms are complete controlled. This period still needs to maintain the highest drug dose at the acute stage. If early to reduce the dose of the drug or drug withdrawal, the risk of resurgence is very high, and this period is called a period of consolidation. The goal of consolidation therapy is to prevent the resurgence of psychiatric symptoms, consolidate curative effect, prevent and control of post-schizophrenia depression, obsessive-compulsive symptoms, and dutch act. Consolidation therapy promotes the recovery of social function, prepares for returning to society, and prevents common side effects such as endocrine disorders, weight gain, drowsiness, heart and kidney dysfunction caused by long-term medication.

Specific measures for consolidation treatment: maintain the treatment dose in the acute phase, the patients can be treated outside the hospital. If there is no discomfort, patients can gradually restore their social function, so as to prevent long-term hospitalization which can result in social function withdrawal of patients. The period of consolidation treatment is generally 3-6 months. In this period doctors should inform the patients and their families regular outpatient review, remind patients need to continue treatment, prevent withdrawal, observe side-effects. Unless the obvious adverse reactions affect the patient's life and work, try not to adjust the dose.

● Maintenance treatment

After consolidation treatment, the patient enters a relatively stable phase and becomes a maintenance period. The goal of maintaining treatment is to prevent recurrence of psychiatric symptoms, improve social function and quality of life. The maintenance treatment can effectively reduce the rate of recurrence, recurrence of symptoms will directly affect the patient's work and learning function, reduce the recurrence is conducive to the maintenance of patients' social function. The duration of maintenance period: the maintenance period of the first episode is 1-2 years, and the recurrence is at least 5 years. The guidelines for the prevention and treatment of schizophrenia in China stipulated that the length of maintenance period should be determined according to the patient's condition, generally not less than 2-5 years. For patients with suicide attempt, violent behavior and aggressive behavior, the treatment of maintenance period should be extended appropriately.

Principle of drug dose adjustment in maintenance period: the maintenance period can slowly reduce the dose of the drugs, reduce 20% of the original dose every 6 months, until the minimum effective dose. Daily single dose administration can increase the treatment compliance of patients. Long acting injection has certain advantages in the maintenance of treatment, intramuscular injection 1 times every 1-4 weeks. It reduces the burden of administration, and intramuscular injection can ensure the drug into the body to play a therapeutic role.

20.2.2.4　Adverse reactions and treatment

Treatment and prevention of adverse drug reactions are as important as the treatment of primary diseases.

（1）Extrapyramidal reaction

The most common neurological side effects of antipsychotic drugs include the followingfour manifestations: acute distonia, akathisia, symptoms like Parkinsonismand and tardive dyskinesia(TD).

1）Acute dystonia

Men and children are more common than women. It appears early, which shows involuntary and peculiar features, including the eyes upturn, torticollis, retrocollis, facial grimacing, twisted, tongue, trismus, opisthotonos and scoliosisetc. Patients often go to the emergency department, which can be easily misdiagnosed as tetanus, hysteria, and history of taking antipsychotic medication help to make the diagnosis.

Treatment: intramuscular injection of scopolamine 0. 3 mg can relieve the symptom immediately. Sometimes it need to reduce the dose of the drug or oral anticholinergic drug such as trihexyphenidyl hydrochloride, or take drugs with low extrapyramidal response.

2）Akathisia

It often appears 1−2 weeks after the treatment, the incidence rate is about 20%, which shows uncontrollable agitation, restlessness, inability to sit, move repeatedly and mark time. It is easy to be misdiagnosed as psychotic agitation or mental illness, so sometimes the dosage of antipsychotic drugs is mistakenly increased to worsen the symptoms.

Treatment: taking benzodiazepines or β−receptor blockers such as propranolol hydrochloride(propranolol), etc. Sometimes we need to reduce the dose of antipsychotic drugs or choose drugs with low extrapyramidal response.

3）Symptoms like Parkinsonism

It often appears in the treatment of the first 1−2 months, the incidence is as high as 56%, and women were more common than men. The elderly are common and misdiagnosed because of apathy, depression or dementia. The manifestations can be classified as movement disorder, tremor, muscle tension increased and autonomic nerve dysfunction. It begins to show slow movement, tremor of the hands and feet, and muscle tension increased. In severe cases, it shows the loss of coordinated movement, stiff, bent posture, festination, mask face, coarse tremor, salivation and seborrhea.

Treatment: anti−cholinergic drug, such as trihexyphenidyl hydrochloride, antipsychotics should slowly increase the dose or use the lowest effective dose. Anticholinergic drugs do not prevent the development of extrapyramidal symptoms, but it can produce anticholinergic side effects. Therefore, if anticholinergic drugs are given, they should be discontinued in a few months.

4）Tardive dyskinesia

It often appears 1−2 years after the treatment, the annual incidence rate is 3%. A few can also appear in a few months, the longer the medication time of use, the higher the incidence. The elderly and organic diseases are more common. TD is characterized by involuntary, rhythmic, stereotyped movements. It disappears during sleep and aggravates when patients are agitated. The earliest sign of TD is slight tremor around the tongue and lips. The patients with long history of TD can appear limb involuntary, aimless twitch, such as dance like strokes, refers to the action, hands like throwing upper limb or lower limbs kept jumping. Some patients appear hypotonia(paralysis), such as unable to straighten the waist, convex, neck soft can't rise head. It also appears some trunk movement coordination, patients showed peculiar posture, such as curved caster and opisthotonos. At present, there is no effective drug treatment in TD. The key is prevention, close observation, the use of the lowest effective dose or replacement of drugs that cause extrapyramidal reaction easily such as risperidone. Anticholinergic drugs may promote the occurrence and exacerbation of TD, and minimize the use of anticholinergic drugs.

Treatment: haloperidol is effective for TD after withdrawal. It can be used at appropriate dosage and gradually reduced to discontinuation. For severe TD, promethazine can be used 25–50 mg, intramuscular injection 1 time per day; or 25 mg, 3 times per day. Patients with severe anxiety can use anxiolytic drugs, such as clonazepam 0.5–1.0 mg or diazepam 2.5–5.0 mg, oral 2–3 times per day, can stabilize the mood, relieve symptoms. Antioxidant vitamin E can also be used, and 5–HT antagonist is effective for some patients.

(2) Other side effects of nervous system

1) Malignant syndrome

Malignant syndrome is a rare and serious adverse reaction with high mortality. Its clinical features include disturbance of consciousness, muscle rigidity, persistent high fever, autonomic nervous instability, and cardiovascular symptoms. Laboratory examination showed elevated white blood cells, elevated levels of muscle phosphate kinase (CPK), transaminase and lactate dehydrogenase, and myosin urine, etc. High fever, sweating, dehydration can caused peripheral circulatory failure which caused death. This disease is still lack of specific treatment method, mainly by early detection, taking comprehensive measures, which included immediate withdrawal, fluid infusion, correct acidosis and electrolyte disorders. Some people use the skeletal muscle relaxant dantrolene sodium is effective in the treatment of malignant hyperthermia. It has been found that the drug for the treatment of antipsychotic induced malignant syndrome. 1 mg/kg of dantrolene sodium were rapidly administered intravenously, and then orally, 4–8 mg/kg per day. Hepatic dysfunction should not be used. In addition, the use of bromocriptine mesylate, 7.5–60 mg/d, has good curative effect. Anticholinergic drugs should not be used because they can affect perspiration and cause higher body temperature.

2) Epileptic seizures

Antipsychotic drugs can reduce seizure threshold and induce epilepsy, mostly in the treatment of chlorpromazine, clozapine andthiazidine. Haloperidol and perphenazine may be relatively safe in the treatment of psychiatric patients with epilepsy.

(3) The side–effects of autonomic nerve

The side–effects of anticholinergic drugs include dry mouth, blurred vision, dysuria and constipation. Serious side–effects include urinary retention, paralytic ileus and oral infection, especially when antipsychotic drugs are combined with anticholinergic drugs and tricyclic antidepressants. Alpha adrenergic blockade is characterized by orthostatic hypotension, reflex tachycardia, delayed ejaculation, or inhibition. Orthostatic hypotension is common in beginning of treatment, and chlorpromazine is more likely to occur during injection. Patients can appear syncope, falls or injuries when in the seat suddenly stand up or get up. Therefore, patients should get up or stand up slowly. Patients with cardiovascular disease increase dose slowly. Once the occurrence of postural hypotension, let patient keep the head low and feet high in a recumbent position, severe patients should be given infusion of norepinephrine or aramine etc. But the epinephrine is disable.

(4) The side effects of metabolism and endocrine

Prolactin levels are increased more often, and estrogen and testosterone levels change are also reported. Women have common diarrhea, amenorrhea and sexual pleasure impairment. Phenothiazine can produce false positive results in pregnancy. Males are more likely to appear lose sexual desire, erection difficulties and ejaculation suppression. Growth hormone levels were decreased, but there was no growth retardation in children treated with phenothiazine or a sustained drug therapy. Abnormal secretion of antidiuretic hormone has also been reported. Chlorpromazine, clozapine and some other drugs can inhibit insulin secretion, resulting in elevated blood sugar and urine glucose positive.

Increased weight gain is associated with increased appetite and decreased activity. The mechanisms are complex, including histamine receptor blockade, changes in glucose tolerance and insulin release mediated by the hypothalamic mechanism. Patients should be abstemious diet. The effect of weight gain of haloperidol is weaker than phenothiazine.

(5) The side effects of mental events

Many antipsychotic drugs produce excessive sedation, and it usually disappears quickly due to tolerance. Dizziness and dullness are often caused by it. Thiazide, benzamide and risperidone have mild activation or stimulation, which can produce anxiety and agitation. The effects on cognitive function in schizophrenia are intertwined with cognitive deficits in the disease itself. Strong sedative phenothiazine tends to inhibit psychomotor and attention, but generally does not affect advanced cognitive function. If anticholinergic drugs are added, memory function may be temporarily affected.

It is not clear whether antipsychotic drugs can cause depression. Whether the drug is administered, schizophrenic patients can exhibit significant emotional fluctuation. Depression can occur in both early and recovery stages of schizophrenia, and suicide is common in schizophrenia. Extrapyramidal side-effects, such as motor failure, may be mistaken for depression. Drugs with strong anticholinergic activity like clozapine and chlorpromazine, are more likely to have withdrawal reactions, such as insomnia, anxiety and restlessness, which should be paid attention to.

(6) Other side effects

Antipsychotic drugs also have many unusual side-effects. The effect of antipsychotic drugs on the liver is alanine aminotransferase (ALT) increased. It is mostly transient, and generally no conscious symptoms. And light patients do not have to stop medication, can be combined with liver treatment. Severe or jaundice patients should immediately stop medication, strengthen liver protection treatment. Biliary obstructive jaundice is rare, sometimes leading to biliary cirrhosis. Other rare allergies include drug eruptions, asthma with fever, edema, arthritis, and lymph node disease. Serious drug eruption may be occurred exfoliative dermatitis, should immediately stop medication and actively deal with.

The incidence of agranulocytosis is rare. Clozapine resulted in a higher incidence of agranulocytosis, while chlorpromazine and thioridazine lead to incidental episodes. Thiazide, thioxanthene and butyl benzene have been no reported. If the white blood cell count is low, clozapine, chlorpromazine, and thioridazine should be avoided. Blood examination should be routinely performed when antipsychotic drugs are used.

The results showed that phenothiazine, especially thioridazine is prone to abnormal ECG, such as prolongation of P-Q interval, decrease of ST segment, change of T-wave, prolongation of QRS and QT interval, and the incidence rate is 30% -70%, which might be the result of changing potassium channel in myocardial layer. Especially in the elderly, drug induced arrhythmias are more frequently, and sudden death can occur in severe cases.

Chlorpromazine and other phenothiazine can form purple gray pigmentation on the cornea, lens and skin, and they are more common in the areas with strong sunlight and women.

(7) Overdose poisoning

Patients with schizophrenia often attempt to commit suicide with excessive use of antipsychotic drugs. Accidental overdose is mostly seen in children. Antipsychotic drugs are less toxic than barbiturates and tricyclic antidepressants, and have low mortality. The earliest signs of excess are agitation or clouding of consciousness. Sometimes dystonia, epilepsy and seizures are seen. The EEG showed prominent slow - waves. Severe hypotension, arrhythmia and hypothermia are often present. Anticholinergic effects (especially in the treatment of thioridazine) can worsen the prognosis, and physostigmine can be used as a detoxifying agent. Extrapyramidal reactions are usually not apparent due to anticholinergic effects of excess drugs. The treatment is basically symptomatic treatment, including a large amount of fluids, attention to maintain normal body temperature and the use of antiepileptic drugs to control epilepsy. Because of the high protein binding rate of most antipsychotics, hemodialysis is not often used. Anticholinergic effect delayed gastric emptying, so gastric lavage should be performed after several hours of overdose. Due to hypotension is caused by blocking alpha and beta adrenergic receptors, pressor agents acting on alpha receptors such as aramine and noradrenergic can only be used. The epinephrine is disable.

20.2.2.5　Drugs interaction

Plasma concentrations of tricyclic antidepressant can be increased by the antipsychotic drugs, which can induced epilepsy, intensified anticholinergic side effects, aggravated the anticholinergic side-effects of anticholinergic drugs, reversed the pressor effect of epinephrine, weaken the antihypertensive effect of antihypertensive drug like guanethidine, increased the blood concentration of beta blockers and calcium channel blockers caused hypotension, strengthen effect of other CNS depressants such as alcohol and diuretic. Antacids affect the absorption of antipsychotic drugs. Smoking can reduce the plasma concentration of some drugs, such as clozapine. Carbamazepine can decrease the plasma concentration of haloperidol and clozapine by inducing liver drug metabolizing enzymes, which can worsen the psychiatric symptoms and it also can increase the risk of granulocyte deficiency in clozapine. Some selective serotonin reuptake inhibitors(SSRIs) such as fluoxetine, paroxetine, and fluvoxamine can inhibit liver drug metabolizing enzymes and increase the plasma concentration of antipsychotic drugs, which can lead to adverse reactions or exacerbation.

20.2.2.6　Antipsychotic drugs

The frequency of drugs used varies in different periods and regions, and the use of atypical antipsychotics are more often be used in developed countries.

(1)First generation antipsychotic drugs

1)Chlorpromazine

Chlorpromazine is the first generation of antipsychotic drugs.

Pharmacokinetics: oral taken or injection is easy to absorb, single oral peak time is 2-4 hours, half-life is 17 hours, 5-10 days reach the level of blood steady state, and the half-life is 30 hours. Intramuscular injection can avoid the first pass effect of liver metabolism, and the bio-availability is about 3 times as much as that of oral administration. The blood brain barrier and placental barrier are easily passed. It is metabolized by the liver, 70%-80% through the kidneys, 10%-30% excreted from feces, a small amount discharge from the human milk, and have an influence on babies.

Function and application: chlorpromazine is D_1 and D_2 receptor blocker. It has high affinity to 5-HT6 and 5-HT7 receptors. It has not only strong sedative effect, but also anti hallucination, delusion, thinking form disorder, hostility, strange behavior and psychomotor excitability. It can be used for the treatment of paranoid schizophrenia and hebephrenia, and can also be used for mania and psychogenic mental disorder. It can quickly and effectively control the patient's excitement and acute psychotic symptoms.

Usage and dosage: the starting dose is 25-50 mg when oral administration, 2-3 times per day. The therapeutic dose was 200-600 mg/d. Intramuscular injection: patients who were excited or uncooperative could receive intramuscular injection of chlorpromazine in 25-50 mg combined with promethazine in 25 mg. Chlorpromazine also can intravenous infusion, chlorpromazine 100-200 mg, plus 5% glucose 500 mL, 60 drops/min. The maintenance dose was 100-300 mg/d.

Adverse reactions: the side-effects of therapeutic dose include lethargy, weakness, prone to orthostatic hypotension, extrapyramidal reactions, anticholinergic reactions(such as dry mouth, constipation, tachycardia), seizures, elevated prolactin levels, lactation, sexual dysfunction, male breast feminization, menstrual change, rash and so on. This drug can cause liver dysfunction, jaundice, pigmentation of skin, visceral and retinal. Sometimes it also can cause granulocyte reduction and anemia. Combination of lithium or antanum can decrease the concentration of chlorpromazine in serum. Combination of alkaline drugs such as aluminum hydroxide can affect the absorption of chlorpromazine. It should be carefully used for organic mental disorders or in the elderly.

2) Perphenazine

Perphenazine is the first generation of antipsychotic drugs.

Pharmacokinetics: after oral administration, it distributes to the whole body. It is excreted by bile, partly absorbed in the intestine, and the half-life is 9 hours. It can be passed through the umbilical cord into the fetus and can be excreted from the mother's milk. It has high lipophilicity and protein binding rate. The metabolism and excretion of this drug decreased significantly in children and old people.

Function and application: perphenazine is high titer DA blockers. Its sedative effect is weak, has a good effect on paranoid schizophrenia and chronic schizophrenia. It's visceral toxicity is small, and it is suitable for the elderly, patients with organs (such as heart, liver, kidney, lung) lesions or somatic disease patients.

Usage and dosage: the starting dose is 8-12 mg/d, gradually increased to 20-60 mg/d, 2-3 times per day. The maintenance dose is 10-20 mg/d.

Adverse reactions: extrapyramidal reaction is the most common, such as tremor, rigidity, bradykinesia, salivation, akathisia, and acute dystonia. Long term and large dosage administration can cause tardive dyskinesia, and may cause an increase in plasma prolactin levels. The possible symptoms related to increased prolactin level arediarrhea, gynecomastia, menstrual disorders and amenorrhea. The side effects also include dry mouth, blurred vision, fatigue, dizziness, tachycardia, constipation, sweating and so on. Rare adverse reactions include orthostatic hypotension, neutropenia and toxic liver damage. Allergic skin rash and malignant syndrome are rare.

3) Haloperidol

Haloperidol is one of the first generation of antipsychotic drugs.

Pharmacokinetics: it is easily to absorb orally. The peak time is 3-4 hours, and the peak time of intramuscular injection is 30 minutes. The half-life is 12-36 hours, 92% is combined with plasma protein, and the effective blood concentration range is 4-20 ng/L. It is metabolized by the liver and excreted from urine and feces.

Function and application: haloperidol has strong DA receptor blocking effect, weak anticholinergic action and anti-adrenergic action. It is one of the drugs for the treatment of excitatory schizophrenia, which is evident in hallucinations and delusions, and is also used in the treatment of acute mania. It is also has curative effect for some of the involuntary movements (such as chorea, torsion spasm) and Tourette disease. Sedation and antiemetic effect are strong. It can also be used in cerebral organic mental disorders. It is no obvious effect on blood pressure and cardiovascular. Injection is often used to deal with emergency problems in the psychiatric department. It is also suitable for elderly people with agitation and agitation with physical diseases.

Usage and dosage: the starting dose is 2-4 mg/d, gradually increased to 10-40 mg/d, 2-3 times per day. The treatment of Tourette and other behavioral disorders is 2-4 mg/d and 2 times per day. The injection dose is 3-5 mg for the first time. After 30-40 minutes without adverse reaction, the dose can be increased to 5-10 mg.

Adverse reactions: the main symptoms were extrapyramidal side effect. The extrapyramidal side effect of long effect preparation is lighter than that of oral administration. Long term application may cause tardive dyskinesia. A few people can have dizziness, fatigue, dry mouth, and rash. Patients with heart, liver, kidney, lung disease and patients with glaucoma, epilepsy, hyperthyroidism are carefully used. This medicine is generally does not combine with lithium carbonate to avoid irreversible brain damage.

4) Sulpiride

Sulpiride is one of the first generation of antipsychotic drugs.

Pharmacokinetics: it is absorbed from the stomach and intestines. The peak time of blood drug concentration is 2 hours. After 48 hours, 30% of the oral dose is discharged from the urine, and some of which is excreted from the dung. The plasma half-life is 8-9 hours. Animal experiments show that the product can enter the umbilical cord blood circulation through the placental barrier. This product is mainly excreted by the kidney. It can be discharged from breast milk.

Function and application: it has a good effect on hallucinations, delusions, symptoms of tension, and some negative symptoms such as passivity and lack of thinking. It has a good effect on schizophrenia patients with depressive symptoms. It has good treatment effect on neurotic vomiting and anorexia nervosa. Small doses can be used for the treatment of gastric and duodenal ulcers. The treatment of schizophrenia requires a high dose.

Usage and dosage: low dose(200-600 mg/d) had antidepressant effect. 200-600 mg/d, intravenous drip(dissolved in normal saline) of 7-10 per day can relieve the symptoms of tension in patients.

Adverse reactions: the main side effects were weight gain, lactation, male breast development, amenorrhea, and hypogonadism. Extrapyramidal reaction canbe occurred at large doses. Patients with hypertension and pheochromocytoma are not used, serious cardiovascular disease and liver damage are used carefully.

5) Penfluridol

Penfluridol is high titer antipsychotic drugs and oral long-acting preparations.

Pharmacokinetics: although oral administration can be absorbed through the gastrointestinal tract, the peak value of the blood is reached after oral administration of 12 hours. The steady state concentration can be measured at 7 days after taking. This product can be stored in the adipose tissue after oral administration and then release slowly. The main metabolites are excreted with feces, and only a small amount of metabolites is discharged from the urine.

Function and application: it is effective for all types of schizophrenia. The patients take the medicine once per week. The drug has a therapeutic effect on hallucinations and delusions.

Usage and dosage: the oral dose ranged from 20 to 120 mg, once a week. It should start from 10 to 20 mg every week and gradually increase by 10-20 mg per week or 2 weeks. Usually, the amount of treatment was 30-60 mg a week. After the symptoms disappeared, the original dose continued to be consolidated for 3 months, and the maintenance dose was 10-20 mg for 1 week.

Adverse reactions: the main adverse reactions were extrapyramidal reactions, such as sedentary failure, acute dystonia, and Parkinson's disease. Long-term use can lead totardive dyskinesia, as well as somnolence, fatigue, dry mouth, menstrual disorder, milk, anxiety and depression. Some patients have allergic rash, abnormal electrocardiogram, granulocytic deficiency and neuroleptic malignant syndrome.

(2) Second generation antipsychotic drugs

1) Clozapine

Pharmacokinetics: the half-life of the oral administration is 3.6-14.3 hours, and the effect lasted for more than 24 hours. The steady blood concentration reaches in 7-10 days, and the effective blood concentration is 300-600 μg/L. It is metabolized by CYP2D6 and CYP1A2, the activity of metabolites is low. 80% of the metabolites is excreted from excrement, and 20% is excreted from the urine.

Function and application: because of its strong D_1 and 5-HT2A receptor blocking effect, clozapine has strong antipsychotic effect. The drug directly act on the mesencephalic reticular activation system, and has a strong sedative and hypnotic effect. It is effective for negative symptoms and positive symptoms of schizophrenia, especially for positive symptoms such as agitation, hallucination, delusion, etc. Clozapine is still effective in cases of ineffective treatment of other drugs. For acute mania, combined with lithium carbonate, the symptoms can be improved for first weeks. However, the combined dosage of the two are small, because clozapine could increase the sensitivity of the patients to lithium carbonate.

Usage and dosage: at the beginning, the amount of oral administration is 25-75 mg/d and 2-3 times per day, and then the amount is gradually added (generally plus 25 mg/d). The dose could increase to 200-500 mg/d, and the maintenance amount is 50-200 mg/d.

Adverse reactions: the application of this medicine is prone to excessive sedation, orthostatic hypotension, tachycardia, constipation, dysuria, salivation, nausea, vomiting, constipation, intestinal paralysis and fatigue. Obvious weight gain can cause hyperlipidemia and diabetes. There are reports of fever, seizures, malignant syndrome, and cardiomyopathy. The fatal granulocytic deficiency is rare, and most scholars argue that it should not be used as a first-line drug.

2) Olanzapine

Pharmacokinetics: olanzapine is easy to be absorbed orally, not affected by food. The peaktime is 4.9 hours, and the average peak concentration is 11 mg/L. It was widely distributed in the tissues, with a large volume of distribution (10.3-18.4 L/kg). It is metabolized in the liver, and the main metabolic enzymes are CYP1A2 and CYP2D6. There are at least 10 kinds of metabolites, all of which are inactive and are mainly excreted by urine. The half-life of is cleared 21-30 hours, and the elderly can reach 54 hours.

Function and application: olanzapine has a high affinity for 5-HT2, M and H_1 receptors. Even small doses of 5 mg/d, the occupancy of 5-HT2 is more than 90%, which is greater than that of D_2 receptor. The occupancy of D_2 receptor was larger than that of clozapine, and similar to risperidone. It is mainly used to treat schizophrenia and a variety of mental and behavioral disorders, including psychic depression, mania, old age and children's mental and behavioral disorders. It may be effective for refractory cases, but it is not as good as clozapine.

Usage and dosage: the initial dose is 5-10 mg/d, and the dose increased by 5 mg. The treatment dose is 10 mg/d, and the negative symptom is 15 mg/d. The dose of refractory people should be slightly larger. The dose of maintenance is 5 mg/d. Olanzapine is easily inactivated by oxidation, and it should be taken immediately after cutting or breaking. Because of CYP1A2 metabolism, CYP1A2 inducers and smoking can reduce the concentration of blood.

Adverse reactions: the main adverse reactions were dizziness, drowsiness, tachycardia, constipation, dry mouth, anxiety, insomnia, tremor, akathisia and mild EPS. Increased appetite and weight gain were more common, about 40% patients increased more than the weight of 7%. There were also elevated aminotransferase levels in a few cases, mostly in the first 1-2 weeks of treatment. It was reported that prolactin increased in 22%-46% of the long term medication patients. The patients with hypotension, cardio cerebral vascular disease, liver function damage and epileptic patients are used carefully.

3) Quetiapine

Pharmacokinetics: the half-life of quetiapine is about 7 hours, and 83% of quetiapineis combined with plasma protein. About 73% of the active metabolites are excreted from the urine and 21% are excreted from the feces.

Function and application: it can be used for the treatment of positive psychotic symptoms, negative symptoms, cognitive symptoms, unstable emotions and attack symptoms. It can be used for the treatment of schizophrenia, acute mania(monotherapy or in combination with lithium or valproate), and other psychiatric disorders such as the maintenance treatment of bipolar affective disorder, behavior treatment of dementia, Parkinson's disease, Louis's dementia behavior disorders, the behavioral problems of children and adolescents, disease associated with impulse control disorders.

Usage and dosage: dose range: 150–750 mg/d in the treatment of schizophrenia, 400–800 mg/d in the treatment of acute bipolar mania. The initial dose is 25 mg/d, 2 times per day, and increased by 25–50 mg/d.

Adverse reactions: the drug is well tolerated and has fewer adverse reactions. The common side effects are diabetes, lipoprotein abnormalities, dizziness, sedation, taste and weight gain. There are no motor system adverse reactions and prolactin increase. Severe adverse reactions are rare, include hyperglycemia, neuroleptic malignant syndrome and epilepsy.

4) Risperidone

Pharmacokinetics: it is easy to absorb by orally taken. It is metabolized by CYP2D6. Its active metabolite is 9-hydroxyrisperidone. Its half-life is 27 hours, 70% excreted from urine, and 14% excreted from the feces.

Function and application: risperidone antagonized D_2 and 5-HT2A receptors strongly and evenly, which are effective for negative symptoms, positive symptoms, emotional symptoms and cognitive dysfunction of schizophrenia. The effective dose of risperidone is small, whose extrapyramidal reaction is slight, the anticholinergic action and sedative effect are weak. It is suitable for patients with acute and chronic schizophrenia, and has good therapeutic effect on schizophrenia and Tourette syndrome. Because of the minor side-effects, it is also suitable for elderly people with organic and functional mental disorders. It is also used as an emotional stabilizer. The effect of risperidone is fast.

Usage and dosage: the treatment dose is 2–6 mg/d, and it is taken 1 or 2 times per day. The dosage is generally not more than 6 mg/d, and the larger dose can have an extrapyramidal reaction.

Adverse reactions: side effects include headache, dizziness, shock, insomnia and so on. The extrapyramidal reactionis less, and obviously when it is increased at 6 mg/d. The liver function and electrocardiogram can be abnormal in a few.

5) Ziprasidone

Pharmacokinetics: the absorption of ziprasidone is complete after oral administration. If it is taken with food, the bioavailability could reach 100%. The half-life is about 7 hours, and 30% of drug is metabolized by the CYP3A4 of liver. The dose can be adjusted appropriately for severe liver injury.

Function and application: ziprasidone has a high affinity for 5-HT2A receptor and low affinity for D_2 receptor. Ziprasidone is also a 5-HT1A receptor antagonist, 5-HT and norepinephrine reuptake inhibitors. Ziprasidone has a therapeutic effect on positive symptoms, negative symptoms, emotional symptoms and cognitive functions of schizophrenia.

Usage and dosage: the initial dose is 20–40 mg/d, and the treatment recommended dose is 120–160 mg/d. The bio-availability is increased while taking food at the same time. A short-effective injection of ziprasidone can be used in patients with acute agitation and psychiatric symptoms. The symptoms can be controlled in 15–30 minutes after injection.

Adverse reactions: ziprasidone has few adverse reactions, good tolerance and low incidence of EPS. Some patients can suffer from fatigue, drowsiness and drowsiness at the early stage. Some patients have gastrointestinal reactions at the beginning of their medication, such as nausea and vomiting, which can be quickly tolerated and disappear. Ziprasidone rarely causes weight gain and increased blood sugar. It is possible that ziprasidone may prolong the QT interval, and should be used carefully for the obvious prolongation of the QT interval. The prolongation of QT interval was greater than 500 ms, and ziprasidone should be stopped immediately. Intravenous magnesium sulfate is given when necessary.

6) Aripiprazole

Pharmacokinetics: the oral bio-availability is 87%, and the binding rate of plasma protein is higher than 99%. 25% of the dosage are excreted by the kidney(including less than 1% of the original drug), and another 55% are excreted with feces(18% of the original drug).

Function and application: aripiprazole is a partial agonist of D_2 receptor. It can improve positive symptoms, cognitive symptoms, negative symptoms and emotional symptoms. Aripiprazole can be used for the treatment of schizophrenia, maintenance treatment of schizophrenia, the maintenance treatment of bipolar disorder, depression(adjuvant therapy), dementia behavior disorder, children and adolescents with behavioral disorders, the problem associated with impulse control disorders.

Usage and dosage: the treatment dose is 15-30 mg/d. Starting from a small dose of 5-10 mg/d, which can alleviate the side-effects.

Adverse reactions: common adverse reactions include dizziness, insomnia, sedentary and activation, nausea and vomiting. Occasionally, orthostatic hypotension, constipation and drowsiness can occur when patients taking drugs in the early period.

7) Amisulpride

Pharmacokinetics: the plasma protein binding rate of amisulpride is about 16%. Amisulpride is excreted from the urine with the original form, whose renal clearance rate is about 330 mL/min. There is little metabolism in the liver, so there is no need to adjust the dose for the patients with liver function. Patients with renal insufficiency should be used carefully.

Function and application: amisulpride is a selective dopamine D_2 and D_3 receptor antagonist, and it can bind with limbic system D_2 and D_3 dopamine receptor selectively. Low dose amisulpride mainly block presynaptic receptor, which can be used for the treatment of negative symptoms. High dose amisulpride mainly block postsynaptic receptors, and can be used for the treatment of positive symptoms.

Usage and dosage: the treatment dose is 200 mg/d. Low dose(less than 300 mg/d) is effective for schizophrenia with predominantly negative symptoms, and high dose(greater than 400 mg/d) is more effective for positive symptoms.

Adverse reactions: amisulpride mainly block mesolimbic dopaminergic neurons in the middle. However, the inhibition of dopaminergic neurons in the striatum is weak, so amisulpride has a stronger anti-psychotic effect and less adverse reactions in the extrapyramidal system. But it can increase the secretion of prolactin.

20.2.3 Antidepressant

20.2.3.1 Classification of antidepressant drugs

Antidepressant is a kind of drug that treats all kinds of depressive symptoms and does not improve the mood of normal people. For the pathogenesis of depression and all kinds of depressive disorders, it is generally accepted that the function of monoamine neurotransmitter function in the central nervous system is decreased. Therefore, most kinds of antidepressants used in clinic are based on this hypothesis. The mechanism of action is to increase the concentration of monoamine neurotransmitters in neuron synaptic gap through different way.

Antidepressant drugs can be divided into the following categories according to the different mechanisms (Table 20-2) : ①tricyclic antidepressants(TCAs) , including heterocyclic developed on this basis and tetracyclica ; ②monoamine oxidase inhibitors(MAOIs) ; ③selective 5-HT reuptake inhibitor(SSRIs) ; ④5-HT reuptake inhibitors combined with heterogeneous point ; ⑤5-serotonin and norepinephrine(NE) reuptake inhibitor(SNRIs) ; ⑥5-HT2A and 5-HT reuptake inhibitors ; ⑦NE and DA reuptake inhibitors ; ⑧selective NE reuptake inhibitors ; ⑨NE and specific 5-HT antidepressants ; ⑩atypical antidepressants and herbal medicine.

Table 20-2   Classification and dose range of commonly-used antidepressants

Classification of drug	Initial dose/(mg/d)	Dosage range/(mg/d)
(1) SSRIs		
Fluoxetine	20	20-60
Paroxetine	20	20-60
Sertraline	50	50-200
Fluvoxamine	50-100	100-300
Citalopram	20	20-60
Escitalopram	10	10-20
(2) SNRIs		
Venlafaxine	37. 5-75	75-375
Duloxetine	60	60-120
(3) Norepinephrine and dopamine reuptake inhibitors(NDRIs)		
Bupropion	150	300-450
(4) Selective norepinephrine reuptake inhibitor(NRIs)		
Reboxetine	4	8-12
(5) 5-hydroxytryptamine block and reuptake inhibitors(SARIs)		
Trazodone	150	150-300
(6) α_2-adrenergic receptor blocker		
Mianserine	30	30-90
Mirtazapine(NaSSA)	15	15-45
(7) Melatonin receptor agonist		
Agomelatine	25	25-50
(8) TCAs		
Imipramine	25-50	100-300
Clomipramine	25-50	100-300
Amitriptyline	25-50	100-300
Doxepin	25-50	100-300
Maprotiline	75	300-600
(9) MAOIs		
Moclobemide	150	300-600

20.2.3.2   General principles of clinical application

(1) Indications: antidepressants are suitable for all kinds of depressive disorders, with an effective rate of 60% –80%.

(2) Early diagnosis and early treatment, avoid the chronicity.

(3) The treatment principle of the whole course of disease should be followed for the treatment of depression, which are the treatment of the acute period, the consolidation period and the maintenance period. In acute phase, it takes 1–3 months to use antidepressant drugs enough to relieve symptoms as thoroughly as possible. The consolidation period is treated for 4–9 months, and the original effective drug and the original effective dose were maintained. The maintenance period depends on the patient's condition for 1–5 years.

(4) Target symptoms and drug selection: appropriate antidepressant drugs are selected according to the symptoms of the patients and the characteristics of the drug.

(5) Dose titration and choice of therapeutic dose: a variety of new antidepressants are well–tolerated, and the initial dose is the treatment dose. The patient is gradually added to the effective dose according to the patient's symptom relief and tolerance.

(6) Drug combination: depression first onset is usually treated with a single drug. If the patients are poor efficacy or adverse reactions, it can be replaced by another antidepressant drug with different mechanisms. For the treatment of refractory depression, the combination of emotional stabilizers or new antipsychotics should be considered.

20.2.3.3   Factors affecting the safety of antidepressants

(1) Adverse reactions associated with the role of neurotransmitter receptor: the receptors of antidepressant effect are very much, which can cause some adverse reactions in the treatment, such as anxiety, agitation, insomnia, headache, drowsiness, blurred vision, dry mouth, sexual dysfunction, decreased appetite, gastrointestinal reactions and so on. Activation of alpha receptor can increase blood pressure, and inhibition of alpha receptor can cause orthostatic hypotension.

(2) Drug interactions and adverse reactions related to pharmacodynamics.

(3) Drug interactions and adverse reactions associated with pharmacokinetics: most antidepressants are metabolized by liver cytochrome P450 enzyme. Some of them, such as SSRIs, have strong inhibitory effects on these enzymes. The degradation of drugs may be slow down that are combined with them for a long time, and increase the blood concentration, resulting in adverse reactions. There are large individual differences in the function of P450 enzyme, and these adverse reactions are more likely to occur in some patients with slow metabolism rates.

(4) The toxic effect of overdose: the new antidepressant drugs are safer than previous drugs, and excessive use generally has no serious adverse reactions. But overdose of tricyclic antidepressant drugs can cause arrhythmia and death.

(5) Abstinence syndrome: after long–term application of antidepressant drugs, the adaptability of the nerve is reduced. After the drug stopped, the receptor is unable to adapt to the change immediately. The withdrawal symptoms of tricyclic drugs include diarrhea and headache, and the withdrawal symptoms may also occur after SSRIs withdrawal. The longer the drug use and the shorter the half–life of the drug, the more vulnerable the patient is to be abstinence symptoms.

20.2.3.4　Tricyclic antidepressant

（1）Pharmacokinetics

Tricyclic antidepressant(TCAs) is one of the most commonly used drugs in the clinical treatment of depression. It is mainly metabolized by the liver. The cytochrome enzymes(CYP) involved in metabolism are 1A2,2D6,3A4. After oxidation,the metabolites generally combine with glucuronic acid to form inactive terminal metabolites,which are excreted through urine or feces. Most studies suggest that there is a linear positive correlation or an inverted U curve relationship between the TCAs steady-state blood concentration and the clinical response. It is generally believed that the type of disease,age,the race,the body disease, the environmental factors and the drug combined at the same time can affect the relationship between the concentration of blood and the curative effect. TCAs can make about 70% of the depression patients get a good relief,about 50% completely remission. But it has obvious anticholinergic side-effects,many patients can't tolerate and reduce the treatment compliance. Heart toxicity and overdose can endanger life. Generally,it takes more than 2 weeks to start effective.

（2）Mechanism of action

TCAs blocked the reuptake of NE and 5-HT by NE and 5-HT nerve endings,which increase the concentration of monoamine neurotransmitters in the synaptic gap and improve depressive symptoms. The inhibitory effect of antidepressants on the reuptake of neurotransmitters is immediately. However,long term use can reduce the sensitivity of the receptor(down-regulation),which is closely related to the delayed clinical effect of antidepressants(2-3 weeks). The blockage of NE reuptake increases the concentration of endogenous NE in the synaptic gap,and then decreases the sensitivity of the presynaptic membrane alpha-2 adrenergic receptor. The long-term use may also reduce the number of central alpha-2 adrenergic receptors. The first step of inhibition of 5-HT reuptake is also to increase the concentration of endogenous 5-HT in the synaptic gap of the cell body. By decreasing the 5-HT1A receptor on the membrane of the presynaptic cell body,it can increase the peripheral release of 5-HT,and finally achieve the antidepressant effect. TCAs also have a strong blocking effect on the 5-HT2A receptor. In addition to blocking NE and 5-HT reuptake,tricyclic antidepressants have M1,alpha-1 and H_1 receptor blocking effects. The clinical manifestations are dry mouth,constipation,blurred vision,dizziness,orthostatic hypotension,sedation,drowsiness and weight gain.

（3）Clinical application

1）Indication

Tricyclic antidepressant drugs are used in treatment of various mental disorders with depressive symptoms,such as endogenous depression,dysthymia,reactive depression,bipolar depression and organic depression. It also can be used for the treatment of generalized anxiety disorder,panic disorder and phobia. Clomipramine is commonly used in the treatment of obsessive-compulsive disorder.

2）Contraindications

Severe heart and liver disease,granulocytic reduction,glaucoma,prostatic hypertrophy,and the first 3 months of pregnancy are forbidden. The patients with epilepsy and the elderly are used carefully. For the depressive symptoms associated with schizophrenia,the treatment should be prudent,and TCAs may aggravate psychotic symptoms.

3）Drugs selection

Clomipramine's sedation is weak,which is suit for melancholia,enuresis of children and obsessive-compulsive disorder. The sedative and anxiolytic effects of amitriptyline are strong,which is suitable for intense type of depression. The antidepressant effect of doxepinis relatively weak,but sedative and anxiolytic effectsare strong, which is commonly used in the treatment of dysthymia and chronic pain.

4) Usage and dosage

Start from small doses, and gradually increase to the maximum effective dose in 1-2 weeks. If the dose is sufficient, the treatment for 6 weeks is not effective or the effect is notobvious, change medicine may be considered. Because the half-life of tricyclic antidepressants in the body is long, they can usually be taken one times a day before bedtime, so as to avoid excessive sedation and anticholinergic side effects during daytime.

After the acute stage of antidepressant treatment, the symptoms of depression have been relieved. At this time, effective treatment dose should be continued for 6 months, then enter the maintenance stage. The maintenance dose is usually lower than the effective dose, and the dosage is gradually reduced in view of the patient's condition and side-effects, usually for 6-9 months or longer. Patients with repeated frequent episodes should be maintained for a long time to prevent recurrence.

(4) Adverse reactions

1) Anticholinergic side-effects

It is the most common side-effects in the treatment of TCAs, which is earlier than the time for the antidepressant effect. It is characterized by dry mouth, constipation, and blurred visual, which can be gradually reduced with the continuation of the treatment. Severe patients can have urinary retention and enteroplegia. The principle of treatment, the dosage of antidepressant drugs should be reduced and the cholinergic agent should be added to counter side effects when necessary.

2) Side effects of the central nervous system

Most TCAs have sedative effect, which is parallel to its histamine receptor binding force. If there is tremor, we can reduce the dose of antidepressant or use the beta blocker instead, such as propranolol. TCAs can induce epilepsy. TCAs can lead to drug-induced confusion or delirium, which is easy to occur in elderly patients and is closely related to the concentration of blood drugs. The abnormality of electroencephalogram induced by TCAs is also closely related to the concentration of blood drug. Some reports have found that TCAs also induces hallucinations before bedtime, psychosis and mania.

3) Cardiovascular side-effects

Cardiovascular side-effects are the main side-effects, such as orthostatic hypotension, tachycardia, and dizziness. Quinidine-like action of TCAs may be associated with arrhythmias induced by drugs. TCAs can also cause prolongation of P-R interval and QRS time, causing II and III degree conduction block, and therefore they can't be used in patients with cardiac conduction block.

4) Side-effects of sex

Because depression and antidepressant drugs can cause sexual dysfunction, it is necessary to inquire about the history of the disease in detail, which is in order to find out whether it is the manifestation of the disease or the side effects of the drug. Sexual dysfunction associated with tricyclic antidepressants includes impotence, ejaculation disorder, loss of sexual desire, and reduced sexual pleasure. Sexual dysfunction can be improved with the improvement of depressive symptoms and the decrease of the amount of drug.

5) Gain weight

It may be related to the blocking of histamine receptor. In addition, some patients have peripheral edema, and salt intake should be restricted at this time.

6) Anaphylaxis

After medication, there is a mild rash, which could continue to be used after treatment. In the case of a serious rash, the drug should be gradually reduced and stopped. Further treatment should avoid the use of drugs that have already been allergic. Even the occasional granulocyte deficiency occurs, and once it appears, the drug should be stopped immediately, and is also forbidden in the future treatment.

7) Excessive intoxication

Excessive use can lead to serious toxic reactions, which have high mortality. The clinical manifestations include coma, seizure and arrhythmia. It can also include hyperthermia, hypotension, enteroplegia, mydriasis, respiratory depression and cardiac arrest. The anticholinergic effect could be alleviated by using physostigmine, and repeat the drug for 1-2 mg per 0.5-1 hours. Other measures include timely gastric lavage, infusion, active treatment of arrhythmia, and control of epileptic seizures. The anticholinergic action of tricyclic drugs can cause gastric emptying to be delayed, and gastric lavage measures can still be taken even after a few hours after overdose.

(5) Drug interaction

Carbamazepine, alcohol, tobacco, oral contraceptives, phenytoin and phenobarbital can induce drug metabolizing enzymes, which can lead to the metabolism of TCAs increased and the blood concentration decreased. While cimetidine, ritalin, chlorpromazine, haloperidol, thyroid hormone, estrogen can inhibit the metabolism of TCAs, which increase the blood concentration. TCAs have an effect on other drugs. They can antagonize the antihypertensive effect of guanethidine and clonidine, increase central inhibition of alcohol and sleeping pills. Combined with sympatheticomimetic can lead to hypertension, seizures, enhance anticholinergic drugs and anticholinergic side effects of antipsychotic drugs, and promote the central nervous toxicity of monoamine oxidase.

(6) Commonly-used tricyclic antidepressants

1) Amitriptyline

Amitriptyline is a representative drug of TCAs. The drug has definite antidepressant effect and good sleeping effect, and has a definite effect on chronic pain. It is the most commonly-used drug in TCAs.

Pharmacokinetics: it is easy to absorb orally. The peak time of the plasma concentration is 8-12 hours, the half-life is 9-25 hours, and the half-life in the elderly above 72 years old is 37.3 hours. The effective plasma concentration is 120 ng/mL, and the plasma protein binding rate is 96%, which is mainly metabolized in the liver. The active metabolites are nortriptyline, 70% of which is excreted from the urine, and 22% is excreted from the feces. It can pass the placental barrier and be secreted in the milk.

Function and application: it is a central presynaptic NE, 5-HT reuptake inhibitor, which also acts on the H_1 receptor and the M receptor, and has a strong anticholinergic and sedative effect. It can effectively improve the mood of the patients with depression, and improve their thinking difficulties, slow action, loss of appetite, insomnia and general malaise. It also has a good anti-anxiety effect. It has good effect on endogenous depression, climacteric depression and somatoform disorder.

Usage and dosage: the first dose is 12.5 mg, 2 times a day, and gradually increased to 150-300 mg/d, which is divided into 2-3 times. The maintenance dose is 50-150 mg/d.

Adverse reactions: ①digestive system: dry mouth, constipation, nausea, vomiting, diarrhea, abdominal distention, paralytic intestinal obstruction, oral odor, liver toxicity and gastroesophageal reflux. ②Blood system: aplastic anemia, leukocytopenia, thrombocytopenia, acid granulocytosis, granulocytic deficiency and myelosuppression. ③Cardiovascular system: occasionally arrhythmia, ECG changes, ventricular tachycardia, palpitation, myocardial infarction, cardiomyopathy, hypotension, and malignant hypertension. ④Nervous system: drowsiness, vertigo, dyskinesia, epileptic seizures, tardive dyskinesia, fatigue, upset, tinnitus, excitement, confusion, mental confusion, ophthalmoplegia, myasthenia gravis and delirium. ⑤Endocrine and metabolism: lactation, hyperthyroidism, hypoglycemia, hyperglycemia and vasopressin secretion abnormality.

⑥The reproductive/urinary system: sexual dysfunction, dysuria and enlargement of testis. ⑦The allergic reaction: allergic dermatitis, angioedema. ⑧The other: fever, sweating, blurred vision, weight gain, increased intraocular pressure and chest pain.

2) Clomipramine

Pharmacokinetics: it is easy to absorb orally. The peak time of the plasma concentrationis 2−6 hours, the bioavailability is 20%−78%, and the protein binding rate is 97%. The parent drug production has a half−life of 19−37 hours, whose metabolite is desclomipramine and its half−life is 54−77 hours. It is metabolized in the liver, its active metabolite are desclomipramine and 8−hydroxy desclomipramine. 51%−60% are excreted by urine and 24%−32% are excreted by feces.

Function and application: it is the central presynaptic NE/5−HT reuptake inhibitor, but the reuptake of 5−HT is greater than the reuptake of NE, so it has a good anti−obsessive−compulsive effect. The anticholinergic action is medium, and it also has anti−anxiety and sedative effects. Combined with SSRIs has an enhanced anti−compulsive effect. Small doses can be used to treat premature ejaculation.

Usage and dosage: oral: anti depressive and compulsive dose is 12.5 mg for the first time, 2 times a day, and can be increased to 150−250 mg/d, 2−3 times a day in a week. The maintenance dose is 50−100 mg/d.

Intra−muscular injection: the first dose of antidepressant and compulsion is 25−50 mg/d, and then can be increased to 100−150 mg/d. After the symptom relieves, it can be changed to oral maintenance.

Intra−venous drip: the first dose of antidepressant and obsessive−compulsive is 25−75 mg/d, which is dissolved in 250−500 mL 0.9% sodium chloride or 5% glucose, once a day. After the effect, continue to drip for 3−5 days, then it can be changed to oral maintenance.

Adversereactions: there are side effects of the digestive system, the endocrine and metabolic system, the nervous system, and the cardiovascular system.

(7) Tetracyclic antidepressants

1) Mapratiline

Pharmacokinetics: the oral absorption is slow but completely. The peak time of plasma concentration is 4−16 hours, and the half−life is 27−58 hours. The binding rate of plasma protein is 88%. The concentration of the lungs, adrenal glands and thyroid glands are high, but the brain, spinal cord and nerve tissue are low. At two hours after intravenous injection, the concentration of CNS was the highest in the hippocampus, followed by the brain, cerebellar cortex, thalamus and midbrain. There was a linear relationship between the concentration of blood and the dose. The main metabolites are finally combination with glucuronic acid, which are excreted from urine and feces.

Function and application: it is a NE reuptake inhibitor which mainly inhibits NE reuptake of the presynaptic. It has a strong antidepressant effect, and also has moderate anticholinergic and sedative effects. It is used for all kinds of depression and other depressive disorders characterized by anxiety and irritability. It is also effective for the depressive state of schizophrenia.

Usage and dosage: oral administration: 75−150 mg/d, once or twice per day. Severe patients can be added to 200 mg/d, and individual can be added to 300 mg/d.

Intravenous injection: 25−100 mg/d.

Adverse reactions: there are mainly dry mouth, fatigue, blurred vision, sleep disorder, and occasional drop of blood pressure and tachycardia. Large dose application can cause T wave inversion and conduction block, and can also cause convulsions. Patients with liver and kidney function damage, glaucoma, dysuria, heart dysfunction, skin allergy, epilepsy are carefully used. Pregnant women and breast−feeding women are forbidden. It can enhance the cardiovascular effects of NE, epinephrine, central depressant and anticholinergic drugs, and should be used carefully. It is forbidden to combine with monoamine oxidase inhibitor (MAOIs).

2) Mianserin

Pharmacokinetics: it is easy to absorb orally. The time to reach plasma peak is 3 hours, the effective blood concentration is 15-75 mg/d, and the plasma protein binding rate is 96%. The metabolism in the liver is mainly excreted from the urine, the half-life is 14-33 hours in young adults, and the old people are 18-48 hours. Long term use does not damage the conduction of the heart, and does not affect the myocardial contractive power.

Function and application: it can be used to improve all kinds of depressive symptoms, including dysthymia and anxiety disorders. It also has some effect on the relapse of psychoactive substances abuse, and it is effective for posttraumatic stress disorder and pain.

Usage and dosage: the effective dose is 30-90 mg/d. The first suitable dose is 15 mg/d. Once taken before retiring, sleep can be improved. The maintenance dose is 15 - 30 mg/d. The maximum dose is 120 mg/d. The dose of controlled drinking is 30-60 mg/d.

Adverse reactions: includes sleepiness, dry mouth, constipation and blurred vision. Leukopenia and leukocyte deficiency occur occasionally, and it can be recovered after stop the medicine. Mianserin may exacerbate the inhibitory effect of alcohol on the central nervous system, so patients can't be drinking during medication. Patients with glaucoma, prostatic hypertrophy, epilepsy, diabetes, and cerebral organic diseases are carefully used.

20.2.3.5 Monoamine oxidase inhibitor(MAOIs): moclobemide

Pharmacokinetics: it is easy to be absorbed orally. After a single oral dose of 50-300 mg, the peak plasma concentration is 0.3-2.7 g/mL, and the peak time is 1-2 hours. The bioavailability is positively related to the dose and repeated use of drugs. The binding rate of plasma protein was about 50%, and the apparent volume was 75-95 L/kg. The drug is widely distributed in the body. It is metabolized by the liver, with a half-life of 2-3 hours. The average retention time of the patients with liver cirrhosis is prolonged, so this patient needs to be reduced by half. Patients with moderate renal impairment generally do not need to do a dose titration. This product can be secreted by milk.

Function and application: monoamine oxidase inhibitors play an important role in the treatment of depression by inhibiting monoamine oxidase activity, reducing monoamine neuro-transmitter degradation and increasing the effective neurotransmitter level of synaptic gap. Monoamine oxidase(MAO) is a microsomal enzyme that degrades monoamine NE, 5-HT and DA, which have important physiological functions. There are two kinds of MAO, and they are MAO-A and MAO-B. The new generation of MAOIs is MAO-A inhibitor, whose antidepressant effect is obvious, and the improvement rate is 72% -88%. MAOIs have a good effect on atypical depression with excessive sleep, appetite, and weight gain. It also have a good effect on bulimia, social phobia, panic attacks, mixed state of depression and anxiety.

Usage and dosage: the initial dose of moclobemide treatmentis 300-450 mg/d, 3 times per day. The dose increased gradually from second weeks. The maximum daily dose is not more than 600 mg/d.

Adverse reaction: this kind of drug should not be combined with tricyclic. If the TCAs are invalid first, the MAOIs can be added after the discontinuation of TCAs, and the period of cleaning is not necessary. If MAOIs is ineffective first, TCAs are used after 1-2 weeks of MAOIs withdrawal. It is forbidden to combine with the 5-HT reuptake inhibitor, and it should not be used with the sympathomimetic amines drugs such as adrenalin and amphetamine. It should also avoid combine with dextromethorphan and pethidine.

20.2.3.6　Selective 5-HT reuptake inhibitors

(1)Mechanism

Selective 5-HT reuptake inhibitors(SSRIs) selectively inhibits the recovery of the 5-HT of the presynaptic membrane,which has little effect on the NE,and does not affect the recovery of DA.

(2)Classification

There are six kinds of SSRIs widely used in clinic,include fluoxetine,paroxetine,sertraline,fluvoxamine,citalopram and escitalopram.

(3)Clinical characteristics

The antidepressant effect is equivalent to TCAs,but the effect on severe depression is probably less than that of TCAs. The half-life is long,most of them only need one times a day,and the curative effect is gradually disappearing after a long time of stopping medicine. Cardiovascular and anticholinergic side-effects are mild,and prostatic hypertrophy and glaucoma patients can also be used.

(4)Adverse reaction

They mainly include nausea,diarrhea,insomnia,unease and sexual dysfunction,and the most common side-effects are short,transient and tolerable.

(5)Drug interaction

They combined with other antidepressants often enhance the curative effect,but does not combine with MAOIs,it may lead to a patient with 5-HT syndrome when it is combined with MAOIs.

(6)Commonly-used SSRIs drugs

1)Fluoxetine

Pharmacokinetics:it is easy to absorb orally,and does not affect by eating. The peak time is 4-6 hours. The half-life is the longest,the half-life of the single-dose is 48-72 hours,and the half-life of the multiple dosing can reach 132 hours. The half-life of the active metabolite is norfluoxetine,whose half-life can reach 7-15 days. It is metabolized by the liver,and liver disease can significantly prolong its clearance time. 80% of the metabolite was excreted by urine and 15% from feces. Fluoxetine has inhibitory effect on CYP2D6,CYP2C and CYP3A4.

Function and application:it has high specificity and selective 5-HT reuptake inhibition. It has no affinity for cholinergic receptor,alpha receptor and histamine receptor,so it has no sedation,hypotension and anticholinergic side effects. Fluoxetine is mainly applicable to a variety of depression,social phobia,bulimia,obsessive compulsive spectrum diseases,depression with obesity and diabetes. It can also be used as an adjuvant abstinence therapy for psychoactive substances abuse.

Usage and dosage: the ideal dose is 20 mg/d,and the side-effects are increased as the dose increased. In the treatment of obsessive-compulsive disorder,bulimia and lose weight,dose is relatively large,which generally is 60 mg/d.

Adverse reaction:it can cause weight loss,anxiety,shock,and insomnia. It also has side effects of nausea,diarrhea and anorexia. It can inhibit platelet aggregation and reduce dosage of anticoagulant drugs when combined with anticoagulant drugs. The side-effects of central nervous system include nervousness,insomnia,tremor,anxiety,dizziness,occasional akathisia,and some patients can have sexual dysfunction.

2)Paroxetine

Pharmacokinetics:it is easy to absorb orally. The peak time is 4 to 6 hours,and the half-life is 24 hours. It is metabolized by the liver,and most of its metabolites are excreted from the urine,then other parts are excreted from the feces.

Function and application:paroxetine is a powerful 5-HT recovery blocker. It has high affinity for NE and cholinergic receptor, so it is more suitable for depression accompanied by anxiety. It has a good effect on depression, anxiety disorder(especially for panic disorder), phobia, chronic pain, eating disorder and alcohol dependence. It also has good therapeutic effect on premenstrual syndrome, premature ejaculation and post-traumatic stress disorder. The drug can inhibit nitric oxide synthase, which make nitric oxide synthesis less, and affect the activity of guanylate cyclase. Guanylate cyclase influence the formation of cyclic guanosine monophosphate, and weaken the excessive erectile function. So paroxetine can be used for the hypersexual of depression and compulsive sexual behavior.

Usage and dosage: the initial dose is 20 mg/d. According to the patient's condition, add 10 mg each time, usually not more than 50 mg/d.

Adverse reaction: paroxetine has anticholinergic effects, treatment dose on the elderly may cause constipation. Paroxetine is a nitric oxide synthase inhibitor, which can cause impotence, ejaculation delay, orgasm delay, and sexual desire deficiency. Paroxetine had strong inhibitory effect on CYP2D6, and can inhibit its metabolism. In the late stage of withdrawal, the inhibition of enzyme disappeared and the concentration of blood decreased rapidly, and the symptomatic rebound appeared easily. The use of paroxetine can have an extrapyramidal side reaction, and should be paid attention to. Patients with prostatic hypertrophy and glaucoma should not be used.

3) Sertraline

Pharmacokinetics: it is easy to be absorbed orally. The peak time is 6-10 hours, and the half-life is 26 hours. There is a positive correlation between the concentration of blood and the dose. It is metabolized by the liver, and the metabolites are excreted from urine and feces. Patients with liver dysfunction can prolong the half-life to 52 hours, and those with renal damage have little influence.

Function and application: sertraline is applicable to all kinds of depression, obsessive-compulsive disorder, panic disorder, post-traumatic stress disorder. It is especially suitable for the elderly depression, and can significantly improve the elderly patients with depression mood, cognitive, psychomotor and sexual function. It has a good effect on anorexia, social anxiety disorder, panic attack and obsessive compulsive disorder. It can be used for the treatment of cocaine dependence and withdrawal syndrome. Sertraline does not affect the blood pressure and volume ejection of the heart, and it can be used for the depressive symptoms associated with coronary heart disease.

Usage and dosage: the daily dose of antidepressant treatment is 50 mg, which could be increased to 100-200 mg/d after 1-2 weeks. In the treatment of obsessive-compulsive disorder, the dosage of the drug is increased.

Adverse reaction: the common side effects are nausea, somnolence, diarrhea, dry mouth, insomnia, and occasional hypotension. Patients with epilepsy, liver and kidney dysfunction, pregnancy, lactation should not be used.

4) Citalopram

Pharmacokinetics: it is easy to be absorbed orally. The half-life is 33 hours, and the drug concentration of blood reached a peak at about 4 hours after a single-dose of 40 mg citalopram. The bio-availability of citalopram is 80%, and the absorption is not affected by food. The distribution volume of citalopram is 12 L/kg.

Function and application: citalopram is a powerful reuptake inhibitor of 5-HT, which has high affinity to H_1 receptor and easy to induce sedation. The indication is similar to other SSRIs. The effect of citalopram on the cytochrome P450 enzyme of liver is the smallest in SSRIs, so there is almost no pharmaceutical incompatibility.

Usage and dosage: the daily oral dose of adults is 20 – 60 mg, once per day. The initial dose is 20 mg/d, and can be increased to 60 mg maximum daily dose according to the severity of the disease and the response of the patients. In order to prevent recurrence, the treatment should be lasted for at least 6 months. Patients over 65 years old and patients with liver function injury are half the dosage, and the daily dose is 10–30 mg. The initial dose is 10 mg daily, the recommended dose is 20 mg daily, and the maximum dose is 40 mg/d.

Adverse reaction: it is nontoxic to the heart, but can cause weight gain. Some patients can have dry mouth, headache, uroschesis, constipation, tremor, insomnia, and hypotension. It is not suitable to be used with MAOIs.

5) Fluvoxamine

Pharmacokinetics: it is easy to be absorbed orally. The drug concentration of blood reached a peak at 3. 5–8 hours after a single-dose of 100 mg fluvoxamine. The half–life of the single–dose is 15 hours, and the half–life of the multiple dosing can reach 22 hours. The concentration of the organs in the liver, kidney, lung and adrenal gland were higher than that of the blood drug. The steady state blood concentration is generally reached in 10 days. It is metabolized by the liver, and its metabolites have no pharmacological activity. The 90% of drug is excreted from urine, and the pharmacokinetic parameters of the elderly are similar to those of young people.

Function and application: it is suitable for all kinds of depression, especially for suicidal attempts. Depression with glaucoma, prostatic hypertrophy, and heart disease can be used. It has a good effect on anxiety, panic disorder, obsessive–compulsive disorder, body dysmorphic disorder and bulimia nervosa. It also has a good therapeutic effect on kleptomania, pathological gambling and shopaholic. Fluvoxamine can alleviate anxiety, insomnia and wine search behavior after alcohol withdrawal. The enzyme inhibitory effect of fluvoxamine can reduce the dose of alprazolam, triazolam, and midazolam, and it can be treated the drug resistance and dependence.

Usage and dosage: the first dose can be 25 mg at night, and increased gradually without obvious side effects. The treatment dose is 100–200 mg/d, and the maximum dose is 300 mg/d. When the daily dose is greater than 100 mg, it can be divided into 2 times.

Adverse reaction: the most common–side effects in the early stages are nausea, vomiting, somnolence, constipation, anorexia, fatigue, hypokinesia, tremor, and occasional thrombocytopenia. After taking a period of time, some side effects can disappear. The patients with epilepsy, liver and kidney dysfunction are carefully used. The therapeutic dose even can cause sexual dysfunction, which has a low incidence of about 10%, and has no effect on ejaculation.

6) Escitalopram

Escitalopram is the mainactive ingredient of citalopram, which is the dextroisomer of citalopram.

Pharmacokinetics: it's easy to be absorbed orally completely. The time to reach the plasma peak concentration is 4 hours after oral administration. The binding rate of plasma protein is 80%, and the half–life is 30 hours. Escitalopram is mainly metabolized by the liver P450 enzyme CYP2C19, but CYP3A4 and CYP2D6 are also involved in the metabolism of the drug. It is mainly excreted from the kidney in the form of metabolites. Drug metabolism in elderly patients is slower than young people.

Function and application: the indications of FDA approval are depression(over 12 years of age), generalized anxiety attacks, social anxiety disorders, and panic disorder. The indications approved by SFDA in China are depressive disorder and panic disorder. It is not used for children.

Usage and dosage: the therapeutic dose is 10–20 mg/d, the maximum daily dose is 20 mg, and taking

2－4 weeks can show the curative effect. The elderly start with half the dose, the therapeutic dose is generally not more than 10 mg/d. There is no need to adjust the dose of mild to moderate renal dysfunction. Severe renal dysfunction should be used carefully. The patients of liver dysfunction are recommended from 5 mg. The dose is adjusted to 10 mg/d according to the patient's individual response in two weeks.

Adverse reaction: escitalopram is well tolerated and has few adverse reactions. The side－effects are similar to other SSRIs drugs. The common side－effects are nausea, insomnia and gastrointestinal adverse reactions. Escitalopram did not have a significant impact on weight.

20.2.3.7　Selective 5－HT and NE reuptake inhibitors

（1）Venlafaxine

Pharmacokinetics: the half－life is 7 hours and metabolized by the liver, whose metabolites have high pharmacological activity. It is excreted from the kidneys, and the half－life is 4－5 hours. The clearance rate is affected by the function of liver and kidney. In the case of liver cirrhosis, the clearance rate decreased by 33% and the half－life of clearance increased by 2 times. The clearance rate of renal failure is reduced by 55%. The clearance rate of elderly people is lower than young people, and the half－life is prolonged.

Function and application: it strongly inhibits the reuptake of 5－HT and NE in the presynaptic membrane, and also weak inhibits DA's reuptake function. It also has a rapid down－regulation of adrenergic beta receptor. So venlafaxine is called 5－HT and NE reuptake inhibitor(SNRI). Low dose only had 5－HT reuptake blocking effect, and middle and high doses had 5－HT and NE reuptake blocking. Very high doses had DA,5－HT and NE reuptake blocking effect. Middle to high doses are used in patients with depression, severe depression, and refractory depression. Quick effect and good tolerance are its advantages. Low dose can be used for sluggishness, excessive sleep, weight gain, and atypical depression. It has good curative effect on refractory depression, anxiety disorder, attention deficit hyperactivity disorder, dysthymic disorder and chronic pain disorder. It is especially good for back pain, muscle pain, heavy sense of extremities and fatigue.

Usage and dosage: the fast release dosage form is used for mild to moderate depression with an initial dose of 25 mg each time,2－3 times per day, and the drug dose is adjusted according to the condition of the disease. Suicidal depression should be added to 200 mg/d within per week, and the maximum dose is 375 mg/d. The initial dosage of sustained－release dosage form is 75 mg/d. It can be increased to 225 mg/d necessary, the average dose is 105 mg/d. The shortest interval is less than 4 days.

Adverse reaction: the side－effects of low dose are nausea, agitation, sexual dysfunction and insomnia. The side－effects of middle and high dose are severe insomnia, agitation, nausea, headache and hypertension. Venlafaxine can lead to 5－HT syndrome. When combined with MAOIs, this serious reaction is more likely to occur and even death. The dose of patients with liver and kidney dysfunction should be reduced, and the patients with epilepsy and blood diseases are used carefully. Patients should avoid drinking during the period of drug use.

（2）Duloxetine

Pharmacokinetics: the half－life of duloxetine is about 12 hours, and the pharmacokinetic parameters are proportional to the dose. The steady state blood concentration reached 3 days after taking the medicine. Duloxetine is mainly metabolized by liver and involves two kinds of P450 enzymes which are CYP2D6 and CYP1A2.

Function and application: duloxetine has a strong inhibitory effect on the reuptake of 5－HT and NE in the presynaptic membrane, which can increase the concentration of 5－HT and NE in the brain and CSF, improve the depressive symptoms and the body's tolerance to pain. Duloxetine can improve somatization caused by depression, such as muscle pain, abdominal pain, headache and other symptoms. The improvement of anxiety symptoms also has a good effect. It is used to treat the symptoms of major depression disorder (MDD), diabetic peripheral neuropathy(DPN) and women's urinary incontinence. It can quickly and broadly relieve the emotional and physical symptoms of depression(especially painful somatization).

Usage and dosage: duloxetine is used only for oral administration. The initial dose of antidepressant treatmentis 40−60 mg/d, generally not more than 60 mg/d. In the treatment of panic disorder, the initial dose is 60 mg/d, and it can be added to the maximum dose of 120 mg/d according to the patient's tolerance.

Adverse reaction: common adverse reactionsare nausea, dry mouth, constipation, increased fatigue, lack of appetite, lethargy and sweating. Other adverse reactions are diarrhea, nausea, weight loss, dizziness, tremor, hot flashes, blurred vision, anxiety, loss of libido, sexual satisfaction decreased, erectile dysfunction, and delayed ejaculation dysfunction. The effect of duloxetine on blood pressure and QTc interphase are no significant clinical significance.

20.2.3.8　5−HT2A receptor antagonist and 5−HT reuptake inhibitor: trazodone

Pharmacokinetics: it is easy to absorb orally. The peak time is 6−10 hours, and the time of steady state blood drug concentration is 4−7 days. The half−life is 5−9 hours. It is metabolized by the liver and the active metabolite is m−chlorobenzperazine(m−CPP), which is discharged from the urine in the form of dissociation and binding.

Function and application: the pharmacological effects include blocking the 5−HT2 receptor, selectively inhibiting the reuptake of 5−HT and blocking the 5−HT2A. The metabolite m−CPP is produced by CYP2D6 enzyme. M−CPP is a 5−HT1A, 5−HT1B, 5−HT1C and 5−HT1D receptor agonist. Trazodone acts on adrenaline, which has a weak presynaptic alpha−2 receptor blockage, a relatively strong postsynaptic alpha−1 receptor antagonism, and H_1 receptor blocking action. It is suitable for the patients with anxiety, intense and sleep disorder. It has a good effect on organic, drug−induced, psychogenic impotence, and can improve sleep quality, increased deep sleep, reduced sleep latency, reduce awakening. It also has a good therapeutic effect on nightmare.

Usage and dosage: the initial oral dose is 25−50 mg per night, and it can be added to 100−150 mg/d in 5−7 days. If the dose is more than 100 mg/d, it can be taken 2 times per day. The maximum dose is 300 mg/d.

Adverse reaction: the common adverse reactions include drowsy, fatigue, dizziness, insomnia, intense, nausea, and postural hypotension. Trazodone has a strong sedative effect(blocking H_1 receptor) and can also cause priapism and pain. Patients with hypotension and ventricular arrhythmia are forbidden.

20.2.3.9　NE and DA reuptake inhibitor: bupropion

Pharmacokinetics: oral bupropion is absorbed rapidly, and the peak time of the plasma concentration is 3 hours. The binding rate of plasma protein is 85%. Drug elimination is divided into two phases, the first phase is 1.5 hours and the second phase is 14 hours. 87% of the drug is excreted by urine and 10% from feces.

Function and application: it has the inhibitory effect of DA reuptake and the effect of agitating DA. Long−term large dose can down−regulated the beta adrenergic receptor. It is applicable to hysteresis depression, excessive sleep, pseudo dementia, and those who are ineffective or intolerant with SSRIs. It can also be used for attention deficit disorder, chronic fatigue syndrome, smoking cessation, the abstinence and craving of stimulants.

Usage and dosage: the initial dose of the fast release dosage form is 100 mg, twice per day, and 3 days after the dosage can be added to 100 mg,3 times per day. The initial dose of the sustained−release dosage form is 150 mg/d,and after 4 days the dose can be added to 150 mg,twice per day.

Adverse reaction: the common adverse reactions are fidgeting, insomnia, headache, nausea and sweating. There are reports of epileptic seizures,so patients with a history of epilepsy are carefully used. Individual can also cause psychosis.

20.2.3.10   Selective NE reuptake inhibitor: reboxetine

Pharmacokinetics: the half−life of reboxetine is 12−16 hours, and the elderly is 15−24 hours. The binding rate of reboxetine with plasma protein is high,and 97% is combined with alpha−1−acid glycoprotein. Therefore,the change of protein level in blood will affect the pharmacokinetics of reboxetine. The concentration of alpha−1−acid glycoprotein in the plasma is increased in the elderly due to lung diseases, which can lead to the increase of blood drug concentration and the decrease of renal clearance of reboxetine.

Function and application: reboxetine is an inhibitor of CYP2D6 and CYP3A4,which has a good effect on all kinds of depression,and it is obviously better than fluoxetine in the recovery of social function.

Usage and dosage: the dose is 8 mg/d,and 4 mg/d in the elderly.

Adverse reaction: the common adverse reactions include dry mouth,constipation,hypotension,tachycardia,abnormal pulsation of the atrium,abnormal ventricular pulsation,abnormal skin sensation and urinary incontinence. It does not have a sedative effect,does not affect cognitive function,and does not interact with alcohol. It can increase the latent period of REM.

20.2.3.11   Noradrenergic and specific serotonergic antidepressant(NaSSA): mirtazapine

Pharmacokinetics: it is easy to take orally and quickly absorbed. The peak time is 2 hours,the half−life is 20−40 hours,and the time of reaching the blood steady concentration is 3−5 days. The rate of plasma protein binding is 85%,and the bio−availability is 50%. It is metabolized by the liver,and the hepatocyte P450 enzyme CYP2D6 and CYP1A2 are involved in the formation of hydroxylated metabolites. The metabolites are excreted by urine(85%) and feces(15%). Patients with liver dysfunction may reduce their clearance rate,prolong the half−life by 40%,and patients with renal dysfunction also reduce the clearance rate. It does not inhibit CYP2D6,CYP1D2,CYP3A,and no enzyme induction. Carbamazepine is CYP3A4 enzyme inducer which can reduce the blood concentration of mirtazapine by 60%,so mirtazapine is not suitable to be used with carbamazepine.

Function and application: it is the first choice of antidepressant drugs for moderate and severe depression with anxiety,intense,insomnia and long−term treatment. It also has a good effect for the somatoform disorders with long−term insomnia,poor appetite,and systemic wandering pain. It is suitable for somatoform disorders with gastrointestinal disorders,irritable bowel syndrome,loss of appetite,abdominal distension, belching. Mirtazapine can improve the compliance of alcohol addicts and improve the clinical symptoms,depressive symptoms and cancer patients' life quality.

Usage and dosage: mirtazapine's method of taking is 15−45 mg/d,once before bedtime,and the recommended amount of the elderly is the same as the adult. After the patient's condition was completely relieved,the patient continued to take 6−9 months. The pregnancy is forbidden.

Adverse reaction: common adverse reaction include sedation and weight gain. But the sedation will gradually disappear as the treatment continues. Weight gain may be associated with improvement in appetite,so the patients with obesity and gluttony should be used carefully. The drug rarely affects sexual function,and it can improve sexual function.

20.2.3.12　Atypical antidepressant: deanxit

Deanxit is a mixture of small dose flupentixol and melitracen. Each tablet contains 0.5 mg of flupentixol and 10 mg of melitracen. Its characteristics are rapid-onset, less side effects and safe. It is combined with tricyclic, tetracyclica and SSRIs antidepressant drugs can enhance the efficacy.

Pharmacokinetics: it is absorbed quickly by oral administration. The time for flupentixol to reach the peak concentration of the plasma is 4 hours, and the half-life is 35 hours. It is metabolized by the liver, 60% of the drug is excreted from the feces, and 15% to 20% is excreted from the urine. The time for melitracen to reach the peak concentration of the plasma is 3.5 hours, and the half-life is 19 hours. The small part of the metabolism is excreted from the feces and most of them are excreted from the urine. Only a small amount of the two are secreted by the placenta and milk.

Function and application: deanxit has the effect of blocking the 5-HT2A receptor and enhancing the effect of 5-HT1A, so it can play an anti-anxiety and anti-depressant effect. Melitracen can inhibit presynaptic membrane reuptake norepinephrine and 5-HT. It improves the content of monoamine transmitters in the synaptic gap, and plays the antidepressant and anti-anxiety effects, which also has the antihistamine effect and can play a sedative effect. Deanxit is mainly used for anxiety and depressive symptoms caused by depression, anxiety, physical disease, organic diseases of the brain, stress and substance withdrawal. It has good effects on neurasthenia, somatoform disorders (somatization disorder, somatoform autonomic dysfunction, somatoform pain disorder).

Usage and dosage: the usage of adults is 1 tablet in the morning and 1 tablet at noon, but 1 tablet in the morning for the elderly. The amount of maintenance is 1 tablet per day.

Adverse reaction: some patients can have a slight dry mouth, occasional insomnia and uneasiness. Patients with serious heart diseases such as early recovery of myocardial infarction, bundle branch block, and narrow angle glaucoma are forbidden. Pregnant and lactation women are used carefully. It is forbidden to be used with monoamine oxidase inhibitors.

20.2.3.13　Herbal medicine: neurostan

The content of hyperforin is not less than 9 mg, and the total content of hypericin is not less than 0.4 mg. In addition, there are many ingredients such as flavonolglucoside, procyanidin and so on. Neurostan is a pure plant antidepressant.

Pharmacokinetics: the patients are given a single dose of 300 mg of Saint John's Wort extract, three times a day, the plasma concentration reached the peak value after 3.6 hours, and the blood steady concentration is reached after 4 days. The half-life of the important components of hyperforinis 9.5 hours. It is mainly metabolized by the liver, and the metabolites are excreted by the kidneys through urine.

Function and application: it inhibits the reabsorption of epinephrine (NE), 5-serotonin (5-HT) and dopamine (DA) in the presynaptic membrane, and increase the concentration of three kinds of neurotransmitters in the synaptic gap. It can down-regulate the function of hypothalamus-pituitary-adrenal axis (HPA) and hypothalamus-pituitary-thyroid axis (HPT), and effectively improve the depressive symptoms. By increasing the formation of melatonin at night, it increases slow wave sleep and improves the quality of sleep. Neurostan is suitable for mild, moderate, severe depression, and depression caused by physical disease. Neurostan has a good therapeutic effect on cerebral dysfunction, depression and memory impairment caused by cerebral ischemic disease, especially for patients with depression caused by cerebrovascular diseases. It has a therapeutic effect on the memory and depression of brain degeneration, such as Alzheimer's disease, and it can also delay the progress of the disease.

Usage and dosage: the amount of adults and children over 12 years old is once 300 mg, 2-3 times a day. When necessary, the dose can be adjusted to 2 tablets each time, 3 times a day.

Adverse reaction: there is a rare side effect. There are few gastrointestinal discomforts, anaphylaxis (such as skin red, swollen, itching), fatigue or uneasiness.

20.2.4   Mood stabilizers

Mood stabilizers, also known as anti-manic drug, are drugs that treat mania, prevent manic or depressive episodes. They include lithium (lithium carbonate) and some antiepileptic drugs such as carbamazepine, valproate etc.

20.2.4.1   Lithium carbonate

Lithium carbonate is the most commonly used anti-manic drug.

(1) Pharmacokinetics

The half-life is 12-24 hours, and the steady state blood concentration needs 5-7 days. Lithium ion is not combined with plasma and tissue protein, which is distributed throughout the body with the body fluid, and the concentration of thyroid and kidney are the highest. Lithium does not change in the body. 95% of the drug is excreted from the urine, and a small amount is excreted from feces, sweat and milk. The absorption of lithium in the proximal convoluted tubule and sodium is competitive, so the rate of excretion is related to the sodium salt intake.

(2) Function and application

The mechanism of lithium salt has not yet been elucidated, and they were mainly concentrated in several aspects of electrolytes, central neurotransmitters, and cyclic adenosine. Lithium salts can replace sodium ions in cells and reduce the excitability of cells. It can also interact with potassium, calcium and magnesium ions to change the distribution of the cells inside and outside, and replace some of the physiological functions of these ions. Lithium can inhibit the synthesis and release of norepinephrine, dopamine and acetylcholine in the brain, and increase the reuptake of norepinephrine and 5 – serotonin in presynaptic membrane. Lithium salt can promote the synthesis and release of 5-serotonin, inhibit adenylate cyclase, and reduce the production of second messenger cyclic adenosine monophosphate (cAMP), which reduce the physiological effect of target cells.

Lithium carbonate is the drug for the treatment of mania, and has preventive effects on mania, bipolar disorder and depression. Schizophrenia with emotional disorders, excitement and agitation can be used as an enhanced therapeutic drug for antipsychotic therapy.

(3) Usage and dosage

The usual specification of lithium carbonate is 250 mg per pill, and it is used orally after meals. The general initial dose is 250 mg per time, 2-3 times a day. The dose can be gradually increased to the effective dose range of 750-1,500 mg/d, occasionally up to 2,000 mg/d.

The poisoned dose of lithium salt is close to the dose of treatment. It is necessary to detect the concentration of lithium in blood, adjust the dose and determine whether there is any poisoning. When treating acute cases, the concentration of blood lithium should be 0.8-1.0 mmol/L. It is easy to cause toxic reactions over 1.4 mmol/L, especially in elderly patients and organic diseases. The onset time of lithium salt treatment is generally 7-10 days. Lithium is suitable for maintenance treatment of bipolar disorder and mania recurrently. Lithium salt can reduce the number of recurrence and reduce the severity of the diseases.

(4) Adverse reaction

Lithium is reabsorbed in the kidney with sodium competition, and the deficiency of sodium or kidney disease may lead to the accumulation of lithium in the body. Side-effects are associated with the concentration of blood lithium. The common occurrence time is $1-2$ weeks, and some appear later. Often drinking light salt water can reduce side effects. Side effects are generally divided into early side-effects, late side-effects and poisoning omen.

1)The early side-effects mainly include weakness, fatigue, somnolence, tremor of fingers, anorexia, abdominal discomfort, nausea, vomiting, dilute stool, diarrhea, polyuria, and dry mouth.

2)The later side-effects are caused by the continuous intake of lithium salts. The patient will have continued polyuria, thirst, weight gain, goiter, myxedema, and fine tremor of the finger. The presence of tremor coarse suggests that the concentration of blood is close to the level of poisoning. Lithium interferes with the synthesis of thyroxine, and female patients can cause hypothyroidism. Electrocardiogram changes similar to hypokalemia may also occur, but they are reversible and may be associated with lithium salt in the replacement of myocardial potassium.

3)The precursor of lithium poisoning is vomiting, diarrhea, tremor coarse, twitch, dull, sleepy, vertigo, dysarthria and disturbance of consciousness. The concentration of blood lithium should be detected immediately and the amount of lithium should be reduced when the concentration of blood lithium reaches 1.4 mmol/L. If the clinical symptoms are serious, the treatment of lithium salt should be stopped immediately. The concentration of blood lithium in the patients are higher, the change of electroencephalogram are more obvious. So it is valuable to detect the electroencephalogram.

4)There are many reasons for lithium poisoning, including the decrease of lithium clearance rate, the influence of kidney disease, the decrease of sodium intake, the overdose of patients, the infirmity of old age and the improper control of blood lithium concentration. The symptoms of intoxication include ataxia, disturbance of motor coordination, muscle spasm, barylalia and confusion, which can lead to coma and death. Severe poisoning symptoms can lead to coma and death. Once the symptoms of poisoning occur, lithium salts should be discontinued immediately. A large number of saline or hypertonic sodium salts are given to accelerate the excretion of lithium or carry out artificial blood dialysis.

Patients with acute and chronic nephritis, renal insufficiency, severe cardiovascular disease, myasthenia gravis, the first 3 months of pregnancy, sodium depletion and low salt diet are forbidden. The patients with Parkinson disease, epilepsy, diabetes, hypothyroidism, neurodermatitis, psoriasis and senile cataract were carefully used.

20.2.4.2 Antiepileptic drugs with mood stability

Several antiepileptic drugs can be used as mood stabilizers. Carbamazepine and valproate are commonly used. In recent years the development of some new antiepileptic drugs, such as gabapentin, lamotrigine and topiramateare used for the treatment of affective disorders.

(1)Carbamazepine

Pharmacokinetics: its oral absorption is slow and irregular. The time of blood peak concentration after oral drugs of 400 mg is 4-5 hours, the peak value of blood concentration is 8-12 μg/mL, and the time to reach the steady-state plasma concentration is $8-55$ hours. The bioavailability is between 58% and 85%. The plasma protein binding rate is about 76%. It is mainly metabolized by the liver, which induces the activity of the liver drug enzyme and accelerate the metabolism of their own drugs. Long term use induced drug metabolism, and the half-life decreased to 10-20 hours. Carbamazepine is mainly excreted in urine and feces in the form of inactive metabolites.

Function and application: it is effective in treating acute mania and preventing manic episodes, especially for those who are not effective in lithium treatment, can't tolerate the side effects of lithium salts and have fast circulatory manic patients. Carbamazepine and lithium salt are combined to prevent relapse of bipolar affective disorder,which is better than lithium salt combined with antipsychotic drugs.

Usage and dosage:the initial dose is 400 mg/d,2 times for oral administration,and the dose can be increased by 200–400 mg every 3–5 days. The dose range is 400–1,600 mg/d,plasma levels should be 4–12 mg/L. The increase of the dose is too fast,it can lead to vertigo or ataxia.

Adverse reaction: carbamazepine has anticholinergic effects, which can lead to blurred vision, dry mouth,and constipation. Occasionally,it can cause leukocyte reduction,thrombocytopenia and liver dysfunction. Blood routine should be regularly tested during treatment. The patients with glaucoma,prostatic hypertrophy,diabetes and alcohol dependence are used carefully. Patients with Leukocyte reduction,thrombocytopenia,abnormal liver function,and pregnant women are forbidden.

(2) Valproate

The common valproate salts are sodium valproate and magnesium valproate.

Pharmacokinetics:they are absorbed quickly and completely. The bio–availability is 100%, and the binding rate of plasma protein is 80% – 94%. The time to reach the plasma peak concentration is 3.01 hours,the half–life is 16.9 hours,and it needs 5–7 days to reach the blood steady state. It is metabolized by the liver,which is excreted by the kidneys and a small amount is excreted from the feces.

Function and application:valproate can reverse or prevent the change of brain morphology in patients with affective disorder by activating RET pathway,and it play a role in stabilizing the mood and preventing recurrence. Valproate can also promote the generation,growth and survival of neurons in the cerebral cortex,which can enhance the generation of hippocampal neurons in adult animals. The treatment effect of valproate is the same as lithium. It may be better for patients with mixed episode and rapid circulatory affective disorder.

Usage and dosage:the initial doseis 400–600 mg/d,and it can be taken at 2–3 times. The dose can be increased by 200 mg every 2–3 days,and the dose range was 800–1,800 mg/d. The concentration of treatment should be 50–100 mg/L.

Adverse reaction: the common side effects are sedation, ataxia, tremor and gastrointestinal irritation symptoms such as nausea,vomiting,anorexia. The risen of transaminase is more common,and there are also reports of death in patients. There are few adverse reactions in the hematopoietic system,such as thrombocytopenia,lymphocyte increase. Toxic hepatitis and pancreatitis are rare. Patients with liver and pancreatic diseases are carefully used and pregnant women are forbidden.

(3) Topiramate

Pharmacokinetics:it can be absorbed quickly and completely. The average plasmapeak concentration is reached at 2 hours for healthy subjects with topiramate 100 mg,which is 1.5 μg/mL. Food has no clinically significant effect on the bioavailability of topiramate. Prototype topiramate and its metabolites are mainly excreted by kidney.

Function and application:topiramate is a new antiepileptic drug. It can enhance the activity of the inhibitory neurotransmitter gamma aminobutyric acid and prevent the effect of glutamic acid on the N–methyl–D–aspartic acid(NMDA) receptor. It has a quick effect on the rapid circulation and refractory bipolar affective disorder. The effect of anti–manic effect is better than antidepressant.

Usage and dosage:the low dose began to be used and gradually added to the effective dose. The doseof treatment is 200 mg/d.

Adverse reaction:the side–effects include nausea,diarrhea,somnolence,fatigue,cacesthesia,attention impairment,impaired memory,etc.

(4) Lamotrigine

Pharmacokinetics: lamotrigineis rapidly and completely absorbed in the intestine, and there is no obvious first pass effect. After oral administration, the plasma peak concentration is reached at 2. 5 hours. The peak time of oral administration after feed is slightly delayed, but the degree of absorption is not affected. The binding rate of plasma protein is about 55%. Lamotrigine is mainly metabolized to glucuronic acid combination, and then excreted in urine.

Function and application: lamotrigine directly stimulate the gamma aminobutyric acid-A receptor(GABA-A) receptor, inhibit the metabolism of GABA and reduce the reuptake of GABA by neurons or glia cells. It is safe and effective in the treatment of refractory fast circulatory bipolar affective disorder, which can reduce the frequency of circulation, improve mood and social function. Lamotrigine has antidepressant effect and antipsychotic effect.

Usage and dosage: the initial dose of monotherapy is 25 mg, once a day. The dose is maintained for 2 weeks, then the dose can be added to 50 mg, once a day for 2 weeks. After that, the dose was increased every 1-2 weeks. The maintenance dose of the best curative effect is 100-200 mg/d, and the dose is given 1 time or 2 times a day.

Adverse reaction: the adverse reactions include headache, tiredness, rash, nausea, dizziness, somnolence and insomnia.

20.2.5 Anxiolytic drugs

The anxiolytic drugs are widely used in clinical practice. At present, the most widely used are benzodiazepines, and the others include buspirone, beta adrenergic receptor blocker(propranolol) , some tricyclic antidepressants and antipsychotics. Benzodiazepines are often used as sedative and hypnotic drug, so the phenomenon of abuse is more serious. This section mainly introduces benzodiazepines and buspirone.

20.2.5.1 Benzodiazepines

(1) Mechanism and classification

Benzodiazepines have a wide variety of derivatives, the common species are more than 10. Benzodiazepines drugs act on the complex of gamma aminobutyric acid(GABA) , benzodiazepines receptor and chloride channel. Benzodiazepines can enhance the activity of GABA and further open the chloride channel, which causes the chloride ion enter into the cell, causing the hyperpolarization of the nerve cells, and thus plays a central inhibitory effect. There are four specific pharmacological effects:①the effect of anti-anxiety,②the sedative and hypnotic effects,③the anticonvulsant effect,④skeletal muscle relaxation.

(2) Indications and contraindications

Benzodiazepines drugs are anti-anxiety drugs and sedatives. They are widely used in the treatment neurosis, insomnia and various physical diseases accompanied by anxiety, tension, insomnia and autonomic nervous system disorders. They also can be used to all kinds of mental disorders associated with anxiety, tension, fear and insomnia, as well as the treatment of agitated depression and mild depression. They are also used for the treatment of epilepsy and the replacement therapy of acute withdrawal symptoms of alcohol.

Those patients with severe cardiovascular disease, nephropathy, drug allergy, drug dependence, the first 3 months of pregnancy, glaucoma, myasthenia gravis, use of alcohol and central depressants should be prohibited. The elderly, children, before and during childbirth are used carefully.

(3) The choice of drugs

When choosing drugs, we should be familiar with the characteristics of different drugs and the characteristics of the patients. If the patient has persistent anxiety and somatic symptoms, it is suitable for a long half-life of drugs, such as diazepam and clonazepam. If the patient's anxiety is fluctuating, the drug of short half-life should be selected, such as oxazepam, and lorazepam. Alprazolam has anti depressant effect, and depression patients can use this medicine. For patients with sleep disorder often taking flurazepam, nitrazepam, estazolam, clonazepam, midazolam. Clonazepam has a good effect on epilepsy. Diazepam is the best substitute for alcohol abstinence. Lorazepam, diazepam and nitrazepam can be used to relieve muscle tension. Patients with liver disease can use lorazepam and oxazepam, because they are not metabolized by the liver.

(4) Usage and dosage

Most benzodiazepines have a longer half-life and can be administered one times a day. According to the patient's condition, they can also be administered 2 times or 3 times a day. A small dose of benzodiazepines can be used in the beginning of treatment, and the amount of treatment can be added 3-4 days later. At the beginning of the acute phase, the dose may be slightly larger, or the intravenous dose is given.

(5) Course of treatment

The symptoms of neurosis often fluctuate by psychosocial factors. Therefore, after the benzodiazepines control the symptoms, the patient is not required to use this drug for a long time. Long-term application can't prevent the recurrence of disease, and long-term application is easy to lead to dependence and resistance. The withdrawal of medicine should be carried out slowly.

(6) Adverse reactions

Benzodiazepines have few side-effects, which are generally well tolerated and occasionally have serious complications. The most common side-effects are somnolence, excessive sedation, impairment of cognitive function, impaired memory, and incoordination. The above-mentioned side effects are common in elderly or liver disease patients. The side effects of blood, liver and kidney are rare. Occasionally there are excitement, nightmare, delirium, confusion, depression, attack, hostility. The first 3 months of pregnancy to take this kind of drug, there are reports of cleft lip and cleft palate in the newborn.

The toxic effects of benzodiazepines are very small. People who take an overdose in suicidal purposes can easily lead to death if they take other antipsychotic drugs or alcohol at the same time. People who only take overdose of benzodiazepines often get into sleep with a slight decrease in blood pressure, who can be awakened and often wake up after 24-48 hours. The treatment measures are gastro lavage, infusion and other comprehensive measures. Hemodialysis is often ineffective.

(7) Tolerance and Dependence

Benzodiazepines can cause tolerance. After a few weeks, it is necessary to adjust the dosage to achieve better results. After long-term application, it can generate dependence, including physical dependence and mental dependence, and can be cross-dependent with alcohol and barbiturate. Somatic symptoms often occur for more than 3 months of continuous use. A sudden interruption of drugs will cause withdrawal symptoms. Withdrawal symptoms include anxiety, agitation, irritability, insomnia, headache, dizziness, tremor, sweating, dysphoria, tinnitus, depersonalization and gastrointestinal symptoms (nausea, vomiting, anorexia, diarrhea, constipation). Severe patients may have convulsions, which are rare but can lead to death. Therefore, benzodiazepines should be avoided to long-term application in clinical practice. Drug withdrawal should be gradually carried out slowly.

(8) Commonly-used benzodiazepines

1) Diazepam

Pharmacokinetics: it is absorbed fast and completely orally. The time of plasma peak concentration is about 0. 52 hours, the steady blood concentration is reached after 4–10 days, and the half–life is 20–70 hours. The absorption of the intramuscular injection is slow and irregular, and it is effective for several minutes after intravenous injection. It is metabolized by the liver, whose metabolites include nordazepam and oxazepam, and they have pharmacological activity in different degree. Metabolites are mainly excreted by the kidneys, which can stay in blood for days or weeks. After the withdrawal, the elimination is slow. Drug can enter the fetal body through placenta, and it can enter cerebrospinal fluid and milk. The level of breast milk is tenth of plasma.

Function and application: the diazepam combined with specific nerve cell membrane receptors strengthens and promotes the nerve conduction function of the main inhibitory neurotransmitter GABA in the brain, which result in sedative, hypnotic and anticonvulsant effects. It has central muscle relaxation, and has a strong anti–anxiety effect. It has a good effect on anxiety, fear of insomnia, muscle spasm, tremor, tension headache, epilepsy, convulsion, and can be also used for alcohol abstinence.

Usage and dosage: the oral dose is 2. 5–5. 0 mg before sleep, and the total oral dose is 7. 5–15. 0 mg/d. The dose of intramuscular injection or slow intravenous injection is 10–20 mg, and the children had a dose of 0. 1–0. 3 mg/kg each time. The dosage of the elderly is reduced by half.

Adverse reaction: the common adverse reactions are somnolence, dizziness and fatigue. Large doses can cause ataxia, tremor, even hypotension, respiratory depression, and tachycardia. Rare side effects include excitement, more words, insomnia, and hallucinations. Long–term use can produce drug dependence, and sudden withdrawal can cause withdrawal symptoms, which manifested as excitement or depression, even convulsions, psychotic deterioration. During the medication, the patients should avoid dangerous work such as driving, high altitude, and machine operation.

2) Alprazolam

Pharmacokinetics: it is absorbed fast and completely orally. The plasma peak time is 1–2 hours after a single dose of 0. 5–3. 0 mg, the half–life is 12–15 hours, and the rate of plasma protein binding is 80%. The main metabolites are 3–hydroxyl–three azole diazepam and 3–hydroxyl–5–methylthree azole diazepam. 80% of the metabolites are excreted in the urine and can be excreted through the placenta and milk.

Function and application: it is mainly used foranti–anxiety, or as an anti–phobic drug, and can be used as hypnotic drug.

Usage and dosage: the initial dose of anti–anxiety is 0. 4 mg, 3 times per day for adult. The maximum dose is 4 mg/d. The dose of sedation and hypnosis is 0. 4–0. 8 mg, before bedtime. The elderly and weak patients began to use a small dose of 0. 2 mg, 3 times per day, and gradually increased to the maximum tolerance dose. The anti–fear dose is 0. 4 mg, 3 times per day, and the dose is increased gradually when needed, whose maximum dose is 10 mg/d.

Adverse reaction: adverse reactions are rare, usually including mental disorder, emotional depression, headache, nausea, vomiting and dysuria. After the sudden stop drug, we should pay attention to the possibility of withdrawal symptoms.

3) Buspirone

Pharmacokinetics: it is easy to be absorbed orally. The peak time is 0. 5–1. 0 hours, and the half–life is 2–11 hours. Most of them are metabolized by the liver, 60% of them are excreted from urine and 40% are excreted by feces. The binding rate of plasma protein is 95%, and hemodialys is can't clear the buspirone in the body.

Function and application: buspirone is a new type of anti–anxiety drug of non–benzodiazepines. This drug is a partial agonist of the 5 – HT1A receptor and also reduces the sensitivity of the 5 – HT2A receptor. There is no obvious sedative, hypnotic and muscular relaxation in the normal dose, which does not damage exercise and cognitive function, but can increase vigilance and attention. The patient had no dependence on the drug. It is mainly applied to generalized anxiety disorder, obsessive compulsive disorder with anxiety symptoms, neurasthenia with anxiety, alcohol dependence, impulsive aggression, depression, and chronic physical disease with anxiety or depression. It can also be used for the treatment of anxiety, craving and drug seeking behavior of psychoactive substance abstinence. It has a certain effect on panic attack, but the effect is not as good as tricyclic antidepressant. There is no interaction with other sedative drugs and alcohol.

Usage and dosage: the dose range of anti – anxiety treatment is 15 – 45 mg/d, and is divided into 3 times. The onset time is longer than that of benzodiazepines, and the beginning of the effect is 7 – 10 days. The dose should be larger when it is used for depression, with a dose range of 60–90 mg/d.

Adverse reaction: there are few adverse reactions, such as dry mouth, dizziness, headache, insomnia, and gastrointestinal dysfunction.

20.2.5.2　Sedative and hypnotic drugs of non–benzodiazepines

(1) Zaleplon

Pharmacokinetics: it is absorbed fast and completely orally. The plasma peak concentration time is 1 hour, and the bioavailability is about 30%. There is a clear first pass effect. The half–life is 1 hour, and there is no drug accumulation when once a day. Only 1% of the dose in the urine is the original medicine. Zaleplon is mainly metabolized in the liver to be metabolized to 5 – oxygen – zaleplon, a small amount of them are metabolized to deethylasezaleplon by CYP3A4, and which are quickly metabolized to 5 – oxygen–deethylasezaleplon by aldehyde dehydrogenase. They are transformed into a glycuronic acid compound and are removed in the urine, and all the metabolites have no pharmacological activity. The food is high in fat and difficult to digest can prolong the absorption of zaleplon, but had no effect on the half–life. The pharmacokinetics of elderly people are not different from those of young people. However, the rate of oral clearance is reduced by 70% –87% in the case of liver dysfunction.

Function and application: because of its fast absorption, fast receptor dissociation rate and short half–life, it can quickly play a sedative hypnotic effect, no hangover effect of traditional sleeping pills, has little effect on psychomotor function and memory function, which can be used for short–term treatment of insomnia and can shorten the sleep latency. But it doesn't indicate that it could increase the time of sleep and reduce the number of wakefulness.

Usage and dosage: the oral dose is 5–10 mg, taken before bedtime, and 5 mg is recommended for the elderly, diabetics, and liver dysfunction. The duration of continuous drug used are limited in 7–10 days.

Adverse reaction: the side–effects include mild headache, vertigo, dry mouth, sweating, anorexia, abdominal pain, nausea, vomiting, fatigue, memory difficulties, depression, tremor, standing instability, diplopia and mental disorder.

(2) Zolpidem

Pharmacokinetics: it is absorbed fast and completely orally. The time of the plasma peak concentrationis 0.5–3.0 hours, the oral bioavailability is 70%, and the protein binding rate is 92%. It attenuates the peak concentration of the drug when it is taken with the food at the same time, which is unfavorable to sleep. The average plasma scavenging half–life is 2.4 hours, so there aren't have hangover on the next day and accumulation. It is metabolized by the liver, 60% of the metabolites are excreted from the urine, 40% are excreted from the excrement, and the half–life of the patients with cirrhosis can be extended to 9.4 hours.

Function and application: zolpidem acts on the GABA receptor complex in the brain, so it can shorten the sleep latency, reduce the number of awakening, and increase the total sleep time. It does not affect the total time of REM sleep and improves the quality of sleep. It hardly changes the sleep structure and only increases the 2 phase of the slow wave sleep. About 52% of the patients fall asleep within 15 minutes and 43% of the patients fall asleep within 15−30 minutes. Due to the half−life is only 2.5 hours, the patient did not sleep on the next day, and had less memory and psychomotor damage. It has good therapeutic effect on short term insomnia, long term insomnia and psychosis insomnia.

Usage and dosage: adults take 10 mg once a day. They must be taken before bedtime. When necessary, they can be increased to 15−20 mg. Those who are over 65 years old or have liver dysfunction are 5 mg. Before going to bed, patients under 65 years old take 10 mg every day. The longest time for medication is not more than 4 weeks. The occasional insomnia treatment time should be limited to 2−5 days, and the short term insomnia(such as severe life events) treatment time is less than 2−3 weeks. For excessive use and the patients with long−term use, it can be reduced gradually to reduce the sleeplessness caused by stopping drugs.

Adverse reaction: include fatigue, sleepiness, depression, vertigo, headache, nausea, vomiting, and diarrhea. There are few adverse reactionsinclude gait instability and tremor. There will also be nightmare and irritability in the middle of the night.

(3) Zopiclone

Pharmacokinetics: it is absorbed fast and completely orally. The time of the plasma peak concentrationis 0.5−1 hours, the oral bioavailability is 80%, and the protein binding rate is 45%. The half−life is 3.5−6 hours. The zopiclone and its metabolites can be produced through the placental barrier, secreted into the milk and saliva. It is mainly metabolized by the liver, and about 4%−5% of the drugs are excreted from the urine by the prototype. Patients with renal insufficiency are not affected, while the expulsion time of the patients with liver cirrhosis and the elderly is prolonged. The drug has no effect on the drug metabolizing enzymes.

Function and application: it acts on the GABA receptor and enhances thenerve inhibitory effect of GABA by activating the GABA receptor. There are sedative and hypnotic effects on insomniacs and normal people, which can shorten the sleep latency and improve the quality of sleep, and have no effect on the memory function of the next day. It is suitable for all kinds of insomnia.

Usage and dosage: the oral dose of the adult is 7.5 mg, which must be taken before sleep, and the elderly can be reduced by half.

Adverse reaction: there may be the next morning sleepiness, dry mouth, bitter taste and fatigue. There are also vertigo, dizziness, nausea, stomach pain, irritability, mental disorder and so on. Long−term use of drugs may produce dependence, and the withdrawal system will be occurs when stop the drug suddenly.

20.2.6 Medication of attention deficit hyperactivity disorder(ADHD)

20.2.6.1 Atomoxetine

(1) Pharmacokinetics

It is absorbed fast and completely orally. It is mainly metabolized by P4502D6(CYP2D6) enzyme in the liver. The metabolites in the body are mainly N−noratoroxetine and 4−hydroxy−atomoxetine. About 80% of the metabolites are excreted in the urine and the rest are excreted by the feces.

(2) Function and application

Atomoxetine can be combined with the presynaptic NE transporters, and effectively inhibit the reabsorption of NE. Atomoxetine could increase the concentration of NE and DA outside the prefrontal cortex cells of the rat. Atomoxetine improves ADHD symptoms and has a similar effect in improving attention disorders and hyperactivity. The efficacy of ADHD in the treatment of children and adolescents is the same as that in Ritalin. Atomoxetineis effective in the three subtypes of ADHD(the predominant type of hyperactivity, the main type of attention barrier and the mixed type). After 34 weeks of medication, the patient's symptoms will be further improved.

(3) Usage and dosage

The oral dose is 1.2 mg/(kg · d), usually not more than 1.8 mg/(kg · d).

(4) Adverse reaction

The duration of gastrointestinal tract adverse reaction is short, and it can be relieved by itself. The adverse reaction of gastrointestinal tract can be reduced by taking the food simultaneously. It can rise high blood pressure and heart rate, most of which can be tolerated, but it is used carefully for patients with hypertension and tachycardia.

20.2.6.2   Methylphenidate hydrochloride extended-release tablets

(1) Pharmacokinetics

It can be absorbed fast orally. The time of the plasma peak concentration is 6-8 hours. The metabolites in the body are mainly α-phenylpiperidine acetate.

(2) Function and application

Methylphenidate hydrochloride is a central nervous stimulant. The mechanism of its action in the treatment of ADHD is not clear. Methylphenidate is believed to block the reuptake of norepinephrine and dopamine by presynaptic neurons, and increase the release of these monoamines to the outer neuronal space.

(3) Usage and dosage

The oral dose is 18-54 mg/d.

(4) Adverse reaction

Long-term abuse can lead to tolerance and mental dependence, with different degrees of behavioral disorders. Especially in the parenteral route of drug abuse, it can cause obvious psychotic attack.

20.3   Electroconvulsive therapy

Electroconvulsive therapy is also called electrical shock therapy. It is a way to achieve the purpose of treatment with a certain amount of current passing through the brain, causing loss of consciousness and spasm. At present, traditional electric shock has been eliminated, and modified electric convulsive therapy is used. The patients are given anesthetics and muscle relaxants before electrify, with seizures does not occur after electricity. It is safer and easy to be accepted by patients and family members.

20.3.1   Indications and contraindications

20.3.1.1   Indications

(1) Severe depression, strong autolesion and dutch act attempt, obvious self-accusation.

(2) Server orgasm and dysphoria.

(3) Antifeedant, negativism and catatonic stupor.

(4) Psychotropic drugs are not effective and intolerant for drug treatment.

20.3.1.2 Contraindications

(1) Cerebral organic diseases, such as intracranial space occupying lesions, cerebrovascular diseases, central nervous system inflammation and trauma. The brain tumor or cerebral aneurysm should be paid attention especially, because when the convulsion attacks, the intracranial pressure will increase suddenly, which may cause cerebral hemorrhage, brain tissue damage, or hernia of brain.

(2) Cardiovascular diseases, such as coronary heart disease, myocardial infarction, hypertension, arrhythmia, aortic aneurysm, and cardiac insufficiency.

(3) Osteoarticular disease, especially in recent cases.

(4) Haemorrhagic or unstable aneurysm malformation.

(5) The disease that has a potential risk of amotio retinae, such as glaucoma and high myopia.

(6) Acute systemic infection, fever.

(7) Severe respiratory disease, serious liver and kidney disease.

(8) Reserpine treatment.

(9) Old people, children and pregnant women.

20.3.2 Methods of electroconvulsive therapy

20.3.2.1 Preparation before treatment

(1) Detailed physical examination, including nervous system examination. Laboratory examination and other auxiliary examinations are necessary, such as blood routine, blood biochemistry, electrocardiogram, electroencephalogram, chest and spinal X-ray radiography.

(2) Informed consent.

(3) Stop taking antiepileptic drugs and anti-anxiety drugs for 8 hours before treatment, avoid the use such drugs during the treatment, fasting and no water more than 4 hours. Antipsychotic, antidepressant, or lithium salts used during the period of treatment should be low dose.

(4) Prepare all kinds of emergency medicine and equipment.

(5) The body temperature, pulse and blood pressure should be measured before treatment. If the temperature is above 37.5 centigrade, the pulse is faster than 120 times/min or less than 50 times/min, the blood pressure is more than 150/100 mmHg or lower than 90/50 mmHg, it should be forbidden.

(6) At 15-30 minutes before treatment, atropine is subcutaneously injected with 0.5-1.0 mg to prevent excessively excitability of the vagus nerve and reduce the secretion.

(7) Excreting stool and urinating, remove dentures, unlock the collar button and belt, remove the hairpin etc.

20.3.2.2 Operation method

The patient supine on the treatment table, the extremities maintain the natural straightening posture, and the 2 shoulder blades are equivalent to the middle section of the thoracic vertebra cushion a sand pillow, so as to make the spinal protrusion. In order to prevent bites, the tongue plate, which is wrapped with gauze, is placed between the upper and lower molars on one side of the patient. The therapist hand care patients with mandibular, prevent mandibular dislocation. The assistant protects the patient's shoulder, elbow, knee, and limbs.

(1) Electrodes coated with conductive gel or saline are placed on the both sides of the head of the patient or the non-dominant side of the temporal region. The side effects of non-dominant side is small, and

the effect of bilateral convulsions is better.

(2)In principle, the minimum amount of electricity to cause spasticity is appropriate. The selection of electricity can be selected according to the types of different electric convulsions. For example, the electric convulsion machine in Shanghai usually uses 80–120 mA, and the electrified time is 2–3 seconds. If there is no convulsive seizures or incomplete seizures at 20–40 seconds after power, most of the reasons are not well contacted with electrodes or the time is not enough. They should be repeated for one time as soon as possible under the correct operation. Otherwise, they should be treated with increasing the power of 10 mA or increasing the time of electricity appropriate.

(3)The frequency of treatment is usually 3 times a week and one course is 6–12 times. The manic state is about 6 times, and the hallucinations and delusions need 8–12 times, and the depression is between the two.

(4)Convulsions are associated with age, sex, medication, and past electrical convulsions. In general, men did not take sedative and antiepileptic drugs are more prone to attack. Convulsions are similar to major epileptic seizures, including 4 stages: latentperiod, tetania, spasmodic and recovery periods.

(5)When the convulsions are stopped and the breathing is restored, the patient should be placed in a quiet room, and the patient's lateral position is best. If the breathing is not good, we should make artificial respiration in time. The patient rest at least 30 minutes and have special care. The nurse should observe the vital sign, consciousness recovery and prevent injuries.

20.3.2.3   Complications

Common complications include headache, nausea, vomiting, anxiety, reversible memory impairment, and systemic muscle pain. These symptoms do not need to be treated. Fractures are more common in fourth to eighth thoracic compression fractures, and should be dealt with immediately. The aged patients and patients who had anticholinergic drugs during the treatment period are more likely to have disorder of consciousness and impaired cognitive function. At this time, electrical convulsions should be discontinued. Death is extremely rare, and most of them are associated with potential physical diseases.

20.3.2.4   Modified electricconvulsive therapy

In order to reduce muscle rigidity, convulsion, and avoid the occurrence of complications such as fracture and dislocation of joints, the modified method of electric convulsive therapy has been popularized now. The contraindication of non–convulsive electroconvulsive therapy is less than that of traditional electroconvulsive therapy, and the elderly patients can also be used.

Under the participation of the anesthesiologist, atropine 0.5 mg was injected intramuscularly before treatment. According to the patient's age and weight, the dose of 1.0–2.5 mg/kg induced patients to sleep by 1% thiopental. When the patient is yawned and the corneal reflex is slow, 0.2% chlorinated succinylcholine is given by intravenous injection from 0.5 mg/kg to 1.5 mg/kg and observe the degree of muscle relaxation. When the patient's tendon reflex disappeared or weakened, the facial and whole body muscle fibers trembling, breathing became shallow, and the whole body muscle relaxed(usually about 2 minutes after giving medicine), it could power 2–3 seconds for patients. The slight movements of the angle, the eyes, the fingers and the toes were observed, and the duration of 30–40 seconds is an effective treatment.

The incidence of complications in the treatment of non–convulsive electroconvulsive therapy is lower than that of traditional electroconvulsive therapy, and the degree is lighter. However, anesthetic accident, delayed asphyxia, and severe arrhythmia may occur, and cardiopulmonary resuscitation should be given immediately.

20.4   Transcranial magnetic stimulation

Transcranial magnetic stimulation(TMS) is a new technique for giving magnetic stimulation to a specific part of the brain. Pulsed magnetic field is applied to the central nervous system(mainly the brain), which changes the membrane potential of cortical neurons, induces induced currents, affects the metabolism and electrical activity of the brain, and induces a series of physiological and biochemical responses. In 1985, A. T. Barker and his colleagues developed the first modern TMS instrument in Sheffield, UK, which has been recognized by clinicians. The treatment principle of TMS is to put an insulated coil on the scalp of a specific location. When the strong current around the coil pass through, it will generatethe local magnetic field intensity of 1.5–2.5 T. The local magnetic field passes through the scalp and skull in the direction perpendicular to the coil and enters a certain depth of the surface of the cortex. The rapid fluctuation of initial current intensity will lead to the fluctuation of magnetic field. The fluctuation of magnetic field will cause secondary currents on the cortical surface, which is about 1/10 million of the initial current intensity. The induced currents can affect the function of nerve cells.

The difference between magnetic stimulation and electrical stimulation is that, because of the high resistance of bone, most electric energy can't enter the brain, and through the scalp tissue between two electrodes, but the skull is transparent to the magnetic field. Moreover, the electric field needs the anode and the cathode, and the monopole can produce the magnetic field. These features allow magnetic stimulation to be confined to a range of 5 mm in diameter, and the current from TMS can be concentrated in a certain area and is more accurate.

20.4.1   Repetitive transcranial magnetic stimulation

Repetitive stimulation in a specific location is called repetitive transcranial magnetic stimulation (rTMS), which has been widely applied in the field of clinical psychiatry, neurological disease and rehabilitation.

20.4.1.1   The technical principle of rTMS

Repetitive transcranial magnetic stimulation can achieve the purpose of stimulating or inhibiting the function of local cerebral cortex by altering its stimulation frequency, thereby playing a therapeutic role. High frequency and high intensity rTMS can produce the summation of excitatory postsynaptic potential, which makes the nerve excitability in the stimulation site. The effect of low frequency stimulation is the opposite, and the balance between brain stimulation and inhibitory function is used to treat the disease. The relationship and interaction between the local nerve stimulated by rTMS, and the interaction between the neural networks affect the function of multiple parts. For patients with brain functions, we need to adjust intensity, frequency, stimulus location and coil direction, so as to achieve good therapeutic effect.

According to the different TMS stimulation pulses, there are three main stimulation modes in TMS: single pulse TMS(sTMS), double pulse TMS(pTMS) and repetitive TMS(rTMS). sTMS is operated by manual control of unregulated pulse output and can also stimulate multiple stimuli, but the stimulation interval is longer(for example, 10 seconds) and is used for routine electrophysiological tests. pTMS continuously stimulates two stimuli at the same stimulus site at very short intervals, or applies two stimulator in two different parts, which is used to study the facilitation and inhibition of nerves. rTMS includes two kinds of high frequency and low frequency, which requires the equipment to give low frequency or fast rhythm rTMS at the same stimulus. Each stimulus pattern is related to different physiological bases and brain mechanisms. The new generation of stereotactic TMS integrates fMRI results, greatly improving the accuracy of TMS stimulation site, accurately controlling the depth of the stimulating brain, and accurately adjusting the intensity of stimulation. Repetitive transcranial stimulation is mainly aimed at stimulating or inhibiting the function of the cerebral cortex by changing the frequency of its stimulation.

The therapeutic parameters of rTMS include stimulation site, intensity, frequency, time of stimulation, and course of treatment. The stimulation site is dependent on experience. The treatment of depression includes stimulation of many parts, such as left dorsal prefrontal lobe, right dorsal prefrontal lobe and left prefrontal lobe. The intensity of the stimulation is quantified by the motion threshold. Motor threshold means that the coil is placed in the motor cortex, and gradually increases the intensity of stimulation until the contralateral fingersare moved. The intensity of this motion is the motor threshold. The study of rTMS for mental disorders mostly used the motor threshold of 80% –100%, and the maximum is no more than 120%. The treatment plans include the number of stimuli per minute, the time of treatment per day, the number of times of daily treatment, the number of days of treatment and the total number of stimuli. The average number of stimuli are 40 times per minute, and the shortest rest time is 20 seconds, 20 minutes a day, 5 days a week. A total of 10 working days lasted for 2 weeks.

20.4.1.2 Indications

(1) Depression

rTMS is the most widely used in the treatment of depression. Most studies have confirmed that rTMS has a moderate antidepressant effect on depression. The frequency of stimulation in the treatment of depression is generally 1 Hz, 10 Hz and 20 Hz, and dorsal prefrontal cortex(DLPFC) is the most commonly selected therapeutic target for depression. In October 2008, the US FDA approved the rTMS therapeutic apparatus for the treatment of depression. It also stipulated that the depressive episode of adult depression patients could be treated by rTMS therapy instrument, if the patient has a poor curative effect with minimal dose and course of antidepressant treatment.

(2) Schizophrenia

The study of rTMS for the treatment of schizophrenia is few. The low frequency rTMS for the left temporal lobe in the treatment of schizophrenia showed better effect.

In recent years, the effect of rTMS on anxiety disorder, post−traumatic stress disorder, obsessive−compulsive disorder, autism and delayed dyskinesia has been developed abroad.

20.4.1.3 Contraindication

(1) Patients with a history of epileptic seizures or strong positive family history of epilepsy, especially the high frequency rTMS is needed. There is a study that low frequency rTMS is effective for intractable epilepsy.

(2) Patients with severe physical disease.

(3) Serious alcohol abusers.

(4) Patients with a history of craniocerebral surgery. There were metal implants in the brain.

(5) Patients with implanted cardiac pacemakers.

(6) Women in pregnancy.

20.4.1.4 Therapeutic methods

The operation process of rTMS:

(1) Turn the stimulus knob to the minimum.

（2）Connect the coil to the high frequency magnetic stimulator. It is necessary to make sure that the therapy instrument can be opened after the coil is connected.

（3）Open the exciter, then test the selection item, and select the motion induced magnetic stimulation project.

（4）Turn on the switch.

（5）Determine the intensity of the stimulus.

（6）Patients treated with rTMS can't carry the following items: pacemaker, metal objects, metal implants, cochlear implants, hearing aids, watches, calculators, credit cards, computer floppy disks and tapes.

（7）The rTMS receiver takes the sitting position, the back to the instrument, and the coil on the selected part of the skull.

（8）Select the stimulus frequency on the exciter.

（9）Set the average number of stimuli each time and the stimulus steps.

（10）Press the "trigger" button. If the lamp is on the light, a stimulus is generated when the stimulator triggers the stimulus. If the exciter is in a repetitive mode, the high frequency magnetic stimulator will be triggered at a specific frequency or maximum frequency.

（11）Adjust the intensity of the stimulus until the appropriate response is seen on the screen of the exciter.

（12）When the treatment is finished, the coil should be placed on the hanger. Do not place it anywhere, especially on any metal surface. The metal can pop up or damage the coil.

（13）The high frequency magnetic stimulator should be turned off in time when it is not used.

（14）Make sure someone is present when you start the machine.

20.4.1.5　Adverse reactions

rTMS has high safety and less adverse reactions. Common adverse reactions include headache and epileptic seizures. The nature of the headache caused by rTMS is similar to that of tension headache, and the incidence is 10% −30% , which is due to repeated stimulation of the scalp muscles. The duration is short, and it can be relieved by itself. If the duration is longer or unbearable, it can be symptomatic treatment. The incidence of epilepsy is low. The study shows that epileptic seizures are generally related to excessive frequency and excessive intensity.

Yang Lei ,Niu Qihui

Chapter 21

Psychotherapy

21.1　Introduction

Psychotherapy is the use of psychological methods to help a person change behavior and overcome problems in desired ways. Firstly, psychotherapists are specially trained therapists who are proficient in theories of personality formation and development, as well as behavioral change theories and skills. Secondly, this kind of help is carried out under the professional framework. This means that such professional activities are recognized by laws or regulations, their places and procedures have certain rules, and are regulated by industry norms. The focus of treatment is to help visitors make changes in their psychological behavior and restore or rebuild their impaired mental function.

21.2　Clinical psychotherapy

21.2.1　Overview of psychotherapy

21.2.1.1　Definition

Psychotherapy refers to on the basis of good relationship between therapists and visitors, professional trained therapists use psychological theories and techniques to improve visitors' cognition, emotion and behavior. It can eliminate or alleviate the psychological problems of the visitors, promote their personality maturity and development.

With the transformation of medical mode, doctors exert psychological influence consciously or unconsciously in medical practice to mobilize the enthusiasm of patients, so as to play a certain therapeutic role in diseases. In all clinical subjects, psychotherapy is more widely used as a special technique.

There is no significant difference between psychotherapy and psychological consultation, and it overlaps to a certain extent. They are similar in the nature of the relationship, the change and the learning process, the guiding theory and the purpose of helping people. The difference is mainly in the object and the situation. Psychological counseling mainly follows the educational mode. The content of consultation involves daily life problems, mainly in schools, factories and other groups. The main object of psychotherapy is the patient, and the treatment place is mainly in the clinical and medical situation.

21.2.1.2　History

Psychotherapy has a long history. As early as in the tribal clan society, if a person is sick, the priest or shaman will use "gods" power for the patient to exorcise the demons. Some of the patients were healed, which contains the elements of psychological therapy.

The beginning of modern psychotherapy is the theory of "animal magnetism" proposed by Mesmer, a doctor in Austria in the eighteenth Century. He put the patient into a state of sleep in a dramatic manner. He is the first person who lead hypnotism into the medical field. On this basis, Freud created psychoanalytic therapy, which became a milestone in the history of psychotherapy. In 1940s, Rodgers developed a "non guided psychotherapy". In 1950s, behavioral therapy is rising rapidly and soon became popular. Soon after, cognitive therapy, existentialism and eclectic psychotherapy schools have been rising. Since 1970s, family therapy has become an important treatment system. Then, positive psychotherapy and positive psychological intervention have received much attention and popularization. Psychotherapy has become an effective treatment method and has been widely used and developed.

In theory, more and more research supports that any single theory is not enough to fully explain the causes of mental disorders and the mechanism of treatment. At present, new treatments tend to be integrated, with a more open communication between different schools and flexible application according to the specific circumstances of the visitors. In terms of course of treatment, short course psychotherapy is applied. The number of treatment is generally promoted within 10 – 20 times, and individual cases can reach 40 times. Some scholars also put forward the concept of "Open single treatment". In the field of application, the application of psychotherapy is more and more extensive. Psychotherapy workers are no longer confined to psychiatrist, but also extend to clinical psychologists, social workers and ministers. The scope of treatment is also extended from the initial psychiatric patients to the general mental health problems in various fields, such as various mental disorders, interpersonal relationships, marriage and family problems.

21.2.2　Basic problems of psychotherapy

21.2.2.1　Ethics

(1) The principle of sincerity

The therapist should be sincere, consistent, and active attention to the visitors, so as to establish a good work alliance to ensure the smooth progress of the psychotherapy.

(2) Client confidentiality

Respecting the personal privacy of the visitors is an important principle to be followed in the psychotherapy. The therapist must not make a fuss and tell anyone his privacy. At the beginning of the treatment, the therapist should explain the principle of confidentiality to the visitor, which is conducive to confidence.

(3) The principle of neutral

Therapists should maintain a neutral attitude and position in psychotherapy. They can not take their value orientation as a reference for analyzing problems, otherwise they will hamper the objectivity of event judgement.

(4) The principle of helping self−reliance

The purpose of psychotherapy is to help the visitor grow up by himself, and the therapist should avoid being dependent by the visitor and avoid playing the role of the guide of life.

（5）The principle of restricted relation

Therapists should establish good theraptic relationship with visitors, but not social relationships beyond their professional boundaries, such as romantic relationships.

21.2.2.2　The setting of psychotherapy

（1）Treatment setting

The treatment setting is the therapist's arrangement of psychological treatment, and it is the basic rule that the therapist and the visitor should abide by. Treatment setting is established before treatment and has the characteristics of relative fixity and pattern. Good treatment settings is not only an important guarantee of curative effect, but also an important treatment technique.

（2）Selection and arrangement of psychotherapy room

The psychological treatment should be carried out in a special place(psychotherapy room). The space of the psychotherapy room should be suitable, the light and temperature in the room are moderate and the ventilation is well ventilated. It is not suitable to place the telephone in the room. The number and position of the office furniture are appropriate. All of these will give people a warm, comfortable and safe feeling. The layout of the therapeutic room may be different from the different schools of treatment.

（3）The appointment, frequency and course of psychotherapy

A treatment agreement should be reserved and signed before psychotherapy. The frequency is usually 1−2 times a week, 40−50 minutes each time. The length of the course is decided by the severity of the visitor's problem and the therapeutic methods. Generally speaking, the course of the practical problem is short and the course of the personality problem is long. In addition, psychoanalytic treatment often takes a long time.

（4）The cost of psychotherapy

Psychosocial treatment should be charged according to the occupation standard. If there is no treatment cost, visitors may not cherish the chance of treatment, and the treatment motivation can not be consolidated. Eventually, the treatment can not be systematically and effectively carried out, which will affect the therapeutic effect.

21.2.2.3　Theraputic relationship

（1）Summary

The psychotherapy relationship is a kind of interpersonal relationship between the therapist and client in the treatment process produces, its essence is a kind of work of the alliance, the visitor is changed by supporting factors in the relationship. The relationship of treatment is unique. It is a professional relationship between therapists and visitors. The treatment relationship is established on the basis of the visitors' initiative and voluntariness. The relationship can only occur at a specific time and place(therapeutic room), and the relationship is terminated at the end of the treatment. In the treatment of the two sides, the common concern is the visitor, not the therapist. The psychotherapy relationship is an important factor affecting the curative effect. All kinds of psychotherapy genres pay great attention to establishing and maintaining a good treatment relationship.

（2）Skills of establishing a psychotherapy relationship

1) Listening technology

Listening to the visitors patiently and attentively is the most fundamental and important technique of psychotherapy. Psychotherapist should not only understand the content expressed by visitors' speech and behavior, but also can understand the content which not directly expressed and did not realized by visitors themselves. Listening is the main way to promote the visitors to understand themselves, to develop the treatment relationship and to push the treatment in depth.

2) Questioning technology

Asking questions is the most commonly used method of psychotherapy. The appropriateness of the problem can enhance communication and help the establishment and maintenance of the treatment relationship. If the problem is not good, it can affect communication and even destroy the relationship of psychotherapy. The ways of asking questions include close ended questions and open ended questions. Close-ended questions usually use the "yes" or "wrong" way, and only "yes" or "no" answers. Such questions are used to clarify facts, to gain emphasis or to narrow the scope. Open-ended questions usually asks questions such as "what" "how" "why". It helps the therapist get some basic facts and materials, and promote the self thinking of visitors.

3) Feedback technology

Feedback technology refers to the therapist to reexpress the visitors' main complain, thoughts, feelings, and emotional experiences in language. Timely and accurate feedback helps to improve the relationship of treatment. Feedback on feelings can help the visitors to recognize and identify their emotions.

4) Nonverbal technology

Nonverbal technology is also called body language. It refers to the use of the face, eyes, sound features, body posture, and clothes except language. When the visitor exchange, psychotherapists should through the proper use of the expression change, express positive attention, understanding, respect and empathy for visitors. The therapist's posture will also effect visitors' feeling. It will give people an arrogant, indifferent, and not easy to close feeling by leaning back, alice his legs. The invisible pressure caused by the excessive body forward and thus visitors will not be able to relax and talk freely.

21.2.2.4 Effect and influencing factors of psychotherapy

(1) The curative effect of psychotherapy

In 1982, the American Psychiatric Association analyzed more than 500 studies. They found that 3/4 of the people who met the normal distribution could benefit from psychotherapy. In 1982, Smith conducted a meta-analysis of 475 psychotherapy researches. Compared with those without treatment, 80% patients who received psychotherapy improved significantly. The efficacy of psychotherapy has been recognized so far. The criteria for evaluating efficacy include the most direct clinical effects, the more happiness experience and the improvement of the ability of social life of visitors.

(2) Factors influencing the curative effect of psychotherapy

1) Treatment methods

Although the treatment methods of all kinds of psychological schools are effective, and the overall efficacy is not very different, it doesn't mean that different methods have the same effect on the same visitors. The key to the effect of psychotherapy is to determine the target problems of the treatment and to select the appropriate treatment techniques. The integration trend of psychotherapy is to emphasize the selection of effective treatment methods or techniques for the various special problems of the visitor. In this way, it not only expands the scope of application, but also improves the curative effect and shortens the course of treatment.

2) Therapist related factors

A therapist is a major factor determining the effectiveness of psychotherapy. The quality and ability of a therapist are much more important than any way of treatment, and sometimes even play a decisive role in the treatment. Jennings and Skovholt(1999) studied 10 master therapist, they found that these psychotherapists would have the following characteristics: ①they have an insatiable desire to learn; ②they are healthy, mature, and pay attention to their emotional health; ③they are good at catching and willing to accept others' e-motions; ④they accept the complexity and uncertainty of people's cognition; ⑤they are good at summarizing lessons; ⑥they are familiar with the effects of their emotions on the treatment; ⑦they have outstanding relationship skills; ⑧they trust the therapist−visitor's working union; ⑨they are good at making use of their own advantages.

3) Visitor related factors

Visitors' educational level, personality characteristics, their trust and expectation level of treatment, the type and severity of diseases have great influence on the outcome of psychotherapy.

(3) Side−effects of psychotherapy

On the one hand, there is no theory of psychotherapy which can explain human psychological phenomenon convincingly and comprehensively. Every theory have different foundation, and there are different focuses on the treatment methods based on this. In this regard, the therapist should study a wide range of psychological theories and integrate them in an all−round way. In practice, the therapists should make up for each method and make the most of the effect. On the other hand, the therapist's own characteristics may also lead to side−effects. Therapists' personal experience, personality traits, values, professional backgrounds, and religious beliefs may affect the relationship, communication mode, value recognition with visitors. For example, in the face of a marriage derailment visitor, the therapist's own values may affect the treatment. To avoid this, therapists are required to receive professional training and adequate self−experience and receive professional supervision.

21.2.3　The classification and the main schools of psychotherapy

21.2.3.1　Classification of psychotherapy

(1) According to the object of receiving treatment, it can be divided into individual psychotherapy, marriage treatment, family treatment and group psychotherapy.

(2) According to the theory school, it can be divided into psychoanalysis and analytical psychotherapy, supportive psychotherapy, behavior therapy, cognitive therapy, humanism psychothera, and morita therapy.

(3) According to whether or not to use language, it can be divided into conversation therapy and operation therapy. The latter includes music therapy, painting therapy, sand table therapy, sculpture therapy, and psychodrama.

21.2.3.2　Psychoanalytic therapy

(1) Concept

Psychoanalysis is based on psychoanalysis theory, by using the unique psychoanalysis technology to adjust the unconscious conflict and immature defense mechanism of visitors, so as to relieve symptoms and promote the personality maturity of visitors. These psychoanalytic techniques include free association, empathy and anti empathy, dream analysis, and analysis impedance. It was founded by Freud, a psychiatrist in Austria in the late 19th Century. It is one of the main schools of psychotherapy.

(2) The basic theory of psychoanalytic therapy

1) Unconsciousness theory

Freud divided human mental activities into three levels: consciousness, preconsciousness, subconscious. Consciousness is the surface, and people can perceive mental activity when they are awake. The preconsciousness is shallow, and it is aware of the high concentration or reminding of it. The subconscious is deep, and people can't detect it, but it can be revealed through analysis. Freud believed that human mental activities, including desire, impulse, thinking, fantasy, judgement and decision, happened and proceed in different levels of consciousness.

2) Personality structure theory

Freud believed that the psychological function of human was composed of id, ego and super-ego. Id is the original component of the personality. It requires immediate satisfaction and follows the principle of happiness. Ego is a ID service that follows the principle of reality and is a reasonable satisfaction for the desire of the ID. Super-ego is the monitoring organization in the personality, and is also the representative of morality and standards, and it follows the perfection principle. If the three are balanced, the personality development will be normal. On the contrary, if conflicts can not be solved well, other disorders such as neurosis can be caused.

3) Psychological defense mechanism

The psychological defense mechanism is a self-defense function of ego, which is the ego used to drive out the impulses, desires, and ideas unacceptably. Defense is usually carried out in the subconscious mind, and the individual does not realize that it is playing a role. Common psychological defense patterns are: repression, denial, rationalization, projection, replacement, degenerative, compensation, reverse formation, and transformation.

(3) The basic technology of psychoanalytic therapy

1) Free association

Free association requires visitors to lie on a recliner and talk about all the thoughts, emotions, and memories. No matter how ridiculous these contents are, how insignificant they feel, or whether they violate the existing moral norms, visitors should have no hesitation and constraint to express all the contents that appear in the mind.

2) Transference and counter-transference

Transference refers to the visitor projecting the emotional relationship with an important object in the past on the therapist. The counter-transference is divided into two kinds of narrow sense and broad sense. The narrow sense of the counter-transference refers to the empathy response of the therapist to the visitor. The generalized counter-transference refers to all of the emotional response of the therapist to the visitor, including the response to the phenomenon of empathy. The modern viewpoint believe that counter-transference, like transference, is inevitable in treatment. Not only doesn't it impede the process of psychotherapy, but on the contrary, it is a tool for the therapist to understand the subconscious of the visitor.

3) Resistance

Resistance refers to the resistance of the visitor to the treatment. It is the force that counteracts the treatment. It is the process of the subconscious. It is not easy to identify and deal with resistance, and it is an important clue to the discovery of the psychological defense mechanism of visitors.

4) The interpretation of dreams

Freud thinks that dreams are the way to the subconscious, representing impulses or aspirations that are suppressed in the subconscious. A dream that can be recalled is called a manifest dream, and a metaphor is behind the dream. The analysis of the dream is to uncover the layers of the dream and seek its true meaning.

(4) Indications

In general, the indications of psychoanalysis include neurosis, somatization, psychosomatic disease, and some personality disorders. The psychoanalysis should not be used for severe mental disorders, such as schizophrenia, major depression, mania, etc. For impulse disorder, serious material dependence, marginal personality disorder and so on, psychoanalysis is also difficult to obtain good curative effect.

21.2.3.3   Supportive psychotherapy

(1) Concept

Supportive psychotherapy refers to therapists using persuasion, inspiration, encouragement, support and persuasion to help visitors to develop their potential abilities and improve their ability to overcome difficulties, so as to promote psychosomatic rehabilitation. It is a basic psychotherapy method, and its principles can be used in all kinds of treatment patterns.

(2) The basic theory of psychoanalytic therapy

Supportive psychotherapy is based on stress theory to play an effective role. Any environmental change in life, such as promotion, conversion, lovelorn, and death of a loved one, may bring a physical and psychological reaction to an individual as a source of stress. The severity of stress, the number of support, the individual's perceptions of frustration and the potential ability to cope with difficulties can all affect the degree of individual stress response.

(3) The basic technology of psychoanalytic therapy

1) Listening

The therapist listens carefully to the visitors, which makes the visitor feel that the therapist is concerned about their pain. It can eliminate the visitor's concerns and feelings of loneliness, and reliance on the therapist, which is also conducive to emotional catharsis.

2) Explanation and suggestion

Based on the establishment of good relationship, therapists explain the problem of visitors in a way that is easy to understand, and put forward suggestions for solving problems.

3) Encouragement and assurance

Therapists actively encourage the potential strengths of visitors to enable them to give full play to their initiative, inspire potential abilities and enhance confidence in coping with crises. The guarantee is a therapist's commitment to visitors, often used in suspicious and emotional people. The guarantee should be appropriate and practical in order to prevent it from destroying the visitors' confidence in the treatment.

4) Emotional release

The therapist helps the visitors to vent their emotions in the treatment environment, which helps the therapist to feel the inner world of the visitor in the early treatment and gain the trust. However, repeated emotional release does not benefit.

5) Use resources wisely

Therapists help visitors examine their own internal or external resources and make full use of them. Visitors are encouraged to accept support and help from family, friends, society, or various institutions. This therapy is especially suitable for the following situations: visitors encounter serious accidents or trauma, visitors are weak or immature in their ability, and need long-term psychological support from others. They are not suitable for psychoanalysis or other special psychotherapy.

(4) Indications

Supportive psychotherapy is a basic psychotherapy model in the clinic, and it is also the most widely used treatment method.

21.2.3.4   Behavioral therapy

(1) Concept

Behavioral therapy is a method based on experimental behavior science to help visitors eliminate certain behaviors or establish certain behaviors, so as to achieve therapeutic effect. Based on the theory of behavior, it aims to change people's behavior, emphasizing on current behavior, environment and events, and not too much about past experience. With the development of cognitive psychology, behavioral therapy gradually draws on and introduces the theory and technology of cognitive change. It combines cognition and behavior in treatment, also known as cognitive behavior therapy.

(2) The basic theory of psychoanalytic therapy

1) Classical conditioned reflex

The classic conditional reflex, discovered by Pavlov, is the most important theoretical cornerstone of behavioral therapy. When a neutral stimulus(such as light) is accompanied with food for many times, the neutral stimulus itself will also cause the saliva secretion of the dog, just like food. Pavlov called this acquired reflex behavior to a neutral stimulus as conditioned reflex. He studied the laws of generalization and differentiation of conditioned reflexes, and used these experimental results to explain the reasons for the establishment, change and retreat of behavior. For example, if you are often criticized and reprimanded in a conference room, you will feel nervous amd and unpleasant when you are approaching or entering this conference room.

2) Operant conditioning

Operant conditioning was first studied by Thorndike and then put forward by Skinner. In the experiment box designed by Skinner(Skinner box), rats press the lever to get food in the box, that is, by rewarding food, the action of pressing lever is increased. The above process is "rewarding learning". The Skinner box explains the principle of behavior enhancement. Skinner proposed that through positive or negative strengthening, the behavior can be changed in the expected direction, thus creating new behavior patterns. For example, when the husband sends flowers, if the wife gives praise immediately, the behavior will be strengthened and sustained.

3) Learning theory

Wahson observed the role of learning in a rat run labyrinth experiment. He believes that no matter how complex human behavior is the result of learning, behavior can be controlled by learning and training. He proposed that learning follows the following rules: when other conditions are equal, the more practice a certain behavior is, the quicker it becomes a habit; When the reaction occurs frequently, the latest reaction is more likely to be strengthened.

(3) The basic technology of psychoanalytic therapy

1) Relaxation training

Relaxation training is a way to enhance the self control ability of the actor through the body's active relaxation. The main types are progressive muscle relaxation, and independent training. Progressive muscle relaxation requirements gradually alternating tension or relax each muscle group, you tense a group of muscles as you breathe in, and you relax themas you breathe out. Relaxation training has a special effect on coping with anxiety, fear and stability. For example, you can do some relaxation exercises for a few minutes when you are experiencing tension and anxiety in the exam.

2) System desensitization therapy

System desensitization therapy refers to a kind of behavioral therapy that gradually eliminates anxiety, fear and other discomfort through a gradual process. It is by the Volpe initiative, which mainly consists of three steps: relaxation training; to help visitors to establish anxiety table, this table is in accordance with the severity of anxiety arranged in ascending order; desensitization: first, let the patients go into the relaxed state, then they will be desensitized according to the level of anxiety until the patients are no longer anxious about the event. For example, if a visitor does not dare to take a plane, we can let them start desensitization from the picture of the aircraft.

3) Implosive therapy

Implosive therapy is also called flooding therapy. Contrary to the system desensitization therapy, it directly exposes the visitor to the stimulus situation, thereby eliminating the fear. The therapist should introduce the situation in detail before the treatment, and make the visitor carefully consider whether to choose the therapy. In addition, major physical diseases should be excluded before treatment. It has a short course of treatment and fast effect, which is often used to treat anxiety and phobia. But it will make the visitors suffer great pain and should be used carefully.

4) Aversion therapy

Aversion therapy refers to the unpleasant or punitive stimulus provided by therapists when visitors have bad behaviors, the stimulus causes them feel aversion or psychological reaction, and ultimately reduce or abandon the behavior of visitors. For example, alcohol addicts take alcohol after taking abstinence, which can cause nausea, headache, anxiety, chest tightness and heart rate. It can build up the disgust of the visitors and eventually stop drinking. This method has a certain effect on alcohol dependence, obsessive–compulsive disorder, and exhibitionism.

5) Positive reinforcement procedures

Positive reinforcement procedures refers to training the appearance of an act or increasing its frequency by strengthening(or rewarding). The method is to give the fortified immediately and train again and again when the expected behavior appears. This method is mainly used for the treatment of chronic schizophrenia, childhood autism, mental retardation, and anorexia nervosa. We need to be aware of the reinforcement should be liked by the visitors. If you want the a child to like to play the piano, then take him to the playground after the piano class.

(4) Indications

Behavioral therapy can be widely used in a variety of individuals with abnormal behavior, including phobia, anxiety disorder, obsessive–compulsive disorder, hysteria etc.; attention deficit and hyperactivity disorder, tic disorder, child conduct disorder, etc.; psychosomatic disease; sexual dysfunction, parasexuality.

21.2.3.5　Cognitive therapy

(1) Concept

Cognitive therapy was born in the 20th Century 60–70 era. It is based on the theoretical hypothesis of cognitive process affecting emotion and behavior, and it is a general term to change or rebuild the psychological therapy of bad cognition through cognitive and behavioral technology. The use of contemporary cognitive therapy should be attributed to the work of Baker and Alice in the 60 years of the 20th century.

(2) The basic theory of psychoanalytic therapy

1) The basic viewpoint of cognitive therapy

Cognitive process is the mediator of behavior and emotion. Maladjusted behavior and emotion is associated with maladjusted cognition. The main task of therapists is to identify these maladaptive cognition with visitors, and to provide learning or training methods to correct these cognition. With the correction of cognition, the psychological block of visitors is also improving.

2) Cognitive theory of emotional disorder

● Negative automatic thoughts

"Negative" means that these ideas are always unpleasant, and "automatic" is that they often appear automatically without logical reasoning. The content of negative automatic thoughts can be negative interpretations of past events, negative perceptions of present conditions, or negative expectations of the future. Negative automatic ideas lead to emotional disorders, and emotional disorders make negative automatic thoughts more frequent and intense, and eventually form a vicious cycle.

- Underlying dysfunctional assumptions

Underlying dysfunctional assumptions refers to all kinds of assumptions that a patient set up from his early experience to himself, and the world, which influences individual's thoughts and behaviors. It exists in the unconscious and is hard to perceive. Some of these assumptions are rigid, extreme and negative, and are characterized by dysfunction. Some assumptions are fragility. For example, some people think that a person's request for help is a sign of weakness. Some assumptions are perfectionism or compulsivity. For example, someone thinks a person must be smart, beautiful, rich, and creative, or it's hard to be happy. The potential underlying dysfunctional assumptions can be initiated by future stress events, and a large number of negative automatic thoughts will be produced once it is started.

- Cognitive distortion

The negative automatic thought is the manifestation of cognitive distortion, and the therapist should help the visitor to identify the logical errors contained in the negative automatic thoughts: the absolute thinking of all or nothing; arbitrary inference, lack of factual basis, and a hasty conclusion; overgeneralizations; excessive extension, the patient will make a conclusion on the value of the whole life on the basis of a small mistake; patients may exaggerate and oversize, exaggerate their mistakes, defects, and degrade their achievements and advantages; injectivity attack, they take responsibility initiatively for the fault or or misfortune of others.

(3) The basic technology of psychoanalytic therapy

1) Beck cognitive therapy

The goal of Beck cognitive therapy is to change the distorted perception of the visitor, thus improving the maladjusted mood and behavior of the visitors. Its basic process is: distinguishing the negative automatic thoughts; testing the negative automatic thoughts, it is the core of cognitive therapy; distinguishing the underlying dysfunctional assumptions. Dysfunctional assumptions are usually more difficult to perceive than automatic thoughts. Therapists can ask visitors to generalize automated ideas to extract their underlying beliefs; questioning the dysfunctional assumptions. Therapists help visitors to change the potential dysfunctional assumptions and reduce the risk of recurrence.

2) Rational-emotive therapy

This method holds that emotional disorders are formed by irrational beliefs, absolute thinking and erroneous evaluation. Therapists should change their irrational beliefs and replace them with reasonable beliefs. With the disappearance of irrational beliefs, tension begins to eliminate, and a new and positive way of behavior is produced.

3) Chinese taoist cognitive therapy

The therapy is founded by Chinese scholars Desen Yang, and Yalin Zhang. The therapy advocates the main ideas of the Taoist school.

(4) Indications

Cognitive therapy is widely-used in many mental and psychological problems, including depression, anxiety, social phobia, eating disorders, sleep disorders, sexual dysfunction, migraine, addictive diseases or drug abuse, delusion of some schizophrenics.

21.2.3.6 Person-centered psychotherapy

(1) Concept

Person-centered psychotherapy was founded by American psychologist Karl Rogers for the first time, he advocated "people-oriented" "client-centered" concept. The therapy is centered on the creation of harmony, acceptance and sincerity, and is considered to be the third school of thought following psychoanalysis and behavioral therapy.

(2) The basic theory of person centered psychotherapy

1) A basic view of human nature

Person centered psychotherapy has great confidence in people and emphasizes the value and dignity of everyone. It believes that people are rational and can be responsible for themselves and have a positive direction of life; people have the nature to pursue a good life and strive for it; people are social, they are trustworthy and can cooperate with them; people have potential to solve life problems effectively; people have the ability to guide themselves and move towards self fulfillment.

2) The concept of self

Different from the meaning of "ego" in psychoanalysis, Rodgers's self concept refers to a person's experience of his own existence, which is the self realized by himself. It includes a person's understanding of himself through his own experience, introspection and feedback from others. Rodgers also suggested that every person has two selves in his heart: one is the real self, that is, the real feeling that the individual obtains in real life; the other is the ideal ego, namely the ideal state of self image. The growth of personality lies in the full realization of the harmony between the ideal self and the real self, and the conflict of the two leads to the psychological disorder.

(3) The basic technology of person centered psychotherapy

Rodgers thinks that visitors have the ability to self actualization. As long as we can create a suitable environment and establish effective therapeutic relationship, visitors can explore their inner feelings and help them develop their potential, and then we can promote personal growth and change of visitors. Rodgers attached great importance to the establishment of good treatment relationship. He suggested that there should be three kinds of personal traits in the treatment relationship, which are sincere and unanimous, unconditional positive regard and empathy.

1) Sincere and unanimous

It means to express their own feelings and attitude of the therapist open to visitors in the treatment, including not only positive, but also the negative feelings and attitudes, to be the same outside and inside. Positive attention means recognition, attention, acceptance and unconditional positive attention to visitors, which means that the therapist accepts visitors unconditionally.

2) Unconditional positive regard

Positive attention refers to the therapist's recognition, attention, and acceptance of visitors. Unconditional positive regard refers to the unconditional admission of visitors to the therapist. No matter what the visitor's feelings are, the therapist should understand and respect it without value judgment. This enables visitors to feel a safe atmosphere, and then express their feelings freely, without worrying about losing the therapist's acceptance.

3) Empathy

Empathy means the therapist goes deep into the spiritual world of the visitor, that is, "put yourself in the place" and "have the same feeling". Rodgers believes that this is a temporary life in other people's lives, giving up their values, without criticizing, and experiencing the feelings and conflicts of visitors from the perspective of visitors.

4) Therapeutic strategies

Person centered psychotherapy is mainly treated with non-guiding effects, including listening, respect, observation, clarification, emotional reflection, and self-disclosure.

(4) Indications

Person centered psychotherapy is suitable for the treatment of various psychological problems and is applicable to all people in principle, including healthy people and patients with mental disorders. The treatment is also applied to areas other than treatment, such as education, medical care, business, social work, and management.

21.2.3.7 Morita therapy

(1) Concept

Morita therapy was founded in 1920s by Professor Morita Masama of Japan. He called it "special treatment for neuroticism".

(2) The basic theory of psychoanalytic therapy

1) The theory of neuroticism

The indication of Morita's therapy is called "neuroticism", roughly equivalent to neurosis in the current diagnostic classification, but contains less than neurosis.

2) "The desire of birth" and "the fear of death"

"Desire for life" is a common desire of human beings to develop themselves. Morita thinks that the desire for survival of neurotic people is too intense, and the corresponding fear of death is more intense than that of ordinary people.

3) Hypochondriacal quality

Morita thinks that neurotic people are sensitive and introspective, because they worry too much about their mind and body. So it is easy to think of the feelings and emotions of normal people as morbid.

4) Psycho interaction

Neurotic patients are often overstressed with some common discomforts, such as anxiety and annoyance, and they feel that these feelings are abnormal and they are distressed by it. When they focus on these discomfort, they make the feeling stronger or even fixed, causing tension and anxiety to become more obvious and form a vicious circle.

5) Let it be, as by what is

This is the treatment principle of Morita therapy. It is rich in philosophic and oriental culture. It means to face the emotions and symptoms in a calm way, focus on their life goals, live actively with symptoms, break the mental interaction, and finally recover the healthy life condition.

(3) The basic technology of psychoanalytic therapy

1) Hospitalization

It is suitable for patients with obvious symptoms. Its treatment process is: ①absolute bed period, in this period, a single person is required to be alone and prohibit entertainment for about 1 weeks. ②Little work period, except for night rest time, patients should not stay in bed. They can do some cleaning in the early morning and chores indoors. They write diary every night, usually for 1 weeks . ③Heavy work period, this stage will arrange heavier outdoor activities (digging and mowing) according to physical strength. Most of them will experience fresh, pleasant and comfortable feelings. This stage usually lasts for 1 - 2 weeks. ④Back-to-society period, this phase relieves most of the patient's limitations, making the patient's depressed desire gradually met in the first few periods, generally lasting for 2 - 4 weeks.

2) Ambulatory treatment

Ambulatory treatment can be used for patients who are not eligible for hospitalization but are well guided. The key to the treatment is to live like a healthy person, no matter how the patient's symptoms and feelings change. As long as the patient is able to act and live in a healthy way, even a simple outpatient treatment can achieve quite a good effect.

(4) Indications

Morita therapy indications include not only various neurosis, but also achieved satisfactory curative effect in the hysteria, the recovery period of depression and schizophrenia and some psychosomatic diseases.

21.2.3.8 Family therapy

(1) Concept

Family therapy is a kind of psychological therapy to the family as the treatment object, it focus on the relationship between family members, but not too much attention to the individual psychological structure and mental state. It believes that the change of the individual depends on the change in the family. Family therapy originated in 1950s, Ackerman was one of the founders of family therapy, Bowen put forward the family system theory(family systems therapy), Minuchin emphasizes the effect of family structure on family relations, Parra Zoli and his colleagues founded the system of family therapy. After 1980s, family treatment has developed rapidly, and there is a trend of integration among different schools.

(2) The basic theory of psychoanalytic therapy

1) Family system

The family system is composed of several subsystems, each subsystem has its functions. They interact with each other, restrict each other, and jointly develop the whole function of the family. The family system operates under the family rules, and it has experienced the conflict and adjustment of the balance mechanism and the change mechanism.

2) Family life cycle

Family life is a continuous process. It has priority, such as independent adult, marriage, child raising, child growth, empty nest and late life. Every family will experience these stages. The process of changing is often the cause of the outbreak of the family's symptoms. For example, the mother/daughter relationship is too close in the family, if the child went away to college, or exile marrying the daughter, the mother may have anxiety, depression or physical discomfort and other symptoms, parents will also re adaptation.

3) Trigonometric relations

Bowen believes that the cornerstone of family emotional system is triangular relationship. When under internal pressure or external pressure, participants in the two person relationship will get involved in third triangles to form a triangle relationship in order to reduce tension and anxiety and get stability again. However, the third who is involved is often a vulnerable injured person. The identification of triangulation and de triangulation is the two core technology in family treatment.

(3) The basic technology of psychoanalytic therapy

1) Structural family therapy

This mode holds that family has its inherent organization or structure, and family structure produces stable maintenance and regulation through the interaction between its subsystems. Subsystems are distinguished by boundaries. Structural family therapy focuses on family organization, relationship, role and power implementation. The treatment strategy is to use various specific methods to correct family structure problems and promote family function.

2) Systematic family therapy

This mode introduces modern scientific methodology such as system theory, cybernetics and information theory into family therapy. It considers the family patterns and rules which constituted by members' interaction modes in family system are the main causes of patient's symptoms. The principle of treatment can be summed up as "hypothetical−cycle−neeutrality". The hypothesis means that the therapist speculates on the reasons for the maintenance of the symptoms; circular questioning is a kind of therapist's ability to understand and communicate information by asking questions to the family; neutrality means that therapists remain neutral in the causes of psychological problems and dispute resolution. Therapists will be allied with family members, but they are not partial to any side.

3) Strategic family therapy

According to the theory, the symptoms of individuals originate from the function of the whole family system, and the problem is the real problem. The therapist must put forward a set of strategies to solve it. Strategic family therapy believes that the problem can be solved by changing the current way of communication, and it does not pay attention to the past. The therapist's task is to make clear goals for the situation, to design a set of interventions, and to arrange specific treatment strategies.

(4) Indications

Family therapy is suitable for all kinds of families with mental or psychological problems, including adolescent mental disorders, poor parent−child relationship, marriage and emotional conflict, various stress events on the family and the family of patients with chronic schizophrenia

21.2.3.9　Group psychotherapy

(1) Concept

Group psychotherapy is a psychotherapy that provides psychological help to team members. The first attempt at group form therapy was Platt, an American physician in 1905. In 1950s, the research and practice of group psychotherapy increased significantly, and became an important force in psychotherapy.

(2) The basic theory of psychoanalytic therapy

The basic mechanism of group psychotherapy is not to be guided, but to achieve the goal of treatment through interpersonal interaction in the group. It is through the interaction of members to help them improve their self−understanding, self−development and self−fulfilment.

The therapeutic change of group is a very complex process, and it is generated by the interaction of various complex experiences of human beings. This interaction can be called the therapeutic factor. The therapists of different schools and different theoretical orientations have different views on the curative effect factors of grouptherapy. It is generally believed that the mechanisms of group therapy include emotional support, hope remolding, universality, information transmission, altruism, behavior simulation, interpersonal learning and group cohesion.

(3) The basic technology of psychoanalytic therapy

1) The settings of group psychotherapy

The nature of the group: it is divided into structural and non structural groups according to the degree of treatment, or it can be divided into open and closed groups according to the fixed degree of the participants

The time and frequency of group treatment: group duration is too short or too long will all affect the treatment effect of group. Generally speaking, group psychotherapy is suitable for 8−15 times, 1−2 times a week, 1.5−2.0 hours per time.

The place for group treatment: group treatment should have enough space for safety, comfort and no interference.

2) The role of the therapist

Active mobilization and encouragement: the therapist should mobilize the enthusiasm of the members, encourage people to open and communicate, and discuss actively.

Moderate participation and guidance: in the early stage of treatment, therapists participate in activities as members, promote understanding among members, moderate guidance and correction in discussions and communication, and ensure that treatment is carried out in the right direction. The therapist also needs to explain some key questions if necessary.

Create a good atmosphere: in order to better understand and communicate with each other, mutual concern and encouragement, the therapist should create a warm and harmonious atmosphere.

3) The implementation of group psychotherapy

The initial phase: the main goal of this phase is to promote mutual understanding of group members and to develop the goals and directions of treatment.

The transformation phase: the main task at this stage is to promote interaction and mutual trust between group members, encourage members to express and deal with conflicts and emotions.

The working phase: the main objective of this phase is to adopt different activities and techniques based on group programmes to promote interaction and discussion of groups.

The end phase: the main task of this stage is to summarize the treatment, evaluate the growth and change of the group members, and help to apply this transformation to life.

(4) Indications

Indications for group psychotherapy include neurosis, social anxiety disorder, adolescent psychological and behavioral disorders, interpersonal problems, psychosomatic diseases, chronic physical diseases, etc. Not suitable for including in group psychotherapy patients: patients with severe depression and anxiety, patients with acute schizophrenia, paranoid personality disorder, drug addiction or alcoholism.

Lian Nan, Yang Lei

Chapter 22

Rehabilitation and Prevention of Mental Disorders

22.1 Inroduction

22.1.1 The significance of rehabilitation and prevention of mental disorders

Prevention, treatment and rehabilitation are inseparable components of any disease. Because the current treatment of mental disorders is not ideal, many mental disorders are chronic, episodes of disease, and may lead to different degrees of disability. Therefore, prevention and rehabilitation are important links in the process of mental disorder intervention, sometimes it is even more important than treatment.

Mental disorders have multiple determinants, the inefficiency of treatment lead to increase the cost of cure. In term of this, rehabilitation of mental disorder is very important for lightening economical burden. It is reported that almost 450 million people suffer from mental and behavioural disorders around world. About 25% person worldwide will develop 1 or more of these disorders during their lifetime. Among the total Disability Adjusted Life Years (DALYs) lost due to all diseases, neuropsychiatric conditions account for 13% and are estimated to increase to 15% by the year 2020. Among ten leading causes of disability and premature death worldwide, five of them are psychiatric conditions. Mental disorders are not only an immense psychological, social and economic burden to society, but also decline to increase the risk of physical illnesses. Above all, to some extent, effective rehabilitation can reduce DALYs through providing better determination, so that it is very important that developing useful rehabilitation policyand programmes.

Similarly, prevention is also an important part among the disease duration. Effective prevention can reduce the risk of mental disorders. Research about effective prevention is beginning to show significant long-term outcomes. There is a wide range of effective preventive programmes and policies available for implementation to lower risk factors, enhance protective factors and reduce psychiatric symptoms and disability and the onset of some mental disorders. These measures are constantly being revised from an evidence-based perspective. These implementational so better positive mental health, contribute to improve physical health and generate social and economic benefits. In the long run, prevention can be cost-effective due to enhance the patients' social function.

22.1.2　Future development

(1)Implementation about rehabilitation and prevention should be guided by available evidence.

(2)Policies and programmes should be made widely available. Making effective policies and programmes widely available would provide organization with a series of preventive tools to tackle mental disorders.

(3)Further efforts should be needed to expand the spectrum of effective rehabilitation and preventive interventions, to improve their effectiveness and cost−effectiveness in difference surroundings and to intensify the evidence base.

(4)Governments would invest lots in these implementation.

(5)Actions and policies that improve the protection of basic human rights are a powerful preventive strategy for mental disorders.

22.2　Mental rehabilitation

22.2.1　Overview

22.2.1.1　The concept of mental rehabilitation

Mental rehabilitation is the use of existing facilities and means to ease the mental symptoms of mentally ill patients, improve their self−care abilities, enhance their quality of life, and strengthen the training of their job and life skills. The goal is to restore the patients' social functions, reduce the occurrence of mental disability, and enable them to return to the social process.

Mental rehabilitation includes hospital rehabilitation and community rehabilitation. The trend of development shows that the focus of mental rehabilitation is gradually shifting from hospital to community rehabilitation. The WHO has pointed out that hospital−based rehabilitation can not meet the needs of the majority of people with mental disability, while only the community−based rehabilitation can provide available basic services to most of the disabled.

22.2.1.2　The task of mental rehabilitation

According to the experience of mental rehabilitation during the past decades, the tasks of mental rehabilitation include four aspects: symptom relief; functional training; comprehensive rehabilitation; and social reintegration. Among them, relieving symptoms is the basis and prerequisite for mental rehabilitation, functional training is the method and means, comprehensive rehabilitation is the criteria and guidelines, and social reintegration is the goal and direction.

(1)Symptoms relief

The procedure of the rehabilitation begins with the onset of disease and runs through the entire process of treatment. After the acute onset of psychosis and acute exacerbation of chronic patients, the first thing to do is to diagnose and use psychotherapy, medication, electrical shock and other physical therapies and special care measures to effectively control the psychiatric symptoms, laying a good foundation for further mental rehabilitation and making necessary preparations.

(2)Functional training

After patient's condition improves and the mental illness is relieved, various behavioral trainings, such as:

1) Learning behavioral skills training, start, allowing patients to learn about current events, knowledge about health, history or scientific and technological knowledge.

2) The training of life skills can be carried out in the future as needed, such as grocery shopping, home furnishing, cooking, social etiquette and transportation using.

3) Job skills are trained by simple assignments, handcrafting, and professional labor training, etc., so that mentally ill patients obtain a certain degree of job skills and be ready to return to society.

(3) Comprehensive rehabilitation

In order to lay a good foundation for furtherly return to the society, comprehensive rehabilitation includes mental illness treatment, nursing, recovery, as well as psychological, sociological, and vocational rehabilitation and other aspects of the comprehensive recovery of patients with mental illness. It needs all mental health rehabilitation centers to be equipped with appropriate personnel of various types, such as psychiatrists, psychiatric nurses, psychologists, sociologists (including social workers), and occupational therapy professionals.

(4) Social reintegration

Before a patient return to the society, professionals need to anticipate the possibility of his or her return and reassess the rehabilitation goals according to the patient's conditions, work potential, career plan, family conditions, and economic conditions to determine whether the destination should be a transitional rehabilitation facility or a direct return to society. Analysis will also be processed to determine whether the original job site or place of residence is appropriate, whether job changing should be taken into consideration, and whether there exist any risk factors of stress.

There are many ways to reintegrate into the society. One is that the patient has fully recovered, and temporarily returned to the community in one of the following ways: ① returning to the family; ② returning to the original workplace; ③ living in a convalescent apartment; ④ participating in patient associations; ⑤ work-therapy stations for psychiatric patients.

22.2.2　Hospital rehabilitation

In China, most patients with chronic mental illness live in mental hospitals or psychiatric nursing homes, and some of them adopt close-ended management methods. The range of activities of these patients is limited to the ward, and often they do not meet the requirements for mental rehabilitation. Fortunately, most hospitals have already started rehabilitation departments and are moving from closed management to open management.

Patient rehabilitation should be the most important consideration in the ward management. In rehabilitation wards, a special management team should be set up to classify patients and promote the rehabilitation of wards. In psychiatric area, a hall for the rehabilitation of patients is set up. There are television sets, tape recorders, kriegspiel chess, playing cards, and other entertainment facilities. The wards are equipped with nurses with special skills to organize patients to read newspapers and watch TV, listen to music, sing, dance, play chess, and play cards and other games.

Patients in the ward can also be given token rewards and penalties for self-care items, such as self-care beds, clothing, manners and other comprehensive evaluation, which will play a better role in the rehabilitation of inpatient mental patients. Some areas specialize in setting up a rehabilitation ward, including the medical group, nursing group, social defense group, music therapy group, occupational therapy group, rehabilitation equipment training group. Patients whose psychiatric symptoms have been relieved and self-awareness has recovered have been provided with a rehabilitation training facility before returning to society. The patients are managed in a fully open-ended way to allow them to undergo rehabilitation training while receiving medical treatment and nursing care. For example, in the store, patients can receive training on how to deal with customers, how to market, and how to manage stores. Through these rehabilitation trainings, many patients have returned to society from here, and have re-advanced their studies, employment, and marriage to live a happy life as normal people.

22.2.3   Community rehabilitation

Rehabilitation from the hospital to community rehabilitation is a continuous process. Patients will be placed in transitional facilities after they leave the hospital. These facilities are designed to enable patients to continue to receive certain behavioral rehabilitation training and gradually adapt to normal community life. They are also prepared to return to the society. In addition to certain rehabilitation work conditions, these transitional facilities also need to solve some practical problems. The first is the housing problem, followed by employment, socialization, and entertainment. At present, the country are constantly exploring the best transitional facility implementation programs. The main forms that have been developed are the following types.

22.2.3.1   Transitional hospital facilities

Day hospitals(daycare stations) or night hospitals are set up in psychiatric hospitals or mental health centers. If the patient's family has a good living condition and is willing to accept the placement, the patient can continue to receive certain medical care or behavioral rehabilitation training during the day in the day hospital. For those who lack the family's living conditions, if the condition permits, they will return to work in the community during the day. The original work unit will provide special arrangements or let the patients enter a shelter factory, and they will be accommodated at night hospitals at night, and will receive necessary medical and rehabilitation training.

22.2.3.2   Transitional residential facilities

The purpose is to help patients solve their housing problems. The transitional boarding (or halfway house) is often set up by public or individuals and is managed by specially trained staff to accommodate those who can be discharged but lack the ability to live independently or who are homeless. These facilities are mainly used to help the patients cope with the daily life and the rehabilitation of their occupational activities, and the patients are gradually sent to day hospitals or places of employment as much as possible.

22.2.3.3   Transitional employment facilities

This is to set up transitional employment places that are closer to real life. These facilities, such as sheltered factory or farm, are mainly used to cultivate the work habits of the patients and train their professional skills so as to prepare for the next step of re-employment. In addition to receiving various industrial labor or agricultural skill training, their life is also interspersed with some rehabilitation measures and social entertainment activities. These facilities can also be equipped with necessary basic medical facilities.

22.2.3.4   Transitional social entertainment facilities

At present, some countries and regions have also set up social entertainment venues specifically to gradually enhance the social functions of people with mental disabilities in the community, in order to train their social activities and enrich their cultural life and improve quality of life. Participants are mainly mentally disabled persons who reside in transitional homestays and some scattered families. Social clubs are set up within the community, with special management, certain cultural facilities, and encouragement and initiation of normal volunteers to participate in the work of assistance to enhance the training effect.

After the above transitional arrangements and a period of training, the facilities should try to send the people who are stable and meet the rehabilitation requirements gradually back to the community. The stable people would be guide to participate in normal social activities and employment, then finally reach fully regained social rehabilitation goals.

22.2.4 Community mental health services

A community is a group of social groups(such as families, clans) or social organizations(such as institutions and groups) that gather in a certain geographic area and form an interconnected group in life. Its characteristics are: ①the composition of the community is based on certain production relations and social relations; ②the community has certain geographical boundaries; ③the residents in the community have specific behavioral norms and lifestyles; ④the residents emotionally have local concepts in the community.

At present, community mental health service organizations in China include the following.

22.2.4.1 Inpatient treatment institutions

Inpatient treatment institutions include community mental health stations in the health system, psychiatric departments in general hospitals, veteran psychiatric hospitals in the civil affairs system, psychiatric patient sanitariums, and psychiatric management hospitals in the public security system.

22.2.4.2 Part of hospitalization institutions

Some hospitalization institutions include day hospital and night hospital.

22.2.4.3 Outpatient services

Community mental health clinics can provide a number of services such as diagnosis, treatment, consultation, psychotherapy, clinic visits.

22.2.4.4 Emergency services

When an emergency occurs, the emergency department can provide medical services.

22.2.4.5 Consultation and contact mental health services

It provides consultation and co-management services for mental health in clinical departments of general hospitals.

22.2.4.6 Asylum or farm

Patients are trained in industrial labor or agricultural labor skills with care.

22.2.4.7 Wellness apartment

One or more healthy people take care of patients close to the psychiatric hospital or in a building where all patients gather. The patient takes care of his or her own life. Medical work is regularly done by doctors from the hospital.

22.2.4.8 Patient associations

A group of discharged patients voluntarily gather together to help each other and manage themselves. The size of the group is uncertain. They regularly receive guidance from the hospital and often carry out various forms of social activities such as concerts, dances, symposiums, art exhibitions, and group travel.

22.2.4.9 Home visits

Community mental health workers regularly visit their homes within the jurisdiction of the area to keep abreast of the patient's condition, prevent recurrence, and reduce the rate of readmissions.

22.2.4.10　Psychiatric workplace treatment station

The psychiatric patients' workplace treatment station, referred to as the treatment station, is a rehabilitation measure taken by the streets, townships, and factories. The treatment station organizes the chronic mentally ill patients with stable conditions and a certain ability to work in their own jurisdictions to participate in some simple labor with in their capacity, and carries out various forms of recreational and sports activities to promote their community rehabilitation.

22.2.4.11　The care network of psychiatric patients

Neighborhood committee cadres, retirees, neighbors or volunteers are selected around the patient. After training with professional knowledge, they will publicize the knowledge of mental illness prevention and protect the patient from discrimination, assist the patient's family members in urging patients to attend clinics and take medications on time, take care of patients, and prevent relapse.

22.2.4.12　Family beds

Patients who can not stay in the hospital can be regularly visited by grass-root prevention and treatment doctors and treated at home.

22.3　Prevention of mental disorders

The prevention of mental disorders is increasingly and closely watched by medical scientists. Preventive psychiatry is an important component of clinical psychiatry. What many countries are doing is to combine different social systems, cultures, and ethnic characteristics, and to work together in a comprehensive way to prevent mental disorders.

In 1964, Caplan elucidated new points for the prevention of psychiatry and proposed a three-level prevention model for mental illness, which had a tremendous impact on the practice of psychiatry. From then on, the prevention of mental disorders has been mainly conducted from these three aspects.

22.3.1　Tertiary prevention of mental disorders

The three level prevention means: ①to reduce the occurrence of mental illness in the community (primary prevention); ②to shorten the course of the disease in persons with mental disorders (secondary prevention); ③to eliminate or reduce disability caused by mental disorders (tertiary prevention).

The 3 levels of prevention of specific mental disorders include the following.

22.3.1.1　Primary prevention

The primary prevention of mental disorders is aimed to promote mental health of healthy people, avoid and eliminate pathogenic factors, and achieve the goal of preventing and controlling the occurrence of mental illness. The primary prevention of mental illness can be carried out in the following three aspects.

(1) Maintain mental health from a biological perspective and prevent the onset of mental illness, including: ①prenatal care services to prevent mental disorders or intellectual impairments caused by factors such as nutritional deficiencies and viral infections; ②perinatal health care, prevention of hypoxia, birth injury, infection; ③childhood planed immunization, health care; ④eugenics and premarital examinations to prevent the occurrence of genetic diseases.

(2) Maintain mental health from a psychological perspective, including: ①to promote breastfeeding, maternal care of infants and young children, affection fostering, and enjoyable motherhood; ②to support

emotionally when encountering life events; ③to self-cultivate, such as cultivation of good personalities; ④to strengthen mental health care in special periods such as adolescence, marriage, childbirth, employment, and retirement; ⑤to strengthen psychological counseling and crisis intervention.

(3) Maintain mental health from the perspective of sociology, including: ①to deal with all kinds of interpersonal relationships (including within the family); ②to strengthen production, life and health care measures, improve social and environmental conditions (such as economic, cultural, labor, production, living conditions), reduce mental disorders caused by poisoning, infection, trauma, malnutrition, and other social environmental factors.

22.3.1.2 Secondary prevention

The goal of secondary prevention is early detection, early diagnosis, early treatment, shortening of the disease course, and prevention of relapse. These can be done from the following aspects.

(1) Popularize mental health knowledge, improve the ability to identify mental illness, and achieve early detection, early diagnosis, and early treatment.

(2) Popularize knowledge of mental illness prevention at all levels of medical institutions, increase the level of psychiatric diagnosis and treatment, and develop a practical screening scale.

(3) Conduct epidemiological surveys of mental illnesses to find out people with mental illness in the population, understand the related factors of the situation, the distribution of mental illness patients, and the distribution of impact, so as to explore the causes and epidemiological patterns, and formulate prevention and control methods to check the effect of prevention and treatment.

(4) Carry out medical surveillance on high-risk groups and high-incidence families to detect mentally ill patients as soon as possible.

(5) Improve the personnel's capacity to promote the diagnostic accuracy, enhance efficacy, and reduce residual symptoms.

(6) Add psychiatry departments to the community medical institutions, expand prevention and control networks, carry out various forms of medical services, and maintain treatment.

(7) Encourage the family, hospital, and society to conduct crisis interventions to reduce and eliminate the psychological and social factors that cause relapse, consolidate curative effects, and prevent the recurrence of mental illness.

22.3.1.3 Tertiary prevention

With the purpose of slowing down the functional deficits caused by mental illness (including the loss of ability caused by mental illness and the low ability to cause residual symptoms after treatment), we must prevent and relieve diseases, promote health, and focus on community rehabilitation. The following aspects should be worked on.

(1) Stress in-hospital work as inpatient treatment is the beginning of rehabilitation. The hospitalization time should be shortened as much as possible and the patients transferred to community rehabilitation as soon as possible.

(2) Strengthen publicity and education so as to achieve the cooperation of the family, society, and medical staff to protect against disability and enhance recovery.

(3) Make full use of community-based rehabilitation facilities such as day hospitals, patient apartments, and sheltered factories (farms) to prevent disuse defects and promote community rehabilitation.

22.3.2 Establish a mental disorder prevention network

The establishment of a mental disorder prevention and control network is one of the main contents of the prevention and treatment of mental illness. It is of equal importance to the general investigation of mental illnesses, the training of prevention and control personnel, the promotion of mental health knowledge, and the implementation of various forms of prevention and treatment equivalence. It is essential for the prevention and treatment of mental illness.

Establishing a network for the prevention and treatment of mental disorders must be conducted under the leadership of health administrative departments at all levels, through specializing the measures according to local conditions, mobilizing relevant departments and all positive factors, and conducting prevention and treatment of mental illness. In larger cities, a three-level control network for cities, districts and sub-districts can be established to take charge of the prevention and treatment of mental illness in the city. City-level psychiatric hospital is the city's psychiatric prevention and control center. In addition to outpatients, wards, and other departments, certain institutions, such as the community control department or community control office, should be set up to supervise the out-of-hospital prevention and treatment of districts and streets. District- or county-level mental hospitals should also establish out-of-hospital prevention and treatment institutions, such as community prevention units or community prevention teams. The street mental disease prevention and control station is a grassroots prevention and treatment institution responsible for the prevention and treatment of all patients in the street. Small cities and the vast rural areas can establish three-level control networks for cities, counties and townships.

22.3.3　The prevention of mental disorders

22.3.3.1　Prevention of organic mental disorders

This kind of mental disorder is based on the organic diseases of the brain. It should pay attention to the health of the whole body and reduce the occurrence of organic and physical diseases of the brain, including: ①strengthening exercise, enhancing physical fitness, increasing the body's resistance and immunity to reduce various diseases caused by acute and chronic infections; ②strengthening traffic management, preventing traffic accidents, reducing brain injury, and preventing mental disorders caused by brain injury; ③extensive and in-depth preventing and controlling somatic diseases, parasitic diseases, sexually transmitted diseases, endemic diseases, infectious diseases, changing unhealthy lifestyles, preventing hypertension, hyperlipidemia, diabetes, etc. The aim is to avoid the occurrence of somatic diseases and central nervous system diseases.

22.3.3.2　Mental disorders caused by psychoactive substances and prevention of mental disorders caused by non-addictive substances

Publicity campaigns on drug knowledge are often carried out among community groups to enable people, especially the young, to understand the types of drugs and the dangers of drug use, and to guide them on how to cope with the luring of other people. Drug addicts are voluntarily or obliged to abstain from drugs, while social and psychological rehabilitation training is conducted to improve their social functions. Strengthening occupational protection and labor protection and reducing the occurrence of toxic diseases such as heavy metals, organic matter, carbon monoxide, and organophosphorus pesticides can prevent and reduce mental disorders caused by non-addictive substances.

22.3.3.3　Prevention of schizophrenia and affective disorders

At present, the major goals are early detection, early diagnosis, and early treatment so as to strive for good results. It is essential to adhere to systematic and reasonable maintenance treatment, reduce and prevent relapse, reduce the harm caused by the disease and mental disability because both of these diseases have familial aggregation. Although they are not completely or clearly classified as genetic diseases, they have a certain genetic predisposition, Therefore, counseling should always be provided actively. If both the husband and the wife suffer from these conditions, they should avoid childbirth, so should patients whose symptoms have not relieved. When looking for a spouse, the family with a diagnosed patient should try to avoid marriage with another person who also has a family history.

22.3.3.4　Prevention of neurosis

Preventing neuroses begins from childhood, such as fostering good character, and learning to deal with peer relationships and various social skills. Once symptoms of neurosis are manifested, psychotherapy, social support, and medication should be considered to promote the improvement of the condition and prevent the deterioration of the symptoms. Patients with neurosis should pay attention to rehabilitation to prevent the occurrence of sickness and promote the recovery of social functions.

22.3.3.5　Prevention of stress disorders and adaptive disorders

This is a group of mental disorders caused by psychosocial factors. Their occurrence is not only related to the intensity, duration, and body state of the predisposing factors, but also closely to the patient's premorbid personality characteristics. Mental health, in addition to being influenced by social culture, is closely related to the balance and flexibility of each person's high−level neurological processes. The training of a person's temperament, even of the strong and imbalanced people to constantly train their internal inhibition, develops the individual's ability to endure, self−discipline, and maintain, so that they can be flexible and eliminate excessive excitability to promote their excitement and suppression with balance. As for the weak type, we must eliminate their excessively passive and defensive responses and make them gradually become stronger. It is also possible to increase the flexibility of the nerve process through personality exercises to prevent the rapid changes in the peripheral environment or social psychological factors, which would result in higher neurological disorders.

On the other hand, the functional status of the individual's nervous system is also important. When high−level neural activities are weakened, such as insomnia, fatigue, exhaustion, etc. , it is easy to trigger certain stress disorders and adaptation disorders. Therefore, sleep, work and rest, strengthen cultural and sports activities should be attended in the daily life; the patients should also maintain a delighted mood, enhance physical fitness, to prevent the occurrence of stress disorders and adaptive disorders.

22.3.3.6　Prevention of mental retardation

Mental retardation is a kind of neuropsychiatric disorder symptom group, mainly caused by intellectual retardation and difficulty in social adjustment. To prevent mental retardation, we must first actively carry out maternal and child health care. Pregnant women should prevent infections, poisoning, trauma, malnutrition, and teratogenic drugs to avoid affecting the fetus. Prenatal care should be strengthened to prevent fetal hypoxia and birth injury. The occurrence of infectious diseases and traumatic brain injury in infants and young children should also be precluded. Second, we must actively prevent and treat endemic diseases, such as early prevention and treatment of endemic goiter, prevention of endemic gnosis, potassium iodide consumption during pregnancy in the prevalent areas, and so on. Third, genetic counseling work should be actively carried out because genetic factors are the root of certain mental retardation, especially the incidence of hereditary diseases in children born by close relatives. Therefore, the close relatives should be avoided. Those with a history of inheritance should undergo amniocentesis at 12−16 weeks of gestation and be checked for chromosome aberrations to determine whether to terminate the pregnancy. Fourth, children's behavior and life should be actively guided, and even be provided with special education to improve their self−care ability and minimize their disability.

22.3.3.7 Prevention of personality disorders

The conditions for the formation of personality are complicated, including innate factors and acquired factors. Inappropriate education methods, ill-fated family life, and poor environmental influences are the main causes of personality disorders. Therefore, to prevent personality disorders, we must first attach importance to the physical and mental health of children and adolescents. Special attention should be paid to the children's family education issues, the family's living environment, the family's relationships, and the parents' education methods. In addition, families should coordinate with schools to provide ideological and moral education to children and prohibit their contact with corrupted groups, inappropriate films, televisions, literature, and illegal video games in order to cultivate their moral values and healthy lifestyles, with magnanimity, honesty, bravery, and cheerful optimism to prevent the occurrence of personality disorders.

Liu Fang

Chapter 23

Mental Illness and Legal Issues

23.1 Introduction

Mental illness refers to a wide range of mental health conditions — disorders that substantially impairs a person's thought, perception of reality, emotional process, or judgment; or grossly impairs behavior as demonstrated by recent disturbed behavior. Examples of mental illness include anxiety disorders, mood disorders, schizophrenia, eating disorders, and addictive behaviors. These disabilities in patients can cause various legal and ethical issues. In order to secure the rights of patients with mental illness and safeguard social justice, there are forensic psychiatry and mental health law.

Forensic psychiatry is a branch of psychiatry, a borderline between psychiatry and law. Forensic psychiatry deals with issues at the interface of penal or criminal law as well as with matters arising in evaluations on civil law cases and in the development and application of mental health legislation. It is a medical subspecialty that includes research and clinical practice in the many areas in which psychiatry is applied to legal issues.

(1)Narrowly, it is applied to the branch of psychiatry that deals with the assessment and treatment of mentally abnormal offenders.

(2)Broadly, the term is applied to all legal aspects of psychiatry, including the civil law and laws regulating psychiatric practice.

Modern forensic psychiatry has benefited from four key developments: ①the evolution in the medico-legal understanding and appreciation of the relationship between mental illness and criminality; ②the evolution of the legal tests to define legal insanity; ③the new methodologies for the treatment of mental conditions that provide alternatives to custodial care; ④the changes in public attitudes and perceptions about mental conditions in general. These four aspects underlie the expansion recently seen in forensic psychiatry from issues entirely related to criminal prosecutions and the treatment of mentally ill offenders to many other fields of law and mental health policy.

An expert in psychiatry and/or psychology can provide invaluable input into the assessment of competency to waive competency to confess, competency to represent oneself in court, competency to stand trial, competency to be sentenced, competency to be executed, and competency to waive death penalty appeals. Competency assessment involves the thorough assessment of the specific skills and knowledge required for a given function that has legal ramifications.

Forensic psychiatrists must have knowledge of courtroom activity and possess an ability to communicate their findings clearly under the difficult situation of cross examination. The knowledge in psychiatry and law defines the subspecialty of forensic psychiatry and provides the ethical foundations for its practitioners.

23.2　The crimes and assessments of offenders with mental disorder

23.2.1　Forensic psychiatric evaluation

A forensic assessment may be required for an individual who has been charged with a crime(usually a violent crime), to establish whether the person has the legal competence to stand trial. If a person with mental illness is convicted to an offense, a forensic report may be required to inform the Court's sentencing decision, as a mental illness at the time of the offense may be a mitigating factor. A forensic assessment may also take the form of a risk assessment, to comment on the relationship between the person's mental illness and the risk of further violent offenses.

The forensic psychiatric examination of competence follows the general principles of other assessments and includes a thorough psychiatric assessment, with an interview and a mental status examination, if possible, and an examination of collateral information. An exploration of how psychiatric diagnosis and symptoms may interfere with any or all of the types of competence is essential.

The psychiatrist makes a diagnosis based on the patient presents signs and symptoms and formulation to help the patient understand the symptoms, with a view to treatment that will help to resolve thesymptoms. In forensic psychiatry, the situation may be complicated by the attempt to apply specific signs and symptoms to legal criteria. Furthermore, evaluees in forensic contexts may exaggerate or minimize their symptoms, for example, to maximize their injury in civil cases or to minimize their involvement or culpability in criminal cases. Forensic psychiatrists are concerned with the accuracy of the received information that forms the basis for their conclusions. Consequently, in performing assessments, they are particularly concerned about dissimulation and malingering of symptoms and disorders.

Physicians have an obligation to assist in the administration of justice. Forensic psychiatrists are physicians who are trained to diagnose and treat patients within the ethics principles embedded in the theraputic relationship. The role of the forensic psychiatrist in assisting court and other agents sometimes demands that the psychiatrist step outside of the theraputic relationship. The psychiatrist is primarily serving the interests or needs of the court, the retaining attorney, or another third party, but their interests may or may not serve those of the evaluee. Therefore, the forensic practitioner strives for objectivity in seeking to answer a psycho-legal question.

Forensic psychiatrists are expected to perform the tasks listed below.

(1) Define the referral questions—Forensic psychiatrists should clarify the referral questions with the attorney/judge prior to accepting the case.

(2) Determine the scope of the assessment—Forensic psychiatrists should determine which legal criteria are relevant for consideration in a forensic psychiatric evaluation.

(3) Translate legal criteria into psychological constructs—Forensic psychiatrists are expected to discuss

with the referral source(judge, attorney) the objective(s) of the evaluation and possible uses of the evaluation results. Based on this information, forensic psychiatrists can then determine what psychological constructs are pertinent and applicable to the case.

(4)Use psychological tests and methods—Forensic psychiatrists should employ valid, reliable, and generally accepted methods of accessing constructs.

(5)Communicate with the referral source—Forensic psychiatrists must maintain contact with the referral source and make modifications to the evaluation purposes and process as needed.

(6)Apply the results of psychiatric research—Forensic psychiatrists are expected to have up-to-date knowledge of research relevant to the forensic issues.

(7)Communicate the results—Forensic psychiatrists should communicate the results of his/her evaluation with legal professionals and decision makers.

The record can also document common manifestations of an intermittent illness, such as the patient's typical manifestation of manic, psychotic, or depressive symptoms.

Psychiatrists are called on by the legal system to provide testimonies in criminal and civil cases. In criminal cases, forensic psychiatrists may be asked to comment on the competence of a person to make decisions throughout all the phases of criminal investigation, trial, and punishment. These include the competence to stand trial, to plead guilty, to be sentenced, to waive appeal, and to be executed. In civil cases, forensic psychiatric experts are asked to evaluate a number of civil competences, including competence to make a will or contract or to make decisions about one's person and property. Psychiatrists are also called on to testify about many other issues related to civil cases. Forensic psychiatrists who work with children and adolescents are frequently involved in evaluations and testimony concerning juvenile delinquency, child custody, termination of parental rights, and other issues.

23.2.2　Criminal responsibility assessment

23.2.2.1　Criminal responsibility

Criminal responsibility is a term in medical jurisprudence where an accuser's mental capacity to understand the charges against him and may have no knowledge of the crime. It is the obligation in law to answer for infractions committed and to suffer the punishment provided by the legislation that governs the infraction in question.

Unlike civil liability, the obligation to answer for damage one has caused, either by repairing it or paying damages, criminal responsibility implies legal recourse for the state against a disturbance of the peace, including:

(1)Participation in a criminal offense.

(2)Forms of criminal responsibility.

(3)Exceptions to criminal responsibility.

In the criminal justice system, a competency evaluation is an assessment of the ability of a defendant to understand and rationally participate in a court process.

23.2.2.2　Determination of criminal responsibility

A forensic psychiatrist frequently requires to deliver expert testimony that can help the court determine criminal responsibility. This evaluation determines intent and causality. Did the individual really intend to commit the offense or was it a consequence of other circumstances or an accident?

Criminal responsibility evaluations are difficult because of their retrospective nature, and because we can never know what was in someone else's mind, especially when that person may have understandable reasons to distort the facts.

Forensic psychiatry must work within the framework of the law, and because the law has a major interest in the nature of responsibility, important areas of forensic psychiatric endeavor, such as forensic neuropsychiatry, must also deal with the nature of responsibility. The purpose of the insanity defense is to permit the exoneration of those individuals whom society believes should not be held morally responsible for their acts. Their lack of responsibility for criminal acts may stem from an absence of free will in their behavior, or the ineffectiveness of punishment in deterring their behavior. Nevertheless, mental disease alone does not exculpate a defendant from responsibility for his criminal acts. Something more must be evident.

"Diminished capacity" is a defense based on impairment of the mind. It supplements, rather than replaces, the insanity defense, allowing evidence of any interference with the normal functioning of the mind to be introduced to prove that the defendant did not have the ability to formulate one of the specific mental elements required for the crime charged.

23.2.2.3   Criminal responsibility assessment

(1) Mental illness or psychiatric disorder

1) In any prosecution for an offense, it is an affirmative defense that, at the time of the conduct charged, as a result of mental illness or serious mental disorder, the accused lacked substantial capacity to appreciate the mistake of the accused's conduct. If the defendant prevails in establishing the affirmative defense provided in this subsection, the trier of fact shall return a verdict of " not guilty by reason of insanity".

2) If it is proved that at the time of the alleged act the accused suffers from a serious mental disorder affecting his or her mind, despite the physical ability, the factual entity should return to its sentence of guilty, but mentally ill.

3) It shall not be a defense under this section if the alleged insanity or mental illness was proximately caused by the voluntary ingestion, inhalation or injection of intoxicating liquor, any drug or other mentally debilitating substance, or any combination thereof, unless such substance was prescribed for the defendant by a licensed health – care practitioner and was used in accordance with the directions of such prescription. As used in this chapter, the terms "insanity" or "mental illness" do not include an abnormality manifested only by repeated criminal or other antisocial conduct.

(2) Rules to prescribe procedures for psychiatric examination, testimony of psychiatrist

1) The procedures for examination of the accused by the accused's own psychiatrist or by a psychiatrist employed by the circumstances under which such an examination will be permitted may be prescribed by rules of the court having jurisdiction over the offense.

2) A psychiatrist testifying at trial concerning the mental condition of the accused shall be permitted to make a statement as to the nature of the examination. A psychiatrist diagnosis of the mental state of the accused at the time of the alleged offence. At the same time, the psychiatrist assesses the ability of the accused to conduct an assessment or to assess whether a particular mental state, which is an element of a crime, has been impaired as a result of a mental illness or serious insanity. The psychiatrist shall be permitted to make any explanation reasonably serving to clarify the diagnosis and opinion and may be cross–examined as to any matter bearing on the psychiatrist's competence or credibility or the validity of the diagnosis or opinion.

Criminal responsibility addresses the condition at the time the crime was committed. A person is mentally incompetent, if he commits an offense when he is suffering from a mental impairment and his mental condition gives rise to the offence. ①Anyone does not know the nature and quality of the conduct. ②Anyone does not know that the conduct is wrong. ③Anyone is unable to control the conduct.

According to the *Criminal Law of the People's Republic of China*, capacity of identification and control are the 2 key points for assessing the criminal responsibility after the diagnosis of mental illness.

If a patient with mental disorder causes harmful consequences at a time when he is unable to recognize or control his own conduct, upon verification and confirmation through legal procedure, he shall not bear criminal responsibility, but his family members or guardian shall be ordered to keep him under strict watch and control and arrange for his medical treatment. If necessary, the government may compel him to receive medical treatment. Any one whose mental illness is of an intermittent nature shall bear criminal responsibility if he commits a crime when he is in a normal mental state. If a patient with mental disorder who has not completely lost the ability of recognizing or controlling his own conduct commits a crime, he shall bear criminal responsibility; however, he may be given a mitigated punishment. Any intoxicated person who commits a crime shall take criminal responsibility.

23.2.3　Civil liability

Civil liability is the obligation to answer for damage one has caused, it refers to the legal requirement to compensate another party for causing them some form of bodily injury or property damage. It is a potential responsibility for payment of damages or other court-enforcement in a lawsuit, as distinguished from criminal liability, which means open to punishment for a crime. If you intentionally or even just mistakenly injure someone or damage someone's property, you could end up being responsible for paying for the other person's losses. This is known as civil liability.

23.2.3.1　Information-gathering in civil assessments

Personal-injury cases involving psychic trauma generate a frequently encountered type of civil assessment. In such cases, important areas of inquiry regarding the evaluee's claim include a detailed description of the alleged precipitating factors and their time course; the duration and amount of exposure to any alleged trauma; and the evaluee's thoughts, feelings, and behavior before, during, and immediately after the traumatic event. Reviewing the evaluee's specific claims outlined in the complaint and other legal documents may assist in addressing the concerns that are the focus of the litigation. In addition, a spouse or significant other, family members, or witnesses to the event can provide additional information on the evaluee's alleged exposure to trauma. This information can be obtained through direct interviews, depositions, or other available records. Any discrepancies in the evaluee's account of circumstances may be clarified through collateral records or statements.

23.2.3.2　Content of assessment: civil(psychic injury)

After gathering the evaluee's account, the psychiatrist should take a detailed history regarding the emotional impact, if any, of the alleged incident or trauma and the reasons for the evaluee's disability, if any. The effects of the incident can be reviewed in the immediate period(from the day to a month after the incident); the medium term(more than one month to one year after the incident); and the long term(more than one year after the incident). When evaluating the claimed psychological effects of the alleged incident, the evaluator should carefully review collateral records(such as psychiatric, medical, and rehabilitation records or newspaper accounts), to evaluate the symptoms, the severity, and the course. Questioning the evaluee about incidents and inconsistencies in the collateral contribution may aid in coming to conclusions. Areas to be covered include psychological and pharmacological treatments, adherence to treatment recommendations, reported treatment failures, adverse consequences of treatment interventions, factors that precipitate or aggravate symptoms, and measures that have been successful in relieving symptoms. Disability assessments generally require an evaluation of how the claimed psychological symptoms (such as a depressed mood or impaired concentration) affect the person's ability to work.

Forensic psychiatrists are often retained to assess the psychiatric competence or capacity of an evaluee to engage in a specific act. In general, there are essential elements that should be considered, including the evaluee's awareness of the situation, factual understanding of the problems involved, appreciation of the likely consequences, ability to manipulate information rationally, ability to function in his own environment, and ability to perform the tasks demanded of him. Specific competence entails four elements, some of which are the same as general competence: communication of a choice sustained long enough to implement it, factual understanding of the problems involved, appreciation of the situation and its consequences, and rational manipulation of information.

Some of these specific competence assessments may involve consent to treatment, guardianship evaluations, testamentary capacity, financial competence, and competence to enter into a contract.

Competence to consent to or refuse treatment involves an assessment of whether the evaluee can give informed consent. This evaluation includes whether the evaluee understands information regarding the risks, benefits, and alternatives to treatment. Further, it is important to assess whether there is a mental disorder that interferes with the evaluee's decision – making capacity. Finally, the consent must be voluntary. This process requires that the treatment team disclose sufficient information to the evaluee.

An assessment of an evaluee's competence to manage financial affairs requires questioning about his awareness of his financial situation, as well as broader questioning about areas that may be affected by specific psychiatric symptoms. For example, a delusion that some organization is trying to steal an evaluee's money may affect financial decision–making. Having established the presence of delusions, it would still be necessary, as in this example, for the psychiatrist to identify a clear link between the delusion or other psychopathology and the financial decision–making task.

Evaluations for testamentary capacity (competence to compose a will) are generally retrospective, since the evaluee in most cases is a decedent whose will is being contested postmortem. The evaluator should make note, if writing a report or testifying, of the inability to conduct a personal interview and the resulting limitations of the assessment. The assessment relies on a retrospective assembly of information concerning the evaluee's mental state at the time of writing the will. It is important to attempt to assess whether the individual had the capacity to be aware of the value of the estate. A pertinent question is whether the evaluee was having delusions, which could directly affect his capacity to compose a realistic will. Another concern is whether the testator was subjected to undue influence: that is, was directly and deliberately manipulated or deceived by a third party. The evaluator may comment on whether a psychiatric condition or symptom (s) made the testator susceptible to manipulation that could legally constitute undue influence.

Psychiatrists and other mental health specialists are often required to conduct assessments with a view to determine the presence of mental or emotional problems in one of the parties. These types of assessments are needed in multiple situations, ranging from examinations to specify the impact of injuries on a third party involved in a motor vehicle accident, to evaluations of the capacity to write a will or contracts, to psychological autopsies in order to assess testamentary capacity in suicidal cases or sudden death, or evaluations for fitness to work and, of late in many countries, evaluations to determine access to benefits contemplated in disability insurance. In most of these situations, the issue at hand is a determination of capacity and competence to perform some function, or the evaluation of autonomous decision making by impaired persons. A determination of incapacity leading to a finding of incompetence becomes a matter of social control that is used to legitimize the application of social strictures on a particular individual. This imposes on clinicians an increased ethical duty to make sure that their decisions have been thoroughly based on the best available clinical evidence.

Ordinarily, there is a presumption of capacity and, hence, that a particular person is competent. A person is assumed to be competent to make decisions, unless proven otherwise. The presence of a major mental or physical condition does not in and of itself produce incapacity in general or for specific functions. In addition, despite the presence of a condition that may affect capacity, a person may still be competent to carry out some functions, mostly because the capacity may fluctuate from time to time, and because competence is not an all or none concept, but it is tied to the specific decision or function to be accomplished. In addition, a finding of incapacity should be time-limited; that is, it will have to be reviewed from time to time. For example, a stroke may have rendered a person incapacitated to drive motor vehicle and hence the person will be deemed incompetent to drive, but the person could still have the capacity and be competent to enter into contracts or to manage personal financial affairs. With time and proper rehabilitation, the person may be able to regain capacity and competence to drive. Ordinarily, a person has to consent to an assessment of incapacity or a legal order has to be obtained to make the person cooperate to the assessment or to proceed to collect information otherwise. It is advisable to use a screening test of capacity and conduct a full assessment only if the person fails the screening. This will prevent imposing an onerous burden on the person subject of the assessment if the screening test is easily passed.

23.2.4　Competency to stand trial

A forensic psychiatric assessment may be required for an individual who has been charged with a crime, in order to establish whether the person has the legal capacity to stand trial. This is the competency evaluation to determine that a defendant has the mental capacity to understand the charges and assist their attorney. In the United States, this is seated in the Fifth Amendment to the United States Constitution, which ensures the right to be present at one's trial, to face one's accusers, and to have help from an attorney. In English and Welsh law, a similar concept is that of "fitness to plead".

Competency can be raised as an issue by a party, or based on the judge's observations of the defendant. If there is a reasonable basis to believe competency is at issue, the court has an absolute duty to order an evaluation. Based on the outcome of the evaluation, the judge will determine whether the defendant is competent to stand trial. When evaluating competency, the judge will consider the defendant's mental state at the time of the legal proceeding and trial.

The following tripartite definition of competence to stand trial is used in most jurisdictions worldwide.

(1) The defendant must understand the nature of the charges against him.

(2) The defendant must understand the purpose of court proceedings.

(3) The defendant must be able to cooperate with an attorney in his own defense.

A person is mentally unfit to stand trial on a charge of an offence if the person's mental processes are so distorted or impaired.

(1) The person is unable to understand, or to respond rationally to the charge of the allegations on which the charge is based.

(2) The person is unable to exercise or to give rational instructions about the exercise of procedural rights (for example, the right to challenge jurors).

(3) The person is unable to understand the nature of the proceedings, or to follow the evidence or the course of the proceedings.

Competency to stand trial is generally determined via a pretrial evaluation of the defendant's overall mental status and mental state at the time of the examination. This evaluation aims to provide sufficient information to allow a judge to rule on the competency of the defendant should a motion to that effect be made by either the prosecutor or defense attorney. A judge may also directly rule a defendant incompetent to stand trial without receiving a motion to that effect from counsel.

A defendant who has been deemed incompetent to stand trial may be required to undergo mental health treatment, including court-ordered hospitalization and the administration of treatment against the defendant's wishes, in an effort to render the defendant competent to stand trial.

Competency is determined by whether the defendant can understand the nature and consequences of the criminal proceedings against him. Specifically, the Supreme Court has held that the defendant must: ①have the sufficient present ability to consult with his or her lawyer with a reasonable degree of rational understanding; ②he or she must have a rational as well as a factual understanding of the proceeding against him or her. Competency determines whether a defendant will be able to appear at trial and understand the proceedings. If a defendant is found not competent to stand trial, he will never be found guilty(or not guilty, for that matter) because no trial would be held in the first place. In other words, you can be declared legally competent and also legally insane. However, you can not be declared legally insane unless you are also legally competent.

23.2.5   The civil liability for damages of the criminally insane

As a rule, mentally ill patients are held to be responsible for their acts just like everyone else. Notwithstanding, the law contains special rules which distinguish individuals with mental illness from other people. The instructions in the Penal Law empower the court to release a defendant from criminal responsibility. To do this the following criteria must be met that:

(1) The accused was mentally ill.

(2) He was in a psychotic state at the time he performed the felony.

(3) His mental illness deprived him of his abilities in at least one of the 2 following areas: ①on the intellectual-cognitive level, he could not understand what he was doing, or the forbidden nature of the act; ②on the level of volition, he was incapable of preventing himself from carrying it out. When the court finds the defendant still mentally ill at the time of the trial, it will decide — in accordance with the law — whether to rule that the patient be admitted to a psychiatric hospital or receive compulsory out-patient treatment. Liability for damages will be imposed upon an individual whenever the prerequisites to define a tort are met, even if the mental requisite is an outcome of one's mentally ill state. The District Court determined that an individual who intended to inflict harm is guilty of assault, even though the intent was an outcome of his mental state. Lack of volition due to one's inability to refrain from action does not constitute a defense for assault. In this case liability for damages was imposed on the defendant. The Court related to the issue of justice according to which an innocent person's damages should not remain uncompensated, and the assailant was required to pay damages to the victim. The question dealt with in the case discussed below is as follows: is it possible to claim civil damages from a mentally ill patient who committed a tort, when it has been established that he could not be held criminally responsible for the same acts for reasons of insanity as defined in the penal law? The process of civil law is not identical to that of criminal law and the civil liability someone who is mentally ill may carry is not necessarily identical to his criminal responsibility. The mentally ill person should be required to pay compensation like any other culprit, in cases where he is found to have the basis of the tort he has committed even if the basis is derived from mental illness or a mental de-

fectiveness from which he was suffering at the time of injury. Therefore, if the patient was not able to be aware that his actions were wrong, it suffices that his actions were intentional from his point of view in order for him to be deemed responsible for the damage caused by his actions. The concept of intention should be interpreted in its simple form: did the person causing the injury want to act in the way that he acted? The question of what motivated him to do this — his character, illness or external forces — does not belong to the area of the concept of volition.

The law of torts has different aims than those of the penal law. One of these aims and one of paramount importance is restitution for the victim. The law of torts does not have an explicit position about the civil responsibility related to torts committed by a legally insane person.

The conclusion that may be reached from the above is that in order for a mentally ill person to be held accountable to make compensation for a tort of assault that he had committed, he needs to be in possession also of the special mental element of "intent". In the event that it is established that this element was present in the accused, he can not take recourse in the defense that the "intent" arose from his mental illness. At the same time, if it becomes evident that he was lacking in volition, he may be exempted from bearing responsibility for his damaging behavior. Thus, when the Court is faced — when making a civil ruling against an assailant who is mentally impaired — with a decision made previously in criminal proceedings, according to which he is not responsible due to insanity, it needs to ask according to which alternative this decision was arrived at. A mentally ill person who caused bodily harm will not be exempted from responsibility solely on the grounds that his mental illness revoked his cognitive abilities. If it adopts the ruling of the Magistrate's Court, the Court may find that an offender who is mentally ill is exempted from responsibility for making restitution only if there was meaningful damage to his ability of volition as a result of his mental illness, to the extent that at the time he carried out the damaging act he was not able to prevent himself from doing it — insane automatism. If it follows the opinion expressed by the District Court, it may grant exemption only when the offender acted while under sane automatism. The legal community does not find a contradiction when the accused is not found guilty of a specific crime but is obligated to pay damages for the same deed, because two separate systems, the criminal and the civil, are involved.

23.2.6　Risk assessment

Forensic psychiatrists are often asked to conduct risk assessments. The most frequent assessment are for risk of violence, inappropriate sexual behavior, and criminal recidivism.

Risk assessment takes place in a variety of contexts. Risk assessments are also used in other tribunals in which future dangerous is a significant factor. It include criminal sentence hearing, probation or parole assessments, death penalty aggravation or mitigation, child custody, disposition assessments involving people found insane or not criminally responsible because of mental illness, hospital civil commitment proceedings, threat assessments, and assessment of potential violent self-harm.

It is important to ensure that all parties understand the type of risk that is being appraised, the methods used, and limitations of the assessment. Clarifying the question is often an important preliminary step in conducting an assessment. Risk assessments usually include appraisal of what could happen, under what circumstances, and over how long a time. Offering an opinion about management interventions and whether they may change risk is often part of the task.

Violence is a major social problem. Assessing and managing violence risk is a key ole of professionals working within the field of mental illness and personality disorder. In the last 30 years it has been a dramatic shift in violence concept and violence risk assessments. Today risk assessments are a composite of empirical knowledge and clinical/professional expertise. The systematic risk assessment is made by referring to a checklist of factors that have been demonstrated to have a relationship to violence based on empirical research. They emphasise prevention rather than prediction and are designed to guide clinicians in determining what level of risk management is needed, in which contexts, and at what points in time.

Many past offenders and suspected or potential future offenders with mental health problems or an intellectual or developmental disability, are supervised in the community by forensic psychiatric teams made up of a variety of professionals, including psychiatrists, psychologists, nurses, and care workers. A forensic assessment of a violent criminal may also take the form of a risk assessment, to gain insights on the relation between the individual's mental condition and the risk of further violent crimes. Risk assessments are the proper concern of mental health professionals to the extent that they initiate corrective interventions that directly or indirectly benefit the individual evaluated. The aim is not so much to predict as to prevent violence. Hence, forensic psychiatrists have dual responsibilities: to promote both the welfare of their clients and the safety of the public. The aim is not so much to predict as to prevent violence, by means of risk management.

23.2.7 Treatment for offenders with mental health issues

Those found to have been not guilty by reason of mental disorder or insanity are generally then required to undergo psychiatric treatment in a mental institution, except in the case of temporary insanity.

23.2.7.1 Treatment recommendations

The psychiatrist should determine and describe any treatment the evaluee received before the forensic assessment, the evaluee's adherence to treatment, and the evaluee's response to treatment. The forensic psychiatrist also may have to determine the treatment necessary to improve the evaluee's level of functioning and whether additional or different treatment is likely to help. This analysis could be appropriate in a variety of civil (e. g. , disability, fitness for duty) and criminal (e. g. , sentence mitigation, risk for recidivism) evaluations.

The outlook may depend on the evaluee's willingness to undergo treatment. Sometimes a consultant has to report that further improvement of the evaluee's physical or emotional symptoms is unlikely unless the evaluee is able and willing to enter psychiatric treatment. This is frequently indicated when an evaluee is immobilized by anger or depression.

23.2.7.2 Treatments

Treatments for people with forensic mental health issues include:

(1) Medication—such as antidepressants, antipsychotics and other medications to control some of the symptoms of particular mental illnesses or mental disorders.

(2) Counselling—one-on-one or group therapy.

(3) Rehabilitation—involvement in a program directed at enabling people to live safely within the community.

Indeed, as with psychiatric treatment in general, medication treatment alone is unlikely to reduce risk of violence in people with mental illness. Interventions ideally should be long-term and contains include a range of psychosocial approaches, including cognitive behavioral therapy, conflict management, and substance abuse treatment.

On entering into the legal system, three major areas need consideration: fitness to stand trial, insanity regulations and dangerousness applications. The major developments on the issue of fitness to stand trial pertain to rulings that defendersfound not fit to stand trial are sent to psychiatric facilities, with the expectation that their competence to be tried is to be restored: the question for clinicians revolves on what parameters to use to predict restorability of competence, which should be based on an adequate response to treatment. Insanity regulations pertain to legal tests used to decide whether the impact of mental illness on competence to understand or appreciate the nature of a crime could be used to declare an offender "not criminally responsible because of a mental condition", "not guilty by reasons of insanity" or any other wording used in different countries. Applications to declare a person a "dangerous offender" usually demand a high level of expertise on the part of forensic experts, who are expected to provide courts with technical and scientific information on risk assessment and prediction of future violence.

23.3　The association between mental disorder and crime

A causal relationship between mental disorder and crime is difficult to show empirically, especially if the type of crime is not defined. The finding that mentally disordered individuals are over-represented in prison does not necessarily mean that their mental disorder caused them to offend. Nor is criminal law-breaking an indicator in itself of mental disorder, no matter how heinous or bizarre the behaviour.

23.3.1　Substance dependence and crime

The use of alcohol and drugs can negatively affect a person's life, impact their family, friends and community, and cause an enormous burden on society. One of the most significant areas of risk with the use of alcohol and drugs is the connection between alcohol, drugs and crime.

23.3.1.1　Alcohol

Because alcohol use is legal and pervasive, it plays a particularly strong role in the relationship to crime and other social problems.

Alcohol, more than any illegal drug, was found to be closely associated with violent crimes, including murder, rape, assault, child and spousal abuse. Among violent crimes, with the exception of robberies, the offender is far more likely to have been drinking than under the influence of other drugs.

Alcohol is often a factor in violence where the attacker and the victim know each other.

23.3.1.2　Drugs and crime

The relationship between drugs and crime is complex. Many illegal drug users commit no other kinds of crimes, and many persons who commit crimes never use illegal drugs. However, at the most intense levels of drug use, drugs and crime are directly and highly correlated and serious drug use can amplify and perpetuate preexisting criminal activity.

There are mainly three types of crimes related to drugs. ①Use-related crime: these are crimes that result from or involve individuals who ingest drugs, and who commit crimes as a result of the effect the drug has on their thought processes and behavior. ②Economic-related crime: crimes which an individual commits a crime in order to fund a drug habit, including theft and prostitution. ③System-related crime: crimes that result from the structure of the drug system. They include production, manufacture, transportation, and sale of drugs, as well as violence related to the production or sale of drugs, such as a turf war.

(1) Voluntary intoxication

Voluntary drug intoxication may not be used to exonerate a defendant completely. This does not mean that voluntary drug intoxication has no impact on a defendant's criminal responsibility.

Most jurisdictions sharply distinguish between settled insanity and temporary insanity caused by voluntary intoxication and do not allow the latter to be used as a defense to criminal activity. A few jurisdictions, however, appear to differentiate between drug-induced psychoses and other forms of drug-induced mental incapacity. Although the law is sometimes murky, these jurisdictions seem to follow the rule that, although voluntary drug intoxication is no defense to a criminal act, temporary insanity caused by voluntary drug intoxication may sometimes be a valid defense. Examples include a temporary insanity induced by the voluntary use of drugs that does not necessarily subside when the drug intoxication ends and a unique latent mental illness that remains dormant most of the time, but can be triggered by the voluntary use of drugs. Voluntary intoxication could be used to negate specific intent but was not, by itself, grounds for an insanity defense.

（2）Involuntary Intoxication

The practice of excusing criminal responsibility committed while in a state of involuntary intoxication extends back to the earliest days of common law. In addressing the issue of involuntary intoxication, the courts have defined it in essentially the same terms as insanity. Like insanity, involuntary intoxication potentially excuses a defendant from culpability because intoxication affects the ability to distinguish between right and wrong. Thus, the mental state of an involuntarily intoxicated defendant is measured by the same test of legal insanity as used for other mental disorders. There is no comprehensive definition for what constitutes involuntary intoxication. In the past, it has been said that the only safe test of involuntary intoxication is the absence of an exercise of independent judgment and volition on the part of the accused in taking the intoxicant. There are instances when intoxication is deemed involuntary despite the fact that the accused exercised appropriate judgment and had volition in taking the intoxicant.

23.3.2   Organic mental disorders

Delirium is occasionally associated with criminal behaviour, because of the associated confusion or disinhibition. Diagnostic problems may arise if the mental disturbance improves before the offender is examined by a doctor.

Dementia is sometimes associated with offences, although crime is otherwise uncommon among the elderly, and violent offences are rare. Violent and disinhibited behaviour may also occur after traumatic damage to the brain following head injury. It may be difficult to distinguish the effects of post-traumatic neurological difficulties from post-traumatic psychological disorder.

Only a few Alzheimer's disease patients had unintentionally committed some type of crime. Most often, it was a traffic violation, but there were some incidents of violence toward other people. Regardless of the specific behavior, though, it should be seen as a consequence of a brain disease and not a crime.

Those with the frontotemporal dementia had the highest rate of criminal behavior. Theft, traffic violations, trespassing and inappropriate sexual advances were among the most common incidents in patients' medical records.

23.3.3   Schizophrenia and related disorder

People with schizophrenia and related disorders are at an increased risk of adverse outcomes, including conviction of a violent offence, suicide, and premature mortality. A new study out of Australia showed that: people with schizophrenia are 3-5 times more likely to commit crimes than those without the mental illness. Violence by people with severe mental illnesses is an issue.

People with schizophrenia are far more likely to harm themselves than be violent toward the public. Violence is not a symptom of schizophrenia.

In public perception, schizophrenia is often associated with violence. This view is reinforced each time there are media reports of violent acts by purported mentally ill persons. Most people with schizophrenia, however, are not violent but are withdrawn and prefer to be left alone. Drug or alcohol abuse raises the risk of violence in people with schizophrenia, particularly if the illness is untreated, but also in people who have no mental illness. When violence does occur, it is most frequently targeted at family members and friends, and more often takes place at home.

Schizophrenia is a heterogeneous clinical syndrome and individuals with this disorder will vary extensively on variables related to violent action. Aggressive behavior per se is also heterogeneous in origin, which makes it challenging to deal with both in research and in clinical practice. Clinicians consider many contributory factors in evaluating a patient for risk of becoming violent, including personality traits, history of violent acts, paranoid beliefs, content of auditory hallucinations, substance abuse, impulsivity, suicidal acts, agitation, excitement, social circumstances, and age and sex. Prediction of a singular violent event is very challenging. More commonly, however, the problem relates to a more continuous pattern of hostility, accusatory comments, and verbal aggression that must be dealt with more or less continuously by the closest social group. In the family, this can create a stressful environment that erodes the quality of life for parents and siblings. It can be very difficult to manage in many living situations leading to altercations with other residents. On the street, in hospitals and in jails, the risk of escalation is great. Therapeutic approaches are often limited. A safe and low stress environment is usually difficult to arrange. Antipsychotic drugs have efficacy for some of the contributing factors, but adherence is a problem. Long actingantipsychotic injections reduce covert nonadherence, but these agents are not used as widely as oral agents.

Substance abuse(i. e., street drugs and alcohol) significantly raises the rate of violence in people with schizophrenia, as is also the case with people who do not have any mental illness. People with paranoid and psychotic symptoms, which can become worse if medications are discontinued, may also be at higher risk for violent behavior.

It is important to provide better services to people with schizophrenia to reduce the incidence of violence, and could probably reduce crime by 5%–10%.

23.3.4 Schizophrenia and violence

Violence is the most commonly examined offence category in relation to schizophrenia. However clinical opinion on a causal link between schizophrenia and violence has fluctuated. Two decades ago it was suggested there was no increased risk for violence in individuals with schizophrenia and other psychoses(Monahan and Steadman, 1983). Since then numerous large population–based studies have shown a modest association between violence and schizophrenia. Studies suggest there is an increased risk of violence in those with schizophrenia with males suffering from schizophrenia being found to be between four and eight times more likely to be violent and females between three and 23 times more likely to be violent than those without reference. In examining these figures, however, there is one important caveat; the overwhelming majority of persons with mental illness are not dangerous and not violent. The presence of delusions has been thought to increase the risk of violence, however this connection, is not universally accepted nor supported conclusively by research. Research that has reported increased risk of violence in people with schizophrenia does not prove a main causal link between violence and schizophrenia. Any link is likely to be mediated partially or fully by other variables such as substance misuse, co – morbidity, family circumstances, and deprivation. More research is needed to take into account the wider social context surrounding individuals with schizophrenia in order to understand more fully the association between schizophrenia and violent offending and also to aid future risk assessment.

23.3.5　Posttraumatic stress disorder

Posttraumatic stress disorder(PTSD) may follow exposure to an extreme traumatic stressor involving direct personal experience of an event that involves actual or threatened death or serious injury, or other threats to one's physical integrity; or witnessing an event that involves death, injury, or a threat to the physical integrity of another person; or learning about unexpected or violent death, serious harm, or threat of death or injury experienced by a family member or other close associate. Its characteristic symptoms include re-experiencing the trauma, persistent avoidance of things associated with the trauma, emotional numbing, and persistently increased arousal.

Post-traumatic stress disorder may be related to offending in 3 ways.

(1)PTSD patients may abuse drugs and alcohol.

(2)PTSD is associated with increased irritability and decreased affect regulation.

(3)PTSD patients may rarely experience dissociative episodes involving violence, especially in circumstances resembling their original trauma. This is often hard to determine retrospectively.

PTSD has been the basis for psychiatric defences to homicide. Especially in cases of battered women with a history of prolonged trauma, occasional acts of retaliatory violence are not uncommon.

23.3.6　Mood disorder and crime

23.3.6.1　Violence and aggression

Persons with bipolar disorder are at significantly increased risk for violence, with some history of violent behavior ranging from 9.4% to just under 50%, often in the presence of comorbid diagnoses. Bipolar patients are prone to agitation that can result in impulsive aggression during manic and mixed episodes. However, depressed states can involve intense dysphoria with agitation and irritability, which can also increase the risk of violent behavior. Bipolar patients may have chronic impulsivity during euthymia, predisposing them to aggression.

Impulsive aggression(as opposed to premeditated aggression) is most commonly associated with bipolar and other affective disorders.

23.3.6.2　Assessing violence risk

In many ways, the assessment of violence risk in patients with bipolar disorder is similar to risk assessment in any patient. Certain data from the patient's history and mental status examination are universally important.

(1)A history of violent acts, especially recent ones and especially if there were any legal consequences.

(2)The extent of alcohol and drug use, because there is a strong association between substance abuse and risk of violence.

(3)Trauma history has a unique relationship with bipolar disorder, and it should be assessed in all patients to determine the risk of violence. Trauma is associated with increased aggression in adults in general, regardless of whether an affective disorder is present.

(4)Other important historical data include demographic information(young men of low socioeconomic status who have few social supports are the most likely to be violent) and access to weapons.

(5)In the mental status assessment, it is important to note psychomotor agitation as well as the nature, frequency, and severity of violent ideation.

(6) Use of an actuarial instrument, such as the Historical, Clinical, and Risk Management–20 (HCR–20) violence assessment scheme, can help integrate systematic inquiry about evidence–based risk factors into assessment of the clinical scenario.

Pay special attention to violent behavior that may have occurred when the person was manic. If at all possible, obtain collateral information about the history of violence. Patients may minimize previous violent actions or not remember them, especially if they were in the midst of a manic episode.

Patients with bipolar disorder are most prone to violence during manic or mixed states — when maximum behavioral dyscontrol is combined with unrealistic beliefs. Patients with dysphoric mania and mixed states may be at especially high risk; the assessment for concurrent depression in a manic patient should therefore be a priority.

23.3.6.3　Specific associations between mood disorders and violence

(1) Depression and homicide–suicide

Homicide–suicide describes the situation when a person kills someone (often a spouse or relative) and then takes their own life. Homicide–suicide has been commonly associated with depression.

(2) Depression and infanticide

Infanticide is the killing of a child by its mother before its first birthday, very common in the context of post–partum depression. It may be distinguished from neonaticide (a baby being killed within the first day of life) and filicide (the killing of a child on or after its first birthday). Two motivational profiles have been identified: mothers who committed neonaticide were mostly troubled by psychosis and social problems; and mothers who committed filicide were defined as severely depressed, with a history of self–directed violence and a high rate of suicide attempts following the filicidal offence.

(3) Association between mood disorders and violence

Affective states, particularly anger and irritability, play a role in aggressive behaviour and are influenced by serotonergic mechanisms. Extensive literature dating back to the 1960s has suggested a link between decreased serotonin function and aggression, probably mediated through impulse control, affect regulation and social functioning. The evidence relating to a clinical association between mood disorders and violence may consider the rate of violence in relation to in–patient treatment of depression, the rate of depression in violent or offender populations and the rates of co–occurring depression and violence in the community.

23.3.7　Personality disorders and crime

Personality disorders are commonly identified in people who commit violent crimes. Recent research also shows that the type of crime committed–sexual or nonsexual–can be linked to the type of personality disorder the offender suffers, such as antisocial personality disorder and borderline personality disorder.

Personality disorders that we often see in offenders who have committed violent crimes include:

23.3.7.1　Conduct disorder

It is a behavioral/emotional disorder that is diagnosed in childhood. Children with conduct disorder display antisocial behaviors that can be violent and destructive. These children may be highly irritable, suffer from low self–esteem and tend to repeatedly violate the norms of society.

23.3.7.2　Antisocial personality disorder

It is characterized in adults as the tendency to have complete disregard for the feelings of others. Adults with antisocial personality disorder may appear to be callous and cynical. These individuals do not typically conform to social norms, and are often deceitful and impulsive. They react in irresponsible, reckless and aggressive ways.

23.3.7.3   Borderline personality disorder

It is characterized in adults by pervasive mood instability. Individuals who experience borderline personality disorder will struggle with anxiety, impulsive aggression, drug and alcohol abuse, and distorted thinking patterns.

Persons committing murder and other violent crime are likely to exhibit a personality disorder (PD). Essentially any personality disorder can be associated with violent crime, with the possible exception of avoidant PD. This includes those described in DSM as well as other disorders such as sadistic PD and psychopathy. The latter two, along with antisocial and paranoid PDs, are the most common personality accompaniments of violent crime. Narcissistic traits[if not narcissistic PD(NPD) itself] are almost universal in this domain, since violent offenders usually place their own desires and urges far above those of other persons. While admixtures of traits from several disorders are common among violent offenders, certain ones are likely to be the main disorder: antisocial PD, Psychopathy, Sadistic PD, Paranoid PD and NPD. Instrumental (as opposed to impulsive) spousal murders are strongly associated with NPD. Men committing serial sexual homicide usually show psychopathy and sadistic PD; half these men also show schizoid PD. Many murderers usually show strong paranoid traits.

The research suggests that there is a link between personality disorder and violent offending, especially with regards to Cluster B personality disorders including anti-social, narcissistic, and paranoid personality disorder.

A relationship between personality disorder and offending had been reported, relating to both violent and sexual crimes. In particular, a link between Cluster B disorders such as antisocial, borderline, histrionic and narcissistic has been shown, as these are the most prevalent within offender samples.

23.3.8   Impulse-control disorder

Impulse-control disorders(ICD) involve self-defeating, strange, socially unacceptable, or self-destructive behavior. Others involve legal, but socially unacceptable acts which escalate to an inability to comply with the law when impulses take over. The law is very complex or whether the law is obvious and known to all, a serious impulse control disorder will be commonly associated with criminal acts.

A simple definition of an impulse disorder is one where the individual can not resist an impulse to behave in a certain way or can not stop repeated behavior, even when they know that the behavior must stop. In some cases, the individual has repeatedly tried and failed to stop the behavior. In many cases, the behavior can go on for years without diagnosis or capture. The categories can be simply defined as violent, fire starting, self-harming, sexually inappropriate or illegal, stealing or gambling.

With fire starting for example, the impulse can cause individuals to start fires in ways that cause property damage and death. In these cases starting fires is either for personal gratification or tension relief. In some cases the status of "hero" or center of attention accrues when the fire setter responds to the fire in a professional capacity. In this case, the term "arsonist" is both descriptive of a psychiatric disorder and a legal criminal classification. But not all arsonists have the impulse control disorder and will set fires for psychologically unrelated reasons, such as revenge, as an act of terrorism, or for monetary gain.

Fire starting is one of the common behaviors in the profiles of serial killers, who generally have other psychiatric disorders along with the impulse control disorders.

Kleptomania is another term which is used interchangeably in the psychiatric and legal fields. Kleptomania is the act of stealing as the result of an impulse to steal things without paying for them, whether they are valuable or not. Stealing is against the law, therefore, kleptomania sufferers are criminals, whether they are caught and prosecuted or not. In some cases, especially where the theft is minor, individuals are caught and processed without the legal system being aware that they suffer from the impulse control disorder. In other cases, the behavior is so profound that a forensic psychologist is ordered to evaluate the individual. In still other cases, the thefts are "enabled" by friends and family members who refuse to confront the individual.

When excessive and problematic gambling develops into an impulse control disorder, there can be restoration of financial losses through criminal acts. Embezzlement, theft, check kiting, professional malfeasance, illegal loan sharking, and other crimes are a result of gambling losses that become catastrophic because the person can not stop gambling. These activities can have been identified as problematic and can go on for a time before the person is caught and the disorder is related to the crime.

Explosive control disorder is a non interchangeable term where physical violence to persons or property are the criminal acts that are the very nature of the disease. In explosive control disorder, there is simply a lack of control over temper, whether the eruption is over something minor or is something that occurred at another time. In these cases, physical violence and property damage are considered to be of such serious harm to the community and to individuals, that the law is compelled to act quickly and aggressively to deal with the individual. As a result, the criminality that relates to explosive impulse control disorder can cause the identification of the problem to happen more quickly than in other impulse control disorders.

23.3.8.1 Pyromania

Pyromania is characterized by impulsive and repetitive urges to deliberately start fires. Because of its nature, the number of studies performed for fire-setting are understandably very few. However studies done on children and adolescents suffering from pyromania have reported its prevalence to be between 2.4% – 3.5% in the United States. It has also been observed that the incidence of fire-setting is more common in juvenile and teenage boys than girls of the same age.

23.3.8.2 Kleptomania

Kleptomania is characterized by an impulsive urge to steal purely for the sake of gratification. In the US the presence of kleptomania is unknown but has been estimated at 6 per 1,000 individuals. Kleptomania is also thought to be the cause of 5% of annual shoplifting in the US. If true, 100,000 arrests are made in the US annually due to kleptomaniac behavior.

23.3.9 Mental illness and violence

Taken together with the previous studies, they painted a more complex picture about mental illness and violence. They suggest that violence by people with mental illness — like aggression in the general population — stems from multiple overlapping factors interacting in complex ways. It includes family history, personal stressors (such as divorce or bereavement), and socioeconomic factors (such as poverty and homeless). So, substance abuse often hard to tease apart the influence of other less obvious factors.

23.3.9.1 Assessing risk of violence

Highly publicized acts of violence by people with mental illness affect more than public perception. Clinicians are under pressure to assess their patients for potential to act in a violent way. Although it is possible to make a general assessment of relative risk, it is impossible to predict an individual, specific act of violence, given that such acts tend to occur when the perpetrator is highly emotional. During a clinical session, the same person may be guarded, less emotional, and even thoughtful, thereby masking any signs of violent intent. And even when the patient explicitly expresses intent to harm someone else, the relative risk for acting on that plan is still significantly influenced by the following life circumstances and clinical factors.

23.3.9.2   History of violence

Individuals who have been arrested or acted violently in the past are more likely than others to become violent again. Much of the research suggests that this factor may be the largest single predictor of future violence. What these studies can not reveal, however, is whether past violence was due to mental illness or some of the other factors explored below.

23.3.9.3   Substance use

Patients with a dual diagnosis are more likely than patients with a psychiatric disorder alone to become violent, so a comprehensive assessment includes questions about substance use in addition to asking about symptoms of a psychiatric disorder.

One theory is that alcohol and drug abuse can trigger violent behavior in people with or without psychiatric disorders because these substances simultaneously impair judgment, change a person's emotional equilibrium, and remove cognitive inhibitions. In people with psychiatric disorders, substance abuse may exacerbate symptoms such as paranoia, grandiosity, or hostility. Patients who abuse drugs or alcohol are also less likely to adhere to treatment for a mental illness, and that can worsen psychiatric symptoms.

Another theory, however, is that substance abuse may be masking, or entwined with, other risk factors for violence.

23.3.9.4   Personality disorders

Borderline personality disorder, antisocial personality disorder, conduct disorder, and other personality disorders often manifest in aggression or violence. When a personality disorder occurs in conjunction with another psychiatric disorder, the combination may also increase risk of violent behavior.

23.3.9.5   Nature of symptoms

Patients with paranoid delusions, command hallucinations, and florid psychotic thoughts may be more likely to become violent than other patients. For clinicians, it is important to understand the patient's own perception of psychotic thoughts, because this may reveal when a patient may feel compelled to fight back.

23.3.9.6   Age and gender

Young people are more likely than older adults to act violently. In addition, men are more likely than women to act violently.

23.3.9.7   Social stress

Poor or homeless people, or those with low socioeconomic status, are more likely than others to become violent.

23.3.9.8   Personal stress, crisis or loss

Unemployment, divorce, or separation in the past year increases a patient's risk of violence. People who were victims of violent crime in the past year are also more likely to assault someone.

23.3.9.9   Early exposure

The risk of violence rises with exposure to aggressive family fights during childhood, physical abuse by a parent, or having a parent with a criminal record.

Moreover, the personality, dignity, and personal and property safety of the patients with mental disorders are inviolable. *The Mental Health Law of the People's Republic of China* is formulated for purposes of developing the cause of mental health, regulating mental health services, and protecting the lawful rights and interests of patients with mental disorders.

Wang Yuan

References

[1] ANTONIO B F, GILLBERTO P L, MIRIAM M R, et al. Prevalence of hyperandrogenism and polycystic ovary syndrome in female to male transsexuals [J]. Endocrinología y nutrición (English Edition), 2014, 61(7):351-358.

[2] APPELBAUM, PAUL S, THOMAS G, et al. Clinical Handbook of Psychiatry & the Law [M]. Philadelphia: Lippincott Williams & Wilkins, 2006.

[3] HENK A, ERIK J G, JOS A J M, et al. A long-term follow-up study of mortality in transsexuals receiving treatment with cross-sex hormones [J]. Eur J Endocrinol, 2011, 164(4):635-642.

[4] BABA T, ENDO T, IKEDA K, et al. Distinctive features of female-to-male transsexualism and prevalence of gender identity disorder in Japan [J]. J Sex Med, 2011, 8(6):1686-1693.

[5] BERRY J K M, DRUMMOND P D. Psychological generators of stress-headaches [J]. Journal of behavioral medicine, 2018, 41(1):109-121.

[6] BERTOLOTE J M, FLEISCHMANN A. Suicide and psychiatric diagnosis: a worldwide perspective [J]. World Psychiatry, 2002, 1(3):181-185.

[7] BJÖRKLUND A, DUNNETT S B. Dopamine neuron systems in the brain: an update [J]. Trends Neurosci, 2007, 30(5):194-202.

[8] BUNCAMPER M E, VAN DER SLUIS W B, VAN DER PAS R S D et al. Surgical Outcome after Penile Inversion Vaginoplasty: A Retrospective Study of 475 Transgender Women [J]. Plast Reconstr Surg, 2016, 138(5):999-1007.

[9] BRUSCOLINI A, SACCHETTI M, LA CAVA M, et al. Quality of life and neuropsychiatric disorders in patients with Graves' Orbitopathy: Current concepts [J]. Autoimmun Rev, 2018, 17(7):639-643.

[10] CODISPOTI V L. Pharmacology of sexually compulsive behavior [J]. Psychiatr Clin North Am, 2008, 31(4):671-679.

[11] CONRON K J, SCOTT G, STOWELL G S, et al. Transgender Health in Massachusetts: Results From a Household Probability Sample of Adults [J]. American Journal of Public Health, 2012, 102(1): 118-222.

[12] COUMANS J M J, DANNER U N, INTEMANN T, et al. Emotion-driven impulsiveness and snack food consumption of European adolescents: Results from the I. Family study [J]. Appetite, 2018, 123:152-159.

[13] COWEN P, HARRISON P, BURNS T. Shorter Oxford Textbook of Psychiatry [M]. 6th edition. London: Oxford University Press, 2012.

[14] DAVE K P. Field of Psychiatry: Current Trends and Future Directions: An IndianPerspective [J]. Mens Sana Monogr, 2016, 14(1):108-117.

[15] DECUYPER M, DE BOLLE M, BOONE E, et al. The relevance of personality assessment in patients with hyperventilationsymptoms [J]. Health Psychol, 2012, 31(3):316-322.

[16] DZIEGLELEWSKI S F. DSM-5 inaction [M]. 2nd edition. New Jersey: John Wiley & Sons, Inc., Hoboken, 2010.

[17] FALCONE M, GARAFFA G, GILLO A, et al. Outcomes of inflatable penile prosthesis insertion in 247 patients completing female to male gender reassignment surgery [J]. BJU int, 2018, 121(1):139-144.

[18] FITCH W L. AAPL Practice Guideline for the Forensic Psychiatric Evaluation of Competence to Stand Trial: an American legalperspective[J]. J Am Acad Psychiatry Law,2007,35(4):509.

[19] GELDER M,MAYOU R,COWEN P. Oxford Psychiatry[M]. London:Oxford University Press,2001.

[20] HESS J,ROSSI N R,PANIC L,et al. Satisfaction with male-to-female gender reassignment surgery [J]. Deutsches Ärzteblatt International,2014,111(47):795-801.

[21] HOLVOET L,HUYS W, COPPENS V,et al. Fifty Shades of Belgian Gray:The Prevalence of BDSM-Related Fantasies and Activities in the General Population[J]. J Sex Med. 2017,14(9):1152-1159.

[22] JOYAL C C,CARPENTIER J. The Prevalence of Paraphilic Interests and Behaviors in the General Population:A Provincial Survey[J]. J Sex Res. 2017,54(2):161-171.

[23] LI D,HE L. Meta-analysis supports association between serotonin transporter (5-HTT) and suicidal-behavior[J]. Molecular Psychiatry,2007,12(1):47-54.

[24] MANIKANDAN S,NILLNI Y I,ZVOLENSKY M J,et al. The role of emotion regulation in the experience of menstrual symptoms and perceived control over anxiety-related eventsacross the menstrual cycle[J]. Arch Womens Ment Health,2016,19(6):1109-1117.

[25] MANN JJ,CURRIER D,STANLEY B,et al. Can biological tests assist prediction of suicide in mood disorders? [J] International Journal of Neuropsychopharmacology,2006,9(4):465-474.

[26] MANN JJ,CURRIER D. A review of prospective studies of biologic predictors of suicidal behavior in mood disorders? [J] Arch Suicide Res,2007,11(1):3-16.

[27] VELEMA M S,DE NOOIJER A H,BURGERS V W G,et al. Health-Related Quality of Life and Mental Health in Primary Aldosteronism:A Systematic Review[J]. Horm Metab Res,2017,49(12):943-950.

[28] OTTO C,BARTHEL D,KLASEN F,et al. Predictors of self-reported health-related quality of life according to the EQ-5D-Y in chronically ill children and adolescents with asthma,diabetes,and juvenile arthritis:longitudinal results[J]. Qual Life Res,2018,27(4):879-890.

[29] PALACIOS J,KHONDODER M,MANN A,et al. Depression and anxiety symptom trajectories in coronary heart disease:Associations with measures of disability and impact on 3-year health care costs[J]. J Psychosom Res,2018,104:1-8.

[30] PHILIPPS M R,LI X Y,ZHANG Y P. Suicide rate in China,1995-99[J]. Lancet,2002,359(9309): 835-840.

[31] PHILIPPS M R,YANG G H,ZHANG Y P,et al. Risk factors for suicide in China:a national case-control psychological autopsy study [J]. Lancet,2002,360(9347):1728-1736.

[32] PIERCE R C,KUMARESAN V. Themesolimbic dopamine system:the final common pathway for the reinforcing effect of drugs of abuse? [J]. Neurosci Biobehav Rev,2006,30(2):215-238.

[33] PIERZ K A,THASE M E. A review ofvilazodone,serotonin,and major depressive disorder[J]. Prim Care Companion CNS Disord,2014;16(1):PCC. 13r01554.

[34] PREISS K,BRENNAN L,CLARKE D. A systematic review of variables associated with the relationship between obesity and depression[J]. Obes Rev,2013,14(11):906-918.

[35] SADOCK B J,SADOCK V A. Concise textbook of clinical psychiatry[M]. New York:Lippincott Williams & Wilkins Press,2008.

[36] SHER L. Forensic psychiatric evaluations:an overview of methods,ethical issues,and criminal and civilassessments[J]. Int J of Adolesc Med Health,2015,27(2):109-115.

[37] VAN DAMME S,COSYNS M,DEMAN S,et al. The Effectiveness of Pitch-raising Surgery in Male-

to-Female Transsexuals:A Systematic Review[J]. J Voice,2017,31(2):244. e1-244. e5.

[38]SIMONSEN R K,HALD G M,KRISTENSEN E,et al. Long-Term Follow-Up of Individuals Undergo-ing Sex-Reassignment Surgery:Somatic Morbidity and Cause of Death[J]. Sexual Medicine. 2016,4 (1):e60-e68.

[39]TAKTAK Ş,YILMAZ E,KARAMUSTAFALIOGLU O,et al. Characteristics of paraphilics in Turkey:A retrospective study-20years[J]. Int J Law Psychiatry,2016,49:22-30.

[40]CLARK T C,LUCASSEN M F,BULLEN P, et al. The Health and Well-Being of Transgender High School Students:Results From the New Zealand Adolescent Health Survey (Youth´12)[J]. J Adolesc Health,2014,55(1):93-99.

[41]DE VRIES A L,MCGUIRE J K,STEENSMA T D,et al. Young adult psychological outcome after pu-berty suppression and gender reassignment[J]. Pediatrics,2014,134(4):696-704.

[42]VUJOVIC S,POPOVIC S,SBUTEGA-MILOSEVIC G,et al. Transsexualism in Serbia:a twenty-year follow-up study[J]. J Sex Med,2009,6(4):1018-1023.

[43]WHITE HUGHTO J M,REISNER S L. A Systematic Review of the Effects of Hormone Therapy on Psychological Functioning and Quality of Life in Transgender Individuals[J]. Transgend Health, 2016,1(1):21-31.

[44]WIEPJES C M,NOTA N M,DE BLOK C J M,et al. The Amsterdam Cohort of Gender Dysphoria Study (1972-2015):Trends in Prevalence,Treatment,and Regrets[J]. J sex Med,2018,15(4):582-590.

[45]WIRTHMANN A E,MAJENKA P,KAUFMANN M C,et al. Phalloplasty in Female-to-Male Trans-sexuals by Gottlieb and Levine´s Free Radial Forearm Flap Technique-A Long-Term Single-Center Experience Over More than Two Decades[J]. J Reconstr Microsurg,2018,34(4):235-241.

[46]YULE M A,BROTTO L A,GORZALKA B B. Sexual Fantasy and Masturbation Among Asexual Indi-viduals:An In-Depth Exploration[J]. Arch Sex Behav,2017,46(1):311-328.

[47]ZHANG S,MELLSOP G,BRINK J,et al. Involuntary admission and treatment of patients with mental disorder[J]. Neurosci Bull,2015,31(1):99-112.